Handbook of
Disaster Research

Handbooks of Sociology and Social Research

Series Editor:
Howard B. Kaplan, *Texas A&M University, College Station, Texas*

HANDBOOK OF COMMUNITY MOVEMENTS AND LOCAL ORGANIZATIONS
Edited by Ram A. Cnaan and Carl Milofsky

HANDBOOK OF DISASTER RESEARCH
Edited by Havidán Rodríguez, Enrico L. Quarantelli, and Russell Dynes

HANDBOOK OF DRUG ABUSE PREVENTION
Theory, Science and Prevention
Edited by Zili Sloboda and William J. Bukoski

HANDBOOK OF THE LIFE COURSE
Edited by Jeylan T. Mortimer and Michael J. Shanahan

HANDBOOK OF POPULATION
Edited by Dudley L. Poston and Michael Micklin

HANDBOOK OF RELIGION AND SOCIAL INSTITUTIONS
Edited by Helen Rose Ebaugh

HANDBOOK OF SOCIAL PSYCHOLOGY
Edited by John Delamater

HANDBOOK OF SOCIOLOGICAL THEORY
Edited by Jonathan H. Turner

HANDBOOK OF THE SOCIOLOGY OF EDUCATION
Edited by Maureen T. Hallinan

HANDBOOK OF THE SOCIOLOGY OF EMOTIONS
Edited by Jan E. Stets and Jonathan H. Turner

HANDBOOK OF THE SOCIOLOGY OF GENDER
Edited by Janet Saltzman Chafetz

HANDBOOK OF THE SOCIOLOGY OF MENTAL HEALTH
Edited by Carol S. Aneshensel and Jo C. Phelan

HANDBOOK OF THE SOCIOLOGY OF THE MILITARY
Edited by Giuseppe Caforio

Handbook of
Disaster Research

Edited by

Havidán Rodríguez
University of Delaware
Newark, Delaware

Enrico L. Quarantelli
University of Delaware
Newark, Delaware

Russell R. Dynes
University of Delaware
Newark, Delaware

With Forewords by

William A. Anderson
Patrick J. Kennedy
Everett Ressler

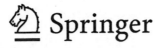 Springer

Havidán Rodríguez
Disaster Research Center
University of Delaware
Newark, DE 19716
havidan@udel.edu

Enrico L. Quarantelli
Disaster Research Center
University of Delaware
Newark, DE 19716
elqdrc@udel.edu

Russell R. Dynes
Disaster Research Center
University of Delaware
Newark, DE 19716
rdynes@udel.edu

ISBN: 978-0-387-73952-6   e-ISBN: 978-0-387-32353-4

Library of Congress Control Number: 2007932796

Printed on acid-free paper.

9 8 7 6 5 4 3 2 1

springer.com

Dedicated to Those Who Contributed to the Beginnings of Disaster Research

Charles Fritz

Kitao Abe

Ritsuo Akimoto

Allan Barton

Fredrick Bates

George Van Den Berghe

Enzo Biginatti

Rue Bucher

Lowell Carr

Charles Chandessais

Roy Clifford

Fred Cuny

William Form

Irving Janis

Barclay Jones

James Kerr

Lewis Killian

Alcira Kreimer

Herb Kunde

Cornelis J. Lammers

Harry Moore

Roy Popkin

John Powell

Samuel Henry Prince

Pitirim A. Sorokin

P.C. Stanissis

Burke Stannard

Shirley Star

James Thompson

Richard Titmuss

Steve Tripp

Ralph Turner

James Tyhurst

Brian Ward

Gilbert White

Harry Williams

Foreword

In case we needed any additional reminders, recent disasters, such as the 2004 Sumatra earthquake, the Indian Ocean tsunami, and the series of 2005 disasters, including Hurricanes' Katrina and Rita, the Pakistan earthquake, and the Central America floods once again demonstrate that we live in a very hazardous world. They also indicate that human societies worldwide have much to learn about the actions to take and to avoid in order to reduce the likelihood that hazardous conditions will result in disasters. In addition, these events make clear that hazards in both developed and developing countries can result in disasters of catastrophic proportions, as was the case with the Sumatra earthquake and the Indian Ocean tsunami, which led to hundreds of thousands of deaths in several developing countries in the region, and Hurricane Katrina, which was the costliest natural disaster in U.S. history.

These recent disasters, and the hazardous conditions that provided the context for them, are also further reminders of the importance of social science hazards and disaster research for extending our understanding on how human society copes with risks and actual events when they occur. It is important that social scientists from all relevant disciplines continue to systematically gather such knowledge on the full range of natural, technological, and human-induced disasters using the best methodologies and guided by the most robust theories and models. Topics related to mitigation, preparedness, response, and recovery should be at the forefront of these social science investigations to not only produce knowledge that is of interest to the research community but also to provide the basis for science-based decision making by planners, emergency managers, and other practicing professionals. A significant start has already been made by the social science community in investigating the Sumatra earthquake and the Indian Ocean tsunami, Hurricanes Katrina and Rita, and other recent disasters, promising needed new understanding on the impact of hazards and disasters on human society.

In recognition of the global reach of hazards and disasters and the fact that an international social science disaster research network has emerged to sort out the complexities and challenges involved in such risks, scholars from around the world contributed to the *Handbook of Disaster Research*. Also, many of the social science disciplines are represented among the contributors, reflecting both the breadth of subjects covered in the *Handbook* as well as the fact that various disciplinary perspectives are required to advance knowledge in the field. In addition, given the needed linkage between the social science disaster research community and practitioners in the field, it is appropriate that several practicing professionals are among the authors of the volume.

Representing the rich tapestry of the field, then, this diverse group of experts has not unexpectedly produced a document with much subject-matter variety, touching on important theoretical, empirical, and applied issues that are related to both the challenges of today and those anticipated in the future. Thus, collectively, the contributions to the *Handbook* provide a benchmark for current social science hazards and disaster research and applications and a vision for where the field should be in the future. This approach is welcomed because of how much remains to be learned regarding the relationship between human society and hazards and disasters as well as about how to further the effective application of existing knowledge given the continuing vulnerability of communities in developed and developing countries alike. With contributions from outstanding scholars and professionals and edited by three of the most prominent leaders in the field, this book is a major addition to the literature in the field of social science hazards and disaster research and applications.

William A. Anderson
National Research Council
U.S. National Academies

Foreword

Since the attacks of September 11, 2001, my office has been actively working to develop legislation to help communities better protect themselves from future disasters. While much has been said and money invested in meeting the technological challenges associated with disasters, very little public attention has been given to the complex social dynamics around them. The *Handbook of Disaster Research* strikes a fitting balance in discussing our nation's need for technology and the efficiency it brings, with the importance of preserving and enhancing the social capital inevitably created in the wake of critical incidents.

Disasters are in fact as much a social event as they are a physical one. Our day-to-day routines are suddenly and violently broken, the social confinements of our culturally defined roles are shattered, and social capital rises as self-organizing social networks emerge. These networks are bands of citizens, who would normally be socially disconnected, coming together for the common pro-social purposes of facing adversity as a group and working to bring back a sense of normalcy to their environment.

As unwanted as disasters are, they do provide unique opportunities for societies to mend their frayed and neglected social fabric, as well as reaffirming a community's collective sense of values. By taking advantage of the spontaneous formation of social networks, and allowing these networks to have responsibilities in disaster response and recovery efforts, we can draw strength from one another while developing meaning from the issues at stake.

When it comes to dealing with disasters there is neither a Republican way nor a Democratic way; there is only the right way. The science is out there and it is incumbent upon us, particularly in government, to learn it. As a member of the United States Congress, I am grateful to Drs. Russell Dynes, Henry Quarantelli, and Havidán Rodríguez, their colleagues, and other distinguished contributors for providing a comprehensive analysis of the research on various disaster-related topics. Only by furthering our knowledge of disasters can policymakers craft legislation that sensibly brings science to service.

Patrick J. Kennedy
Member of Congress

Foreword

Every emergency reaffirms our limited understanding of hazard management—prevention, reduction, preparedness, and response; the need for systematic social science research has never been greater. From a comparative international perspective, we need to identify those factors that exist in the physical world and the social environment that lead to potentially disastrous situations. To achieve this, disasters must be interpreted not so much as problems in themselves, but as a result of other problems in the socioeconomic and ecological context. Globally, insufficient attention is being paid to disaster preparedness and response and to the social context and social factors that impact disasters. Thus, it is necessary to redress the balance between investment in research in the physical sciences and investment in the social sciences. The all-important social factors that contribute to disaster vulnerability, the definition of disaster, and response to emergencies, unfortunately, have been undervalued.

Whether knowledge gained of human behavior in more developed countries is pertinent to the explanation of disaster phenomena in developing nations becomes less critical with the ongoing effects of globalization. Indeed, it would seem that the evidence indicates that cross-cultural similarities in disaster behavior may be greater than the differences. The editors of this handbook have encouraged their contributors to think in cross-cultural and international terms. Given that encouragement, global programs, such as those supported by UNICEF, which operate around the world with the aim to benefit the most vulnerable, can also benefit from this knowledge.

Everett Ressler
UNICEF, Geneva

Editors' Introduction

Disasters create difficulties, even for those who study disasters. Much of that difficulty stems from the necessity to deal with concepts, which have popular meanings, and some of those meanings evoke moral and emotional reactions. Conceptual discussions about disaster related activities could evoke charges that researchers miss the point. Also, interest in disasters cuts across disciplinary lines so that one's own disciplinary interests are considered critical while the interests of others are interesting but marginal.

Quarantelli (2005) has recently described the social context in which the social scientific study of disaster has emerged, most of which is barely half a century old. He described the first sociological efforts to study disaster and how the Cold War, after World War II, began to raise questions about how American communities might react to enemy attacks. The larger social context prompted the initial efforts to look at peacetime disasters and indirectly led to the support of the Disaster Research Center. The idea of the Disaster Research Center and, subsequently, what came to be known as DRC, was independently created by sociologists at The Ohio State University.

The outline of this *Handbook* and the topics selected for attention draw heavily from the perspective of the DRC. This is less because the editors are from DRC, but more from the fact that much of the earliest social science disaster research was done at DRC. Some attention to disasters had of course preceded the Center's existence, ranging from Prince's doctoral dissertation (1920) on social change and disasters to Sorokin's theoretical treatise (1942) to the first systematic field studies undertaken by the National Opinion Research Center (1949–1954) to the series of studies done at the National Academy of Sciences (1952–1960). However, for about two decades after those works, DRC undertook the only continuous and systematic research in the area, and produced the bulk of the publications that were written. Thus, the early history of disaster studies is to a large extent the history of DRC and its early graduates.

As background, the book *Organized Behavior in Disaster* (Dynes, 1970) provides a description of the early work of the DRC and a review of prior disaster research. That review noted that there were four common usages of "disaster": as an agent description, such as a hurricane, an explosion, a flood and, more recently, a terrorist attack; as physical damage, in terms of both structures and people; as social disruption, creating a series of problems for communities and nations; and finally, perhaps the most common usage, as negative evaluation, describing situations and people as being confused, bad, as well as unlucky, and any other combination of these evaluations possible. In many discussions, different meanings can occur interchangeably within the same sentence. For our purposes here, the central meaning of disaster is social disruption.

Organized Behavior in Disaster was based on the literature available at that time. Of course, some literature was of greater value than others. It was noted then that there were three types of existing literature: (1) popular, (2) official, and (3) professional and scientific, which we summarize below.

POPULAR LITERATURE

It is perhaps legitimate to term media presentations as "literature." It can be recorded, re-run, and archived. With the advent of cable TV, with hours to fill with visual content, disaster film becomes staple content; both heroes and victims can be incorporated into the story. The best shots are of the physical damage and asking victims whether they have received help and how they feel. The major program themes center on the physical destruction, victimization, and lack of assistance, with the intent of portraying a state of "chaos or anarchy" following the disaster.

These same themes are also central to the motion pictures version of disaster, except movies can provide a more coherent story and better visual effects. There is also a literature on survivors and eyewitnesses to major disasters in the past. While none of these sources provide much useful information about disaster behavior per se, their activity and participation in disaster occasions are worthy of examination (see the chapters by Webb and by Scanlon in this volume).

OFFICIAL LITERATURE

Official documents of governmental and quasi-governmental agencies, security agencies, and nonprofit assistance agencies include reports often filled with descriptive statistics and descriptions of their involvement in various phases of disasters. Often, such reports can be considered to be a form of "public relations;" efforts to justify past activities and to convince themselves and others as to their value in the past and their need in the future. Government documents often provide valuable information not necessarily about the disaster occasion but about the political stand and dynamics concerning disasters at a particular time period.

PROFESSIONAL AND SCIENTIFIC LITERATURE

Most of the sources quoted throughout the various contributions in this *Handbook* would fall into this category. While there is a tradition within the physical and biological sciences as well as various engineering disciplines to study disaster agents and to understand physical damage, the concern here will be with the social sciences. In the research reviewed in *Organized Behavior in Disaster*, it was noted that almost all previous research had been opportunistic, in the sense that, given their proximity to a particular crisis event, social scientists realized that such events provided a unique research opportunity. Therefore, they hurriedly developed research plans and assembled research teams that were convenient but not necessarily competent. At times, such contrived studies made creative contributions but often were duplicative and explored unproductive leads. A potential solution for that problem was suggested in the final pages of

Organized Behavior in Disasters and it provides the starting point for the contributions that are included in the *Handbook of Disaster Research*.

The *Handbook* suggests a new approach, which might overcome the research limitations of earlier research. The previous approach was conditioned not only by the review of the previous literature but also by the focus on ongoing activities at DRC. The Center was initiated in 1963 at the Ohio State University with an initial and primary focus on organizations and on the emergency period, which had been neglected in large part because of the logistical and financial problems of organizing quick response research. It continued to be difficult to convince research funders that the Center did not know when and where we were going to do research; although we could certainly study the events, we could not necessarily predict where and when they would happen. Our first major field trip was in 1963 in the United States as the result of a propane explosion during the Ice Show at the Indiana State Fair Coliseum. Given the high death and injury rates, this event provided the opportunity to look at the "processing" of victims by rescue and medical organizations. It occurred at the same time that another DRC field team was in Italy where a landslide produced a dam overflow and created severe damage to the village at the bottom of the dam. These events provided the opportunity to contrast different national disaster systems. Also, several months after the founding of the Center, a major earthquake occurred in Alaska, affecting the largest city, Anchorage, as well as several native villages. The size of Anchorage and the research efforts of various DRC field teams allowed us to understand the patterns of response for a variety of municipal and state agencies. Several months later, an earthquake of similar intensity affected Niigata, Japan allowing us to contrast Japanese and U.S. response to a disaster agent of similar intensity. Thus, our review of the earlier disaster literature was not a review in the conventional sense, but looked at previous research in the context of our own ongoing fieldwork. Some of the authors in this handbook were part of that collective process.

At the end of our review in *Organized Behavior in Disasters*, a series of ideas were put forth for future research on disasters, as indicated in the following section.

1. A research organization must be developed that has, on standby, experienced field teams that can be mobilized immediately given that new researchers are often preoccupied with the novelty of the situation and find it difficult to sort out the unique from the novel.
2. Future research should be centered on macro rather than micro levels. This is certainly a reflection of the disciplinary "bias" of the founders of the Center and the subsequent directors. But it was also a warning of a cultural bias in American society, which tends to reduce all explanations to the individual level, isolated from any social context.
3. Research must become comparative in the fullest sense. Three types of comparisons were recommended—among crisis events, organizations, and sociocultural systems.

It is useful to comment on some of the ways that those initial recommendations have been implemented. The DRC has maintained field team capabilities since 1963, both at the Ohio State University and when it moved to the University of Delaware in 1985. The primary focus is still on organizations but the research interests have expanded to include research on mitigation, preparedness, and recovery. The focus on comparisons among crises events continues. The more than 650 different field trips taken over that time include the full range of possible disaster occasions.

The effort to look at disasters in different sociocultural systems has taken a number of different forms. One of the first initiatives of the Center was to make contact with English,

French, and Dutch researchers as well as notifying international agencies in Geneva, such as the United Nations and the League of Red Cross Societies of our research plans. There were other strategies used to increase the interest and effort among disaster researchers in other parts of the world. Central to that effort was the development of workshops for researchers in specific countries or regions. This was done with Japanese social scientists in Ohio; with Italian researchers in Delaware and in Italy; with South Asian researchers at the Asian Disaster Preparedness Center in Thailand; with Central American and Caribbean researchers in Costa Rica; with Russian researchers in Moscow; and with Indian researchers in Patna, Bihar. International contacts were enhanced by the participation of various DRC staff members at research workshops in more than 25 countries. These contacts were furthered by the creation of a research committee on disasters in the structure of the International Sociological Association and the creation of the *International Journal of Mass Emergencies and Disasters*. That organizational location did not preclude nonsociologists from participation. The growth of this international network prompted a number of researchers to come to the Center for extended stays on Fulbright and Winston Churchill fellowships, on various government-funded fellowships, and on sabbatical leave from academic institutions; many more have come on shorter visits.

Perhaps the most inclusive example of cooperative activity occurred in the 1985 Mexico City Earthquake. Soon after the earthquake, a researcher from the Instituto de Investigación de la Comunicación, a survey research center in Mexico City, arrived looking to develop research questions regarding the earthquake response for their regularly scheduled survey of the Mexico City population. A second visitor from the Secretaría de Gobernación, which had been given expanded responsibility in the post-earthquake period, came to the Center to discuss disaster issues. This resulted in one of the directors going to Mexico City to talk with the Secretaría staff. As a result of these visits, DRC initiated a joint research project with the Institute to do another survey on the first anniversary of the earthquake and developed another project with La Facultad Latinoamericana de Ciencias Sociales (FLACSO) to study the organizational response of the municipal government. In this part of the project, the two groups jointly developed the research strategies and DRC personnel went to Mexico City to train interviewers in DRC field research operations. Certainly, that effort was an optimum situation in collaborative research and it suggests that, at times, it is possible. To this day, DRC continues to engage in international research on disasters and to collaborate with international researchers in the field.

While we have included some comparative research efforts in this volume and encouraged our contributors to make an effort to seek it out in their own analysis, we recognize that it is easier to deal with materials that are culturally familiar. We are aware, however, of very significant research activities in Australia and Japan as well as programmatic work at the Asian Disaster Preparedness Center at the Asian Institute of Technology in Thailand dealing with disaster planning in large Asian cities. There is a growing group of researchers centering around El Centro de Investigación y Estudios Superiores en Antropología Social in Mexico and a network of researchers in Latin America called LA RED. Also, there has been a disaster research tradition in England, The Netherlands, France, Spain, Germany and Italy. In those countries, there has been a continuing focus on floods, which has been an enduring problem, and there has been an emphasis on disasters in developing countries. In Sweden, there has been important work on risk with comparative studies of different emergency response systems in the Baltic States. A disaster research tradition has also emerged in Russia and in several Eastern European nations, especially the Czech Republic. To the editors, these developments are gratifying and we recognize that we have not fully represented the importance of those contributions here. It is noteworthy that the importance of comparative research is not just to take into account differences in response to disaster, but also to emphasize the similarities as well as the creative solutions, which can be identified around the world.

In addition to the value of comparative studies, research on disasters has come from a variety of disciplines and areas of study, including Geography, Psychology, Economics, Political Science, Communications, Operations Research, Decision Theory, Public Administration, Anthropology, and others that are somewhat difficult to classify by discipline. Two research traditions deserve special notation. Natural hazards research generally uses a human ecological perspective dealing with the interaction of human and nonhuman factors in relation to risk. Gilbert White is generally credited with initiating research on hazards with his 1942 dissertation on human adjustment to floods. In 1976, he became the Director of the Natural Hazards Research and Applications Center at the University of Colorado, which over the years has become an important location for sharing information focusing on the mitigation of natural disasters. Another research tradition, which developed more recently, has been risk analysis. Drawing from a number of disciplines, it has been concerned with the identification, measurement, and evaluation of risk. Such research has been the basis for the creation of occupational titles such as risk managers and risk analysts. More central to our concerns here is the notion that risk is socially defined (for more details on the scope and origins of the natural hazards and risk traditions, see Kirby 1990.)

The *Handbook of Disaster Research* focuses on disasters as social phenomena. While there are occasional references in different chapters to hazards as physical phenomena and their possible relationship to disasters, the hazard perspective is not very explicitly or at length addressed in most of this work. As some scholars have noted (Alexander 2000; Mitchell 1990) the field of hazards studies had an origin separate from disaster research, often studied different topics, and has used different theoretical frameworks. Of course, some hazard scholars, such as Gilbert White, have contributed to both fields of studies.

POPULAR IMAGES OF DISASTER BEHAVIOR

In our earlier review of the disaster literature, while our goal was to develop ways to study the functioning of organizations in emergencies, we continued to be amazed as to the popular images of what happens to individuals, organizations, and communities as compared with the picture obtained from reading the research literature. In fact, Quarantelli and Dynes (1972) wrote an article, published in the popular social science journal *Psychology Today,* that contrasted the mass cultural view of disaster behavior with research evidence. For most individuals, disaster experience is so rare that most of our "knowledge" comes from stories and pictures from the mass culture, and now, with cable television in many countries, those images are available 24 hours a day. Those who produce such images use their own vision of what should be pictured. Those persistent images, however, are not necessarily a reality but assume what problems disasters create and what needs to be done.

It is useful to contrast two sets of images, one drawn from the mass culture—that of confused victims—and another that fits the research literature much better—that of active survivors. These images have to be placed in the context that, after the disaster impact, there is the "conviction" that disasters create social chaos. This "chaos" is signaled by a rapid increase in irrational social behavior—panic is the term used most frequently—or by the perception of people being "stunned" and not being able to respond to emergency or crisis situations. These effects are seen to result in "victims" with severely hampered decision-making capacity whose long repressed criminal and antisocial tendencies surface. It is assumed that these antisocial traits emerge since traditional social control mechanisms have now lost their effectiveness. In addition, traditional forms of pre-disaster social organizations (families, community organizations, local government) are seen as ineffective since they are now populated with confused victims. The confused victim image suggests that extraordinary measures need to be initiated. Since disaster problems stem from the confusion of their victims and the ineffectiveness of the pre-disaster social structure, the logical policy response is to establish "command" over the chaos and regain "control" over the disorganized, confused victims. This means that outside assistance is necessary to establish authority and generate correct decisions to replace those confused. Therefore, in general, policy directions establish "command and control" and perhaps provide some therapy for "confused victims."

As noted earlier, there is a different view that can be inferred from the research evidence and from careful observation—that of the active survivor. The designation of "active" suggests that "victims" do respond actively to the prospects and impacts of disaster—in making preparations for family members and for others in their community; by giving attention to warnings and to danger; and by seeking out information about risk potential. Such actions cannot be described as "panic." Some community members will make bad decisions, just as they have before the disaster. The preoccupation with possibilities of antisocial behavior shifts attention away from the increase in altruistic behavior and volunteerism, which always emerges after a disaster. We also know that most search and rescue is done by friends and neighbors, not by what are now called "first responders." The problems created by disasters are usually those that existed before: poor land use, unenforced building codes, lack of attention to mitigating community risks, poverty, inadequate medical care, and substandard housing, among others. The best way to understand disaster effects is to know what the community was like prior to the disaster event.

The image of active survivors, rather than confused victims, is important for future research. It means that knowledge, rather than command and control, is more important in reducing the negative consequences of disasters in all types of social structures. Some of the problems created by disasters are of larger magnitude but they can be solved by usual community decision-making. However, many of these problems cannot be solved by a quick fix of technology. The goal should be to understand how people, organizations, and communities can adapt and improve their decision-making and problem-solving skills. Understanding how, cooperatively, they can bring together human and material resources to "solve" the new and different problems is more important than creating artificial authority. These skills can be enhanced within any impacted community so that those communities do not become dependent on outside "assistance."

STRUCTURE OF THE HANDBOOK

It is best to view the organization of the *Handbook of Disaster Research* in terms of a model of a library rather than as a lengthy novel. Since the focus is on disaster research, we have given attention to conceptual issues dealing with the word "disaster" and on methodological issues relating to research on disasters. We include a discussion of Geographic Information Systems as a useful research tool and its implications for future research; of how research is being used in the growing number of courses in emergency management; and an examination of how research is useful in dealing with emergency operations.

Since disasters are not random, equal-probability events, we included several essays on various types of vulnerabilities. There are many losers in disasters but there are also some winners. Many of the selections are centered on the central problem solving unit—the community, which is a universal social form cross-culturally. Some of these discussions are centered on the resources, which communities utilize in problem-solving in disasters. In addition, we look at a series of community processes that are evoked by disasters, including warnings, search and rescue, coordination, and organizational adaptation, as well as dealing with death and injury, and recovery. We then moved to a consideration of nation-states' emergency systems, including those such as Russia's, which has been undergoing significant change. We also look at the relationship between disaster and development, which is of central concern for foreign assistance programs and international financial agencies. We then move to a discussion of new dimensions of research as well as several projections of disasters into the future, in terms of an increasingly urban, diverse, industrialized, and technology connected world, focusing on what Furedi has termed "the growth of a market of fear," or in Perrow's terms, "Disasters Evermore."

It should be noted that certain contributions that we originally anticipated could not be realized. First, we have no extensive discussion focusing on international disaster assistance programs and the more recent and important efforts of the World Bank. We have no extensive discussion of what might be called the potential for mega-disasters in a world where massive urban settlements contain an increasing proportion of the world population. We have no extensive discussion of mitigation. We have not given attention to the importance of emergency medical services and to the problem that emerges when disaster agents, such as tsunamis, impact an area where different religious and cultural traditions affect the handling of disaster victims. Unfortunately, some of our good intentions in planning the *Handbook* were not realized. We did ask our contributors to address future research priorities and possibilities in an attempt to generate the beginnings of an agenda for a new generation of disaster researchers.

It is important to note here that the editors do not see disaster research as the study of deviance or of social pathology but as an attempt to understand a variety of types of social systems having to deal with complex and often unexpected problems. Disasters allow the opportunity for social scientists to study human behavior in which adaptation, resilience, and innovation are often more clearly revealed than in "normal" and stable times. The fact that traditional social units such as families, organizations, and communities have grappled with disaster over centuries indicates that "solutions" are possible. This means that problem solving abilities can be improved and disaster research can contribute to that understanding.

Unfortunately, nation-states' disaster planning seldom considers local communities as capable of problem solving and they develop plans suggesting the necessity of instituting social control. Using inept analogies from the past, national planning is often predicated on a model of "enemy" attack and considers local communities as fragile and disorganized. Disaster "victims" are seen as either passive or paralyzed by fear. Based on those assumptions, nation-states often plan to supplement or replace local decision-making, using the rationale of patriotic paternalism.

Certainly, disasters disrupt conventional social routines and structures but to describe this as social chaos is incorrect. Emergencies do not reduce the capacities of individuals to cope but they present new and unexpected problems to solve. It is wise to remember that in the social history of some of the most dynamic world cities are episodes of successful coping with major emergencies - New York, Washington, Chicago, San Francisco, Tokyo, London, Mexico City, Berlin, and many others. Conventional social structures should be seen as the key resources for problem solving, not as the key location of confusion. Efforts to understand disasters should lead to using the abilities of various social units to more effectively solve the problems, which emergencies create. It has been noted that the conventional Chinese symbol for disaster is a combination of two different characters, one symbolizing "danger" and the other "opportunity." Henceforth, the discussion is focused on opportunity.

Havidán Rodríguez
Enrico (Henry) L. Quarantelli
Russell (Russ) R. Dynes
Disaster Research Center
University of Delaware
Newark, Delaware

Acknowledgments

Editing a book of this nature is truly an art form. As many artists know, developing a "masterpiece" requires an extensive amount of time, hard work, and, most importantly, patience and perseverance. Even when the work of art is "finished" and displayed in (hopefully) some prominent and inviting place, you reflect on it and wished you had added some supplemental colors, included other images or scenery, or eliminated some of those pastel types of colors. But, alas, the work is done, and with a great deal of pride combined with a great dose of humility and satisfaction, you thank all those who made this project possible. Although the final product is extremely important, it was the process that was essential and made the project worth pursuing. It allowed us to interact with our colleagues, share ideas, learn about new initiatives, and become a bit more familiarized with the work of leading scholars and researchers from a diverse set of disciplines and from a number of countries. Yes, at times, it seemed a long and tedious process, but, at the end, we all became better (or, at least, more informed) social scientists and disaster researchers. We sincerely appreciate the help, collaboration, contributions, and recommendations of all those who made the *Handbook of Disaster Research* possible.

There are always many individuals involved in a project of this magnitude, ranging from the authors of the different chapters included in the *Handbook*, to those who provided very critical and insightful (although not always welcomed) reviews, to those who worked endless hours planning, organizing, and compiling all the information requested by the editors and the publisher. All the authors will make important contributions to the field of disaster research with the chapters that they submitted for inclusion in this *Handbook*. We appreciate your thoughtfulness and your critical perspectives regarding how the different topics included in the diverse chapters of this *Handbook* have evolved, where we are currently in this particular area of study, and the future propositions for the field. We hope that these contributions will serve to expand the disaster field both substantively and methodologically; that they will encourage many researchers to pursue some of the areas of study proposed by many of the authors of this *Handbook*; and will also encourage funding agencies to provide the necessary funds in order to allow them (e.g., researchers) to engage in these research initiatives, many calling for multi- or interdisciplinary and cross-national collaborations.

We are extremely grateful to Pat Young (Coordinator for the Research Collection at the Disaster Research Center) for all her hard work in the development of this *Handbook*. Pat was instrumental in the final (and most difficult) stages of putting the *Handbook* together. She integrated all the chapters, collected all types of information from the authors, edited parts of the *Handbook*, and was very willing and eager to help and contribute to this important endeavor. As is generally the case with these projects, a number of students (both graduate and undergraduate) also played a key role in this process. Students at the Disaster Research Center worked extremely hard in gathering an extensive amount of information, putting together and editing the reference section of the *Handbook*, and providing the much needed help in order to complete this project in a timely manner. Our most sincere thanks go to Gabriela Wasileski, Michael (Mike) B. Clark, Letitia C. Jarmon, Michelle Moses, and Lauren M. Ross.

Finally, we also want to thank Teresa Krauss and other staff members at Springer who were very supportive and provided the needed assistance in order to allow us to engage in this work and complete *The Handbook of Disaster Research*.

Havidán Rodríguez
Enrico (Henry) L. Quarantelli
Russell (Russ) R. Dynes
Disaster Research Center
University of Delaware
Newark, Delaware

Contributors

Benigno E. Aguirre, University of Delaware, Disaster Research Center, Department of Sociology and Criminal Justice, Newark, Delaware. Professional interests include social power, social conflict, and inequality in disasters.

J. M. Albala-Bertrand, Queen Mary, University of London, Department of Economics. Research interests focus mainly on the political economy of hazards and its macroeconomic effects as well as on structural change in developing countries vis-à-vis globalization policy models.

Lauren E. Barsky, University of Delaware, Department of Sociology and Criminal Justice, Newark, Delaware. Professional interests include disaster mythology, mass media, and collective behavior.

Arjen Boin, Leiden University, Department of Public Administration, The Netherlands. Professional interests include crisis and disaster management, public leadership, and public institutions.

Bob Bolin, Arizona State University, School of Human Evolution and Social Change, Tempe, Arizona. Research interests include hazards and environmental justice issues in urban settings. Work also focuses on drought, social vulnerability, and water resource issues.

Susan Lovegren Bosworth, College of William and Mary, Associate Provost for Planning and Assessment, Williamsburg, Virginia. Professional interests include applying theoretical and methodological tools used to investigate hazards and disasters to instances of change in higher education.

Linda B. Bourque, University of California School of Public Health, Department of Community Health Sciences, Southern California Injury Prevention Center, Center for Public Health and Disasters, Los Angeles, California. Professional interests include impacts of disasters on communities and community response to disasters; ophthalmic clinical trials on refractive corneal surgeries; design, administration, and analysis of questionnaires and surveys.

Neil R. Britton, Earthquake Disaster Mitigation Research Centre, National Research Institute for Earth Sciences and Disaster Prevention, Kobe, Japan. Professional interests focus on disaster risk management development and application.

Nicole Dash, University of North Texas, Department of Sociology, Denton, Texas. Professional interests include evacuation decision-making and how social vulnerability relates to disaster impact, preparedness, and recovery.

Richard A. Rotanz, Emergency Manager, Nassau County Emergency Management, Nassau County, New York and Adelphi University, Department of Anthropology, Garden City, New York. Professional interests include emergency management, response and preparedness analysis.

Jenniffer M. Santos, University of Delaware, Disaster Research Center, Department of Sociology and Criminal Justice, Newark, Delaware. Academic interests include: sociological theory, race and ethnicity, social movements, mass media, geographic information systems, and vulnerability to natural disasters.

Joseph Scanlon, Carleton University, Director of the Emergency Communications Research Unit, Ottawa, Canada. He has been doing disaster research for 35 years.

Judith M. Siegel, University of California, Los Angeles, Department of Community Health Sciences, School of Public Health, Los Angeles, California. Professional interests include health promotion, stress and coping, psychological aspects of disasters.

Gavin P. Smith, Program Manager, Risk and Emergency Management Division, PBS&J. Professional interests include sustainable disaster recovery, hazard mitigation, post-disaster policy analysis, and linking research and practice. Dr. Smith is currently serving as the Director of the Office of Recovery and Renewal in the Governor's Office of the State of Mississippi.

Barbara Vogt Sorensen, Oak Ridge National Laboratory, Oak Ridge, Tennessee. Professional interests include risk communication, decontamination and emergency response, social equity and vulnerability issues.

John H. Sorensen, Oak Ridge National Laboratory, Oak Ridge, Tennessee. Professional interests include warning systems and response, emergency evacuation, and simulation modeling.

Robert A. Stallings, University of Southern California, Los Angeles, School of Policy, Planning, and Development, Los Angeles, California. Professional interests include the social construction of risk and sociological theories of disaster.

Deborah S.K. Thomas, University of Colorado at Denver and Health Sciences Center, Department of Geography and Environmental Sciences, Denver, Colorado. Professional interests include hazards, health, vulnerability, and GIS.

Kathleen J. Tierney, Director, Natural Hazards Center and Professor, University of Colorado Boulder, Department of Sociology and Institute of Behavioral Science, Boulder, Colorado. Research interests include the conceptualization and measurement of disaster resilience, business and economic impacts of disasters, crisis-related collective behavior, disaster response networks, and the analysis of emergency management and homeland security policies and programs.

Tricia Wachtendorf, University of Delaware, Disaster Research Center, Department of Sociology and Criminal Justice, Newark, Delaware. Professional interests include organizational improvisation, transnational disasters, and community-based approaches to disaster mitigation, response, and recovery.

William L. Waugh, Jr., Georgia State University, Andrew Young School of Policy Studies, Atlanta, Georgia. Primary areas of disaster research are organizational analysis and policy evaluation. He has studied national responses to terrorist violence for thirty years.

Gary R. Webb, Oklahoma State University, Department of Sociology, Stillwater, Oklahoma. Research interests include organizational responses to disasters, improvisation during crises, and the cultural dimensions of disasters.

Dennis Wenger, Texas A&M University, Department of Landscape Architecture and Urban Planning, Hazard Reduction and Recovery Center, College Station, Texas. Professional interests include organizational, community, and multidisciplinary studies of natural, technological and human-induced disasters.

Michele M. Wood, University of California, Los Angeles, School of Public Health, Department of Community Health Sciences, Los Angeles, California. Professional interests include natural hazards, terrorism, and HIV/AIDS.

Yang Zhang, University of Illinois, Springfield, Department of Environmental Studies, Springfield, Illinois. Professional interests include environmental planning, natural disasters, land use, GIS, and quantitative methods.

Contents

CHAPTER 1

What Is a Disaster?

RONALD W. PERRY

Fieldwork is stimulating, challenging, and provides immediate rewards for the researcher. Although contemplating theoretical and paradigmatic issues in one's office may be less exciting by comparison, it is important to deal with such tasks. Devising a definition of disasters or assessing consensus on a definition is not only a part of sound theory and methodology (Bunge, 1998) but also contributes to a clearer vision of the field of study, and on a very practical level, helps to sort out apparent anomalies in research findings and sets the stage for a progression from simple description toward the social scientific tasks of explanation, prediction, and control (Homans, 1967).

This chapter does not propose a new or unique definition of disasters, but rather recounts efforts to define disasters by social scientists, particularly sociologists. This is accomplished in several phases. First, attention is given to issues associated with definitions, including clarifying the goal of defining disasters and the type of definition of interest. The task of presenting definitions from the literature is tackled next. Finally, the definitions are reviewed to assess levels of consensus and the presence of common themes.

WHAT KIND OF DEFINITION?

Seeking or proposing definitions of disaster can be a complex task that brings out the pedantic in scholars and may create considerable frustration (Cutter, 2005a). Some of the complexity and frustration can be addressed by specifying the purpose and audience for definitions of disasters. Such definitions must be placed into a meaningful context that clarifies the essential goal of the definition and the uses to which the definition is to be put. At the outset, it must be acknowledged that the goals in creating definitions vary and that there is no single legitimate purpose or content for definitions. Further, one must clarify whether disaster is being defined as a concept or as an area of study, although there is an inevitable overlap between the two approaches.

To attack the latter issue first, concern in this chapter is with the definition of disaster less as a concept than as an area of study. Of course, the two ideas are not completely separable and they clearly overlap. Certainly for methodologists and philosophers of science, the term concept has a very specific meaning in the theoretical lexicon. However, while defining an area of study has implications for theory and theory construction, the direct aim is more meta-theoretical in that one seeks to introduce parameters on what is to be studied. At this stage, one can avoid becoming immersed in the challenge of creating nominal and operational definitions that pertain largely to concepts and the conceptualization process.

Hempel (1952) makes a useful distinction between *real* and *nominal* definitions. A real definition, also called a connotative definition (Cohen, 1980, p. 143), is a statement that specifies or identifies the critical properties or features of the concept that is being defined. For Hempel, this type of definition is in effect a class term intended to capture—with a degree of openness or ambiguity—phenomena within an umbrella of meaning. The example he uses is a chair defined as "... a separate movable seat for one person" (Hempel, 1952, p. 2). On the other hand, a nominal definition may be seen as an expression of detailed characteristics that are tied to a given term, which usually represents a given concept. Zetterberg (1965) emphasizes the inductive nature of nominally defining a concept in his example that low levels of opportunity, substandard housing, and deficient medical care are *observables* that reflect the *term* poor, and are captured in the *concept* of poverty. The nominal definition forms the "meaning framework" for a concept that is scrutinized when developing operational definitions to initiate an inductive or deductive research process, and research is ultimately aimed at or used for theory construction.

The notion of real or connotative definition leads down a different path, one more dependent on the philosophy of science—whether one emphasizes a positivist, modified positivist, or non-positivist approach (Martindale, 1979, p. 21). While there has been much criticism (Masterman, 1970) and revision (Kuhn, 1970; Ritzer, 1979) of the sociological use of paradigm over the years, it remains a useful—if still loosely used—idea. Thus, Ritzer (1979, p. 26) sees a paradigm as the most fundamental picture of scientific subject matter, as the feature that defines "what should be studied, what questions should be asked..." From this perspective, defining an area of study overlaps the problem of identifying a paradigm. Equally important, paradigms and areas of study are consensus based, and providing definitions is not an empirical task but an intellectual exercise resulting in an abstract construction (Kaplan, 1964). What is sought, in the context of this chapter, are definitions of disaster that address concerns of paradigm and do so by identifying critical features or characteristics of disasters.

WHO DOES THE DEFINING?

This discussion prefaces another distinction in defining disaster. Who has the "right" to propose such definitions? In reality anyone has the right to propose a definition of disaster, and the definition proposed depends on the purposes or interests of the definer. Kroll-Smith and Gunter (1998) embrace what they call an interpretive voice and emphasize the notion that sociologists should look for the definition of disaster among those who experience it (and are studied by sociologists). Buckle (2005) notes that government develops "mandated" definitions of disaster to determine the boundaries of emergency management and response; in the United States, Presidential Disaster Declarations use these types of definitions. Britton (1986b) argues that emergency managers have a specific perspective on what constitutes a disaster and are often forced to simultaneously deal with definitions that differ between levels of government and between specific policy audiences. Shaluf, Ahmadun, and Mustapha (2003) describe the role of regulatory agencies in defining technological disasters. Others who propose and use definitions of disaster include journalists, historians, and social scientists.

Quarantelli (1987b) has argued that there is no basis in logic and little hope in practice that a single definition can be devised that meets and is universally accepted and useful.

Indeed, "heart attack" may convey to a victim all that he or she needs to know and at the same time be only a vague description of an ailment to a cardiologist. It is necessary to recognize that disaster will always mean many things to many people, and the description will serve many different purposes—thus there will be many definitions. What becomes important is the specification of the audience for the definition, bearing in mind the use to which that audience will put the definition. Quarantelli (2005a) emphasizes that as social scientists—sociologists in particular—defining disasters, we need to devote attention to the sociological context and tradition, attending in particular to delimiting the phenomenon to become a focus for the processes of social science. This chapter follows Quarantelli's admonition.

The definition of disaster of interest here is one to be used by social scientists to delineate an area of study and in so doing set the stage for knowledge accumulation and theory construction. This is not to say that citizen perceptions of disasters—or the definition of disasters generated by any other collectivity for that matter—are less important. All are entitled to their definition and each is legitimate and most likely serves an intended purpose. For sociologists, the content and patterns of such definitions are even a reasonable focus of research. However, the goal here is to deal with definitions of disaster proposed by social scientists for social scientific purposes.

THE CONTEXT OF DEFINITION ISSUES

Even when the type of definition, its purpose, and audience are specified, a challenge remains in devising—or recounting—definitions of disaster. One issue is that, even if we limit scrutiny to social science, several definitions are available at any one time, not to mention a large number of empirical studies—some executed with an explicit definition in mind, most not—with which to contend. Thus, when one proposes a definition of disaster, it may be an abstract and nonempirical exercise, but there is certainly reason to reflect on previous definitions and research. Social science cannot be conducted in an intellectual and empirical vacuum. If one assumes that the definitions were proposed and the research carried out in good faith and with professionalism, then each represents a legitimate attempt to either capture the meaning or operate within the meaning of disaster. Consequently, prior definitions and studies at least have the potential to inform current visions for definitions.

The challenge in using this information rests in the diversity of expression as well as within the changing contexts in which disaster research has been undertaken. There is some consensus that Samuel Prince's (1920) dissertation on the Halifax explosion was the first systematic study of disaster. A decade later, Carr (1932) addressed issues of substance, definition, and sequence in disasters. In so doing, Carr was the first to describe disasters as inherently rooted in social change. However, the real growth in disaster studies began in the early 1950s, accelerated with the founding of the Disaster Research Center in 1963, and the field has virtually exploded since the mid-1970s (Tierney, Lindell, & Perry, 2001). Indeed, in his seminal review of disaster findings in 1986, Drabek found about one thousand empirical studies and the rate of research has expanded since then. Interestingly, only a very small number of these researchers dealt much with the definition of disasters. In fact, defining disasters became a widespread concern only since the publication of Quarantelli's (1987b) Presidential Address to the International Research Committee on Disasters and much of that attention is testimony to Quarantelli's perseverance.

In the early decades of disaster research, definitions of the phenomenon were commonly left implicit or partial, a state of affairs observed not just in disaster research or among sociologists, or in the social sciences for that matter. For example, Carr identified a disaster as a product of its consequences, arguing that if the walls withstand the earthquake and the dam retains the water, there is no disaster. Instead, he looks at disaster as the "collapse of the cultural protections" (Carr, 1932, p. 211). The implicit definition that a disaster is any event that generates significant negative consequences seems to have resulted in identification of disasters with events in the natural environment (floods, earthquakes, severe storms, etc.), technological incidents, and wartime incidents (Dombrowsky, 1981). This "disaster as negative, agent-caused event" approach can still be found in spite of early work distinguishing disasters from other events (civil disturbances and wars, for example) associated with negative consequences (Barton, 1963; Quarantelli, 1966; Warheit, 1972). Quarantelli (1982b) was among the first scholars to aggressively question this practice of defining disasters by surface characteristics of the agent. The early 1960s saw a formally proposed social scientific definition of disasters by Charles E. Fritz, first in a chapter on disasters in a social problems textbook (1961a) and subsequently in a social science encyclopedia (1968). These definitional efforts were followed closely by Barton's seminal examinations of disasters and creation of a typology in 1963.

The point here is that when one proposes a definition of disasters, one does not start from scratch. As much as it might be appealing to focus solely on the intellectual abstract task, we are influenced by, and need to acknowledge, our reading of the literature. After all, definitions are largely the product of an inductive process. Often, this involves looking backwards and making inferences to classify rather than eliminate research, while at same time exercising intellect in selecting key characteristics. It is likely that many, if not most, of the definitions reviewed in the next section were devised in this fashion.

Finally, definitions often grow convoluted because researchers do not clearly distinguish among causes, characteristics, and consequences of the phenomenon being defined. Indeed, as Stallings (2005) points out, definitions are not intended to be a collection of causal statements. Quarantelli (2005a, p. 333) similarly argues that researchers must separate the conditions, characteristics, and consequences of disasters when developing definitions. The definitions presented below have been selected from the original works to emphasize where possible each author's statement of characteristics.

DEFINITIONS OF DISASTER

Although an effort was made to gather as many formal definitions of disaster as possible, no claim can be made that those presented here exhaust the record. Those selected for inclusion do seem to be among the most visible definitions presented over the decades. Since the mid-1990s, when Quarantelli began assembling groups of disaster scholars to discuss definitions, the task has been made easier by volumes he assembled (Quarantelli, 1998a; Perry & Quarantelli, 2005). In choosing definitions, there was a sense of need to accommodate interdisciplinary study, but also to focus on the issue of disaster as a principally sociological construct.

Several classes of definitions are not included in this discussion. First among these are mandated definitions that are generated as a matter of social or government policy. These are usually used in making decisions about official disaster declarations or resource allocations connected with mitigation, preparedness, response or recovery. The purposes for which such definitions are devised are manifold, but not within a social scientific context. There are at least two excellent discussions of mandated definitions in the recent literature (Britton, 2005; Buckle, 2005). Similarly, hazards are not disasters and hazard-related definitions are included only to the extent that they explicitly address the occasion of disaster. Also eliminated are phenotypic definitions that focus on the surface features of an agent, such as natural versus man-made.

The simple presentation of definitions of disaster also raises a challenge. Chronological time, especially publication dates, is not a particularly effective ordering devise, as it implies serial or sequential development. In practice, many people used a definition for years without publishing it; some never wrote it down or published it only after using it implicitly for years. Many researchers simply adopted another scholar's definition, again explicitly or implicitly. One remedy to this problem is to group definitions by era, with a simultaneous concern for what might be called "paradigm" or "orientation." Certainly the definitions proposed and the studies conducted in the first decade of modern disaster research (1950s) influenced most of the work that followed. But this approach must be tempered to acknowledge that definitional foci have varied over the years. This condition sometimes places the same scholar in different categories at different times. The imperfect solution adopted here is to examine three focal areas: the classic approach and its variants, the hazards-disaster tradition, and the explicitly socially focused tradition. Like all stage or sequence models, these three "traditions" can be seen to overlap in time and to a small extent in content. They are acknowledged to be analytic creations designed to facilitate discussion. There is no guarantee, however, that different observers might not place specific definitions in different places, or for that matter, devise more or fewer categories. Nonetheless, as artificial ordering devices are concerned, they are practicable.

THE CLASSICAL PERIOD AND ITS EVOLUTIONS

The classical period may be seen as beginning the end of World War II and closing with the publication of Fritz's definition in 1961. The influence of the thinking and writing in this period on definitions of disaster , of course, extends to the present day. Three important intellectual and research activities operated early in this period. Studies were conducted of the impact of bombing on European and Japanese cities. The studies from Europe (United States Strategic Bombing Survey, 1947; Ikle, 1951) were systematic and included the reaction of the population as well as the customary examinations of physical damage. In 1951 and 1952, the National Opinion Research Center at the University of Chicago conducted a series of studies of eight disasters (mostly airplane crashes, but also fires and an earthquake). Charles Fritz oversaw the NORC studies and the field teams included E. L. Quarantelli. The third development was the formation of the Disaster Research Group, in 1952, at the National Research Council under the auspices of the National Academy of Sciences (NAS-NRC). This group was charged with conducting a review of the state of disaster research and conducted what has become a classic series of studies (Williams, 1954).

Many of these studies left the meaning of disaster implicit, but the definitions that did arise mentioned an event as catalyst for what now would be described as a failure of the social system to deliver reasonable conditions of life. At a minimum, the data from these studies collectively formed the first systematic (as opposed to journalistic or historical) information about human behavior in disasters. It is important to make two observations about this era. First, while the definitions explicitly mentioned an agent as catalyst (hence the use of the term "event"), most really dealt with the social disruption attendant to the cause rather than the cause or agent itself. Fritz's (1961b) research on the therapeutic community that arose following disasters is an important example of this emphasis on the social. It is easy to criticize these definitions as event centered if one has not actually read and appreciated the human and social variables that were actually studied. Second, the seeds of emergent norm thinking were sown during this period. This framework was ultimately developed by sociological social psychologists (particularly students of Mead's symbolic interactionism), and influenced students of collective behavior (particularly those interested in crowd behavior) and disaster researchers. It was manifest on the definitional side among disaster researchers in the vision that social interactions were supported by norms that might be rendered ineffective by disasters, thereby requiring different norms until the environment began to stabilize again (Gillespie & Perry, 1974). Research following this premise included Anderson's (1969) study of change after the 1964 Alaska earthquake and much later, Stallings' (1998) presentation of "exceptions" and "exception routines" as a perspective on disaster and the social order. Thus, although much of it was not published in the open literature, this era saw a great deal of inductive research, some deductive research, and much thinking that spawned attempts at theory development later. In effect, this period generated the first real "database" for subsequent research and theorizing.

In this active research context, three formal definitions of disaster were published. Anthony F. C. Wallace (1956a, p. 1), in a paper originally given as a committee report to the National Academy of Sciences—National Research Council Disaster Research Group in 1954, characterized disasters broadly as situations that involve not just impact, but the threat of "an interruption of normally effective procedures for reducing certain tensions, together with a dramatic increase in tensions." The social readjustment following these interruptions was also cited as part of the definition of the disaster. This early definition is generic and reflects the general opinion of then contemporary disaster researchers that disasters were events with negative social consequences. The use of the term "extreme situations" prefaced the later concern that disasters may actually be a subcategory of a larger class of events. At about the same time, Lewis M. Killian (1954, p. 67) proposed that disasters disrupt the social order, producing physical destruction and death that becomes important because people must cope by departing "from the pattern of norm expectations." Killian retained the negative dimension as a key feature of disasters as well as the importance of social consequences generated by a need to change normative behaviors. Harry Estil Moore was associated with the Disaster Research Group for some years, generating in the early 1960s what are now classic studies of warning response behavior. As part of his studies of tornadoes in Texas, Moore (1958, p. 310) also emphasized that a defining feature of disasters is that they make people adopt new behavior patterns; however, "the loss of life is an essential element." These three definitions are remarkably consistent with one another. Each characterizes disaster in terms of the impact on social order, and each focuses on negative consequences. Emergent norm thinking is implicit in all: the pattern of interrupted stability, followed by adaptation to the interruption, followed by a resumption (though not necessarily unchanged) of behavior in a stable period. These definitions also share a general or generic quality.

Fritz, working for the most part in the same tradition and on many of the same projects as the first three authors, proposed a definition of disaster in 1961 (and reiterated it in 1968) designed to capture the sociological notion of disaster. Fritz saw disaster as an event impacting an entire society or some subdivision and including the notion of real impact with threat of impact, but emphasized that "essential functions of the society [are] prevented" (1961a, p. 655).

This definition does not depart radically from the previous ones, but it attempts to be more "precise" and detailed. It did specify disaster as an "event" that later critics would argue moved the focus from strictly social and it also explicitly added "time and space" qualifications that one might argue limited disasters to being rapid onset events, although that implication was already implicit in the other definitions. There was also the rather strenuous requirement that a "society or relatively self-sufficient subdivision" be affected. This is interesting because at the time the definition was proposed (and since for that matter), little research was directed at disasters affecting an entire society. For decades later, it appears that the liberal determination of "relatively self-sufficient subdivision" allowed disaster researchers to embrace the definition while studying communities and groups smaller than communities.

Fritz's definition then was generated out of the intellectual context of the major disaster research efforts of the 1950s and the social context of the cold war. The apparent societal and governmental concern regarding a Soviet threat of an external attack came to be reflected in the notion that disasters were both events and external to a focal society or social group. In retrospect, one advantage of the definition was that it seemed to provide an umbrella for much of the increasing number of studies done by a growing multidisciplinary body of disaster researchers. After its publication, for decades many researchers simply adopted it verbatim or pointed to it. Wettenhall's (1975) studies of bush fire disasters; Perry, Lindell, and Greene's flood research (1981); and Perry's study of a nuclear power plant accident (1985) are only a few of many examples of those who adopted Fritz unchanged. Still, into the 21st century, researchers pose definitions that embrace the basic tenets of Fritz work. Buckle (2005, p. 179), speaking of a consensual definition of disasters, that one draws a sense of significant, irreversible loss and damage from disasters, requiring "the need of long term recovery." Similarly, Smith (2005, p. 301) proposed that disasters are events that produce death and damage and cause "considerable social, political and economic disruptions." Even Kroll-Smith and Gunter (1998, pp. 161–163), who clearly consider their thinking not part of "classical disaster sociology," describe incidents to be studied as disasters that largely meet the criteria in Fritz's definition; their argument is more about how and whom to study.

As recently as 2003, Henry Fischer, in accepting the Fritz definition, pointed out that sociologists really study social change under disaster conditions (2003, p. 95). Like Fischer, researchers began to accommodate slight variance from the original definition in what they were studying by adding modifiers to the definition. Thus, over time, small changes began to creep into the Fritz definition, introduced by researchers who largely embraced what they believed was Fritz's meaning. Four examples show this trend lasting well into the 1980s.

Gideon Sjoberg (1962, p. 357) characterized disaster as a "severe, relatively sudden, and frequently unexpected disruption" of a social system resulting from some precipitating event that is not subject to societal control. Thus Sjoberg introduces the notions that the precipitating event is sudden onset, external to the system and not subject to control. On the surface, this approach appears to tie disasters to the state of technology that might define control, but as Mileti (1999) indicated much later, humans can exert control in some cases by simply changing their settlement patterns. In the same year, Cisin and Clark (1962, p. 30) appeared to drop some of Fritz's qualifiers by saying a disaster is any event that "seriously disrupts normal activities." In elaboration, these authors added the explicit qualifier that the disaster may result from a threat that does not materialize as well as from an actual impact. This adds a new dimension to potential disaster studies (threats of destruction or disruption), while at the same time introducing some latitude in the stringent target of disasters set by Fritz by noting the disruption can be of "normal activities" and not specifying the social system.

Barry Turner (1978, p. 83) re-created part of the Fritz definition in defining disaster, but emphasized the notion that there must be a collapse of social structural arrangements that were previously "culturally accepted as adequate." Turner's definition was given in the context of a book on disasters with origins in human forces ("man-made") and adds the notion that disasters take place when precautions that are culturally based fail to allow continuation of "normal" behavior patterns. Drabek (1986, p. 7) adopted Fritz's words verbatim but prefaced

CONSENSUS ON DEFINITIONS

In almost every definition cited in the foregoing section, the author or authors included an elaboration to explain intent and often demonstrated causes and consequences of disasters. These elaborations contain important messages, but space limitations prohibited their presentation here. The following comments on themes often rely on these elaborations as well as my interpretation (right or wrong). In the end, the references are there to be checked by skeptics.

More than three dozen definitions of disaster have been presented in this chapter. It would be unrealistic to expect to find homogeneity among them. But clearly there are similarities and overlap; it can certainly be argued that the three artificially constructed "families" of definitions show considerable similarity within groups. And one would not expect to find common definition in any professional grouping, perhaps especially among social scientists. It is possible, however, to assess levels of general consensus across the definitions as a means of inferring agreement about what disaster researchers see as their field of study.

In this regard, the degree of consensus depends both upon the observer and on the level of specificity demanded to define consensus. Quarantelli (2005a, p. 338) summarizes his assessment by observing that "it would be difficult to deny that there is a substantial lack of consensus" about the meaning of the term disaster. I agree that comparing the detail of each definition (except when multiple authors adopt verbatim the definition of another author) yields an environment of significant differences. Similarly, there are differences in social scientific orientation as well; compare the positivist approaches of Stallings, Kreps, and Dombrowsky with the more interpretive approach of Kroll-Smith and Gunter, versus the almost mystical–phenomenological approach of Jigyasu. At the same time, the task becomes more manageable if the goal is to identify common themes in the definitions.

In discussing what he calls the current paradigm of disaster research, Quarantelli (2005a, p. 339) points out that it is rooted in two fundamental ideas. First, disasters are inherently social phenomena. It is not the hurricane wind or storm surge that makes the disaster; these are the source of damage. The disaster is the impact on individual coping patterns and the inputs and outputs of social systems. Second, the disaster is rooted in the social structure and reflects the processes of social change. It is from these features of the social system that we find vulnerability to the particular source. In effect, this vision of the field is reflected in the majority of the definitions reviewed here. Looking for themes is a fruitful way of capturing concepts of the field that might be obscured in the specific language and detail of a comparatively short definition. Of course there is the risk of misinterpretation when making inferences about themes, but social science is filled with such risk and at some point it is more irresponsible to say nothing than to risk being wrong. Kaplan (1964) warned about reconstructed logic (the scientist's "cleaned up" reconstruction of what they do) versus logic in use (what an observer would see a scientist do). Definitions can be seen as a form of reconstructed logic, and by identifying themes one is at least attempting to capture the logic in use.

I view a theme as arbitrarily specified as a common opinion by many (not even most) of the authors of the definitions reviewed. Studying disasters means you look for what? There is wide agreement (outside the classic hazard perspective) that disasters are social, that they are understood in human interaction. The researchers captured here under the rubric of "disaster as a social phenomenon" thereby often use the word occasion rather than event when speaking of disaster. There is also wide agreement that in disaster one finds disruption of the social. Some definitions and elaborations mention the source of the disruption as an event or force, but almost all agree on the social fact of disruption and that people's lives are being disrupted. Many agree that disasters stem not from the agent that causes the disruption, but from the social structure of norms and values, hence the protections. Vulnerability, a part of many of the definitions, is to be found in social structure and disruption is the outcome of vulnerability. There is some consensus, by inference, that the magnitude of a disaster should be measured not in lives or property lost, but by the extent of the failure of the normative or cultural system. Another fairly common theme is the issue of resilience. Some definitions in the classical tradition mark the end of one phase of disasters as the point at which normative stability is restored, while others call this restoration the implementation of emergency measures (norms) or exception routines. The link to emergent norm thinking is unmistakable. Typically, those who emphasize vulnerability include the notion of resilience in some form. Finally, although some authors speak of disasters as social problems, there is a general consensus that disasters are best understood in a context of social change. Carr seems to have originated this thinking in 1932 and it is present in much of the work of the classical era as well as being a staple of those who define disasters as exclusively a social phenomenon. Among the latter, and in some of the recent hazard-disaster definitions, as well as a handful of the definitions that evolved from the classical period, there is an emphasis on defining disasters in social time and space rather than physical time and space. As yet, more disaster researchers ignore social time and space than understand it or incorporate it into their research.

While all these common themes fit well within Quarantelli's exposition of a current disaster paradigm, much disagreement about disasters as an area of study remains. Some of the disagreement about disasters rests in issues that are not exclusively definitional. That is, there is disagreement about how disasters should be studied, how the definitions proposed by different groups (citizens, policy formulators, etc.) should be treated, the nature of social science, even whether disaster research is subsumed by social science, as well as disciplinary differences such as the hazards-disaster distinction. A few differences are based on definition and relate to such issues as the extent to which disasters originate outside a social system, the degree to which social change is emphasized, the centrality of the role of an agent, and how disaster consequences are to be conceived.

Some of the disagreement about disasters seems to stem from what are really taxonomic issues or at least from the typologies or classifications that are produced by taxonomic thinking (Perry, 1989). These are essentially disagreements about what kinds of characteristics should be included in the definition of a disaster and are expressed in different ways. Many of the scholars who authored the definitions have noted that disasters seem to be part of a "larger class of events." Indeed many who have proposed definitions from across the three perspectives included with their definitions a set of dimensions—such as social preparedness, speed of onset, scope and duration of impact—to create categories of disasters. Others have talked about how one can distinguish disasters from events that "look like" disasters. Quarantelli (2005a, p. 333) distinguishes disasters, catastrophes, and crises. Boin, Stallings, and Rosenthal have likewise separated disasters and crises (although using different referents for the latter term). Stallings (1991) and Quarantelli (2005a, p. 336) have proposed that situations involving conflict belong in a category different than "disaster." Similarly, Quarantelli (2005a, p. 335), as well as the authors of several of the definitions reviewed in this chapter, suggest the elimination of slow developing and diffuse events from the category of "disaster."

Quarantelli (1987a) makes a most convincing case for investing effort in taxonomy to create meaningful classification systems. He points out that the many empirical studies of "disasters" have begun to produce anomalous findings; using only one example, we know that serious mental health consequences, rare in most studies based on floods, tornadoes, hurricanes, and earthquakes, appear to be greater in cases associated with conflict situations (see Perry & Mankin, 2004 for a discussion of terrorist attacks). One explanation for such anomalies is classification error, comparing two things that are similar in phenotype, but are different genotypes. Classification systems are a way of sorting occasions and findings to make appropriate comparisons based on genotype. Quarantelli argues that disaster researchers need a classification system based on general dimensions that not only distinguish among different disaster agents, but also specify differences within one category of agent (1987a, p. 26). Drabek (1986, p. 6) stressed nearly 20 years ago that taxonomy is the "most pressing issue confronting the field at this time."

Certainly many disaster researchers have felt this need. Proposals for dimensions for classification schemes have historically accompanied efforts at definition since the earliest days. Two comprehensive typologies have been devised. Barton (1963, 1969, 2005) created a host of categories in a typology of collective stress situations, and Kreps (1989) devised an intricate system by looking at domains, tasks, resources, and activities (DTRA). There have consequently been many varied attempts to start disaster research down the taxonomic path, but with mediocre success. For the most part, those who conduct and interpret disaster research have neglected existing typological systems and rarely have chosen to qualify their findings in terms of the dimensions that are common in the literature: speed of onset, scope, and duration of impact and the like. The confusion and apparent anomalies that derive from this practice are likely to continue until researchers begin to document such qualifications or to operate within some typology. The explosion of disaster studies described at the beginning of this chapter will only exacerbate the problems.

The real challenge and danger is for the growth of disaster research as a field of study. As Hank Fischer indicated, most disaster research is not about the meaning of disaster. Descriptive studies can be (and long have been) generated with little attention to issues of theory or paradigm for that matter. However, as Drabek (1989) has warned, the creation of models and the production of viable explanations, predictions, and efforts at control move well beyond the descriptive task. To assemble a meaningful body of knowledge about disasters (Perry, 2005), it is absolutely critical that disaster researchers pursue Quarantelli's admonition not just to develop greater consensus regarding the meaning of the term, but also begin scrupulous use of typologies. Failing that, the field will continue to amass a disconnected collection of descriptive research that cannot be linked via existing conceptual tools.

AN AGENDA FOR FUTURE RESEARCH

The critical issues raised in this chapter do not focus on further research. The call here is for thinking, not for more doing. Research can and will continue, but sociologists must renew and revitalize their focus on conceptual matters. As indicated in the previous section, there are already hundreds of studies of individual, organizational, and institutional behavior in the literature that describe, and in a few cases attempt to explain, actions during times of "disaster." The problem is that a variety of views co-exist—some differing significantly—of the defining features of disaster. As Quarantelli and others have argued, the research record has accumulated under these varying definitions of disaster and has begun to produce apparently conflicting findings, when there may or may not be real differences. The reports of "looting behavior" in New Orleans following Hurricane Katrina (Quarantelli, 2005b) again underscore that more attention needs to be paid to the social context of the behavior (e.g., conflict or abandonment) than just to its characterization as taking place following a "disaster." Indeed, the problem of "what is a disaster" will never be solved by more fieldwork.

The real work to be done with respect to definitions of disaster has to do first with conceptualization; one needs to decide what disaster means. More specifically, each researcher needs to decide. This is not an empirical task. One must decide on fundamentals such as whether disasters are social phenomena or are the events with which they are often associated or even some natural or technological process. The stream of definitions recounted in this chapter seeks a starting point by identifying areas of consensus in what might be seen as a sea of differences. The differences count too. A significant point is that this practice of making explicit our definition of disaster has begun to take hold, although there is much more to be done.

The second part of the work to be done focuses on dialog among sociologists and disaster researchers. It is no longer appropriate to expect that a researcher can continue to do studies without specifying what constitutes a disaster. Further, the task of defining disasters should no longer be treated as an unnecessary abstraction that occupies the minds of a few senior (old) disaster researchers. There needs to be a serious engagement on the definition issue. A concern with taxonomy—the reasoning that underlies typologies or classification systems—should logically evolve out of this dialogue or engagement. Clearly, as other disciplines (such as botany and zoology) have found, we need to further specify our subject matter. This work too has seen a modest start. Taxonomic thinking cannot be characterized as the "easy work." It demands that one carefully understand the growing field of findings, appreciate the meaning of disaster in conceptual terms, and engage in both inductive and some deductive reasoning to support the creation of classification systems. The plural use of systems is an operative and indicative term here. There need not be a single typology; many can coexist. But there must be one or some typologies and they must be widely scrutinized by the disaster community. The more scrutiny, the more likely and quickly consensus at some level will begin to emerge.

Perhaps most critical, researchers will need to characterize their ongoing research in terms of one or more typologies. "Where does this study fit in the disaster cornucopia?" should be asked with each piece of research. At the same time, a need arises to consider the disaster findings of days (decades) past. When we cite those findings we must begin to group them into one or more of today's typologies. In this way, it would be routine to separate findings about looting behavior in situations that do and do not involve conflict. One practical outcome of the use of typologies is that we can reduce the potential ambiguity associated with interpreting our findings across events and at the same time present a clearer and more precise picture to those who may be using our findings to devise social policy. We will never "research" our way out of this problem. Such a tactic will only bury the field further in a kind of intellectual and conceptual muddle that will produce obfuscation and confusion.

CHAPTER 2

A Heuristic Approach to Future Disasters and Crises: New, Old, and In-Between Types

E.L. Quarantelli, Patrick Lagadec,
and Arjen Boin

Disasters and crises have been part of the human experience since people started living in groups. Through the centuries, however, new hazards and risks have emerged that have added to the possibilities of new disasters and crises arising from them. Only a very small fraction of risks and hazards actually lead to a disaster or crisis, but they are usually a necessary condition for such surfacing. New types have emerged while older ones have not disappeared. The development of synthetic chemicals in the 19th century and nuclear power in the 20th century created the risk of toxic chemical disasters and crises from radioactive fallouts. Ancient disasters such as floods and earthquakes remain with us today. This chapter raises the question of whether we are at another important historical juncture with the emergence of a new distinctive class of disasters and crises not seen before.

Our goal is twofold. First, we seek to describe and analyze these possibly new phenomena. Our second aim is to categorize all disasters and crises into a systematic conceptual framework. The newer disasters and crises are additions to older forms; they recombine elements of old threats with new vulnerabilities. In the future, we will concurrently see new types of disasters and crises, along with continuing manifestations of old ones, as well as mixed forms that in some respects have characteristics of older types mixed in with newer elements. In short, as we move further into the 21st century, risks and hazards will have more heterogeneity than ever before with their occasional manifestations in disasters and crises. This differentiation will present very complicated and challenging problems in planning for and managing such negative occurrences.

We offer here a heuristic approach to understanding the disasters and crises of the future. The chapter is presented primarily as a guide to further inquiry, hopefully stimulating more investigation on conceptions of disasters and crises in the past, present, and future. Unlike concepts in some areas of scientific inquiry, in which definitive conclusions can be reached (e.g., about the speed of light), the phenomenon we are discussing is of a dynamic nature and subject to change over time. The answer to the question of what constitutes a disaster or crisis has evolved and will continue to do so. Perry, in his chapter in this handbook, provides an impressive analysis of how scholarly discussion has been trending toward a more generic viewpoint, while also showing that most formulations can be categorized as one of three kinds.

NOT NEW SOCIAL PHENOMENA

Human societies have always been faced with risks and hazards. Earthquakes, very hostile inter-and intragroup relationships, floods, sudden epidemics, threats to take multiple hostages or massacre large numbers of persons, avalanches, fires, tsunamis, and similar relatively quickly appearing phenomena have marked human history for centuries if not eons. Some of these have been the source of disasters and crises.

These explicitly recognized negative social phenomena requiring a group reaction go back to the times when human beings started to live in stable communities, approximately 5,000 to 6,000 years ago (see Lenski, Lenski, & Nolan, 1991). However, recent archeological studies suggest that humans started to abandon nomadic wanderings and settled into permanent sites around 9,500 years ago (Balter, 2005), so community-recognized disasters and crises might have an even longer history.

The earliest occurrences are described in legends and myths, oral traditions and folk songs, religious accounts, and archeological evidence from many different cultures and sub-cultures around the world. For example, a "great flood" story has long existed in many places (Lang, 1985). These prehistorical indications of disasters and crises have of course been added to considerably by the development of history with descriptive accounts of contemporary occurrences, as well as examinations of past ones.

As human societies have evolved, new threats and hazards have emerged as well. New dangers have been added to existing ones; for example, risks from chemical, nuclear, and biological agents have been added to natural hazards.

Intentional conflict situations have become more damaging, at least in the sense of involving more and more victims. The last 90 years have seen two world wars, massive air and missile attacks by the military on civilians distant from battle areas, many terrorist attacks, widespread ethnic strife, and so forth. Just in the last decade, genocide may have killed one million persons in Rwanda, and millions have become refugees and tens of thousands have died in Dafur in the Sudan in Africa; similar attacks have occurred in Indonesia. Also, although terrorism is not a new phenomenon, its targets have expanded considerably.

Also, although we will discuss it only in passing here, a case can be made that there has been a progressive quantitative increase, especially in the last two centuries, of new risks and hazards (e.g., chemical and nuclear). In fact, some scholars and academics have argued that the very attempt to cope with increasing risks, especially of a technological nature, is indirectly generating new hazards. As the human race has increasingly been able to cope with securing such basic needs as food and shelter, some of the very coping mechanisms involved (such as the double-edged consequences of agricultural pesticides) have generated new risks for human societies (Beck, 1999; Perrow, 1999;). For example, in 2004 toxic chemicals were successfully used to eradicate massive locust infestations affecting 10 Western and Northern African countries. But at the same time, those very chemicals had other widespread detrimental effects on humans, animals, and crops (IRIN, 2004). Implicit in this line of thinking is the argument that double-edged consequences from new innovations (such as the use of chemicals, nuclear power, and genetic engineering) will continue to appear (Tenner, 1996).

Given all of this, is it possible to say how many disasters and crises have occurred? For a variety of theoretical and practical reasons discussed elsewhere (see Quarantelli, 2001b) any attempt to obtain exact quantification is fraught with major difficulties. Nevertheless, the Centre for Research on the Epidemiology of Disasters (CRED) has reported that from 1900 to 2004 there have been slightly more than 14,000 disasters (but all crises involving conflict as well as famines were not included in this statistical compilation, although droughts and very extreme temperature variations were counted). In addition, the CRED figures indicate an upward trend in occurrences of this nature. (For more on CRED and its statistics, visit its Web site, http://www.unisdr.org).

On the other hand, Alexander (2005, p. 25), citing some of the same data sources used by CRED, has written that there are about 220 natural catastrophes, 70 technological disasters, and 3 new armed conflicts each year. He also states that disasters are increasing. The cited numbers are not consistent with the CRED statistics and the figures he reports for technological disasters are far higher than Cutter (1991) found in her international survey of evacuations in chemical disasters. Still other numbers advanced by other sources vary even more (e.g., Glickman, Golding, & Silverman, 1992; the many chapters in Ingleton, 1999; the annual World Disasters Reports issued by the Red Cross and Red Crescent Societies, and the listing of current disasters in every issue of *The Disaster Prevention and Management Journal*).

What can we make of these inconsistent observations? We can probably accept without too much difficulty that "disasters" from a purely numerical viewpoint are not rare, isolated events. We might also tentatively assume that disasters and other crises are increasing, given that it can be shown that hazards and risks have increased. But we should also note two other things. Clearly, any statistics about numbers rest heavily on the definitions used. For example, just including or excluding "famines" can massively skew any statistical count because we would be speaking of hundreds of occurrences and millions of people (Quarantelli, 2001b). These different figures also raise questions about future occurrences. Can we really say, as some of us have (e.g., Quarantelli, 1991b), that the future will bring more disasters, if we have no reliable statistics on prior happenings as a baseline to use in counting? At present, it would seem safer to argue that some future events are qualitatively different, and not necessarily that there will be more of them in total (although we would argue the last is a viable hypothesis that requires a good statistical analysis).

SOCIETAL INTERPRETATIONS AND RESPONSES

Societies for the most part have not been passive in the face of these increasing dangers to human life and well-being. This is somewhat contrary to what is implicit in much of the social science literature, especially that concerned with disasters. In fact, some of these writings directly or indirectly state that a fatalistic attitude prevailed in the early stages of societal development (e.g., Quarantelli, 2000) as a result of religious beliefs that attributed negative societal happenings to punishments or tests by supernatural entities (the "Acts of God" notion, although this particular phrase became a common use mostly because it served the interests of insurance companies). But prayers, offerings, and rituals are widely seen as means to influence the supernatural. So passivity is not an automatic response to disasters and crises even by religious believers, an observation sometimes unnoticed by secular researchers.

Historical studies strongly indicate that societal interpretations have been more differentiated than once believed and have shifted through the centuries, at least in the Western world. In ancient Greece, Aristotle categorized disasters as the result of natural phenomena and not manifestations of supernatural interventions (Aristotle, 1952). However, with the spread of Christianity about 2,000 years ago came the belief that disasters were "special providences sent directly" from "God to punish sinners" (Mulcahy, 2002, p. 110). Thus, in the Middle Ages, even scholars and educated elitists "no longer questioned the holy origins of natural disasters" (Massard-Guilbaud, Platt, & Schott, 2002, p. 19). Starting in the 17th century, however, such explanations started to be replaced by "ones that viewed disasters as accidental or natural events" (Mulcahy, 2002, p. 110). This, of course, also reflected a strong trend toward secularization in Western societies. Perhaps this reached a climax with the 1755 Lisbon earthquake, which Dynes notes can be seen as the "first modern disaster" (2000b, p. 10).

So far our discussion has been mostly from the perspective of the educated elitists in Western societies. Little scholarly attention seems to have been given to what developed in non-Western social systems. One passing observation about the Ottoman Empire and fire disasters hints that the pattern just discussed might not be universal. Thus while fire prevention measures were encouraged in cities, they were not mandated "since calamities were considered" as expressions of the will of God (Yerolympos, 2002, p. 224). Even as late as 1826, an Ottoman urban building code stated that according to religious writing "the will of the Almighty will be done" and nothing can and should be done about that. At the same time, this code advances the idea that nevertheless there were protective measures that could be taken against fires that are "the will of Allah" (quoted in Yerolympos, 2002, p. 226). Of course incompatibilities between natural and supernatural views about the world are not unique to disaster and crisis phenomena, but that still leaves the distinction important. For an interesting attempt to deal with these two perspectives see the paper entitled "Disaster: a reality or a construct? Perspective from the East," written by Jigyasu (2005), an Indian scholar.

Historians have also noted that the beliefs of educated and professional elitists and citizens in general in almost all societies may be only partly correlated. Certainly this was true in the past. But even recently, an Australian disaster researcher asserted that after the 2004 Southwestern Asian tsunami most of the population seemed to believe that the disaster was "sent either as a test of faith or punishment" (McAneney, 2005, p. 3). As another writer noted, following the tsunami, religiously oriented views surfaced. Some were by "fundamentalist Christians" who tend to view all disasters "as a harbinger of the apocalypse." Others were by "radical Islamists" who are inclined to see any disaster that "washes the beaches clear of half-nude tourists to be divine" (Neiman, 2005, p. 16). After Hurricane Katrina, some leaders of evangelical groups spoke of the disaster as punishment imposed by God for "national sins" (Cooperman, 2005).

However, in the absence of systematic studies, probably the best hypothesis to be researched is that at present religious interpretations about disasters and crisis still appear to be widely held, but relative to the past probably have eroded among people in general. The orientation is almost certainly affected by sharp cross-societal differences in the importance attributed to religion, as can be noted in the religious belief systems and practices currently existing in the United States and many Islamic countries, compared to Japan or a highly secular Western Europe.

Apart from the varying interpretations of the phenomena, how have societies behaviorally reacted to the existing and ever increasing threats and risks? As a whole, human groups have evolved a variety of formal and informal mechanisms to prevent and to deal with crises and disasters. But societies have followed different directions depending on the perceived sources of disasters and crises. Responses tend to differ with the perception of the primary origin (the supernatural, the natural, or the human sphere).

For example, floods were seen long ago as a continuing problem that required a collective response involving engineering measures. Stories that a Chinese Emperor, 23 centuries before Christ, deepened the ever flooding Yellow River by massive dredging and the building of diversion canals may be more legend than fact (Waterbury, 1979, p. 35). However, there is clear evidence that in Egypt in the 20th century B.C., the 12th Dynasty Pharaoh, Amenemher II, completed southwest of Cairo what was probably history's first substantial river control project (an irrigation canal and dam with sluice gates). Other documentary evidence indicates that dams for flood control purposes were built as far back as 1260 B.C. in Greece (Schnitter, 1994, p. 1, 8–9). Such mitigatory efforts indicate both the belief that there was a long-term natural risk as well as one that could be coped with by physically altering structural dimensions.

Later, particularly in Europe, there were many recurrent efforts to institute mitigation measures. For example, earthquake-resistant building techniques were developed in ancient Rome, although "they had been forgotten by the middle ages" (Massard-Guilbaud, Platt, & Schott, 2002, p. 31). The threats from floods and fires spurred mitigation efforts in Greece. Starting in the 15th century, developing urban areas devised many safeguards against fires, varying from regulations regarding inflammable items to storage of water for fire-fighting purposes. Dams, dikes, and piles along riverbanks were built in many towns in medieval Poland(Sowina, 2002). Of course actions taken were not always successful, but the efforts showed that in the face of everyday dangers, citizens and officials were often not passive but proactive as well as reactive. If nothing else, these examples show that organized mitigation efforts have been undertaken for a long time in human history. Trying to prevent or reduce the impact of possible disasters is not an idea, as some seem to think, that was invented by the US Federal Emergency Management Agency (FEMA), which laudably did move in that direction at the end of the last century.

Two other major behavioral trends have persisted that are really preventive in intent if not always in reality. One has been the routinization of responses by emergency-oriented groups so as to prevent emergencies from escalating into disasters or crises. For example, in ancient Rome, the first groups informally set up to fight fires were composed of untrained slaves. But when a fire in 6 A.D. burned almost a quarter of Rome, a Corps of Vigiles was created that had full-time personnel and specialized equipment. In more recent times, there are good examples of this routinization in the planning of public utilities that have standardized operating procedures to deal with everyday emergencies so as to prevent them from becoming disasters. Various UN and other international organizations such as the International Atomic Energy Agency try to head off the development of crises in situations of conflict. In short, societies have continually evolved groups and procedures to try to prevent old and new risks and threats from escalating into disasters and crises.

A second more recent major trend has been the development of specific organizations to deal first with wartime crises and then with peacetime disasters. Civilian emergency management agencies have evolved from roots in civil defense groups created for air raid situations(Blanchard, 2004). Accompanying this has been the professionalization of disaster planners and crisis managers. There has been a notable shift from the involvement of amateurs to educated professionals in societies such as Canada, the United States, Australia, and some Western European countries. Thus, for about a century societies have been creating specific organizations to deal first with new risks for civilians created by changes in warfare, and then improving on these new groups as they have been extended to peacetime situations.

Human societies adjusted not only to early risks and hazards, but also to the newer ones that appeared up to the last century. The very survival of the human race is testimony to the coping and adjustive social mechanisms of humans as they face such threats. Occasionally a few communities and groups have not been able to cope with the manifestations of contemporary risks and hazards, but these have been very rare.

Neither disasters nor crises involving conflict have had much effect on the continuing existence of cities anywhere in the world. Throughout history, many cities have been destroyed. They have been "sacked, shaken, burned, bombed, flooded, starved, irradiated and poisoned" but in almost every case, phoenix-like, they have been reestablished (Vale & Campanella, 2004, p. 1). Around the world from the 12th to the 19th centuries, only 42 cities throughout the world were "permanently abandoned following destruction" (Vale & Campanella, 2004, p. 1). The same analysis notes that large cities such as Baghdad, Moscow, Aleppo, Mexico City, and Budapest and we may add more recently Dresden, Tokyo, Hiroshima, and Nagasaki, all suffered massive physical destruction and lost huge numbers of their populations as a result of disasters and wartime attacks. But all were rebuilt and rebounded; in fact, at the start of the 19th century, "such resilience became a nearly universal fact" about urban settlements around the world (Vale & Campanella, 2004, p. 1). Looking at the earlier mentioned Japanese cities today as well as Warsaw, Berlin, and Hamburg, it seems this recuperative tendency was still very strong at the middle of the last century (see also Schneider & Susser, 2003). Given that, the widespread predictions in 2005 that New Orleans will not recover from the catastrophic impact of Hurricane Katrina are very unlikely to be correct.

SYSTEMATIC STUDIES ARE NEW

Early efforts to understand and to cope with disasters and crises were generally of an ad hoc nature. With the strong development of science in the 19th century, there was the start of some understanding of the physical aspects of natural disasters, and these had some influence on structural mitigation measures. However, the systematic social science study of such negatively viewed occurrences is only about a half-century old. This is not surprising given that the social sciences as a whole are about 100 years old. Thus, social science knowledge for coping with disasters has only recently become available.

Disaster and crisis research of a social nature is a post-World War II phenomenon. That some of the earliest pioneer researchers are still around as of the writing of this chapter is a good indication of the recent origin of this field of study. This history is spelled out in detail, although selectively, elsewhere (see e.g., Fritz, 1961; Kreps, 1984; Quarantelli, 1988a, 2000; Schorr, 1987; Wright & Rossi, 1981).

But if a case is to be made that there are identifiable but new aspects of this in nontraditional disasters and crises, some kind of comparison has to be made. What are the distinctive aspects of the newer disasters and crises that are not seen in traditional ones? To deal with this and to go beyond journalistic sources, we considered what social science studies and reports had found about behavior in disasters and crises up to the present time. We then implicitly compared those observations and findings with the distinctive behavioral aspects of the newer disasters and crises.

To be sure, such accounts and reports as do exist are somewhat selective and not complete. Nevertheless, at the present time, case studies and analytical reports on natural and technological disasters (and to some extent on other crises) number in the four figures. In addition, numerous impressions of specific behavioral dimensions have been derived from field research (for summaries and inventories see Alexander, 2000; Cutter, 1994; Dynes & Tierney, 1994; Dynes, DeMarchi, & Pelanda, 1987; Farazmand, 2001; Mileti, 1999; Oliver-Smith, 1999a; Perry, Lindell, & Prater, 2005; Rosenthal, Boin, & Comfort, 2001; Rosenthal, Charles, & 't Hart,

1989; Tierney, Lindell, & Perry, 2001; Turner & Pidgeon, 1978; Waugh & Hy, 1990). In short, there is currently a solid body of research-generated knowledge developed over the last half century of continuing and ever-increasing studies around the world in different social science disciplines.

DIFFERENT CONCEPTIONS OF DISASTERS
AND CRISES

One issue that has interested researchers and scholars has been on how to conceptualize disasters and related collective crises. Unfortunately, there has been only partial consensus on how to approach the problem. It is not that there have not been major efforts to clarify the important question of what is a disaster or a crisis. What is X? If one wants to plan for X or point out the consequences of X, there has to be at least some minimum consensus about what X is. Otherwise, people will often talk past one another and about different things. As evident in two recently edited volumes on what is a disaster (Quarantelli, 1998; Perry & Quarantelli, 2005). At the practical or operational level the situation is even worse. Methods or procedures that might be advocated will simply make no sense given the different conceptions of disaster or crisis that might be involved (e.g., effective police actions for riot occasions need to be rather different than for consensus situations, as discussed later).

It is true that it is more important to look into what creates or generates something than it is to identify something. But it is very difficult to discuss what generating conditions are, unless one can specify what one is talking about in the first place. In other words, characteristics have to be roughly identified before one can examine the conditions and the consequences. That is our rationale behind specifying characteristics first.

However, there is far from full agreement that all disasters and crises can be categorized together as relatively homogeneous phenomena, despite the fact that there have been a number of attempts to distinguish between, among, and within different kinds of disasters and crises. However, no one overall view has won anywhere near general acceptance among self-designated disaster and crisis researchers. To illustrate we will briefly note some of the major formulations advanced.

For example, one of the very earliest attempts distinguished between natural and technological disasters, although some pioneer efforts such as at the Disaster Research Center (DRC) never accepted that as a meaningful distinction. The basic assumption was that the inherent nature of the agent involved made a difference. Implicit was the idea that technological dangers or threats present a different and more varying kind of challenge to human societies than do natural hazards or risks. But most researchers have since dropped the distinction as hazards have come to be seen as less important than the social setting in which they appear. Thus, in recent major volumes on what is a disaster (Perry & Quarantelli, 2005; Quarantelli, 1998), the distinction was not even mentioned by most of the two dozen scholars who addressed the basic question. But there are still some who say that separating out disasters with a technological base is a worthwhile endeavor (e.g., Picou & Gill, 1996; see also Erikson, 1994).

Other scholars have struggled with the notion that there may be some important differences between what can be called "disasters" and "crises." The assumption here is that different community-level social phenomena are involved, depending on the referent. Thus, some scholars distinguish between consensus and conflict types of crises (Stallings, 1988, tries to reconcile the two perspectives). In some research circles, almost all natural and most technological disasters are viewed as consensus types of crises (Quarantelli, 1998). These are contrasted with crises involving conflict such as riots, terrorist attacks, and ethnic cleansings and intergroup clashes.

In the latter type, at least one major party is either trying to make it worse or to extend the duration of the crisis. In natural and technological disasters, no one deliberately wants to make the situation worse or to create more damage or fatalities. Disputes or serious disagreements regarding natural or technological disasters are inevitable, and personal, organizational, and community conflicts will exist, for example in the recovery phase of disasters, where scapegoating is common (Bucher, 1957; Drabek & Quarantelli, 1967, 1969). In some crises the overall intent of major social actors is to deliberately attempt to generate conflict. In contrast to the unfolding sequential process of natural disasters, terrorist groups or protesting rioters not only intentionally seek to disrupt social life but they also modify or delay their attacks depending on perceived countermeasures.

Apart from a simple observable logical distinction between consensus and conflict types of crises, empirical studies have also established behavioral differences. For example, looting behavior is distinctively different in the two types. In the typical disaster in Western societies, almost always looting is very rare, covert and socially condemned, done by individuals, and involves targets of opportunity. In contrast, in many conflict crises looting is very common, overt and socially supported, undertaken by established groups of relatives or friends, and involves deliberately targeted locations (Quarantelli & Dynes, 1969). Likewise, there are major differences in hospital activities in the two kinds of crises, with more variation in conflict situations. There are differences also in the extent to which both organizational and community level changes occur as a result of consensus and conflict crises, with more changes resulting from conflict occasions (Quarantelli, 1993b). Finally, it has been suggested that the mass media operates differently in terrorism situations and in natural and technological disasters (Committee of Concerned Journalists, 1999, 2001). However, see Fischer (2003) for a contrary view that sees terrorist occasions as more or less being the same as what behaviorally appears in natural and technological disasters).

It is not unimportant to note that both the Oklahoma City bombing and the 9/11 World Trade Center attack led to sharp clashes between different groups of initial organizational responders. There were those who saw these occurrences primarily as criminal attacks necessitating closure of the location as a crime scene, and those who saw them primarily as situations where the priority ought to be on rescuing survivors, a universal disaster response. In the 9/11 situation, the clash continued later into the issues of the handling of dead bodies and debris clearance. At the operational level, although it was not verbalized in those terms, the responders split along the consensus/conflict line. All this goes to show that crises and disasters are always socially constructed, and whether it is by theorists, researchers, operational personnel, or citizens, any designation comes from the construction process and is not inherent in the phenomena itself. This is well illustrated in an article by Cunningham (2005), who shows that a major cyanide spill into the Danube River was differently defined as an incident, an accident, or a catastrophe, depending on how culpability was perceived and who was providing the definition.

Still other distinctions have been made. Some advocate "crisis" as the central concept in description and analysis (see the chapter by Boin in this handbook). In this line of thinking, a crisis involves an urgent threat to the core functions of a social system. A disaster instead is seen as "a crisis with a bad ending." To an extent this is consistent with the earlier expressed idea that although there are many hazards and risks, only a few actually manifest themselves. But the crisis idea does not differentiate among the manifestations themselves as the consensus and conflict distinction does. Also, to some a "crisis" implies immediacy and need for very quick action, but existing hazards and risks infrequently require this. (On the differences between the two ideas, see Boin, 2005.)

Finally, there also have been recent attempts to categorize conflict situations as one type of disaster. Thus, some talk of natural disasters, accidental disasters (mostly with reference to technological disasters), and deliberate disasters. Of course one of the crises we discuss later, computer system failures, can be the result of either mechanical accidents or deliberate insertions of viruses. Many transportation accidents, such as plane crashes or train wrecks, can also be both. The same can be said for forest fires; some result from arson, some from lightning. As a reviewer of an initial draft of this chapter noted, however, "it is difficult to ignore that some of the phenomena that disaster and crisis researchers are interested in, involve intentionality on the part of the social actors involved (e.g., terrorism) and some simply do not have that characteristic (e.g., natural disasters)." Thus "that distinction would seem important to include in any attempt to characterize disasters and/or crises." This reviewer also noted that some crises such as computer system failures do not necessarily involve conflict. Still others have argued that disasters, riots, and terrorist acts should be seen as three different kinds of crises (Peek & Sutton, 2003). More recently there have been attempts to differentiate, in a qualitative sense, disasters from catastrophes (Quarantelli, 2005b).

The preceding observations suggest that it would be far better for researchers to avoid focusing on a possible agent that might be involved and instead to examine the social behavior that appears and is the essence of a disaster or crisis. It would also seem that the intentions of participants in the setting cannot be ignored.

This is not the place to try and settle conceptual disagreements and we will not attempt to do so. Anyone in these areas of study should acknowledge that there are different views, and different proponents should try to make their positions as explicit as possible so people do not continue to talk past one another. It is perhaps not amiss here to note that the very words or terms used to designate the core nature of the phenomena are etymologically very complex, with major shifts in meaning through time (see Safire, 2005 who struggles with past and present etymological meanings of "disaster," "catastrophe," "calamity," and "cataclysm"; also see Murria, 2004, who looking outside the English language, found a bewildering set of words used, many of which had no equivalent meanings in other languages.) We are far from having standardized terms and similar connotations and denotations for them.

NEW KINDS OF DISASTERS AND CRISES

In the last decade or so, a conceptual question has been receiving increasing attention: Have new kinds of crises and disasters begun to appear?

Journalistic accounts of recent disasters raise that question at least intuitively. For example, massive computer system failures have occurred either through the insertions of viruses or as a result of mechanical problems in linked systems. There have been terrorist attacks of a magnitude and scale not seen before, widespread illnesses and health-related difficulties that appear to be qualitatively different from traditional medical problems, financial and economic collapses that cut across different social systems, space satellites and shuttles plunging into the Earth, large-scale serial sniper attacks as well as mass shootings and hostage takings, and animal health emergencies (e.g., mad cow disease) and vector-borne diseases not seen before.

Occurrences that seem to have both traditional and nontraditional features include the recent heat waves in Paris (Lagadec, 2004) and Chicago (Klinenberg, 2002) as well as ice storms such as in Canada (Scanlon, 1998b). Likewise, certain kinds of conflicts such as the recent genocide-like violence in Africa and the former Yugoslavia appear to comprise both old and new features. These mixtures of old and new often catch mass media attention and generate governmental and nongovernmental organization (NGO) actions in ways that are different in major ways from what had been done in previous centuries.

Now it is not the responsibility of social scientists such as us to deal specifically with the most recent news bulletins. Such descriptive accounts are of research use only if they indicate something of a more general nature. One question along that line that can be raised here is whether or not the journalistic accounts are indicating that something of a more basic nature is happening.

The Chernobyl radiation fallout led some scholars and researchers to start asking if there was not something distinctively new about that disaster. The fallout was first openly measured in Sweden, where officials were very mystified in that they could not locate any possible radiation source in their own country. Later radiation effects on vegetation eaten by reindeer past the Arctic Circle in northern Sweden were linked to the nuclear plant accident in the Soviet Union. To some researchers, that raised questions of how local emergency planners and managers could have anticipated, in any risk analysis they might have undertaken, what actually happened. The mysterious origins, crossing of national boundaries, and the emergent involvement of many European and transnational groups, was not something researchers had typically seen in concert in earlier disasters. If this was true, then Chernobyl was a "focusing event," something that calls into question previously held views (Birkland, 1997).

Looking back, it is clear that certain other disasters also should have alerted all of us to the probability that new forms of adversity were emerging. In November 1986, water used to put out fire in a plant involving agricultural chemicals spilled into the river Rhine. The highly polluted river went through Switzerland, Germany, France, Luxembourg, and the Netherlands. A series of massive fire smog episodes plagued Indonesia in 1997 and 1998. Land speculations led to fire clearing efforts that, partly because of drought conditions, resulted in forest fires that produced huge and thick smog hazes that spread over much of Southeast Asia (Barber & Schweithelm, 2000). These disrupted travel, which in turn affected tourism as well as creating respiratory health problems, and led to political criticism of Indonesia by other countries as multination efforts to cope with the problem were not very successful. Both of these occasions had characteristics that were not typically seen in traditional disasters.

We think it would be fair to say that most scholars and researchers interested in disasters and other crises generally agree that at present there are new types of risks and hazards as well as changes in social settings. If the world is increasingly being faced with nontraditional instances, what is the nature of such happenings? We address this question in the next section.

NATURE OF NEW HAPPENINGS

The two prime and initial examples we used in our analysis were the severe acute respiratory syndrome (SARS) and the SoBig computer F virus spread, both of which appeared in 2003. The first involved a "natural" phenomenon, whereas the second was intentionally created. Since much descriptive literature is available on both, we here provide only very brief statements about these phenomena.

The new infectious disease SARS appeared in the winter of 2003. Apparently jumping from animals to humans, it originated in southern rural China, near the city of Guangzhou. From there it moved through Hong Kong and Southeast Asia. It spread quickly around the world because international plane flights were shorter than its incubation period. At least 774 infected persons died. It particularly hit Canada with outbreaks in Vancouver in the West and Toronto far away in the East. In time, of the several hundred persons who became ill, 44 died and thousands of others were quarantined. The city's health care system virtually closed down except for the most urgent of cases, with countless procedures being delayed or canceled. This led to widespread anxiety in the area, resulting in the closing of schools, the cancellation of many meetings, and because visitors and tourists stayed away, a considerable negative effect on the economy (Commission Report, 2004, p. 28). The report notes a lack of coordination among the multitude of private and public sector organizations involved, a lack of consistent information on what was really happening, and jurisdictional squabbling on who should be doing what. Although SARS vanished worldwide after June 2003, to this day it is still not clear why it became so virulent in the initial outbreak and why it has disappeared (Yardley, 2005).

The SoBig computer F virus spread in August 2003. This was hardly the first deliberate insertion of an electronic virus into computer systems. The first occurred in 1981 (see http://www.cknow.com/vtiter/vihistory.htm for a comprehensive history of computer virus episodes). The SoBig worm carried its own SMPT mail program and used Windows® network shares to spread (Schwartz, 2003). Actually this virus was initially only one of a set of others that were circulating at the same time, but it soon became the dominant one in the world. It affected many computer systems and threatened almost all computers in existence. The damage was very costly in terms of use of time, effort, and resources. A variety of organizations around the world, public and private, attempted to deal with the problem. Initially uncoordinated, there eventually emerged in an informal way a degree of informational networking on how to cope with what was happening (Koerner, 2003).

What can we generalize from not only these two cases but also others that we looked at later? At one time, we identified a dozen different dimensions. In our more recent analyses we have reduced them to six. The characteristics we depict are stated in ideal typical terms, that is, from a social science perspective, what the phenomena would be if they existed in pure or perfect form.

First, the phenomena jump across many international and national/political governmental boundaries. There was, for example, the huge spatial leap of SARS from a rural area in China to metropolitan Toronto, Canada. In some instances, the phenomenon may spread to every possible target around the world, like the SoBig computer F virus did. It crosses functional boundaries, jumping from one sector to another, and crossing from the private into public sectors (and sometimes back).

Second, the phenomena spread very fast. Cases of SARS went around the world in less than 24 hours, starting with a person who had been in China and then flying to Canada, quickly infecting persons in Toronto. The spread of the SoBig F virus was called the fastest ever (Spread, 2003; Thompson, 2004). This quick spread is accompanied by a very quick if not almost simultaneous global awareness of the risk because of mass media attention. Despite this speed, however, at the start, the end of the happening's course is not clear cut.

Third, there is no known central or clear point of origin, at least initially, along with the fact that the possible negative effects at first are far from clear. This stood out when SARS first appeared in Canada. There is much ambiguity as to what might happen. Ambiguity is of course a major hallmark of disasters and crises (Tierney, 2005b), but it appears even more drastic in these newer cases.

Fourth, there are potentially if not actual large number of victims, directly or indirectly. The SoBig computer virus infected 30% of e-mail users in China, which is about 20 million people (Survey, 2003) and about three fourths of e-mail messages around the world were infected by this virus (Koerner, 2003). In contrast to the geographic limits of most past disasters, the potential number of victims is often open ended in the newer ones.

Fifth, traditional local community "solutions" are not obvious. This is rather contrary to the current emphasis in emergency management philosophy. The prime and first locus of planning and managing cannot be the local community as it is presently understood. International and transnational organizations are typically involved very early in the initial response. The nation-state may not even be a prime actor in the situation.

Sixth, although responding organizations and groups are major players, there is an exceptional amount of emergent behavior and the development of many informal ephemeral linkages. In some respects the informal social networks generated, involving much information networking, are not always easily identifiable from the outside, even though they are often the crucial actors at the height of the crisis.

We call these phenomena "trans-system social ruptures" (TSSRs). This term is an extension of the earlier label of "social ruptures" advanced by Lagadec (2000). The longer phrase is used to emphasize the fact they jump across different societal boundaries, disrupting the fabric of different social systems.

POSSIBLE FUTURE TSSRS

If a disciplinary approach is worthwhile, it should be able to somewhat predict the future, something that the social sciences studying disasters have little attempted. In this section, we project several possible future scenarios that involve TSSRs. Even though some of the scenarios discussed might seem like science fiction, they are well within the realm of realistic scientific possibilities.

The first scenario is the possibility that asteroids or comets may hit the Earth (Di Justo, 2005). Of course, this has happened in the past, but even more recent impacts found no or relatively few human beings around. There are two major possibilities with respect to impact (McGuire, 2000; Wisner, 2004). A landing in the ocean would trigger a tsunami-like impact in coastal areas. Just thinking of the possibility of how, when, and where ahead of time coastal population evacuations might have to be undertaken is a daunting task. Statistically less likely is a landing in a heavily populated area. A terrestrial impact anywhere on land, however, would generate very high quantities of dust in the atmosphere, which would affect food production as well as creating economic disruption. This would be akin to the Tombora volcanic eruption in 1813, which led to very cold summers and crop failures (Post, 1977). The planning and management problems for handling an event like this that could be of a global nature would be enormous.

In recent times, the Soviet satellite, *Cosmos* broke up over Canada (Scanlon, 2001), and the Columbia space shuttle explosion scattered debris over a large part of the United States. Our brief examination of these more geographically limited instances suggests that they had many of the characteristics of TSSRs as could appear in a comet impact. They would present extraordinary disaster management problems. The space shuttle accident, for example, required that an unplanned effort coordinating organizations that had not previously worked with one another and other unfamiliar groups, public and private (ranging from the U.S. Forest Service to local Red Cross volunteers to regional medical groups), be informally instituted over a great part of the United States (Donahue, 2003). This clearly indicates characteristics of TSSRs if a real comet or asteroid impact occasion arose, with massive crossing of boundaries, very large number of potential victims, no local community "solutions" for the problem, and so forth.

about the future. But perhaps that is asking more of disaster and crisis researchers than is reasonable. After all, social scientists with expertise in certain areas, to take recent examples, failed completely to predict or forecast the nonviolent demise of the Soviet Union, the peaceful transition of blacks taking over the government of South Africa, or the development of a market economy in communist China.

THE DIFFERENTIATED AND CHANGING
SOCIAL SETTING

A disaster or crisis always occurs in some kind of social setting. By social setting we mean social systems. These systems can and do differ in social structures and cultural frameworks.

The extreme differences around the world are not always noted. For instance, at present the lives of some individuals mostly revolve around cyberspace and the high tech world (see any issue of *Wired* Magazine for examples of this). They have every new gadget that can inform them about the world. At the other extreme are the residents of the Andaman Islands who live at a level many would consider "primitive." Thus, at the time of the recent tsunami in Southeast Asia they had no access to modern warning systems. But before the tsunami, members of the tribal communities saw signs of disturbed marine life and heard unusual agitated cries of sea birds. This was interpreted as a sign of impending danger, so that part of the population got off the beaches and retreated inland to the woods and survived intact (Tewari, 2005; http://www.tsunami2004-india.org). Even in the middle of highly urban societies there can be isolated social groups such as the Amish communities close to Three Mile Island who did not learn of the accident at the nuclear plant until many days later.

The social setting is very important. But whose setting is involved? That could be looked at in different ways, but for our purposes here, we will be speaking primarily of differences at the societal level.

There has been a bias in disaster and crisis research toward focusing on specific agents and specific events. Thus, social science researchers are sometimes inclined to say they studied this or that earthquake, flood, explosion, and/or radioactive fallout. At one level that is irrelevant. The terms refer to geophysical, climatological, or physical occurrences, which are hardly the province of social scientists. Instead those focused on the social in the broad sense of the term should be studying social phenomena. Our view is that what should be looked at more is not the possible agent that might be involved, but the social setting of the happening. This becomes obvious when researchers have to look at, for example, the recent Southeast Asia tsunami or locust infestations in Africa. Both of these occasions impacted a variety of social systems as well as involving social actors from outside those systems. This led in the tsunami disaster to sharp cultural clashes regarding how to handle the dead between Western European organizations who came in to look mostly for bodies of their tourist citizens and local groups who had different beliefs and values with respect to dead bodies (Scanlon, personal communication).

That given, there is a need to look at both the current social settings as well as certain social trends that influence disasters and crises. In do not address all aspects of social systems and cultural frameworks or their social evolution, either past or prospective. Instead we will selectively discuss and illustrate a few dimensions that appear particularly important with respect to crises and disasters.

What might these be? Let us first look at existing social structures around the world. What differences are there in authority relationships, social institutions, and social diversity?

As examples we might note that Australia and the United States have far more decentralized governments than do France or Japan (Bosner, 2002; Schoff, 2004). This affects what might or might not happen at times of disasters. For instance, given the research evidence that top-down systems have more problems in responding, it might have been expected, as did occur, that there would be a considerable delay in the central government response to the earthquake in the Kobe area in Japan (see the chapter on national planning and response by Britton in this handbook, where he extensively discusses Japanese disaster planning and managing; see also Nakamura, 2000).

As another example, a mass media system exists in almost all societies, but even with the same technologies this social institution operates in rather different ways in China compared with Western Europe. This is especially important because to a considerable extent the mass communication system is by far the major source of "information" about a disaster or a crisis (see the chapter by Scanlon in this handbook). In major ways, it socially constructs disasters and crises. This is partly illustrated by the fact that in the former Soviet Union even major disasters and overt internal conflicts in the form of riots were simply not openly reported (Berg, 1988). And only late in 2005 did Chinese authorities announce that henceforth death tolls in natural disasters would be made public, but not for other kinds of crises (Kahn, 2005).

Finally, another social structural dimension has to do with the range of social diversity in different systems. Social groupings and categories can be markedly different in their homogeneity or heterogeneity. The variation, for instance, can be in terms of life styles, class differences, or demographic composition. The aging population in Western Europe and Japan is in sharp contrast to the very young populations in most developing countries. Thus, 21% of the population in the United States is younger than 15 years of age, in contrast to Iran where the figure is 30% or India, where it is 36%. This is important, because the very young and the very old disproportionately incur the greatest number of fatalities in disasters. (For class and ethnic diversity in different societies and their effects on disaster preparedness, response and recovery, see the chapter by Bolin in this handbook.)

Human societies also differ in terms of their cultural frameworks. As anthropologists have pointed out, they can have very different patterns of beliefs, norms, and values. As one example, there can be widely held different conceptions of what occasions are designated as disasters and crises. The source can be attributed to supernatural, natural, or human factors as indicated earlier. This can markedly affect everything from what mitigation measures might be considered to how recovery and reconstruction will be undertaken.

Norms indicating what course of action should be followed in different situations can vary tremendously. For example, the norm of helping others outside of one's own immediate group at times of disasters and crises ranges from full help to none. Thus, although the Kobe earthquake was an exception, any extensive volunteering after disasters was very rare in Japan (for a comparison of the United States and Japan in this respect, see Hayashi, 2004). In societies with extreme cross-cultural ethnic or racial differences, volunteering to help others outside of one's own group at times of disasters or crisis is almost unknown.

Finally, much of what is valued can differ substantially. For instance, even the value of doing disaster research and implementing findings from studies varies from one culture to another. This activity is valued very highly in the United States compared to, say, Indonesia, with Russia falling somewhat in between.

Social structures and cultural frameworks of course are always changing. To understand future disasters and crises, it is necessary to identify and understand trends that may be operative with respect to both social structures and cultural frameworks. In particular, for our purposes, it is important to note trends that might be cutting across structural and cultural boundaries.

At the structural level, one notable ongoing change is what has been called globalization. Leaving aside the substantive disputes about the meaning of the term, what is involved is at least the increasing appearance of new social actors at the global level. For example, with respect to disaster relief and recovery there is the continuing rise of transnational or international organizations such as UN entities, religiously oriented groupings, and the World Bank. With the decline of the importance of the nation-state (Guehenno, 1995; Mann, 1997), more and new social actors, especially of an NGO nature, are to be anticipated.

A case can also be made that a variety of informal social networks have developed that globally cut across political boundaries, and that this will increase in the future. A clear example is the popular culture that appeals to the young, with ties and links that cut across most national boundaries. Some anti-American insurgent groups around the world can be seen wearing T shirts or caps that carry the names of music and sport groups in the United States. More important for the disaster and crisis areas is that such informal networks also are increasing in trade, science, and communications, to mention but a few examples (Quarantelli, 2002c). Such networks are creating a social capital (in the social science sense) that will be increasingly important in dealing with disasters and crises.

Among trends at the cultural level is the greater insistence of citizens that they ought to be actively protected against disasters and crises (Beck, 1999). This is part of a democratic ideology that has increasingly spread around the world. It is particularly surfacing in developing countries such as Turkey where recent disasters have evoked popular discontent and demonstrations that were unheard of before.

Finally, the 9/11 attacks, have clearly been a "focusing event" (as Birkland, 1997, uses the term), especially for official thinking not just in the United States but in other countries as well, and changed along some lines, certain values, beliefs, and norms (Smelser, 2004; Tierney, 2005b). There is a tendency, at least in the United States after 9/11, to think that all future crises and disasters will be new forms of terrorism. One can see this in the creation of the U.S. Department of Homeland Security, which is often repeating approaches and methods of thinking that the last 50 years of research have shown to be erroneous (e.g., an imposition of a command and control model, assuming that citizens will react inappropriately to warnings, seeing organizational improvisation as bad managing, etc.; see Dynes, 2003). Some of these problems surfaced during Hurricane Katrina. The changes have been in addition accompanied by the downgrading of FEMA and its emphasis on mitigation (Cohn, 2005). In fact, FEMA now has responsibility only for disaster response, with preparedness being incorporated in a general directorate that will clearly spend more time and effort on terrorism rather than disasters. There is also a growing clash between a disaster focus and a terrorism focus, with the latter leading to actions that will make disasters more likely (Drew, 2005). Whether valid or not, these ideas will heavily influence thinking about disasters and crises, at least in the near future and not just in the United States.

Overall, the existing social structures and cultural frameworks as well as changes going on in both, have to be taken into account in any further thinking about disasters and crises. These dimensions affect the larger social settings in which a disaster or crisis occurs. In saying this we are at least indirectly implying why disasters and crises have changed through time. To go from depicting characteristics to the conditions that generate these characteristics requires going considerably beyond, for example, the growing importance of informal networks or the also increasing expectations of citizens that some organization, such as the state, has responsibility to protect them against threats.

The ideas expressed in the preceding text and the examples used were intended to make several simple points. Given their validity, they suggest, for instance, that an earthquake in

France of the same magnitude as one in Iran will probably be reacted to differently. A riot in Sweden will be a somewhat different phenomenon than one in Myanmar. To understand and analyze such happenings requires taking into account the aspects just discussed. It is hard to believe that countries that currently have no functioning national government, such as Somalia and the Congo or marginally operative ones such as Afghanistan, will have the same reaction to disasters and crises as societies with fully functional national governments. Different kinds of disasters and crises will occur in rather different social settings. In fact, events that today are considered disasters or crises were not necessarily so viewed in the past.

In noting these cross-societal and cross-cultural differences, we are not saying that there are no universal principles of disaster and crisis behavior. Considerable research evidence supports this notion. We would argue, for example, that many aspects of effective warning systems, problems of bureaucracies in responding, and the crucial importance of the family/household unit are roughly the same in all societies. To suggest the importance of cross-societal and cross-cultural differences is simply to suggest that good social science research needs to take differences into account while at the same time searching for universal principles about disasters and crises. This is consistent with disaster researchers and scholars (e.g., Oliver-Smith, 1994) who have argued that studies in these areas have seriously neglected the historical context of such happenings, what we have called the social setting. Of course, this neglect of the larger and particularly historical context has characterized much social science research of any kind (Wallerstein, 1995); it is not peculiar to disaster and crisis studies.

SOCIAL AMPLIFICATION OF DISASTERS AND CRISES

The last section brings us to a consideration of other crises and disasters that only partly share the characteristics of TSSRs. Many crises and disasters have old or traditional characteristics, but nevertheless are new in some important aspects. These represent cases of what we will call the social amplifications of crises and disasters (SACD). Others initially developed an idea about a social augmentation process with respect to risk (see especially Pidgeon, Kasperson, & Slovic, 2003). To them, risk depends not only on the character of the dangerous agent itself but also on how it was seen in the larger context in which it appeared. The idea that there can be social amplification of risk rests on the assumption that aspects relevant to hazards interact with processes of a psychological, social, institutional, and cultural nature in such a manner that they can increase or decrease perceptions of risk (Kasperson & Kasperson, 2005). It is important to note that the perceived risk could be raised or diminished depending on the factors in the larger context, which makes it different from the vulnerability paradigm which tends to assume the factors involved will be primarily negative ones. We have taken this idea and extended it to the behaviors that appear in disasters and crises. Hence besides the development of new agents or hazards or risks as can be seen in TSSRs, there are also the existing social settings as well as changes in them that crucially affect if and how some crises and disasters will occur and be perceived.

Extreme heat waves and massive blizzards are hardly new weather phenomena (Burt, 2004). The historical record as well as contemporary studies on the social aspects of such happenings is surprisingly sparse (Hewitt & Burton, 1971; International Federation of Red Cross and Red Crescent Societies, 2004, p. 37–55; Koppe, Kovacs, Jendritzbky, & Menne, 2004; Sheehan & Hewitt, 1969;). As climatological hazards they have been around as long as the human race, and in that respect, like blizzards and cold waves, they have very old antecedents (for statistical data see Burt, 2004).

Two recent heat waves, however, have contained new elements. In 2003, a long lasting and very intensive heat wave battered France. Nearly 15,000 persons died (and perhaps 22,000 to 35,000 in all of Europe). Particularly noticeable was that the victims were primarily socially isolated older persons. Another characteristic was that officials were very slow in accepting the fact that there was a problem and so there was very little initial response (Lagadec, 2004). A somewhat similar earlier incident occurred in 1995 in Chicago that was not much noticed until reported in a study 7 years later (see Klinenberg, 2002). It exhibited some of the same features, that is, older isolated victims, bureaucratic indifference, and mass media uncertainty.

At the other temperature extreme, in 1998, Canada experienced an accumulation of snow and ice that went considerably beyond the typical. The ice storm heavily impacted electric and transport systems, especially around Montreal. The critical infrastructures that were affected created chain reactions that reached into banks and refineries. At least 66 municipalities declared a state of emergency. Such a very large geographic area was involved that many police were baffled that "there was no scene" that could be the focus of attention (Scanlon, 1998b). There were also many emergent groups and informal network linkages (Scanlon, 1999a).

In some ways, this was similar to what happened in August 2003, when the highly interconnected eastern North American power grid started to fail when three transmission lines in the state of Ohio came into contact with trees and short circuited (Townsend & Moss, 2005). This created a cascade of power failures that resulted in blackouts in cities from New York to Toronto and eventually left around 50 million persons without power, which, in turn, disrupted everyday community and social routines (Ballman, 2003). It took months of investigation to establish the exact path of failure propagation through a huge, complex network. Telecommunication and electrical infrastructures entwined in complex interconnected and network systems spread over a large geographic area with multiple end users. Therefore, localized disruptions can cascade into large-scale failures (for more details, see Townsend & Moss, 2005).

Such power blackouts have recently become very common. They occurred, among other areas, in Auckland, New Zealand in 1998 (Newlove, Stern, & Svedin, 2002); in Buenos Aires in 1999 (Ullberg, 2004); in Stockholm in 2001 and 2002; in Siberian cities in 2001 (Humphrey, 2003); and in Moscow in 2005 (Arvedlund, 2005). All of these cases initially involved accidents or software and hardware failures in complex technical systems that generate severe consequences, creating a crisis with major economic and often political effects. These kinds of crises should have been expected. Even two decades ago, a National Research Council report (1989) forecast the almost certain probability of these kinds of risks in future network linkages.

Blackouts can also be deliberately created either for good or malevolent reasons unrelated to problems in network linkages. Employees of the now notorious Enron energy company, to exploit Western energy markets, indirectly but deliberately took off line a perfectly functioning Las Vegas power plant so that rolling blackouts hit plant-dependent northern and central California, with about a million residences and businesses losing power (Peterson, 2005). In the earliest days of electricity in New York City, the mayor ordered the power cut off when poor maintenance of exposed and open wires resulted in a number of electrocutions of citizens and electrical workers (Jonnes, 2004). One should not think of blackouts as solely the result of mechanical or physical failures creating chain-like cascades.

These examples are not quite TSSRs but neither do they represent the older or more traditional types. It is the social setting in which they occur that determines their characteristics (this is consistent with similar thinking expressed in Wisner, Blaikie, Cannon, & Davis, 2004). The social settings are more complex and differentiated than ever before, so SACDs are more frequent than ever before. In fact, these in-between types may be more common than TSSRs. We believe SACDs can be expected in the future and probably at an accelerating rate.

THE FULL RANGE OF ALL DISASTERS AND CRISES

Where do TSSRs and SACDs fit into the full range of all disasters and crises? We have already indicated that we see TSSRs as adding to the complex of such events rather than replacing them. That said, our view is that we should think of disasters and crises as falling into one of three conceptual categories: old, new, and in-between types. In this section we discuss old ones, making a case that most disasters are still traditional ones.

In the United States in 2004, there were 78 federally declared disasters (as well as 43 fire management assistance declarations). While we did not examine closely all these occurrences, we did look at some very closely.

For example, four major hurricanes hit the state of Florida that year (for an epidemiologic survey of residents in the state, see Centers for Disease Control [CDC], 2005). We saw very little in what we found that required thinking of them in some major new ways, or even in planning for or managing them. The problems, individual or organizational, that surfaced were the usual ones, and how to handle them successfully is fairly well known. More important, emergent difficulties were actually somewhat better handled than in the past, perhaps reflecting that officials may have had exposure to earlier studies and reports. Thus, the warnings issued and the evacuations (one third of those surveyed) that took place were better than in the past. Looting concerns were almost nonexistent and fewer than 10% of people showed possible mental health effects. The pre-impact organizational mobilization and placement of resources beyond the community level was also better. The efficiency and effectiveness of local emergency management offices were markedly higher than in the past. Not everything was done well. Long known problematical aspects and failures to implement measures that research had suggested a long time ago were found. There were major difficulties in interorganizational coordination. The recovery period was plagued by the usual problems. Even the failures that showed up in pre-impact mitigation efforts were known.

From our viewpoint, the majority of contemporary disasters in the United States are resemble most of the earlier ones. What could be seen in the 2004 hurricanes in Florida was rather similar to what the DRC had studied there in the 1960s and the 1970s. As the electronic age advances beyond its infancy and as other social trends continue (e.g., the already mentioned aging of the population), new elements may appear, creating new problems that will necessitate new planning. If and when that happens, we may have new kinds of hurricane disasters, but movement in that direction will be slow.

Apart from the Florida events, we can also report what the senior author of this chapter recently experienced in his local area. As the famous sociologist Herbert Blumer used to say in his class lectures a long time ago, it is sometimes useful to check whatever is theoretically proposed against personal experience. In 2005, an extensive snowstorm led to the closing of almost all schools and government offices in the state of Delaware. This was accompanied by the widespread cancellations of religious and sports events. Air, road, and train service was disrupted across the board. All of this resulted in major economic losses in the million of dollars. There were scattered interruptions of critical life systems. The governor issued a state of emergency declaration and the state as well as local emergency management offices fully mobilized. To be sure, what happened did not rival what surfaced in the Canadian blizzard discussed earlier. But it would be difficult to argue that it did not meet criteria often used by many to categorize disasters. For example, it met two of the criteria the CRED uses to identify a disaster, any one of which is enough for the classification: declaration of state of emergency and 100 persons affected. (But it did not show up in the CRED statistics!) Equally important, what happened was not that different from what others and we had experienced in the past. In short, it was a traditional disaster.

Finally, at the same time we were thinking about the Florida hurricanes and the Delaware snowstorm, we also observed other events that many would consider disasters or crises. Certainly, a BP Texas plant explosion in 2005 would qualify. It involved the third largest refinery in the country that produces about 3% of the U.S. gasoline supply. More than 100 people were injured and 15 died. In addition, refinery equipment was physically destroyed and nearby buildings were leveled. There was full mobilization of local emergency management person-nel (Franks, 2005). At about the same time, there were landslides in the states of Utah and California; a stampede with hundreds of deaths in a Bombay, India temple; train and plane crashes in different places around the world, as well as large bus accidents; a dam rupture that swept away five villages, bridges, and roads in Pakistan; recurrent coal mine accidents and collapses in China; recurrent false reports in Asia about tsunamis that greatly disrupted local routines; sinking of ferries with many deaths; and localized riots and hostage takings. At least based on press reports, it does not seem that there was anything distinctively new about these occasions. They seem to greatly resemble many such prior happenings.

It does not appear to us that TSSRs and SACDs will totally supersede at least the more circumscribed and localized crises and disasters that will continue to have traditional charac-teristics, including the need to be handled at the local community level. Unless current social trends change very quickly in hypothetical directions (e.g., marked changes as a result of biotechnological advances), for the foreseeable future there will continue to be many rather old and traditional local community disasters and crises (such as localized floods and tornadoes, hostage takings or mass shootings, exploding tanker trucks or overturned trains, circumscribed landslides, disturbances if not riots at local sport venues, large plant fires, sudden discoveries of previously unknown very toxic local waste sites, most airplane crashes, stampedes and panic flights in buildings, etc.).

Mega-disasters and global crises will be rare in a numerical and relative sense, although they may generate much mass media attention. For example, recent terrorist attacks on the Madrid and London train systems were certainly major crises and symbolically very important, but numerically there are far more local train wrecks and collisions every day in many countries in the world. The more localized crises and disasters will continue to be the most numerous, despite ever increasing TSSRs and SACDs. Overall, the world is faced with a mixture of old, new, and in-between types of disasters and crises, but numbers of each type are far from equal.

IMPLICATIONS

What are some of the implications for planning and managing that result from taking the perspective we have suggested about crises and disasters? If our descriptions and analyses of such happenings are valid, there would seem to be the need at least for some new kinds of planning for and managing of TSSRs and SACDs. Nontraditional disasters and crises require some nonconventional processes and social arrangements. They demand innovative thinking "outside of the box" as Lagadec (2005) has frequently said (see also Boin & Lagadec, 2000).

This does not mean that everything has to be new. As said earlier, all disasters and crises share certain common dimensions or elements. For example, if early warning is possible at all, research has consistently shown that acceptable warnings have to come from a legitimately recognized source, have to be consistent, and have to indicate that the threat or risk is fairly immediate. These principles would seem to apply also to TSSRs and SACDs, although other measures might be necessary.

Actually, if the older types of risks and hazards and their occasional manifestations in crises and disasters were all we needed to be worried about, we would be in rather good shape. As previously mentioned, few threats actually manifest themselves in disasters. For example, in the 14,600 plus tornadoes appearing in the United States between 1952 and 1973, only 497 involved caualties, and 26 of these occasions accounted for almost half of the fatalities (Noji, 2000). Similarly, it was noted in 1993 that while about 1.3 million people had been killed in earthquakes since 1900 more than 70% of them had died in only 12 occurrences (Jones, Noji, Smith, & Wagner, 1993, p. 19).

That said, we can also say that the older risks and hazards and their relatively rare manifestations in crises and disasters are being coped with much better than they ever were even just a half-century ago. For example, there has been a remarkable reduction in certain societies of fatalities and even property destruction in some natural disaster occasions associated with hurricanes, floods, and earthquakes (see Scanlon, 2004, for data on North America). In the conflict area, the outcomes have been much more uneven, but even here, for example, the recurrence of world wars seems very unlikely.

But given that, are their certain aspects about coping that are more distinctive of SACDs and TSSRs? Certainly all kinds of specific practical questions might be asked. For example, let us assume that a health risk is involved. If international cooperation is needed, who talks with whom about what? At what time is action initiated? Who takes the lead in organizing a response? What legal issues are involved? (For example, if health is the issue, can health authorities close airports?) There might be many experts and much technical information around; if so, and they are not consistent, whose voice and ideas should be followed? What should be given priority? How could a forced quarantine be enforced? What of ethical issues? Who should get limited vaccines? What should the mass media be told and by who and when? (Boin, t'Hart, Stern, & Sundelius, 2005).

Let us move on to a more general level of planning and managing. We briefly indicate, almost in outline form, half a dozen principles that ought to be taken into account by disaster planners and crisis managers. (However, for a much fuller discussion about planning for and managing newer crises see the chapter by Lagadec in this handbook).

First, a clear distinction should be made between the planning and managing processes. As these terms are used in the literature, planning really refers to the strategies that need to be used in a situation. Managing has reference to the tactics that might be used in dealing with contingencies. There is a low correlation between planning and managing in the first place, even for traditional crises and disasters. But in newer kinds of disasters and crises, there are likely to be, for reasons already indicated, far more contingencies present in the situation. That is why even more of a focus on managing is needed.

Second, the appearance of much emergent social phenomena (groups and behaviors) needs to be taken into account. The reason for such emergence is that they arise in response to "unmet demands" in the situation (this happened most recently in the search for the Columbia shuttle pieces as discussed in Donahue, 2003). There are always new or emergent groups at times of major disasters and crises, but in SACDs and TSSRs they appear at a much higher rate.

Networks and network links also have to be particularly taken into account. There is a tendency to think of groups and interorganizational links. That is appropriate for traditional types of disasters. However, in TSSRs and SACDs these are less important than the informal networking that occurs. Research on this topic is considerably helped these days by the existence of a relatively recent body of literature including professional journals (e.g., *Global Networks: A Journal of International Affairs*).

Third, there is the need to be imaginative and creative. SACDs and TSSRs create new and higher level problems as a result of the dimensions and characteristics of these events. Hurricane Katrina, which was more a catastrophe than a disaster, might seem to suggest such challenges are almost impossible to meet. However, that is not the case. A good example is found in the immediate aftermath of 9/11 in New York. In spite of the total loss of the New York City Office of Emergency Management and its EOC facility, a completely new EOC was established elsewhere and started to operate very effectively within 72 hours after the attack. There had been no planning for such an event, yet around 750,000 persons were evacuated by water transportation from lower Manhattan (Kendra, Wachtendorf, & Quarantelli, 2003). These are not minor examples of what can be done.

Fourth, exercises and simulations of disasters and crises must have built-in contingencies (Boin, Kofman-Bos, & Overdijk, 2004). Most such training and educational efforts along such lines are designed to be like scripts for plays. That is a very poor model to use. Many contingencies exist in TSSRs and SACDs; therefore similar unexpected happenings should be built into exercises and training (Perry, 2004). Realistic contingencies, unknown to most of the players in the scenarios, make thinking through unconventional options imperative.

Fifth, planning should be with citizens and their social groups, and not for them. There is no such thing as the "public" in the sense of some homogenous entity (Blumer, 1948). There are only individual citizens and the groups of which they are members. The perspective from the bottom up is crucial to getting things done. This has nothing to do with democratic ideologies; it has instead to do with getting effective and efficient planning and managing of disasters and crises. Related to this is that openness with information rather than secrecy is mandatory. This runs against the norms of most bureaucracies and other organizations. The more information the mass media and citizens have, the better they will be able to react and respond (Wagman, 2003). However, all this is easier said than done. For example, even in modern urban areas, there typically are a variety of "of information receivers" so that all "do not seek information in the same way, using the same language or the same cultural reference frames" (Castenfors & Svedin, 2001, p. 251). Nevertheless, in the United States in 2005 a bill was introduced in Congress, *The Ready, Willing, and Able Act,* which calls for the establishment of a time-limited working group composed of federal government officials and Citizen Corps Council members to establish standards for having citizens work in close collaboration with local government officials, health authorities, emergency managers, and professional responders to develop and modify community based disaster preparedness, response, recovery, and mitigation plans.

Finally, there is a need to start thinking of local communities in ways different than they have been traditionally viewed. Up to now communities have been seen as occupying some geographic space and existing in some chronological time. Instead, we should visualize the kinds of communities that exist today are in cyberspace. These newer communities must be thought of as existing in social space and social time. Viewed this way, the newer kinds of communities can be seen as very important in planning for and managing disasters and crises that cut across national boundaries. To think this way requires a moving away from the traditional view of communities in the past. This will not be easy given that the traditional community focus is strongly entrenched in most places around the world (see United Nations, 2005). But "virtual reality communities" will be the social realities in the future.

LOOKING AT THE FUTURE OF THE FUTURE

Assuming that what we have written has validity, what new research should be undertaken in the future on the topic of future disasters and crises? In previous pages we suggested some future studies on specific topics that would be worthwhile doing. However, in this section we outline research of a more general nature.

For one, practically everything we discussed ought to be looked at from the aspect of different cultures and societies. As mentioned earlier, there is a bias in our perspective that reflects our greater familiarity with and awareness of examples from the West (and even more narrowly Western Europe, the United States, and Canada). In particular there is a need to undertake research in developing as opposed to developed countries, which includes at least some analyses by researchers and scholars from the very social systems that are being studied. The different cultural perspectives that would be brought to bear might be very enlightening, and enable us to see things that we do not see at present, being somewhat a prisoner of our own culture.

Second, here and there in this chapter, we have alluded to the fact that it is more important to study the conditions that generate disasters and crises than it is to specify characteristics of the phenomena that are being studied. But there has to be at least some understanding of the nature of X before there can be a serious turn to ascertaining the conditions that generate X. We have taken this first step in this chapter. Future work should focus more on the generating conditions. A general model would involve the following ideas. The first is to look at social systems (societal, community, and/or organizational ones), and to analyze how they have become more complex and tightly coupled. The last statement would be treated as a working hypothesis. If that turns out to be true, it could then be hypothesized that systems can break down in more ways than ever before. A secondary research thrust would be to see if systems also have developed ways to deal with or cope with threatening breakdowns. As such, it might be argued that what ensues is an uneven balance between resiliency and vulnerability.

In studying contemporary trends, particular attention might be given to demographic ones. It would be difficult to find any country today where the population composition is not changing in some way. The increasing population density in high-risk areas seems particularly important in possible TSSRs and even more so for SACDs. Another value in doing research on this topic is that much demographic data are of a quantitative nature.

Although we have discussed a variety of examples of TSSRs and SACDs, there are other possibilities we have noted only in passing. In particular, we mentioned financial and economic collapses cutting across different systems. A good example would be the collapse in 1998 of the private Long Term Capital Management hedge fund that operated internationally. As a result of a major brokerage house pulling out of the fund, a sudden Russian moratorium on its debt, and other complex financial transactions, a downward chain reaction started. Its deterioration in September of that year threatened to destabilize not only stock markets around the world, but global financial systems in general. To prevent this, a consortium of domestic and foreign banks and brokerage firms, unofficially led by the U.S. Federal Reserve, informally generated three and a half billion dollars in cash to prevent an immediate collapse (Lowenstein, 2004).

How can this financial collapse conceivably be thought of as comparable in any way to natural disasters and crises involving conflict? One simple answer is that for nearly a hundred years, one subfield of sociology has categorized, for example, panic flight in theater fires and financial panics as generic subtypes within the field of collective behavior (Blumer, 1939; Smelser, 1963). Both happenings involve new, emergent behaviors of a nontraditional nature. In this respect, scholars long ago put both types of behavior into the same category. Although disaster and crisis researchers have not looked at financial collapses, perhaps it is time that they did so, and particularly to examine if these are other instances of TSSRs. These kinds of happenings seem to occur very quickly, have ambiguous consequences, cut across political and sector boundaries, involve a great deal of emergent behavior, and cannot be handled at the community level. In short, what must be sought are genotypic characteristics, not phenotypic ones (see the chapter by Perry in this handbook). If whales, humans, and bats can all be usefully categorized as mammals for scientific research purposes, maybe students of disasters should also pay less attention to phenotypic features. If so, should other disruptive phenomena such as AIDS also be approached as disasters? Our overall point is that new research along the lines indicated might lead researchers to see phenomena in ways that are different from the way they had seen these in the past.

Finally, we have said little about the research methodologies that might be necessary to study TRRSs and SACDs. Up to now, disaster and crisis researchers have argued that the methods they use in their research are indistinguishable from those used throughout the social sciences. The methods are simply applied under circumstances that are relatively unique (Stallings, 2002).

In general, we agree with that position. But two questions can be raised. First, if social scientists venture into such areas as genetic engineering, cyberspace, robotics, and complex infectious diseases, do they need to have knowledge of these phenomena to a degree that they presently do not have? We have to confess that at times we have been uneasy trying to understand the SARS phenomena, which we had not experienced in studying disasters associated with earthquakes or chemical explosions. This may suggest the need for interdisciplinary research. Perhaps it also indicates that social scientists ought to expand their knowledge base before venturing to study certain disasters and crises, especially the newer ones. In the sociology of science there have already been studies of how researchers from rather different disciplines studying one research question interact with one another and what problems they have. Researchers in the disaster and crisis area should look at these studies. Even better, research might be conducted along these lines on social scientists that have or are specifically studying TSSRs or SACDs. We are not aware that there has been even one such study done anywhere.

Possibly more important, greater use should be made of the newer technologies that are currently available. Social scientists generally and students of disasters and crises in particular have done very little to take advantage of ever increasing computer and related technologies such as digital cameras and cell phones or electronic journals, to gather, analyze, and report findings. If we are going to study computer system disasters, would it not be appropriate to use computers as much as possible in such studies? (For specific suggestions, see Quarantelli, 2005a, pp. 359–366.)

CONCLUSIONS

Our view is that the area of disasters and crises is changing. In addition to the traditional kinds, we see an ever-increasing number of new and mixed crises and disasters. It is therefore likely that there will be both qualitative and quantitative changes of a negative nature.

Although this might seem to be a very pessimistic outlook, it is not the case. There is reason to think, as we tried to document earlier, that human societies in the future will be able to cope with whatever new risks and hazards come into being. To be sure, given hazards and risks, there are bound to be disasters and crises. A risk-free society has never existed and will never exist. But although this is undoubtedly true in a general sense, it is not so with reference to any particular or specific case. In fact, the great majority of potential dangers never manifest themselves eventually in disasters and crises.

Finally, we note again that the approach in this chapter has been a heuristic one. We have not implied that we have absolute and conclusive research-based knowledge or understanding about all of the issues we have discussed. This is in line with Alexander, who recently wrote that scientific research is never ending in its quest for knowledge, rather than trying to reach once-for-all final conclusions, and therefore "none of us should presume to have all the answers" (2005, p. 97).

In yet another niche—enfolded in the field of communications studies—interesting work is being done on the relationship between crisis actors, (political) stakeholders, media, and civilians (Fearn-Banks, 1996; Seeger, Sellmer, & Ulmer, 2003). This body of research helps us understand why sound decisions may or may not help to manage a crisis, depending on the way they are communicated. It helps us understand how media frames shape crisis reports, which, in turn, affect general perceptions of the crisis and the authorities managing it.

Our *tour d'horizon* would not be complete without mentioning the risk field, itself an interdisciplinary social–scientific venture (Pidgeon, Kasperson, & Slovic, 2003). It studies why and how people act on negligible risks (avoiding flying) while they ignore others (smoking, driving without seatbelts). The steadfast stream in this field tries to calculate risks, which should help policymakers make thorough decisions on baffling issues such as genetically modified food, environmental pollution, or space travel.

The last pillar of thought mentioned here is, of course, the field of disaster research. The crisis approach outlined in this chapter leans heavily on both the empirical and theoretical findings of disaster research. The thorough understanding of collective behavior, disaster myths, and the pathologies of top-down coordination in times of adversity have proved particularly fruitful to understanding crisis dynamics (see the other chapters of this book for the lessons of disaster research).

These perspectives have helped us to better understand the nature of crisis and the dynamics of crisis management. In the next two sections, we present the key insights generated in the crisis field with regard to key questions formulated earlier.

THE UBIQUITY OF CRISIS

Crises were once explained in terms of bad luck or God's punishment, but this view has become obsolete (Bovens & 't Hart, 1996; Quarantelli, 1998; Steinberg, 2000). Crises are the result of multiple causes, which interact over time to produce a threat with devastating potential.

This may be somewhat counterintuitive, as it defies the traditional logic of "triggers" and underlying causes. Linear thinking ("big events must have big causes") thus gives way to a more subtle perspective that emphasizes the unintended consequences of increased complexity (Buchanan, 2000). The approach does not seek to identify specific factors that "cause" a crisis. It proposes that *escalatory processes undermine a social system's capacity to cope with disturbances*. The agents of disturbance may come from anywhere—ranging from earthquakes to human errors—but the ultimate cause of the crisis lies in the inability of a system to deal with the disturbance.

The causes of vulnerability often reside deep within the system. They typically remain unnoticed, or key policymakers fail to attend to them (Turner, 1978). In the process leading up to a crisis, these seemingly innocent factors combine and transform into disruptive forces that come to represent an undeniable threat to the system. These factors are sometimes referred to as pathogens, as they are present long before the crisis becomes manifest (Reason, 1990).

The notion that crises are an unwanted by-product of complex systems has been popularized by Charles Perrow's (1999) analysis of the nuclear power incident at Three Miles Island. Perrow describes how a relatively minor glitch in the plant was misunderstood in the control room. The plant operators initially thought they understood the problem and applied the required technical response. But as they had actually misinterpreted the warning signal, the response worsened the problem. The increased threat mystified the operators (they could not understand why the problem persisted) and invited an urgent response. By again applying the "right" response to the wrong problem, the operators continued to exacerbate the problem. Finally, someone figured out the correct source of the problem, just in time to stave off a disaster.

The very qualities of complex systems that drive progress lie at the heart of most if not all technological crises. As sociotechnical systems become more complex and increasingly connected (tightly coupled) to other (sub)systems, their vulnerability for disturbances increases (Perrow, 1999; Turner, 1978). The more complex a system becomes, the harder it is for anyone to understand it in its entirety. Tight coupling between a system's component parts and with those of other systems allows for the rapid proliferation of interactions (and errors) throughout the system.

Complexity and lengthy chains of accident causation do not remain confined to the world of high-risk technology. Consider the world of global finance and the financial crises that have rattled it in recent years (Eichengreen, 2002). Globalization and ICT have tightly connected most world markets and financial systems. As a result, a minor problem in a seemingly isolated market can trigger a financial meltdown in markets on the other side of the globe. Structural vulnerabilities in relatively weak economies such as Russia, Argentina, or Turkey may suddenly "explode" on Wall Street and cause worldwide economic decline.

The same characteristics can be found in crises that beset low-tech environments such as prisons or sports stadiums. Urban riots, prison disturbances, and sports crowd disasters always seem to start off with relatively minor incidents (Waddington, 1992, refers to flashpoints). On closer inspection, however, it becomes clear that it is a similar mix of interrelated causes that produces major outbursts of this kind.

In the case of prison disturbances, the interaction between guards and inmates is of particular relevance (Boin & Rattray, 2004). Consider the 1990 riot that all but destroyed the Strangeways prison in Manchester (United Kingdom). In the incubation period leading up to the riot, prison guards had to adapt their way of working in the face of budgetary pressure. Inmates did not understand or appreciate this change in staff behavior and subsequently began to challenge staff authority, which, in turn, generated anxiety and stress among staff. As staff began to act in an increasingly defensive and inconsistent manner, prisoners became even more frustrated with staff behavior. A reiterative, self-reinforcing pattern of changing behavior and staff–prisoner conflict set the stage for a riot. A small incident started the riot, which, in turn, touched off a string of disturbances in other prisons. Many civil disturbances between protestors and police seem to unfold according to the same pattern (Goldstone & Useem, 1999; Smelser, 1962; Waddington, 1992).

All this makes a crisis hard to detect. As complex systems cannot be simply understood, it is hard to qualify the manifold activities and processes that take place in these systems. Growing vulnerabilities go unrecognized and ineffective attempts to deal with seemingly minor disturbances continue. The system thus "fuels" the lurking crisis. Only a minor "trigger" is needed to initiate a destructive cycle of escalation, which may then rapidly spread throughout the system. Crises may have their roots far away (in a geographical sense) but rapidly snowball through the global networks, jumping from one system to another, gathering destructive potential along the way.

An intriguing question asks whether modern systems have become increasingly vulnerable to breakdown. One might argue that modern society is better than ever equipped to deal with routine failures: great hospitals, computers and telephones, fire trucks and universities, regulation and funds—these factors have helped to minimize the scope and number of crises that were once routine (Wildavsky, 1988). Others argue that the resilience of modern society has deteriorated: when a threat does materialize (say an electrical power outage), the most modern systems suffer most. Students of natural disasters make a similar point: modern society increases its vulnerability to disaster by building in places where history warns not to build. The costs of natural and man-made disasters continue to grow, while scenarios of future crises promise more mayhem (see the chapter by Quarantelli, Lagadec, & Boin in this handbook).[1]

Before anything can be done to prevent crisis scenarios from materializing, emerging threats must be explicitly recognized as crises. There are at least three reasons why many potential crises fail to gain such recognition.

First, threats to shared values or life-sustaining functions simply cannot always be recognized before their disastrous consequences materialize. As the crisis process begins to unfold, policymakers often do not see anything out of the ordinary. Everything is still in place, even though hidden interactions eat away at the pillars of the system. It is only when the crisis is in full swing and becomes manifest that policymakers can recognize it for what it is.

The second reason is found in the contested nature of crisis. A crisis rarely, if ever, "speaks for itself." The definition of a situation is, as social scientists say, the outcome of a subjective process. More often than not people will differ in their perception and appreciation of a threat. In fact, we might say that crisis definitions are continuously subjected to the forces of politicization (Edelman, 1977). One man's crisis may be another man's opportunity.

Even if consensus would exist that a serious threat is emerging, the status of this new problem is far from assured. Governments deal with urgent problems every day; attention to one problem takes away attention from another. For a threat to be recognized as a crisis, it must clear firmly entrenched hurdles (Birkland, 1997; Bovens & 't Hart, 1996).

Now that we have explored the origins of crisis, let us see how public authorities deal with these forms of emerging adversity. If they fail, the actions of crisis managers will feed straight back into an escalatory process with potentially disastrous consequences.

CRISIS MANAGEMENT: CRUCIAL CHALLENGES FOR LEADERSHIP

Citizens whose lives are affected by critical contingencies expect governments and public agencies to do their utmost to keep them out of harm's way. They expect the officials in charge to make critical decisions and provide direction even in the most difficult circumstances. So do the journalists that produce the stories that help to shape the crisis in the minds of the public. And so do members of parliament, public interest groups, institutional watchdogs, and other voices on the political stage that monitor and influence the behavior of leaders. However misplaced, unfair, or illusory these expectations may be hardly matters. These expectations are real in their political consequences (Thomas & Thomas, 1928).

The challenges of crisis management appear to be rising, not because the mechanisms of crisis have changed (the jury is still out on the issue, as discussed earlier). Crisis management has become more challenging because the democratic context has changed over the past decades. Analysts agree, for instance, that citizens and politicians alike have become at once more fearful and less tolerant of major hazards to public health, safety, and prosperity. The modern Western citizen has little patience for imperfections; he has come to fear glitches and has learned to see more of what he fears. In this culture of fear—sometimes referred to as the "risk society"—the role of the modern mass media is crucial (Beck, 1992).

---

[1] Although much more pronounced today, the tendency to search for culprits following the occurrence of disaster and crisis is age old; see Drabek and Quarantelli (1967) as well as Douglas (1992).

In contemporary Western society, a crisis sets in motion extensive follow-up reporting, investigations by political forums as well as civil and criminal juridical proceedings. It is not uncommon for public officials and agencies to be singled out as the responsible actors for prevention, preparedness, and response failures. Public leaders must defend themselves against seemingly incontrovertible evidence of their incompetence, ignorance, or insensitivity.

Crisis management should not be viewed just in terms of the coping capacity of governmental institutions and public policies; it should be considered a deeply controversial and intensely political activity (Habermas, 1975; Edelman, 1977; 't Hart, 1993). This translates into five critical challenges for crisis management: *sense making*, *decision making*, *meaning making*, *terminating*, and *learning* (Boin, 't Hart, Stern, & Sundelius, 2005). Let us now briefly review these challenges in somewhat more detail.

Sense Making

A crisis seems to pose a straightforward challenge: once a crisis becomes manifest, crisis managers must take measures to deal with its consequences. Reality is much more complex, however. Most crises do not materialize with a big bang; they are the product of escalation. Policymakers must recognize from vague, ambivalent, and contradictory signals that something out of the ordinary is developing. The critical nature of these developments is not self-evident; policymakers have to "make sense" of them (Edelman, 1977).

They must appraise the threat and decide what the crisis is about. However penetrating the events that trigger a crisis—jet planes hitting skyscrapers, thousands of people found dead in mass graves—a uniform picture of the events rarely emerges: Do they constitute a tragedy, an outrage, perhaps a punishment, or, inconceivably, a blessing in disguise? Crisis managers will have to determine how threatening the events are, to what or whom, what their operational and strategic parameters are, and how the situation will develop in the period to come. Signals come from all kinds of sources: some loud, some soft, some accurate, some widely off the mark. But how to tell which is which? How to distill cogent signals from the noise of crisis?

Research findings suggest that crisis managers often have a hard time meeting this challenge. The bewildering pace, ambiguity, and complexity of crises can easily overwhelm normal modes of situation assessment. Stress may further impair sense-making abilities. The organizations in which crisis managers typically function tend to produce additional barriers to crisis recognition. In fact, research shows that organizations are unable to detect even the most simple incubation processes with few factors, interacting according to standard patterns and taking a long lead time (Turner, 1978).

It is not all bad news. Some groups of people are known for their ability to remain their cool and to stay clear-headed under pressure. They have developed a mode of information processing that enables competent performance under crisis conditions (Flin, 1996; Klein, 2001). Veteran military officers, journalists, as well as fire and police commanders are known for this. Senior politicians and bureaucrats are generally veterans too—veterans of countless political and bureaucratic battles during their rise to the power. Those who make it all the way to the top of the hill in competitive political-administrative systems tend to have relatively well developed mechanisms for coping with stress.

Some researchers also point to organizations that have developed a proactive culture of "looking for problems" in their environment. These so-called high-reliability organizations have somehow developed a capacity for thorough yet fast-paced information processing under stressful conditions. The unresolved question is whether organizations can design these features into existing organizational cultures (Weick & Sutcliffe, 2002).

Making Critical Decisions

Responding to crises confronts governments and public agencies with pressing choice opportunities. These can be of many kinds. The needs and problems triggered by the onset of crisis may be so enormous that the scarce resources available will have to be prioritized. This is much like politics as usual except that in crisis circumstances the disparities between demand and supply of public resources are much bigger; the situation remains unclear and volatile; and the time to think, consult, and gain acceptance for decisions is highly restricted. Crises also confront governments and leaders with issues they do not face on a daily basis, for example, concerning the deployment of the military, the use of lethal force, or the radical restriction of civil liberties.

The classic example of crisis decision making is the Cuban Missile Crisis (1963), during which U.S. President John F. Kennedy was presented with pictures of Soviet missile installations under construction in Cuba. The photos conveyed a geostrategic reality in the making that Kennedy considered unacceptable, and it was up to him to decide what to do about it. Whatever his choice from the options presented to him by his advisers—an air strike, an invasion of Cuba, a naval blockade—and however hard it was to predict the exact consequences, one thing seemed certain: the final decision would have a momentous impact on Soviet–American relations and possibly on world peace. Crisis decision-making is making hard calls, which involve tough value tradeoffs and major political risks (Brecher, 1993; Janis, 1989).

Many pivotal crisis decisions are *not* taken by individual leaders or by small informal groups of senior policymakers. They emerge from various alternative loci of decision making and coordination ('t Hart, Rosenthal, & Kouzmin, 1993; McConnell, 2003). In fact, the crisis response in modern society is best characterized in terms of a network. This is not necessarily counterproductive, many leaders have learned, as delegation of decision-making authority down the line usually enhances resilience rather than detracting from it.

An effective response also requires interagency and intergovernmental coordination. After all, each decision must be implemented by a set of organizations; only when these organizations work together is there a chance that effective implementation will happen. Getting public bureaucracies to adapt to crisis circumstances is a daunting, and some say impossible, task in itself. Most public organizations were originally designed to conduct routine business in accordance with such values as fairness, lawfulness, and efficiency. The management of crisis, however, requires flexibility, improvisation, redundancy, and the breaking of rules.

Coordination is not a self-evident feature of crisis management operations. The question of who is in charge typically arouses great passions. In disaster studies, the "battle of the Samaritans" is a well-documented phenomenon: agencies representing different technologies of crisis coping find it difficult to align their actions. Moreover, a crisis does not make the public suddenly "forget" the sensitivities and conflicts that governed the daily relations between authorities and others in fairly recent times.

A truly effective crisis response is to a large extent the result of a naturally evolving process. It cannot be managed in linear, step-by-step, and comprehensive fashion from a single crisis center, however full of top decision makers and stacked with state of the art information technology. There are simply too many hurdles that separate a leadership decision from its timely execution in the field.

Meaning Making

In a crisis, leaders are expected to reduce uncertainty and provide an authoritative account of what is going on, why it is happening, and what needs to be done. When they have made sense of the events and have arrived at some sort of situational appraisal and made strategic policy choices, leaders must get others to accept their definition of the situation. They must impute "meaning" to the unfolding crisis in such a way that their efforts to manage it are enhanced. If they do not, or if they do not succeed at it, their decisions will not be understood or respected. If other actors in the crisis succeed in dominating the meaning-making process, the ability of incumbent leaders to decide and maneuver is severely constrained.

Two problems often recur. First, public leaders are not the only ones trying to frame the crisis. Their messages coincide and compete with those of other parties, who hold other positions and interests, who are likely to espouse various alternative definitions of the situation and advocate different courses of action. Censoring them is hardly a viable option in a democracy.

Second, authorities often cannot provide correct information right away. They struggle with the mountains of raw data (reports, rumors, pictures) that are quickly amassed when something extraordinary happens. Turning them into a coherent picture of the situation is a major challenge by itself. Getting it out to the public in the form of accurate, clear, and actionable information requires a major public relations effort. This effort is often hindered by the aroused state of the audience: people whose lives are deeply affected tend to be anxious if not stressed. Moreover, they do not necessarily see the government as their ally. And preexisting distrust of government does not evaporate in times of crisis.

Terminating a Crisis

Governments—at least democratic ones—cannot afford to stay in crisis mode forever. A sense of normalcy will have to return sooner or later. It is a critical leadership challenge to make this happen in a timely and expedient fashion.

Crisis termination is twofold. It is about shifting back from emergency to routine mode. This requires some form of downsizing of crisis operations. At the strategic level, it also requires rendering account for what has happened and gaining acceptance for this account. These two aspects of crisis termination are distinct, but in practice often closely intertwined. The system of governance—its rules, its organizations, its power-holders —has to be (re)stabilized; it must regain the necessary legitimacy to perform its usual functions. Leaders cannot bring this about by unilateral decree, even if they may possess the formal mandate to initiate and terminate crises in a legal sense (by declaring a state of disaster or by evoking martial law). Formal termination gestures can follow but never lead the mood of a community. Premature closure may even backfire: allegations of underestimation and cover-up are quick to emerge in an opinion climate that is still on edge.

The burden of proof in accountability discussions lies with leaders: they must establish beyond doubt that they cannot be held responsible for the occurrence or escalation of a crisis. These accountability debates can easily degenerate into "blame games" with a focus on identifying and punishing "culprits" rather than discursive reflection about the full range of causes and consequences.[2] The challenge for leaders is to cope with the politics of crisis accountability without resorting to undignified and potentially self-defeating defensive tactics of blame avoidance that only serve to prolong the crisis by transforming it into a political confrontation at knife's edge.

Crisis leaders can be competent and conscientious, but that alone says little about how their performance will be evaluated when the crisis is over. Policymakers and agencies that failed to perform their duties prior to or during the critical stages need not despair, however: if they "manage" the political game of the crisis aftermath well, they may prevent losses to their reputation, autonomy, and resources. Crises have winners and losers. The political (and legal) dynamics of the accountability process determines which crisis actors end up where (Brändström & Kuipers, 2003).

Learning

Political and organizational lesson-drawing constitutes the final challenge. A crisis offers a reservoir of potential lessons for contingency planning and training for future crises. One would expect all those involved to study these lessons and feed them back into organizational practices, policies, and laws.

Lesson-drawing is one of the most underdeveloped aspects of crisis management (Lagadec, 1997; Stern, 1997). In addition to cognitive and institutional barriers to learning, lesson-drawing is constrained by the role of these lessons in determining the impact that crises have on a society. Crises become part of collective memory, a source of historical analogies for future leaders (Khong, 1992; Sturken, 1997). The political depiction of crisis as a product of prevention and foresight failures would force people to rethink the assumptions on which preexisting policies and rule systems rested. Other stakeholders in the game of crisis-induced lesson-drawing might seize upon the lessons to advocate measures and policy reforms that incumbent leaders reject. Leaders thus have a large stake in steering the lesson-drawing process in the political and bureaucratic arenas. The crucial challenge here is to achieve a dominant influence on the feedback stream that crises generate into preexisting policy networks and public organizations.

The documentation of these inhibiting complexities has done nothing to dispel the near-utopian belief in crisis *opportunities* that is found not only in academic literature, but also in popular wisdom (Boin & 't Hart, 2003). A crisis is seen as a good time to clean up and start anew. Crises then represent discontinuities that must be seized upon—a true test of leadership, the experts claim. So most people are not surprised to see sweeping reforms in the wake of crisis: That will never happen again! They intuitively distrust leaders who claim bad luck and point out that their organizations and policy have a great track record.

Crises tend to cast long shadows upon the political systems in which they occur. It is only when we study these longer term processes that we are able to assess the full impact of crises. Unfortunately, such studies are rare (but see Birkland, 1997; Kurtz & Browne, 2004). Most studies of the "crisis aftermath" of emergencies have been about community reconstruction, individual and collective trauma, and legal battles. We need to complement these studies by taking a broader macrosocial perspective that looks at collective "learning" for an entire nation, polity, or society in the aftermath of crisis. It remains an open question if crises tend to serve as triggers of systemic change or if they serve to forestall such change, and to what extent these processes can be channeled by good crisis governance.

CONCLUSION: THE CRISIS APPROACH RECONSIDERED

The crisis approach outlined in this chapter provides a framework for understanding the dynamic evolution of crisis and the prospects for public management of urgent threats. The approach adopts a long time line, which makes it possible to trace a crisis from its early roots to its burial in public memory. It admonishes the research community to complement operational perspectives with political perspectives. Most importantly, perhaps, is its capacity to tease out the interplay between crisis dynamics and response failures.

Two lessons seem of particular relevance to practitioners. First, one should accept that even the richest and most competent government imaginable can never guarantee that major disruptions will not occur. Policymakers cannot escape the dilemmas of crisis response by banking on crisis prevention. Crisis prevention is a necessary and indeed vitally important strategy, but it pertains only to known emergencies—those that happened before. This requires a strategy of resilience (Wildavsky, 1988). This lesson resonates with key insights in the disaster field.

The second lesson reminds us that crisis is a label, a semantic construction people use to characterize situations or epochs that they somehow regard as extraordinary, volatile, and potentially far-reaching in their negative implications. The intensity or scope of a crisis is thus not solely determined by the nature of the threat, the level of uncertainty, or the time available to decision makers. A crisis is to a considerable extent what people—influenced by the inevitable mass media onslaught following an unscheduled event—make of it.

Why people collectively label and experience a situation as a crisis remains somewhat of a mystery. Physical facts, numbers, and other seemingly objective indicators are important factors, but they are not decisive. A flood that kills 200 people is a more or less routine emergency in Bangladesh, but it would be experienced as a major crisis in, say, Miami or Paris. Crises are in the eye of the beholder. It is people's frames of reference, experience and memory, values and interests that determine their perceptions of crisis. A sense of "collective stress" results not just from some objective threat, but also from the intricate interaction between events, individual perceptions, media representations, political reactions, and government efforts at "meaning making."

This process of collective understanding is one of escalation and de-escalation. It is subject to the influence of actors who have a stake in playing up a crisis mood, or playing it down. And this is exactly what happens when unexpected incidents or major disruptions are predicted or actually occur: different political, bureaucratic, societal, and international stakeholders will not only form their own picture of the situation and classify it in terms of threats and opportunities, but many of them will actively seek to influence the public perception of the situation. Once a particular definition of the situation has taken hold in mass media and political discourse, it becomes a political reality that policymakers have to take into account and act upon. Initial definitions tend to be persistent.

An effective crisis response will inevitably require a two-pronged strategy: dealing with the events "on the ground" (whether literally as in civil emergencies or, metaphorically, as in a currency or stock market crisis); and dealing with the political upheaval and instability triggered by these events. Neglecting one or the other is detrimental to any attempt to exercise public leadership in a crisis.

These lessons help us to flag two challenges for further research. First, much work remains to be done on the understanding of crisis dynamics. If crises cannot be prevented, we must learn to recognize them in time. Early warning can work only if it builds on a solid theory of crisis development. Second, researchers need to invest in a better understanding of resilience. Crisis researchers tend to agree (with disaster researchers we should note) that resilience may be one of the key strategies to deal with system breakdowns. Much more systematic work needs to be done on the identification of mechanisms that provide for resilient societies.

Understanding crisis development will contribute to our understanding of disasters. The continued and deepened collaboration between crisis researchers in all their different niches and the field of disaster studies should therefore receive—an easily accomplishable—priority. Our chapter in this book aims to do just that.

CHAPTER 4

Methodological Issues[1]

ROBERT A. STALLINGS

"It's the same, only it's different." This sounds like one of former American baseball player Yogi Berra's malapropisms. Nevertheless, it is appropriate when discussing methods of disaster research. Fifty years ago, Lewis Killian (2002 [1956]) stated it this way: "Basically, the methodological problems of field studies in disasters are those common to any effort to conduct scientifically valid field studies in the behavioral sciences. The disaster situation itself, however, creates special or aggravated problems ..." (p. 49). The basic tools of disaster researchers—a theory, a working hypothesis, an appropriate research design, a plan for selecting cases for study, a strategy for gathering data or recording observations, and a way to extract meaning from the materials collected—are easily recognizable as those used in all of the social sciences. Yet, issues specific to disaster research need to be addressed.

Simply put, the difference in doing research on disasters is the *context* in which it is carried out (Mileti, 1987, p. 69; Taylor, 1978, p. 276). The greater the difference between that context and the everyday world in which the rest of social science research takes place, the more unique are the challenges of disaster research (Stallings, 2002b, pp. 21–22). This means, for example, that studies conducted during the crisis time period (a term from Quarantelli, 2002a) face challenges that research carried out during the late stages of recovery or during pre-disaster mitigation and preparedness phases do not. The latter encounter only the usual difficulties found in all social science research—no more, no less. This chapter focuses on issues that arise in conducting research in settings that are usually far from the day-to-day. Admittedly it is skewed toward methods of disaster research employed by sociologists because the author's background and training are in this field.

No attempt is made in this chapter to discuss the range of methodological issues currently facing the social sciences in general or even sociology in particular. Instead, three issues have been singled out because they seem to comprise the essence of the difference, when it exists, between disaster studies of all types and "everyday" research: (1) *timing*, meaning generally *when* the process of observing or collecting data and other materials takes place in relation to

[1] Special thanks to Jo Karabasz for making sure that the author stayed with this project until it was completed. Conversations with Kathleen Tierney and Dennis Wenger greatly aided the updating of certain aspects of this chapter. Linda Bourque provided information and answered key questions about recent methodological issues in survey research. Each is herewith acknowledged without in any way being implicated in the resulting product. Comments and suggestions from the tri-editors were helpful in improving this chapter and are greatly appreciated, even though not every one of them was followed.

the onset of disaster; (2) *access*, referring especially to researchers' initial contacts with interview subjects, survey respondents, and holders of documents or other relevant materials; and (3) *generalizability*, or what Killian (2002 [1956]) calls the ability to draw "valid conclusions" (p. 54) from disaster studies. While only partial solutions exist for many of these issues, *triangulation*, meaning the emergence of patterns out of the findings from many studies using different methods, seems to offer the most confidence in the "validity of the conclusions drawn" (p. 49) from disaster studies. Of course, the three issues themselves are interrelated: the ability to generalize from the findings of any given piece of disaster research is directly affected by the successful resolution of timing and access issues, and access itself is affected considerably by timing issues.

Three of the most common types of disaster studies are discussed in this chapter: *field research*, often identified as the qualitative case study or simply field studies; *survey research*; and *documentary research*. In the last category I include historical research. Clearly, documentary research, like field studies and survey research, involves dealing with people rather than just written documents. Because so much of the literature is based on field studies, because many of the unique constraints on disaster research are encountered only in carrying out this type of study, and because they are most often conducted during the crisis time period, more space is devoted to this topic than to the other two.

FIELD STUDIES

The prototypical method of disaster research has been the field study.[2] The following is an illustration: A researcher or group of researchers learns of the occurrence of some disaster,[3] most often through the news media. Despite the fact that such initial information is usually far from accurate, arriving on site as soon as possible is generally seen by field researchers as key to the success of their work, so the decision to launch a study needs to be made quickly. In large-scale research operations such as the Disaster Research Center (DRC),[4] especially in its earliest days when a sizable stand-by research capability was maintained, a small (one- or two-person) "reconnaissance team" might be dispatched initially. These teams would attempt to accomplish several things. They would, as nonparticipants, observe activities at locations where important disaster-related tasks were being carried out such as in emergency operations centers (EOCs), field command posts, hospital emergency rooms, temporary shelters, and disaster relief "one-stop" centers. They also would try to informally "interview" (speak with) the people involved or at least set up appointments for later formal interviews "when things have calmed down." If the reconnaissance team judged the situation suitable for a more thorough study, then one or more subsequent field trips would be undertaken. During follow-up visits to the site, formal interviews would be conducted. At all times, researchers would be alert for any documents that they might obtain, which typically would include copies of disaster plans, emergency logs, notes or minutes of meetings, after-action reports, local newspapers, and other relevant records of any kind. After returning from the site, at least one member of the

---

[2] Much of the current research of this type is carried out in the form of Quick Response studies with small grants from the Natural Hazards Center at the University of Colorado. (See http://www.colorado.edu/hazards/qr/).

[3] Exactly what events should be considered disasters for research purposes is a complex issue that will be ignored for the time being. (See Quarantelli, 1998; Perry & Quarantelli, 2005.)

[4] The Disaster Research Center was located at The Ohio State University in Columbus, Ohio, from its formation in 1963 until 1985. Since then, it has been located at the University of Delaware in Newark, Delaware.

field team would write up a preliminary report of the team's findings and conclusions based on field notes, observations, casual conversations as well as formal interviews, and documentary material collected.

Timing

Timing is paramount in disaster field studies. It is frequently discussed in field reports, but details of the decision-making process that leads up to getting to the disaster site in the timeliest manner are usually implicit. The following examples illustrate some of the considerations involved.

One of the earliest studies undertaken by the Disaster Research Center (DRC) during its first years in existence at The Ohio State University was of flooding on the Ohio River at Cincinnati (Anderson, 1965). In its brief introduction, the research note describing this study gives a glimpse of the processes involved:

> Early in March, 1964, the Ohio River Valley was subjected to very heavy rains. After several days of almost continuous downpour the major river in the valley, the Ohio, reached the flood stage of 52 feet at Cincinnati. This signaled the beginning of the worst flood in that city and in the valley in 19 years and was climaxed on March 11 when the water crested at 66.2 feet. Throughout Pennsylvania, West Virginia, Kentucky, Ohio and Indiana, thousands were left homeless as a result of flooding from the river and several of its tributaries. Red Cross officials estimated that about 110,000 persons were directly affected by the floods in the five state area. At least nine deaths were attributable to the high waters, seven in Ohio and one each in Kentucky and Indiana. Total property damage went beyond the 100 million dollar figure. (p. 1)

Researchers typically learn of disasters the way others do—through the news media, especially radio and television. *When* such reports are received relative to the onset of disaster affects the kind of study that can be fielded and to some extent the topics that can be investigated. A meandering off-shore hurricane or a slow-developing flood may enable researchers to select a probable target location and position themselves there in advance of impact (see Quarantelli, 2002a, pp. 106–107).

Initial deployment of a field team based on early news reports, whether just before or as soon as possible after onset, is complicated because the earliest estimates of casualties and damage are notoriously inaccurate (Quarantelli, 2002a, p. 107). The DRC "law" was that estimates of the number of dead varied inversely with distance from the disaster (Dynes, Haas, & Quarantelli, 1967, p. 219). Notice in the first paragraph quoted that the information received was technical: flood-stage river levels had been reached; the river crested at a certain height on a particular date; "worst flood" in a specific period of time; and so forth. In the second paragraph, estimates of the human dimensions of this disaster are described: "thousands" homeless; "110,000 persons" directly affected; at least nine deaths; property damage "beyond the 100 million dollar figure." Based on reports of such estimates, the decision to launch or not launch a field study must be made—and made quickly.

Just how tricky this decision can be is illustrated in another example. The incident was a freight train derailment and resulting toxic fire that caused widespread and prolonged evacuation in the immediate vicinity of Miamisburg, Ohio, south of Dayton. The researcher (Stallings, 1986) was interested in interorganizational relationships among emergency response agencies and was attempting to determine through news reports whether the derailment and fire would provide the degree of interorganizational complexity that would justify a 2,500-mile-trip to the accident site:

> Entry into the field in the Miamisburg case was complicated by the changing nature of the incident, the nature and scale of the evacuation, and the routines of both the [researcher's] normal work week and the phases of the emergency period. First news of the incident reaching the West Coast late Tuesday evening, July 8 [1986], suggested that the accident was more or less "routine." But after the second explosion and subsequent evacuation on Wednesday, it began to appear that the situation fit the research design outlined in the Quick Response proposal, and plans were made to depart for the scene. With the evacuation estimated to last through the end of the week and with the probability that at its conclusion key representatives of disaster-response organizations would take some well-deserved time off, it appeared that the optimal time to begin gathering data would be Monday, July 14. (p. 4)

In the case of the DRC study of the Ohio River flood, the decision was made more easily:

> On Tuesday, March 10, a two-member DRC team went to Cincinnati to conduct a preliminary survey of the situation. Two days were spent on this initial trip interviewing local officials and making general observations. (Anderson, 1965, p. 1)

This field team was able to arrive at the disaster "site" twenty-four hours *before* flood waters crested, that is, during the emergency or crisis time period itself. This was due both to the relatively slow-onset nature of the flood and to the proximity of these researchers to the disaster area (in 1964, the DRC was slightly more than 100 miles from the Ohio River at Cincinnati).

> After the team returned to Columbus, the DRC staff decided that a follow-up trip focusing on organizational preparedness or what will be treated in this paper as an aspect of the "flood disaster subculture" would contribute to an understanding of community response to disasters. With this in mind, a three-man team returned to Cincinnati on March 15 for two additional days of study. (p. 1)

The reconnaissance team had confirmed the impression formed from news reports that this flood disaster was worthy of study, at least relative to the resources required such as the costs of travel to the site. Notice that this is always a relative decision—the nature of the disaster, in particular its magnitude, relative to the resources required to study it. In other words, a similar disaster, especially one comparable in scale, in a more distant location might be judged less worthy of study. The qualifier to this statement of course is the substantive interest of the researcher. For instance, a disaster of otherwise unremarkable characteristics may have damaged or destroyed one or more nursing homes and assisted living facilities. A researcher interested specifically in threats to the elderly in disaster might select such an event for study on substantive grounds. Generally speaking, the decision to undertake a field study of events with unique properties such as the nuclear reactor accident at Three Mile Island, Pennsylvania, or ones of obviously catastrophic magnitude such as the 2004 Asian tsunami and Hurricane Katrina are easier to make, but timing issues remain in these cases as well.

Not discussed in this quoted passage are three important accomplishments of these reconnaissance teams when they are successful and why timing is so important to their success. First, they piece together an overview of what has happened during the pre-impact and crisis time periods, including identifying the principal actors (organizations, in the case of most DRC studies) and any unique aspects of the disaster. Early disaster researchers referred to the former as establishing the *Gestalt* of the overall disaster response (Dynes, Haas, & Quarantelli, 1967, p. 221; Killian, 2002 [1956], p. 69). Second, reconnaissance teams return with a list of key contacts in the groups and organizations most heavily involved in the disaster response. If a follow-up trip were deemed appropriate, appointments for interviews can then be arranged by telephone before the follow-up team departs. (It was standard procedure for one member of DRC reconnaissance teams to be responsible for obtaining a local telephone directory, for example.)

Third, and perhaps most important for the success of follow-up field trips, contacts made by members of reconnaissance teams greatly facilitate later access to informants. Typically, many more people would have been contacted than were formally interviewed, with reconnaissance team members introducing the research project, showing their identification or credential, providing a business card, and leaving contacts with the pledge that subsequent field teams would be getting in touch with them to request a formal interview. These initial contacts usually provide subsequent field teams an "in" with key organizations, differentiating them from later-arriving researchers. They would also establish the identity of field team members as researchers rather than reporters and other representatives of the news media.

In the case of the one-person field study of the Miamisburg train derailment, all three tasks were compressed into one trip to the locale:

> After arrival on Monday morning, contact was first established with the regional emergency response agency, the Miami Valley Disaster Services Authority, headquartered in Dayton. Staff members who were not still at the site of the derailment provided an initial briefing and overview of the organizations involved. A beginning list of the names of key respondents was obtained. The remainder of the first day was spent in touring the cities affected, visiting the crash site, and generally "getting the lay of the land." The second day in the field (Tuesday, July 15) found most key respondents needing time to catch up on work that had piled up during the emergency period, so the day's principal activity consisted of making appointments for interviews during the remainder of the week. Wednesday, Thursday, and Friday were devoted entirely to interviews with key respondents having special insight into the interorganizational relationships that emerged during the emergency. (Stallings, 1986, pp. 4–5)

Also hidden in the passage from the DRC Ohio River flood report is what goes on between the return of the reconnaissance team and the fielding of the follow-up study. Discussions would have been held regarding the issues or problems to be focused on during the follow-up. Interview guides might be written specifically for such a study. In the case cited, the decision was made to concentrate on elements of a "disaster subculture" as they were reflected in the actions of key emergency response organizations. (Organizational and group representatives were interviewed because the focus of DRC's early research was on organized behavior rather than on individuals; see Dynes, 1970, pp. 1–5).

Quarantelli (2002a) makes the case for the earliest possible arrival at the disaster site:

> The value of being on the scene at the height of crises cannot be overstated. It is worthwhile to be in such situations for two basic reasons. First, observations can be made and documents collected that cannot be obtained through later interviewing. The social barriers that normally exist to restrict access to high-level officials and key organizations do not exist. A second reason for being on the scene early [is that it] ensures a high degree of access and cooperation. Victims are typically candid, cooperative, and willing to talk in ways far more difficult to get later. (p. 107)

It is probably fair to say that poor field research results when studies are begun only after disaster has struck. Not only does this increase problems associated with late arrival on the scene, but it also probably means that the researcher is unprepared to take advantage of the opportunity afforded by unfolding events. If the researcher is unfamiliar with the literature on previous disasters, for example, both missed opportunities and "reinventing the wheel" are likely to occur. Unless the event is so compelling as to make any sort of study preferable to no study at all,[5] it is probably better to head to the library rather than to the disaster site. Becoming familiar with the existing literature can be used as an opportunity to create working hypotheses that will be available beforehand when the next disaster strikes, as it inevitably will. Interview guides or rudimentary questionnaires can also be designed and held ready for a future event.

Not all barriers to timely entry to disaster sites are to be found at the sites themselves. Lack of funding can be a major barrier. While there have been occasions when researchers have initiated studies without outside funding (covering the costs of field research "out of pocket," so to speak), most such instances have occurred when the researcher is already in the immediate vicinity when disaster strikes. Fortunately, it is no longer necessary for disaster researchers to begin the months-long process of writing a lengthy and complicated research proposal, submitting it to a large government agency or private foundation for review, then waiting weeks for a favorable decision and eventual receipt of funds, including money for travel and other direct expenses involved in carrying out a field study. Major funders such as the National Science Foundation have created small-grant programs that facilitate researchers' ability to begin research without the usual delays. In addition, the Natural Hazards Center administers "quick response grants" that are available to researchers both on an annual basis (that is, pre-disaster) and in the immediate aftermath of significant disasters, which do not require lengthy proposals and have relatively rapid review and decision times. The primary purpose of these quick-response grants is to provide, as the term implies, a level of support sufficient to enable field researchers to reach disaster sites in timely fashion. In return, the center expects a preliminary report on the study and its findings and makes these available online as Quick Response Reports. (See Note 2 for the link to these reports on the center's Web site.)

Another barrier to timely arrival at the scene of a disaster can arise from the Institutional Review Boards (IRBs) at the researcher's home university. Previously known as human subjects committees, IRBs exercise universities' ethical and legal responsibilities for ensuring that the rights and the physical, psychological, and emotional well-being of research subjects are protected by researchers. This involves requirements that researchers provide subjects with information about the nature of the research and its intended uses, apprising subjects that they have the right to refuse to participate in the research, and assurances about the confidentiality of any information provided by subjects including how that information will be stored, for how long, and who will have access to it. Providing IRBs with the necessary documentation to obtain official approval to carry out the research one has planned can be not only a source of irritation for researchers but also a source of delay in beginning the gathering of data. One solution is to seek, if not prior approval, then at least all the information that will be required for formal approval and to prepare in advance as much of the documentation that will be needed when the time comes. Successfully navigating the IRB process may be another reason to bypass the study of an existing disaster in favor of better planning for a study of the subsequent disasters that are sure to arise.

Access

As noted earlier, the primary reason that researchers who conduct field studies of disasters consider the ability to get to the scene in timely fashion to be so important is that timing

---

[5] On the other hand, if an event is that compelling, then there is a very high probability that veteran disaster researchers, better equipped to take advantage of the situation than novices, are already in the field. The case will therefore probably not be lost to the research field as a whole.

is usually crucial for gaining access to the key people to be interviewed and for acquiring invaluable documentary materials. Both become more difficult if not impossible later in the disaster process. Researchers refer to this as the problem of ephemeral (Quarantelli, 2002, p. 107) or perishable data (Bourque, Shoaf, & Nguyen, 2002, pp. 179–183). Both terms refer to everything from the impossibility of observing personally events after the fact, to obtaining documents that were freely available during the crisis time period but are deemed too sensitive for outsiders after disaster ends, to respondents' personal recall that may be skewed by repeated retelling of their stories to a succession of interviewers.

Tierney (2002b, pp. 359–365) has written expressly on the relationships among timing, access, and generalizability in research where formal organizations are the primary units of analysis: "Virtually all organizations, both public and private, seek a favorable public image, and one means to accomplish this aim is to exercise control over information, including the kinds of information researchers seek. The need for organizational impression management is probably even more marked in disaster situations than during normal times ..." (p. 359). More generally, each successive phase of the disaster process seems to bring about a change in the relationship between researchers and subjects. Drabek (1970, pp. 331–332) observes that, while cooperation may be adequate initially, researchers become increasing suspect as more and more outsiders arrive representing insurance, sales, welfare, and other interests.

One barrier large-scale organizations use to deflect disaster researchers is the Public Information Officer (PIO). Created to handle information requests from the news media, organizational officials frequently try to fend off requests for interviews by steering disaster researchers to PIOs and to press conferences (Tierney, 2002b, p. 360). In fact, researchers are often seen as a threat to the organization similar to that posed by reporters. Tierney notes that these informational-control mechanisms "... promote a 'command post' point of view [see Quarantelli, 1981] that privileges the official information-dissemination function over the perspectives represented by other elements in the disaster management network" (p. 361). By blocking access to the varied individual perspectives on the disaster within organizations, officials are better able to present a single, approved, "orthodox" perspective.

Another situation making access problematic, especially in large-scale, highly publicized disasters, is the "convergence" of researchers. Convergence has been a term used in this field to denote the movement of material, information, and especially people toward the disaster site from outside the area (Fritz & Mathewson, 1957, p. 3). It is a ubiquitous aspect of disasters, most visible in news reports of sightseers converging on the disaster site. High-visibility catastrophes not only attract veteran disaster researchers, who themselves are more numerous now than two or three decades ago, but also spawn novice disaster researchers, who might be veterans in some other research specialty but who are studying a disaster for the first time. While funding agencies and other professional associations can facilitate a certain amount of coordination among researchers and avoid at least the most blatant forms of duplication of effort, nevertheless the presence of a large number of researchers in the field can create competition among them for access to a handful of informants such as a mayor, a police chief, or other individuals who may have unique perspectives on events (Tierney, 2002b, p. 364). At the very least, respondents may feel besieged by multiple requests for formal interviews and decide to grant none. More cooperative respondents may provide rehearsed answers after being interviewed numerous times, making it difficult for later interviewers to probe effectively. Clearly, timing can be especially important in mega-disasters, with the first researchers on the scene enjoying a "competitive advantage" in access to never-to-be-repeated events, to people, and to perishable documents. Having an established reputation in this field such as that enjoyed by the Disaster Research Center, which has been conducting research on disasters continuously since 1963, or the Natural Hazards Center, can also provide a competitive advantage in gaining access.

The issue of access to all members of disaster-relevant organizations is one aspect of a larger issue that Killian (2002 [1956]) refers to as "sampling 'points of observation' " (p. 68). In most social science research, research subjects are *respondents* who are sources of data on their personal attitudes, behavior, and characteristics. In disaster research, especially in field studies, subjects are more often treated as *informants* who describe not only their own actions but also those of people around them. Often the researcher's goal is to obtain a holistic picture of some social process or bundle of processes. Any systematic constraints on access to informants introduce an unknown amount of distortion into the picture obtained.

Ideally, one would like access to organizational informants from different levels in the chain of command and from different subdivisions, the precise determination of which being dictated by the circumstances of the disaster. When officials deny researchers access to specific elements within organizations, a bias is introduced into the "data." Similarly at the individual level, if only subjects from one location within the disaster area are available to interviewers (e.g., those from the least heavily damaged areas), an incomplete picture is likely. This is the case, for example, when researchers are prevented from contacting individuals assumed to have been most traumatized by the disaster (e.g., so-called vulnerable populations such as young people).

Barriers such as these arise not only in the field. University IRBs, perhaps altruistically but also perhaps out of fear of "bad publicity" if not litigation, increasingly but indirectly impose forms of constraints on researchers' access to human subjects. Requirements vary across universities, but overall there has been increasing concern on the part of IRBs for the protection of presumed at-risk human subjects, of whom disaster victims would presumably be a prime example. Many universities require researchers to provide subjects with written documents such as those described in the previous subsection and to obtain signed consent forms before conducting interviews. Also, more precise disclosure is being required about the storage and usage of interview data. (The ever-present threat of third parties seeking to obtain copies of recorded interviews or transcripts through litigation is something that both researchers and potential subjects are usually aware of.) All of these well-intended procedures have had a noticeable effect in making respondents more wary of researchers (Tierney, 2002b, pp. 353–355).

Nevertheless, if approached in an appropriate manner and under the right set of circumstances, most people do not refuse to be interviewed by researchers. The incentives to grant interviewers' requests have been noted over the years. Some respondents are undoubtedly interested in sharing their experiences, good and bad, so that others may learn from them (Killian, 2002 [1956], pp. 71–72). Some seem to find recounting for researchers what they have experienced to be therapeutic, as many DRC field team members frequently noted. Still others may simply be flattered that they have been chosen for an interview or may desire to embellish their actions in the eyes of others.

Generalizability

By generalizability, I am referring to researchers' ability to make empirically grounded statements describing phenomena and relationships among phenomena that hold across all similar events. Generalizability may have a negative connotation to some readers (as in the criticism, "That's a generalization," implying that a statement is suspect because it cannot possibly hold for all cases). However, generalization is the goal of all science, including the social sciences. And the limits of generalization—knowing as precisely as possible the boundary between when such statements hold and when they do not—is as important for understanding as are the statements themselves. This is one reason why the definition of "disaster" itself is such an important issue in this field (see Quarantelli, 1998; Perry & Quarantelli, 2005). Such a definition provides answers to the questions: To what types of events do the generalizations from disaster research apply? And, implicitly or explicitly, to what types do they *not* apply?

Just as timing affects access to subjects, observable acts, and documentary materials, so too does access affect generalizability. Most of the major ways in which this can occur were discussed in the preceding subsection in terms of the selection of subjects and the unique perspectives on disaster that they can provide. These are sampling considerations in the largest sense of that term. But "sampling" in disaster field studies seldom involves population listings and the probabilistic selection of cases. Nevertheless, some sampling plan is followed. Most sampling strategies used in disaster field studies produce what are commonly referred to as nonprobability *purposive samples*. These are samples dictated by the nature of events and people's participation in them. Indeed, when researchers desire the perspectives on disaster of a particular category of actors (women in key response roles, for example; see Enarson, 2000b) purposive samples are the only appropriate device. They clearly are preferable to the *accidental samples* typically used by news reporters (e.g., people who just happen to be at a particular location at the time reporters and camera crews are ready to record a series of interviews).

Before readers dismiss the findings of disaster field studies because at first blush they seem to be "unscientific" based as they are on nonrandom samples, let me hasten to point out that the goal of all sampling strategies is to create a subset (the sample) from a larger set (the universe or population) that is *representative*. The desired end result is a sample whose characteristics are as similar as possible to those of the universe as a whole or whose characteristics differ from those of the universe in ways that are *known*. Random selection of cases is a strategy employed when the researcher *does not know how* to select cases that will be representative of the universe. It is, in effect, a strategy that assumes ignorance. Chance governs selection instead of knowledge of the universe. In the disaster situation, researchers do know something about how different segments of the population-at-large were affected by and how they reacted to events. A sample can be selected purposively to reflect patterns of activity or patterns of victimization.[6] Conversely, a random sample of a disaster-stricken community would have a high probability of failing to produce a sample that includes such key actors as the mayor, the chief of police, and the emergency services coordinator. Each would have the same chance of being selected as any other member of the local population—no more, no less. Hence, purposive sampling and so-called "snow-ball" sampling (wherein informants identify still other informants to be interviewed) are more appropriate for many more types of disaster research than traditional probability sampling techniques.

Another traditional topic associated with sampling needs to be discussed in connection with the issue of the generalizability of the findings of field studies. This is the matter of *sample size*. No matter how many interviews are conducted, whether with organizational informants or individual respondents, and no matter whether the sampling strategies produce probability or nonprobability samples, the resulting field study is in reality a "sample" of one disaster drawn nonrandomly from the (hypothetical) universe of all disasters (Mileti, 1987, p. 67). Mileti's

---

[6] Of course, probability and nonprobability samples in disasters are not mutually exclusive. In organizational research, for example, a purposive sample of informants may be created at the higher ranks (chief, deputy chiefs, division commanders, etc.) while a probability sample may be chosen among rank-and-file police officers.

recommendation is *replication*, specifically, adding to the sample of one field study a second study and then another and another. This is not merely an expansion of the existing literature; it is increasing the sample size, one case study at a time. Confidence in the generalizations from a single study grows as similar patterns of findings appear in subsequent studies.

Another issue involved in the generalizability of findings from disaster field studies is that of *establishing causal relationships*. Whatever specific language is used, researchers are interested in drawing conclusions about one of two things. Most often it is linking behavioral *consequences* to the temporally prior disaster event (i.e., their cause). Sometimes it is linking pre-disaster adjustments as the cause of post-disaster consequences. Regardless of the content of the specific causal hypothesis involved, the logic of cause-and-effect demands multiple cases. Confidence in causal generalizations is further enhanced if some of the cases are *non*-disasters that constitute a *control group*. Mill's (1872 [1843], pp. 451–452, 458–460) Method of Difference and Joint Method of Agreement and Difference demand, respectively, the contrasting of a disaster with a non-disaster and of multiple instances of disasters with multiple instances of non-disasters. In the case of complexes of social processes such as disasters, these requirements are untenable.

As a result, much effort in a disaster field study is expended to identify a *baseline* for purposes of comparison. Typically this baseline is a description of the unit of analysis (e.g., a community, an organization, or even individuals) *prior to* the crisis time period. Descriptions of conditions, procedures, or typical activities before disaster serve as the logical equivalent of a control group. Differences between pre-impact and post-impact patterns are inferred to have been caused by the disaster rather than by some unknown spurious factor. Obviously, such inferences are more readily acceptable when the "change" is the activation of a disaster plan, for example. They become more tenuous when the change is a higher local post-disaster unemployment rate. Did the disaster cause unemployment to rise and remain higher than before the event? Or did some macroeconomic factor produce the downturn in employment, one that would have occurred anyway, even without the disaster? There are ways of dealing with such questions statistically in the case of "social indicators" such as unemployment rates (e.g., Friesema, Caporaso, Goldstein, Lineberry, & McCleary, 1979; Wright, Rossi, Wright, & Weber-Burdin, 1979). However, in the particular instance of field studies, statistical controls, time-series models, and so forth, are not available.

The best approximation to inferring causal relationships in one-shot field studies of disasters is *triangulation*. Partly what is meant by triangulation is the accumulation—metaphorically, the piling on top of one another—of more and more field studies until the common findings that run through all or most of them stand out. These then become generalizations about disasters, "what the research literature has to say" about such events. But triangulation involves more than replication. It also encompasses the consistency of findings across different *types* of research: not just qualitative case studies, but also survey research and the analysis of documents, historical or otherwise. No individual study is without limitations, and different types of research designs are better suited for some research problems rather than others. As in any field of research, when the preponderance of evidence from a variety of different types of studies supports a particular generalization, researchers can claim with some level of confidence that they have a valid conclusion, in Killian's words.

Numerous examples supporting this contention about the efficacy of triangulation for the field of disaster research could be offered. Two will suffice. Much of the conventional wisdom about people's behavior in disasters had been dispelled, at least in the research literature, by the early 1970s. Earliest to fall by the wayside was the belief that people when confronting disaster would panic or otherwise behave irrationally (e.g., Quarantelli, 1954). More generally, the accumulation of research using a variety of research designs destroyed a number of myths about disasters (Quarantelli & Dynes, 1972; Taylor, 1977; Wenger, Dykes, Sebok, & Neff, 1975). In addition, another series of studies of urban riots during the 1960s showed the limits of some of the generalizations about disasters. For example, looting—the mass theft of consumer goods—was so rare as to be almost nonexistent in disasters (despite the recent events in New Orleans after Hurricane Katrina) but was a significant feature of urban civil disturbances (Dynes & Quarantelli, 1968; Quarantelli & Dynes, 1970). This qualification to an accepted generalization led to further evaluation of the findings of field studies of disasters, for example, about the difference in post-disaster norms sanctioning looting in small, insular towns versus large, diverse urban areas—and presumably overwhelmingly catastrophic events such as Katrina.

SURVEY RESEARCH

Field studies typically involve a small number of researchers, often only one, who are in face-to-face contact with the people caught up in disaster and who seek rich qualitative descriptions of disaster-related structures and processes. Most often these studies have been exploratory in nature, with their major objective being the generation of hypotheses rather than hypothesis testing. In contrast, survey research in disasters has both a different type of relationship between researcher and subject and different objectives. As a result, the issues of timing, access, and generalizability take slightly different forms.

Timing

The most explicit examination of these three issues is by Bourque and her colleagues (Bourque et al., 2002). They not only discuss these as well as other issues; more importantly, they evaluate them with empirical evidence from six post-disaster surveys. In evaluating timeliness, the authors first identify three potential impediments affecting the ability to collect post-disaster survey data in a timely fashion: lack of a questionnaire to administer; lack of an already drawn probability sample; and lack of funding (p. 178). The first two can be overcome relatively easily by interested researchers (for one early study, these authors had access to an unused questionnaire constructed years earlier by a colleague; pp. 162–163). Of the three, the biggest barrier is "the high cost involved in moving large numbers of qualified interviewers into an area quickly" (p. 178).

In addressing this question of resources, Bourque et al. raise a more fundamental question: "[H]ow imperative is it [for survey researchers] to enter the area immediately?" (p. 178). They quickly point out that many of the questions about both reactions to and consequences of disasters can only be answered with data collected "... well after the index disaster" (p. 178). Focusing specifically on the psychological impact of disaster on individuals, they note that "... there is no definitive information about when, or if, excessive psychological distress—to the level of post-traumatic stress disorder—occurs" (p. 178). They further note that telephones, used for most contemporary survey research, may be inoperable or their networks overloaded in the immediate post-impact period. (Assuming that phone service is more disrupted the closer the customer is to the impact site, a survey of households selected randomly and carried out before service is fully restored will produce a sample biased toward the *least* victimized households.) Their conclusion is that any delays in carrying out surveys are not automatically "untimely" in so far as collecting post-disaster data at the household and individual levels is concerned.

The question regarding timing in post-disaster surveys then becomes: Are some types of data "'perishable' and subject to memory decay or memory enhancement" (p. 179)? Using three waves of data collected 8, 19, and 24 months after the 1994 Northridge (California) earthquake, Bourque and her colleagues examined responses to the same set of questions included in each and found that "[W]hat is striking about the data is the extent to which all the information tends to remain constant across the three years of data collection" (p. 183). The authors conclude that "... this suggests that social information about disasters may not be as perishable as we sometimes think and that memories about a disaster remain quite stable for at least a substantial period after a disaster" (p. 183).

Because some surveys are done on an annual basis, there are a few instances in the disaster research literature in which a regularly scheduled survey was followed by the onset of disaster that in turn prompted a follow-up post-disaster survey (see Drabek & Key, 1984, esp. pp. 3–4; see also Sweet, 1998). In the following study (Van Willigen, 2001), the disaster occurred while a regularly scheduled survey already was underway:

> This research utilizes data from the Annual Eastern North Carolina Survey conducted by the Survey Research Laboratory, East Carolina University. This survey is an annual event, and questions had been included to assess the well-being of area residents before the hurricane was predicted. Telephone interviews began with a representative sample of households generated by random digit dialing. Once contact was established with the household, a random selection procedure was utilized to select an adult respondent. Seven hundred forty-two respondents had completed the survey when the interviewing was interrupted by the hurricane. A new sample was drawn, and interviews were resumed in early October, approximately two weeks after Hurricane Floyd, and continued for six weeks, through the middle of November. Four hundred nineteen respondents were successfully interviewed after the hurricane. (p. 65)

In general, it is not that timing issues are less important in survey research on disasters as compared with field studies. Rather, the topics that survey research seems best suited to investigate involve less ephemeral phenomena. As in all well-executed research, the idea is to avoid utilizing this type of research design for topics for which it is not well suited. This means, among other things, using survey techniques to collect data on individual- and household-level phenomena that may be expected to persist for a reasonable length of time. Hence, some of the issues of timeliness that are central in field studies are less troublesome in survey research, even when data on crisis time period phenomena are sought.

Access

The ability to access respondents via survey methods in studying disasters requires addressing two separate issues. One is related to the fact that nearly all contemporary post-disaster surveys, at least in the United States, are conducted by telephone. (See Bourque et al., 2002, pp. 160–162 for brief discussions of random digit dialing and computer-assisted telephone interviewing techniques.) Therefore, the distribution of telephone use within the population to be sampled, both in general and in the aftermath of disaster, is of fundamental importance. This issue is discussed in the next subsection in the context of how representative are the samples in post-disaster surveys and the extent to which this affects the generalization of survey results. The other issue discussed here is that of the responsiveness of subjects in post-disaster survey research conducted by telephone.

Bourque and her colleagues (2002) provide the best treatment of this question because they were able to bring data to bear in assessing it. The authors compared the response rates (i.e., the percentage of respondents successfully interviewed out of all those contacted) for the six post-disaster surveys ". . . with response rates obtained in other telephone surveys conducted . . . in southern California during the same calendar periods" (p. 176). They found that the two sets of response rates were on the whole similar. Slight variations among surveys could be accounted for by differences in the resources available for the surveys rather the different settings. The more resources, the greater the number of "callbacks" (repeated calls to the same household) attempted, the higher the response rate.

In the following excerpt, a researcher grapples with problems of access and how they might affect the generalizability of his findings. This 1997 survey (Farley, 1998) involved a random sample in the St. Louis, Missouri, metropolitan area and dealt with earthquake hazard awareness and preparedness in the New Madrid Seismic Zone:

> At least one call was made to a total of 983 households. Due to busy signals, no answer, or answering machines, we were unable over the course of the three evenings [of November 4, 6, and 9, 1997] to reach 412 of these households, despite some attempts at callbacks the second and third evenings. A total of 571 valid households were reached of which 250, or 44 percent, resulted in completed surveys. A total of 56 percent of households reached refused to participate in the survey. While a refusal rate this high is of some concern if a researcher is attempting to estimate population parameters, the primary objective of this survey was to make comparisons to baseline data established through surveys with similar methodologies in the past and with refusal rates that did not differ markedly from the present survey. For example, refusal rates ranged from 44 to 54 percent in the St. Louis metropolitan area in the second, third, and fourth surveys in this series. Thus, while readers should use caution in generalizing precise percentages to the population, the comparability of the samples across time-series surveys suggests that valid inferences can be made about trends over time in responses. (p. 309)

Bourque and her colleagues (2002) summarize the issue of access in post-disaster surveys: "On the basis of these comparisons, we conclude that there is no evidence that persons in households with telephones are any more reluctant to participate in a study after a disaster than they would be at any other time" (pp. 177–178).

Generalizability

The ability to draw "valid conclusions" about disasters from post-event surveys may be evaluated in light of three specific issues: the representativeness of samples surveyed via telephone, the availability of adequate control groups for inferring causal relationships, and the appropriateness of comparisons across different surveys in the aftermath of separate disasters.

Because so much of post-event survey research uses personal interviews conducted by telephone, the most important aspect regarding the representativeness of samples is the availability of telephone services in the aftermath of disaster:

> One concern that has been raised about doing surveys after a disaster is that the sample from which the data are collected is not representative of the population affected by the disaster. Two general objections are raised in this regard. First, it is suggested that telephone surveys will "miss" substantial numbers of persons who do not have telephones or access to telephones *prior* to the index disaster. Second, it is suggested that telephone surveys "miss" those who are dislocated as the result of the index disaster and, therefore, fail to get information on those most affected by the disaster. (Bourque et al., 2002, p. 173; emphasis in the original)

In response, Bourque and her colleagues argue that in urban areas (where most post-disaster survey research is conducted) "...telephone coverage is so pervasive in the U.S. and so quickly reinstated following disasters in the U.S. that the representativeness of any RDD [random digit dialing] sample ... will be as good or better than any other method of data collection ..." (p. 173), provided that survey researchers follow best practices common to telephone-based survey research as a whole. The authors examined the survey conducted following the Loma Prieta earthquake in the San Francisco Bay Area because its critics had charged that this survey underrepresented "...the homeless and those who occupied single-room-occupancy (SRO) hotels prior to the earthquake" (p. 174). Their careful analysis (pp. 174–176) leads them to conclude that a small proportion of the Bay Area population was indeed missed. However, researchers know *who* was missed and *to what extent* and can therefore estimate the likely effects on study results. They reiterate that telephone interviewing does provide "...a dependable overall picture of what happened to an entire community during and after a disaster" (p. 176). The proviso to this statement, of course, is that data from those populations known to be missed by telephone interviewing can only be obtained by other types of sampling (e.g., so-called "snow-ball" sampling of homeless disaster victims) and data collection methods (e.g., face-to-face interviews).

The following excerpts are typical of the narrative in research reports where the researcher discusses the representativeness of the sample drawn. Usually the characteristics of respondents in the sample are compared with some baseline for the population such as the most recent decennial Census of Population, as in this example from Farley (1998):

> Before proceeding with the analysis, I examined the demographics of the sample and compared the sample demographics to the combined demographics of the counties included in the survey according to the 1990 Census.... [T]he sample characteristics are thus close or closer [referring to the margin of error for the size of the sample] to the population characteristics in the overwhelming majority of instances.... [O]ur sample appears in general to be reasonably representative of the population except with respect to socioeconomic status, ... [T]here is no reason to believe that there is any significant impact on the trends over time in earthquake awareness and preparedness, which are the main focus of this paper (p. 310).

In the section on field studies, the question of control groups necessary for inferring causal relationships was discussed. The same challenge confronts survey researchers. As before, interest is in being able to link post-disaster attitudes and behaviors to the disaster experience rather than to some other causal factors. The logic for making such an inferential connection requires comparing disaster victims with nonvictims. In technical terms, this requires some way of measuring respondents' "exposure" to the causal variable, in this case the disaster. Early disaster researchers, following the precedent of ecological models of cities that were a major part of the pioneering Chicago school of urban sociology (see Faris, 1970 [1967], pp. 51–87), developed a spatial model with concentric circles distinguishing areas in terms of the typical disaster-related activity within them (Wallace, 1956b, p. 3). Areas in the model ranged from that of total impact at its center to the outer, undamaged areas from which local and regional aid was supplied (pp. 3–6). These early researchers used this spatial model to identify population strata in disaster-stricken communities and drew probability samples from within each strata, producing an overall sample of households for comparison that were assumed to represent varying degrees of victimization (see Killian, 2002 [1956], pp. 51, 63–67).

Bourque and her colleagues (2002) propose a similar strategy for one particular type of disastrous event, earthquakes:

> There is no way that a researcher can establish randomized control groups in studying responses to disasters, but the existence of population-based samples does allow systematic examination of whether and how experiences and responses differ across groups within the same community who are differentially exposed to the disaster. In earthquakes, the Modified Mercalli Intensities (MMI) provide an approximation of the extent to which an area experienced shaking. Using MMI as an indicator of the extent to which respondents and their homes were "exposed" to the earthquake or the "dose" that they received, we can examine whether reports of damage, injury, and emotional distress differed with the MMI. We expect that these three variables do vary with exposure or "dose" of the earthquake that the respondent experienced. (p. 184)

Their examination of two post-earthquake surveys supports this expectation. Respondents' opinions generally followed the expected pattern (p. 187). In general, the authors conclude:

> The availability of data from probability samples where exposure to the disaster varies enables the researcher to estimate the extent to which proximity to a disaster results in different experiences, behaviors, and attitudes. While not as powerful as an experimental design for examining the impact of a disaster on communities, the use of the concept of dose-response provides a viable proxy or surrogate for a controlled experiment and allows inferences to be made about how the disaster has differentially affected households with, for example, similar household resources. (p. 188)

As was the case in field studies, so too with post-disaster surveys there are strategies for at least approximating the comparisons that form the basis of test and control groups in drawing causal inferences about the consequences of disaster for individuals, households, and communities. Another, more typical example is the following from Ollenburger and Tobin (1999):

> A detailed investigation was undertaken of flood victims in Des Moines, Iowa, in 1993; this cohort was subsequently described as the high exposure group. First, a stratified random sample of flood victims was drawn based on Census records, large-scale maps, and telephone directories and an introductory letter mailed to prospective respondents. An in-depth telephone questionnaire was then administered by trained interviewers from the Center for Family Research in Rural Mental Health at Iowa State University approximately four months after the flood. One hundred and six questionnaires were successfully completed with each interview lasting up to 40 minutes. There was a refusal rate of 15 percent. Three months later, a large-scale control survey was undertaken in Des Moines and surrounding communities. This survey, again conducted by the Center for Family Research in Rural Mental Health, incorporated many of the same items of the original survey as well as further questions concerning psychological morbidity and level of flood exposure. A total of 1,735 surveys were completed; these served as the control group. (pp. 66–67)

Finally, the relatively greater codification of survey research methods makes possible more specific comparisons across separate post-disaster surveys than is possible for multiple field studies. Differences in timing, response rates, sample sizes, sample characteristics, and even question wording can be weighed in comparing findings from one survey to another and the effects such differences may have had on them estimated. This "... allows researchers to compare community behavior across time, events, and locations" (Bourque et al., 2002, p. 169). Bourque and her colleagues, for example, compare household preparedness activities between northern and southern California as well as over time (pp. 169–173). Comparisons of surveys conducted at different points in time are especially useful for identifying trends. Interpreted loosely as similar to an interrupted times series, comparing the results of several surveys done before a disaster such as an earthquake with several conducted on the same population afterward can make as strong a case as possible for inferring the causal impact of disasters on attitudes and behaviors. In addition, superimposing the findings from survey research onto those from field studies, where both deal with the same phenomena, is part of the triangulation process that increases the ability of disaster researchers to draw "valid conclusions."

DOCUMENTARY RESEARCH

The term "documentary research" implies that there is some specific research design or method that distinguishes the analysis of documents from other types of disaster research. This is misleading. With the possible exception of historical research, the use of documents in the research process is usually supplementary or complementary to either field studies or the statistical analysis of secondary data. (For a caution on the use of documents, see Killian, 2002 [1956], p. 81.) As the term is used here, "documents" refers to more than the usual materials collected in disaster field studies such as organizational logs and records, local newspapers, and after-action reports. It includes all materials that exist in either written, printed, or digital form that are obtained by researchers other than through the interview or questionnaire process. I have avoided calling them secondary data as opposed to the primary data obtained via interviewing and questionnaire completion. However, the notion of secondary data does identify what all these materials have in common. They are all physical records regardless of format that were created by someone *other than* the researcher for a purpose *other than that* for which they will be used *by* the researcher.

I have further arbitrarily divided the following subsections into three separate discussions. One deals with contemporaneous documentary materials of an ephemeral nature, meaning that if the researcher does not obtain them at the time of the disaster or very soon thereafter they are not likely to be available or even exist later on. The second deals with documents and records produced in the months and years following a disaster, typically by formal organizations and official agencies, that are usually converted into quantitative data for statistical analysis. The third deals with historical materials, the kinds of documents that over time have passed from the hands of those who created them to others, often either relatives and descendants or archives and libraries.

Quarantelli (2002a) gives the most comprehensive description of documentary materials as the term is used in reference to field studies, noting that

> . . . in the DRC framework the term "document" was used to cover anything of a physical nature that could either be copied or obtained. Thus, for example, it included, at one end, relevant graffiti, signs on buildings, notes placed on EOC bulletin boards, informal organizational logs and group minutes, citizen recordings of the event, and jokes circulating about the occasion (including gallows humor) to, at the other end, official handouts, public proclamations and press releases, written organizational data (e.g., charters, budgets, annual reports, disaster plans, manuals, after-action reports), printed community data (e.g., Chamber of Commerce profiles, telephone books), statistics from emergency-related organizations (with similar data from the previous week and year), and mass communication stories. (p. 116)

While the typical use of documentary materials in field studies is descriptive, that is, to supplement the interviews and observations that are used to construct an overall picture of disaster-related structures and processes, there is nothing inherent in such materials to limit their use to qualitative description alone. Indeed, even the DRC field teams, which specialized in exploratory and qualitative research, were instructed to gather the kinds of materials that could yield quantitative indicators ". . . to identify disruption of community life" (Quarantelli, 2002a, p. 115):

> . . . DRC shall attempt to obtain *statistics, afteraction reports, and whatever other documentary data* are available from the [fifteen types of] listed organizations. The intent is to try to develop measures of a quantitative sort of the disruptions and difficulties a community undergoes as a result of a disaster. Unless otherwise indicated, we should get the statistics on a three-week period around the disaster (assuming an emergency period of one week) and a comparable three weeks a year before. (p. 115; italics in the original)

Documents of exclusively written content also can frequently be used to produce quantitative variables for statistical analysis. This is accomplished either through a formal content analysis of entire documents or through the coding of specific variables from reports or summaries, for example. The former procedure is most often employed in analyses of news reports, especially reports in the print media (see, among many others, Dearing & Kazmierczak, 1993; Emani & Kasperson, 1996; Hiroi, Mikami, & Miyata, 1985; Nimmo, 1984; Seydlitz, Spencer, Laska, & Triche, 1991; Wenger & Friedman, 1986; Wilkins, 1986). Stallings (1979) used such a coding scheme to transform successful and unsuccessful applications for disaster aid into a dependent variable for statistical modeling.

Finally, written documents form the basis for historical research on disasters. (The most interesting and informative source is Scanlon, 2002; see, as an example of historical disaster research, Dynes, 2000b.) These include everything from vintage newspaper clippings to diaries to personal correspondence. Also included are official histories prepared by organizations immediately after disaster, records of testimony at hearings and before investigative bodies, and records and lists of all kinds. Historical disaster research does not deal exclusively with the written word, however. Even an event that occurred as much as 80 years before can yield a surprising amount of oral history, as relatives and descendants of eyewitnesses and survivors recount for researchers stories handed down to them (see Scanlon, 2002, pp. 286–288).

Timing

The issue of timing plays out differently in the case of documents used in each of the three different types of research—the exploratory field study, the explanatory quantitative analysis, and historical research. In the case of field studies where rich description is a major objective, the critical aspect is the ephemeral nature of nearly all types of documentary materials sought. The one-time-only aspect of the materials makes the issues of timing and access one and the same. That is, if researchers are not on site to capture the written material almost at the time it is created then odds are that it will be lost permanently. Consider just a few types mentioned by Quarantelli (above): graffiti scrawled on the standing walls of damaged buildings, soon to be torn down for reasons of both safety and rebuilding; messages and lists written in chalk on backboards likely to be erased as soon as room is needed for newer messages and lists; and scribbled notes taken to record telephone requests for action or instructions tossed in waste baskets as emergency operations are being wrapped up. Unless researchers are physically present at such "data collection" opportunities to capture this type of information, it will never become part of the documentary "evidence" from the disaster. Quarantelli (2002a, p. 106; see also Phillips, 2002, p. 206) has long advocated the use of video cameras in the field to facilitate the capturing of such ephemeral materials. However, cameras and other recording devices such as cellular telephones with built-in digital cameras still must be operated by people who have access to the scene at just the right moment. Further, gaining access often requires that researchers agree not to use any audio, photographic, or video recording devices.

In contrast to the fleeting opportunities to collect the kinds of documentary materials so valuable in field research, the type of documents most valuable for statistical analyses are not likely to exist for months or even years following disaster. These documents either contain or are themselves of such a nature that they can be converted into the secondary data that can be analyzed statistically. Two different types exist, and each has its own dynamic. One type contains data or information that is readily quantifiable and is produced by organizations and agencies directly involved in disaster. The second type consists of all the data produced routinely typically by governmental entities that can be used as statistical "indicators" of either the severity or the consequences of disaster. These include such things as local building permits issued, property taxes collected, unemployment figures, live birth rates, divorce rates, suicide rates per 1,000 population, etc. Research that requires such secondary data obviously cannot be undertaken until they are available, and this could be a year if not years after the crisis time period has ended.

In the case of historical disaster research, the time after disaster when the researcher begins the search for documentary materials will determine the type of material likely to be available. If the disaster occurred within a generation or even two, then there are still likely to be survivors who can be tracked down and interviewed. Loss of memory can accompany the aging process, but as Scanlon (2002) found in his reconstruction of the 1917 Halifax munitions ship explosion: "Disasters are so dramatic that many vividly remember what happened even three-quarters of a century earlier" (p. 267). If the disaster is one that took place a century or two before, letters and memoirs of survivors as well as newspaper clippings are useful:

> One starting point both for getting an overview of what happened and for creating a list for follow-up later was newspapers. While newspapers are notorious for making errors of detail, including errors about disasters . . . , they provide a broad picture of an incident and, because they are dated, help establish a sequence of events. They also provide names of organizations involved . . . While local newspapers are important, newspapers away from the scene are also useful . . . Newspapers also give a sense of the times. (Scanlon, 2002, pp. 272–273)

If the disaster occurred more than two or three centuries earlier, then the main sources of information are likely to be written histories of the period or of the region, published autobiographical materials, and fiction from that era that uses the disaster in some way. As Scanlon (2002) notes: "Dramatic events inspire fiction, some of it autobiographical" (p. 274).

Access

Even though access and timing are so closely connected that this topic was introduced in the preceding subsection, there is another aspect of access to documentary materials that is independent of timing issues. This is the bias that is introduced when researchers are prevented, either intentionally or as a result of unavoidable circumstances (such as the inability to be in two places at once), from gaining access to selective kinds of documentary materials. The sources of selective access are important to identify since the consequences of selectivity affect the generalizability of findings.

In the case of field studies, the greatest potential sources of selective access to documentary type materials are emergency response organizations, especially law enforcement. Often for good reasons but sometimes for self-serving ones, official disaster response agencies frequently try to limit not only researchers' access to personnel for interviews but also to control the written documents that researchers are able to obtain. When they are successful at restricting the flow of official documents and other information to only those that are available to the public-at-large (including the news media), the picture of disaster that researchers are presented with will be biased toward what Quarantelli (1981) has aptly labeled the "command post point of view," meaning the picture of disaster that those in charge would like people to have (Tierney, 2002b, p. 361).

Among more recent developments affecting researchers' abilities to acquire documentary materials is the increasing use of cell phones and PDAs (personal digital assistants) in the field. Organizational communication and record keeping are becoming more and more decentralized as well as more and more ephemeral as a result. E-mail poses a challenge for researchers in general, let alone disaster researchers. Researchers know or suspect that e-mail relevant to disaster operations exists, but organizational, legal, and practical constraints on locating and acquiring it are formidable, if not prohibitive.

In the case of statistical analyses that use documentary materials as sources of secondary data, the problem of selective access is less overt. It is clearly possible that researchers may be denied access to existing data, particularly if those data are proprietary in nature or, more recently, deemed of national security interest. More frequently, the frustration of researchers stems from the fact that the data sought for quantitative analysis are simply not collected or, if collected, they are not held in a single location.[7] In general, the researcher is limited to those items of secondary data in which agencies are interested or are legally charged with collecting. The U.S. Census of the Population is the prototype. All of the criticisms of the Census as a source of secondary data for research purposes can be made of the sources of secondary data for disaster research as well.

An extreme case of selective access to documents is worth recalling because it illustrates how such selectivity can affect the generalizability of findings. The case is the award-winning book on the 1972 Buffalo Creek, West Virginia, dam break and flood disaster, *Everything in Its Path*, by noted Ivy League sociologist Kai Erikson (1976). Erikson, widely known primarily for his widely used book on the sociology of deviance (Erikson, 1966), had not previously been involved in any research on disasters. He was hired soon after the flood by the law firm representing plaintiffs in legal action against the coal company responsible for building and maintaining the dam that had collapsed and thus had access to legal depositions, psychiatric evaluations, and statements and letters written by the survivors to their attorneys. In addition, he conducted interviews and distributed a mailed questionnaire to all the adult plaintiffs in the action with a 90% response rate (Erikson, 1976, p. 14).

Not surprisingly, Erikson found that everyone along Buffalo Creek had been traumatized by the flood disaster, both individually and collectively (pp. 153–155). This finding, however, was at odds with 25 years of research on disasters that had accumulated by that time. A reviewer of the book, one of the pioneers of the field of disaster studies (and one of the editors of this volume), found Erikson's findings "troublesome" and requiring further explanation (Dynes, 1978b, p. 721). One possibility was that the Buffalo Creek flood disaster was so unusual that Erikson's findings were bound to be different from those of others in the field. Erikson himself might not have been aware of this since he was a newcomer (although he does cite several of the key disaster studies available at the time; see in particular Erikson, 1976, pp. 266–267). If this were the case, then the Buffalo Creek disaster would be so unusual as to have only limited generalization to other community disasters (Dynes, 1978b, p. 721). However, Dynes suggests that Erikson's unusual findings are better explained by the nature of the materials to which he had access (p. 722). The motives and

---

[7] The author once sought data on local election outcomes in California counties that had previously experienced a gubernatorially declared disaster. The California Secretary of State is responsible for certifying the outcome of all local elections in the state. However, the author learned that the Secretary of State's office at that time did not physically possess the actual local election results. These instead were in the hands of the individual county clerks. To gather the results would have required contacting each of California's 58 county seats.

interests of plaintiffs in a major class-action lawsuit whose homes had been destroyed and whose lives uprooted seemingly were accepted at face value. The study results overwhelmingly reflected the point of view of individuals knowingly engaged in an adversarial legal action.

Regarding problems of access to documentary materials in historical disaster research, the most complete discussion is that in Scanlon (2002). His experience in revisiting the history of the 1917 Halifax, Nova Scotia, disaster shows the hit-and-miss, serendipitous nature of accessing historical documents:

> Historical research has limitations. Records are lost or destroyed. Some sources are dead. Others are alive but their memories dim. Persons have taken records with them and kept them in private hands. However, there are also advantages. Some records that were private or secret have become public; some persons will produce records or talk about past events, though they would not have been cooperative at the time. In addition, some statistics and comparative data will exist only because time has passed. Sophisticated methods of analysis may reveal things that were not evident years ago. (Scanlon, 2002, pp. 266–267)

Scanlon (2002) suggests as starting points newspapers, books, academic theses, official papers, reports, minutes, logs, and letters (p. 268):

> While much of this material will be found in libraries or archives, it may be far from obvious which libraries and archives are worth visiting. After that, finding material becomes even more challenging. There are private papers ranging from notes written in a scribbler to diaries to typed memos. Tracking these down means poking around in basements or vaults. It also means using unconventional techniques, making one's interests known, and following trails from family, friends, professional colleagues, or even strangers to written sources, then trying to fit the material into a pattern. (p. 268)
> ... Some archives and specialized libraries are very useful, others less so; all have information. However, there are hierarchies of archives. Beginners to historical research should start where there is an interest in their topic. Major archives are more useful to persons who know what they are looking for. (p. 278)

In accessing documents, Scanlon reminds researchers that it is people—living human beings—who possess or at least know about the existence of documents of potential research interest. His tips for those new to historical disaster research are built around this simple fact:

> It is extremely important to tell everyone what you are doing, and that means *everyone*—the [hotel] desk clerk, the hotel maid, the swimming pool attendant, the parking attendant, storekeepers, service station attendants. Incidents like the Halifax explosion are the stuff of legends, and everyone is interested. By telling people about your research, you allow word of your interest to spread.... Publishing findings can also be important. When the author published an article about the role of the railroads, that led to an editorial in a Halifax paper, and that led to a letter to the editor. (Scanlon, 2002, pp. 283–284; emphasis in the original)

Information was also discovered by following a trail, starting with a person, ending with a record. This was done with help from family, friends, and colleagues. Doing this requires conviction that any lead is worth following—and dogged determination. (p. 289)

In summing up his experience, Scanlon (2002) observes: "Not every trail was productive.... [But for] every apparently unproductive trail, there were unexpected discoveries" (p. 292).

My own concluding observation is that the process of gaining access to historical documents is not as random as it might appear. Although researchers' abilities to acquire materials may involve a bit of luck in addition to the dogged determination that Scanlon (a former news reporter) describes, the initial production and subsequent retention of documentary materials, like all source materials for historical analysis, have more to do with wealth, power, and literacy. As the question of selectivity is raised in the general question of "Whose history gets told?" so, too, one might ask "Whose perspectives on the disasters of the past survive?" With the passage of time, the influence of wealth and power plays an increasingly important part in determining which documents are preserved and therefore which documents disaster researchers ultimately will be able to access.

Generalizability

The documentary materials used in disaster research should come with a warning label. Killian (2002 [1956]) described it succinctly half a century ago: "Documents constitute an important source of data in the study of disaster, but they must be used with caution" (p. 81). ". . . [T]he bias of the writers must be kept in mind" (p. 82). Before using any documents, researchers should investigate the people behind them. They should learn as much as possible about a document's creators as well as its preservers, their points of view, their interests, and their motives. This is part of the "leg work" involved in field studies. It should also be part of the statistical analysis of secondary data. A good financial adviser will know the weaknesses of any economic indicator used to evaluate an investment opportunity; a good disaster researcher—indeed, good researchers in general—should have the same knowledge of the variables used in quantitative analyses.

Historiography also addresses the origins and motives behind the documents that historians use. Scanlon (2002), not surprisingly, has thought a good deal about establishing the validity of materials in historical disaster research and offers several suggestions:

> People create records, and the same rules apply for testing validity as apply to checking personal stories. Does the material have internal consistency? Is there any corroboration? Is the account something that reasonably could have been known to the person who created the record? If it is not evident, it is important to ask, "How did you know that?" Sometimes persons will provide information both about things they did or saw *and* about what they heard. It is important to separate observations from second-hand accounts. The first are usually accurate, the second are not. While this is harder to do using documents, it is important to ask, when reading a written account, "How would that person have known that?" It is also important to ask if there is anything which suggests why the person might have been less than truthful or have had a systematic bias. Finally, one must pay some attention to when an account was recorded. As time passes, members of organizations are likely to recall better organization than actually existed. They are also likely to recall that decisions were made at a higher level than was the case. . . . Some stories are easy to verify. . . . Other accounts are credible because one meshes with another. . . . Other accounts do not mesh so easily. . . . Some material is credible because the source has no apparent or conceivable reason for bias. . . . Sometimes material is useful because it helps establish credibility of other accounts. . . . The fact that something is not credible does not make it useless. (pp. 297–299; emphasis in the original)

Although documentary and archival materials may be more often used in disaster studies currently than when Taylor (1978, p. 276) urged researchers to make greater use of them, the same cautions about their use remain nearly 30 years later.

CONCLUSIONS AND PROSPECTS

Disaster Research Outside North American and Western Europe

In bringing this chapter to a close, it is appropriate to note some of its deficiencies as well as some of the topics likely to be major parts of similar undertakings in the future. Most obvious among the former is the applicability of the suggestions offered here to studies of disasters world wide. The bulk of research on disasters to date has been conducted by North American researchers on events in North America. Although research outside this portion of the Western Hemisphere has increased greatly in recent decades, existing discussions of the methods of disaster research, including the present one, are overwhelmingly colored by this geographic, national, and cultural skewing. A few treatments of methodological issues unique to disaster research in the developing world exist. Issues in cross-national comparative research facing nonnative researchers, for example, are discussed by Peacock (2002). Another perspective by a non-North American disaster researcher is provided by Khondker (2002) utilizing his experience in studying disasters in Bangladesh. With examinations such as these as starting points, it is time for a synthesis and an evaluation of research experience outside the developed world. Treatments from two different perspectives would be valuable—that of non-natives based upon their work in countries other than their own; and that of natives studying disasters in their own countries. For now, it must be said that the lessons to be taken from the present chapter may be less useful for researchers operating outside North America.

Some of the key issues that researchers face in conducting research on disasters in developing countries can be noted here at least. Most obvious is the choice of appropriate research design. Field studies remain a mainstay for a variety of reasons (Khondker, 2002, p. 337). Survey research is clearly possible, but the applicability of telephone-based survey techniques in most developing nations remains questionable. And documentary research confronts many of the same problems noted above in addition to those related to language differences and the need for translation skills (for non-natives) not to mention the predominance of oral rather than written traditions in many places where disasters are common.

Other issues that have been identified in the still sparse literature on methods for studying disasters in countries other than one's own include problems of ethnocentrism on the part of researchers and their lack of knowledge or appreciation of local beliefs and customs such as those associated with gender roles. The creation of multinational teams of investigators is one way that researchers have addressed such problems (Peacock, 2002, p. 237), including in such teams individuals, whether native or not, who can perform services such as securing cooperation from local leaders and conducting interviews with indigenous research subjects (Khondker, 2002, pp. 340–341). Another major set of problems is what Peacock (2002, pp. 244–247) calls "equivalence" issues. These include the reliability (i.e., the consistency of measurement from country to country) of social and economic indicators such as crime, divorce, suicides, and economic productivity. Also problematic is the comparability of seemingly similar units of analysis such as "the family." Even the comparability of events is often problematic in ways that differ from much of the current debate about what constitutes a disaster. Khondker (2002, pp. 335–337) notes, for example, that differentiating disasters from the normal state of affairs in many developing countries is sometimes difficult. How, for instance, does one distinguish between a famine and the constant state of mass poverty and malnutrition that are chronic in many parts of the world?

Despite such problems, there is virtually universal agreement that research on disasters occurring outside the developed nations is invaluable, whatever the obstacles. Peacock (2002, pp. 239–240) for one identifies several trends that will continue to facilitate such research: the growing recognition of global issues and processes and how disasters play into these; increased funding for disaster research, especially from international organizations; a growing population of disaster researchers in countries outside North America and Western Europe; and increasing interest in and development of cross-national databases. Perhaps just as helpful, Peacock notes that, based upon his experience in studying the aftermath of Hurricane Andrew in South Florida and various disasters in Latin America, problems associated with disaster research abroad are not all that dissimilar from those encountered in doing similar research in ethnically and culturally diverse U.S. cities such as Miami (p. 236).

Ethical Issues in Disaster Research

In addition to methodological issues in studying disasters in less developed countries, another topic not dealt with explicitly here thus far, yet one also deserving of its own chapter-length treatment, is that of ethical issues in disaster research. The same generalizations with which this chapter began can be repeated for ethical issues in this field: they are unique only in degree, and their uniqueness varies directly with proximity to the crisis time period. Otherwise, the ethics of disaster research are no different from those associated with the social sciences in general. (For an introductory discussion of the latter, see Babbie, 1995, pp. 445–466.)

Ethical issues involve the *consequences* of researchers' actions during as well as after disaster and during the research process as well as after the research is formally concluded. Most prominent are questions regarding the impact of data gathering, whatever form it may take, on the lives of research subjects. The standard for researchers (and for university IRBs) is summed up in the phrase, "Do no harm" (Babbie, 1995, pp. 449–450). But during the crisis time period, researchers are intruding into people's lives at one of the worst possible moments. What special responsibilities do they have when interviewing people who may have lost all their worldly possessions and maybe even loved ones as well? What special responsibilities do they have when observing and perhaps occasionally conversing with disaster responders during the crisis time period?

Disaster researchers commonly justify both forms of intrusion as necessary for accumulating the knowledge that can be used to reduce suffering and improve response in future disasters. Yet the price of this knowledge accumulation—physical, psychological, emotional—is born disproportionately by subjects, not by researchers.[8] How hard should researchers push for an interview with a disaster victim, for example? Should they avoid asking certain questions when they suspect that those questions will be especially difficult to answer, given what they already know about what the subject has experienced? Should they persist to complete an interview with a subject who becomes highly emotional, or should they terminate the interview? Should they try to complete the interview at a later time or simply leave the subject alone? Should researchers refuse to perform an important emergency-related task if asked to do so by response personnel, even if no one else is available to do it?

---

[8] This is not to ignore the price that researchers themselves pay, especially those directly exposed to the human carnage and physical destruction they witness in the immediate aftermath of disaster impact. The crucial distinction is that researchers by and large have voluntarily chosen to expose themselves to the products of calamity while the disaster victims who are their subjects and informants have not. While the former are likely to return to a "normal" existence in a matter of days, the latter will live with the consequences of their victimization for a much longer time, in many cases for the rest of their lives.

available are increasingly required of principal investigators before they can begin collecting data. Without prior approval, timing can be affected. If the effect of such ponderous-appearing preliminaries is to reduce the probability that subjects will agree to be interviewed, then access and ultimately generalizability will be affected.

Organizational self-protection, or its more extreme version, self-preservation, is another pre-9/11 trend that seems to have intensified. The increasing tendency of organizations to manage their public images, including the image that they present to researchers, was noted above (Tierney, 2002b, pp. 359–362). There is a sense among some field researchers that potential subjects' fear of retaliation from their superiors has increased in recent years. To the extent that such concerns actually do inhibit organizational "lower-participants" (from Etzioni, 1964) from agreeing to be interviewed, the more researchers must guard against the "command-post" point of view typically presented by organizational "higher-ups."

One trend seems to have been slowed by the events of 9/11. This is the trend away from field studies of the crisis time period of disasters and catastrophes in favor of topics less temporally connected to impact such as mitigation and recovery. In part this may be attributable to the costs of maintaining so-called standby field teams such as those employed by the DRC for many years (see Quarantelli, 2002a, especially pp. 101–106; for other discussions, see Scanlon & Taylor, 1977; Biderman, 1966). Such a standby capability requires continuity of funding at a certain level in order to train and retain a cohort of graduate research assistants (GRAs) who turn over completely every 4 or 5 years. Too, the priorities of major funding agencies such as the National Science Foundation have changed over time. Giving higher priority in proposal evaluation to multidisciplinary teams of researchers, for example, favors participation by individual disaster researchers over standby teams. The downside of such multidisciplinary efforts is that the specialized interests of social scientists become a lesser priority among those of physical scientists and engineers, or at worst are only afterthoughts. Other funding priority shifts such as greater interest in mitigation and the (usually unspoken) belief that enough is known about the crisis time period further reduce the willingness to fund standby teams and the kind of field studies described earlier in this chapter.

The most obvious and most pervasive effect of 9/11 on disaster research, not surprisingly, has been the greatly increased concern for security on the part of many key emergency response organizations. Security concerns have made all three types of research more difficult. Access to EOCs, where researchers can observe disaster operations first-hand, make initial contacts for later interviews, and collect the most ephemeral of the ephemeral documents, has become more difficult. Obtaining formal interviews in security-conscious organizations is also more difficult. Prior working relationships and a national (and international) reputation for studying disasters can be decisive in overcoming such obstacles in a timely manner. Survey research has become more problematic as well, although this seems to be more the case when organizations are involved, either as objects of study or as sponsors and endorsers than with general surveys of population samples. And document acquisition, not surprisingly given the considerations noted previously, is noticeably more difficult where emergency response organizations are involved. Paraphrasing one veteran disaster researcher, the current climate is one in which "testosterone is everywhere."

Social and Technological Change and the Methods of Disaster Research

The new century has seen a carryover from the previous one of various social changes and trends affecting disaster research. Among the most significant is the continuing growth in the number of social scientists conducting research on disasters and hazards in countries outside Western Europe and North America. Transnational groups such as the International Research Committee on Disasters (Research Committee 39 of the International Sociological Association), LA RED (a multidisciplinary network of disaster specialists in Latin America and the Caribbean), the Disaster & Social Crisis Research Network (a multidisciplinary group interested in the development of disaster-resilient communities in Europe), and more specialized groups such as the Gender and Disaster Network not only serve as links among researchers in different countries but also help to nurture those new to the field. Although the cohort of academics engaged in disaster research on a consistent basis in the United States has not expanded as rapidly as that in other parts of the globe, nevertheless it has seen the training and emergence of a second and now a third "generation" of disaster researchers. Also relevant to disaster research in the United States has been the growing number of undergraduate and graduate degree programs in disaster management that are producing a new cohort of professionally-trained emergency managers (see, e.g., Neal, 2000). These individuals by and large have a better understanding of and appreciation for the value of social science research than many of their colleagues. To the extent that they are able to open doors for researchers, they make the task of studying disasters easier.

New technologies are also affecting disaster research, making the work easier and researchers more efficient in many ways but posing new challenges as well. On the plus side, a variety of portable electronic devices are especially useful in field work, at least when conditions permit. Chief among these are cellular telephones. Cell phones make the coordination among field team members easier and expedite relationships with potential subjects. Along with PDAs and BlackBerries having e-mail, Internet, and Global Position System (GPS) capabilities, they facilitate better, more instantaneous relationships between field teams and their home bases. Cell phones with digital cameras also make it easier to photograph scenes inside EOCs and at other locations that otherwise would take many words to describe. They also can be used to capture ephemeral "documents" such graffiti and erasable scribbling on blackboards. At the same time, camera phones may cause difficulties with organizational officials concerned about privacy, security, and litigation. They also pose ethical questions related to privacy, voluntary participation, and right of refusal such as whether it is acceptable to use them without first seeking permission.

Digital audio recorders in one sense are no different from their more cumbersome ancestors which have been used to record interviews in the field for more than half a century. However, uploaded to a computer with voice recognition software, it is possible to transcribe interviews without having someone listen to the recording and key in everything that was said (although the process of conversion to text remains less than seamless). Voice recognition software and a laptop computer allow field researchers to dictate their handwritten notes, observations, and anything else so that it can be printed out or even e-mailed back to the home base immediately. And camcorders, while also similar to other regular cameras, movie cameras, and video recorders, make it possible to store, transmit, and process pictorial data more quickly and more efficiently. However, the same issues surround their use in the field as with these older devices. In addition to privacy concerns, there is the additional concern that the use of camcorders and other photographic devices might alter in some way the behavior of subjects being recorded.

New technologies in the hands of research subjects offer the possibility of new types and sources of data on disaster and its aftermath. Most obvious are Internet Web sites. These range from existing sites maintained by news organizations that post articles and photos pertaining to the disaster to the sites of emergency and relief organizations to entirely new sites created in the aftermath of a disaster. Blogs (i.e., Web logs), the diary-like personal accounts written by individuals that have proliferated on the Internet, are a potentially rich source of data. So, too, are message boards, newsgroups, and Internet Relay Chat (IRC, or chat, for short). Researchers interested in the popular culture of disasters (see Eyre, Wachtendorf, & Webb, 2000) have an exciting future ahead of them as they mine these new data sources.

A note of caution must be sounded regarding such sources, however. Although the availability of digital documents, particularly official documents on government agency Web sites, can be quite useful, the availability of online documents remains hit-and-miss, raising questions about why some documents are available and others are not. Blogs, message boards, newsgroups, and chat are used by a select segment of the population. Who these users are, what viewpoints they bring to the Internet, and what interests and motives they have should be the subject of separate research. It can be assumed, for example, that such participants are not only among a society's more literate members but also are among its most "technology literate" as well. What implications do these twin characteristics have for the ability to generalize from such data sources?

Other drawbacks of these new technologies have implications for disaster research as well as social science research more generally. Chief among these is increasing cell phone use and its impact on survey research. Apart from issues such as the availability of cellular telephone service in the aftermath of disaster, a new concern is the *disconnect* between cell phone users and their geographic locations. Sampling techniques for telephone-based surveys attempt to compare disaster victims with nonvictims selected randomly with area codes and prefixes identified as high damage and low or no damage areas, respectively. However, cell phone users (and those using VOIP [Voice over Internet Protocol], a computer-based telephone technology) are no longer necessarily located in the same geographic area as their landline-using counterparts. Reaching subjects who use cell phone raises questions about violating the U.S. Telephone Consumer Protection Act (47 U.S.C. 227), about how to compensate subjects for their cell phone usage, about the safety of interviewing subjects without knowing what they are doing while being interviewed (e.g., driving), and about the types of questions that can appropriately be asked if subjects are responding in public places where others are able to hear their replies.

There is also a downside to these new digital media as sources of data on disasters. With cell phones and other hand-held devices capable of sending and receiving text messages, data on interpersonal and interorganizational communications become increasingly more ephemeral in absence of written communication logs. So, too, does e-mail correspondence for those not included on distribution lists. Acquiring copies of such correspondence after the fact may be exceedingly difficult for practical as well as legal reasons. Other examples could easily be cited.

The overall conclusion would seem to be that these new technologies represent a net benefit for disaster researchers, but at the same time they exacerbate existing challenges and create a few new ones as well. Another conclusion is that there needs to be some research on disaster research itself. Shared experiences need to be captured and organized, and a set of "best practices" or at least recommendations formulated. This is especially true for experiences of researchers operating outside North America and Western Europe and of those working with these newer digital media and technologies. This chapter, if it achieves its objective, can serve as a starting point.

CHAPTER 5

The Role of Geographic Information Systems/Remote Sensing in Disaster Management

Deborah S.K. Thomas, Kivanç Ertuĝay, and Serkan Kemeç

Geographic Information Systems (GIS), Remote Sensing (RS), and Global Positioning Systems (GPS) have gained much attention for their applications in disaster management and are increasingly utilized throughout the entire disaster management cycle as a tool to support decision making. GIS is commonly recognized as a key support tool for disaster management (Mileti, 1999). The visualization capabilities of these systems have almost become expected by policymakers, disaster managers, and even the public.

The mapping of hazards and the impacts on people has a long and rich history with roots in many basic cartographic concepts (Hodgson & Cutter, 2001; Monmonier, 1997). For example, daily weather maps were first produced in Europe and then in the 1800s in the United States. The Sanborn Company compiled systematic maps of urban hazards for fire insurance in major U.S. cities starting in the 1870s. The systematic mapping of hazard zones in relation to human settlement patterns for understanding human response can be linked to Gilbert White in the 1960s and 1970s (Burton, Kates, & White, 1993; White, 1974). The real expansion of the application of GIS to disasters began with the advent of ubiquitous computer use, especially affordable desktop computers and software in the late 1980s and 1990s. Along with software and hardware availability, increasing numbers of hazard datasets, both for the United States and internationally, have become accessible and the application of GIS technology has rapidly expanded in both disaster research and practice.

Even though geographic questions have long been of concern to both disaster researchers and practitioners alike, the proliferation of GIS has essentially increased the capacity of those in the disaster community to incorporate geographic approaches. Knowing where hazard zones are located and understanding the relationship to the distribution of people (and subgroups) is fundamental to developing mitigation strategies or creating preparedness plans. Real-time geographic data can improve the allocation of resources for response. Of course, geographic approaches are much more complex than this and extend beyond only the use of GIS, remote sensing, and GPS, but these technologies model geographic aspects of disaster risk and human adaptation to hazards.

Rather than focusing entirely on the technical aspects of these tools, this chapter concentrates on these technologies as part of a spatial (geographic) decision support system for disaster management (SDSS). This encompasses some technical aspects in addition to organizational issues. Key to taking this perspective is that a decision support system is just that; it meets the needs of the practitioner while at the same time integrating current physical and social science approaches. Thus, the SDSS must be firmly based in current research as well as meeting the needs of decision makers who utilized the systems. The first part of the chapter discusses SDSSs, followed by examples of current application in disaster management, and in conclusion presents some directions for future research.

DISASTER SPATIAL DECISION SUPPORT SYSTEMS

Disaster management requires complex coordination between resources, equipment, skills, and human resources from a wide variety of agencies.This multifaceted process thus necessitates strong decision support systems to foster cooperation and assist disaster loss reduction (Assilzadeh & Mansor, 2004; Pourvakhshouri & Mansor, 2003). Interoperability of emergency services is especially necessary during response and relief phases and is supported by an SDSS (Zlatanova, van Oosterom & Verbree 2004). Importantly, an SDSS also plays a vital role in mitigation and planning. Advanced decision support systems must perform sophisticated tasks at the right place and in the right moment, involving problem definition, identification of alternatives, and analyses and evaluation of alternatives followed by selection of the best alternative (DeSilva, 2001). GIS alone cannot fulfill this role, but is an integral piece in a robust system that supports decision makers, whether these are disaster managers, policymakers, first responders, or the public.

Spatial Decision Support Systems

GIS is an interface for handling, collecting, sharing, recording, analyzing, updating, organizing, and integrating spatial (geographic) data, derived from maps, remote sensing, or GPS. In the most basic sense, GIS allows for the mapping of all hazard-related data, transforming it into visual information. Within a GIS, a database is directly connected to the graphical mapped information and so data can be manipulated and mapped, or a user can interact with the map to retrieve data. A GIS also incorporates analytical functions. Thus, GIS are fundamentally used to explore spatial relationships. For instance, by viewing floodplains along with hospitals and roads, a disaster manager could select all of the hospitals in the floodplain or delineate which roads accessing a hospital might flood. Or, the GIS could be used to evaluate which schools are near fault zones or in floodplains for the purpose of prioritizing mitigation strategies or for evacuation planning. In addition to simply compiling inventories of hazard risk, the built environment, infrastructure, and vulnerable populations, GIS can relate these to one another.

The challenge is that GIS technology alone cannot always provide problem-specific model support (e.g., vehicle routing or flood models frequently exist independent of a GIS). Standard GIS software are usually general purpose systems and do not focus on specific problem areas without integrating with other types of software packages. Further, a GIS can only partly model, test, and compare among alternatives to evaluate a specific problem (Pourvakhshouri &

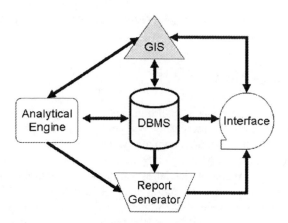

FIGURE 5.1. SDSS diagram.

Mansor, 2003). Consequently, the real aim is a spatial decision support system (SDSS) with GIS integrated into a broader framework that incorporates specialized analytical modeling capabilities, database management systems, graphical display capabilities, tabular reporting capabilities, and decision maker's expert knowledge (see Fig. 5.1). Although design can vary slightly, a SDSS includes analytical tools (to enable data investigation) decision models (to perform scenario investigations), a geographic/spatial database, and a user interface, as well as expert knowledge (Densham, 1991; Fabbri, 1998; Zerger & Smith, 2003). They support both structured and ill-structured problem solving and must be flexible and adaptable for dealing with evolving and dynamic scenarios in disaster management (DeSilva, 2001). Most importantly, the success of an SDSS is most related to how well it supports the needs of the decision maker, not how advanced the technology is (Keenan, 1998; Muller, 1993).

Incorporation of Basic Geographic Concepts

Geographic data have many unique characteristics, such as scale, resolution, and projection. For instance, the scale at which data are collected directly impacts the level of detail included, which in turn affects the types of questions that may be answered or the analytical approach required. Answering a question concerning whether or not a property is in a floodplain illustrates this point. Ideally, one would want very detailed tax maps along with engineering maps of the floodplain to make a determination. Using a statewide roadmap with streams and rivers (smaller scale maps) would not be an adequate option. Scale is but one geographic data consideration. Some others include how often and how recently the data were collected and by whom, the type of sensor for remotely sensed data, the original source, format, and procedures for collecting and processing. Not surprisingly, all of this also translates into data visualization and analysis considerations.

The creation of maps requires special attention because of the way in which people under-stand and interpret maps. Thus, not only do the data impact the output, but people's perceptions and map reading skills should also be considered when creating a map. For example, red is generally interpreted as "danger" and so using green to depict wildfire-prone areas would not be particularly effective. Cartographic (map-making) principles should always be incorporated into the design and implementation of any SDSS interface and visualization capabilities.

In essence, handling and manipulation of geographic data requires expertise beyond a typical understanding of nonspatial data issues. As spatial data, maps, and models become embedded into a broader disaster SDSS, geographic concepts must be addressed and incorporated into the system as well.

Elements of a Disaster SDSS

The level of coordination and scenario-building aspects necessary for a disaster SDSS may seem somewhat futuristic, but the increasing availability of geographic technologies make it more possible than ever to consider an integrated system that supports disaster management to reduce loss (Tung & Siva, 2001). Although they can be described with varying categorization, any disaster SDSS would consist of several essential pieces, including data collection, data management, and the data processing and application development. All of these elements support the incorporation of geographic approaches into the disaster management process.

Data collection comprises a multitude of activities utilizing a variety of sources. Data may be from primary sources (compiled directly from the field using PDA devices, GPS, and cell phones, or even generated from people's decisions or perceptions) or from remote sensing (satellite imagery, aerial photography, or other detection and monitoring devices). Secondary sources are also essential; these should be already available and interoperable with data sharing agreements in place between various groups who hold the data. Ideally, data should be current and timely.

The data management component of the SDSS not only integrates all of the data from various sources, but also makes these data available to appropriate people at different times and places (fixed or mobile). It must be expandable and flexible in order to integrate new sensors, accommodate new actors, and integrate new software applications in the future. Quality control of the data occurs here, as do data security and management of user access.

Analytic tools and models are incorporated into the data processing and application development segment to process data into useful information that can be utilized for decision making. Efficient and reliable hazard forecasting and monitoring should occur here, leading to monitoring/detecting, early warning, and mitigation. Utilizing the full range of tools, vulnerability analyses, risk assessments, and scenario descriptions (varying inputs based on priorities from stakeholders) could all be produced. Data must be converted to information that is meaningful and useful to decision makers and those involved in the disaster management process.

An entirely functional disaster SDSS for multiple hazards supporting decision making in all phases of disaster management is not fully realized, but perhaps is not that far in the future. Certainly, the many ways that geographic technologies are already supporting disaster management illustrate the potential that exists for effective use.

EXAMPLES OF GIS APPLICATIONS TO DISASTER MANAGEMENT

Examples of the use of GIS in disaster management range from relative simple local scale hazard mapping to interactive SDSS. While not necessarily fully incorporated into a disaster SDSS, these applications illustrate the potential for use within a disaster SDSS. Geographic technologies can be utilized for damage assessment, thematic hazard mapping, establishing early warning systems, risk prediction and situational analyses, and prioritization of mitigation alternatives. Table 5.1 summarizes some ways in which GIS has already supported various phases of the disaster management cycle. Many of these activities actually support efforts

TABLE 5.1. Examples of GIS Supporting Disaster Management

Mitigation	Evaluation of mitigation alternatives	Çabuk, A., 2001 (land-use mitigation)
	Prioritization of efforts	Wood & Good, 2004 (community hazard planning)
Preparedness	Environmental monitoring	Lanza & Siccardi, 1995 (evacuation)
	Event mapping (detecting, monitoring, and modeling virtually all different types of individual hazards)	Lindell et al., 1985 (evacuation)
		De Silva et al., 1993 (evacuation)
	Risk assessment	Newsom & Mitrani, 1993 (evacuation)
	Risk communication (public and emergency workers)	De Silva, 2001 (evacuation)
	Evacuation planning	Cova, 1997 (evacuation)
	Identification of vulnerable populations	Cutter et al., 2000 (multihazard and vulnerability assessment)
		Cavallin & Floris, 1995 (groundwater pollution)
		Zerger & Smith, 2003 (flood)
		Lanza & Siccardi, 1995 (flood)
		Hickey & Jankowski, 1997 (erosion modeling)
		Ambrosia et al., 1998 (wildfire detection)
		McKean et al., 1991 (landslide assessment)
Response	Damage assessment	Kohiyama et al., 2004 (early damage estimation)
	Response and relief coordination	Pourvakhshouri & Mansor, 2003 (oil spill)
	Coordination of relief efforts	
	Aid allocation	Kaiser et al., 2003 (humanitarian relief)
	Monitoring of lifeline status	
	Early warning	
Recovery	Resource allocation	Turker & San, 2003 (damage estimation)
	Coordination and monitoring of cleanup	

in multiple stages. For example, risk assessment and hazard mapping are one of the first critical pieces to creating a system in which mitigation alternatives can be assessed. Or, event detection and monitoring are the precursors to an early warning system. Realizing this and the fact that several of the studies could also fit into several of the disaster phases, the categorization presented in Table 5.1 simply provides an overview of GIS applications in disaster management. Most of the studies and examples included go beyond just simple hazard mapping and add some element to the concept of a disaster SDSS.

Evacuation Planning

Evacuation planning highlights the use of an SDSS for a specific purpose within disaster management. So, although this is a relatively specific use, rather than a broader disaster management system, the potential and process are clearly demonstrated. These systems link transportation models with GIS and decision systems in a manner that offers a more improved output than any of the systems could produce individually, a key contribution of a disaster SDSS.

Several early examples were applied to evacuation planning for nuclear power plants. Lindell et al. (1985) created a system that calculated the radius of the area for the evacuation, the delay time between warning and start of evacuation, and the speed of evacuation. In addition,

spatial data along with educational materials (USGS, 2005d, 2005e, 2005f). Many of these are global, not just for the United States. In Europe, the European Mediterranean Disaster Information Network (EU-MEDIN) is an initiative to establish a portal for hazards data in order to foster coordinated access to data before, during, and after a disaster strikes (EU-MEDIN, 2005). An important data repository for understanding hazard impacts at a global scale is the Center for Research on the Epidemiology of Disasters, which maintains an international database on natural and technological disasters by country and region, including deaths, injuries, damages, and impacted people (CRED, 2005).

In addition to the Web data portals and static mapping, there are several examples of actual interactive online mapping projects, giving the user the capability to display and combine data in which he or she is interested. FEMA's Multihazard Mapping Initiative is an interactive Internet mapping service (FEMA, 2005a). Data are incorporated from a variety of sources to drive the system, which displays information selected by the user. NOAA Coastal Services Center also has several Internet mapping projects, including a prototype of the Risk and Vulnerability Assessment Tool for Brevard and Volusia Counties in Florida (NOAA Coastal Services, 2005), illustrating the steps communities can take for risk and vulnerability assessments.

Probably one of the most elaborate examples in terms of being developed explicitly for supporting disaster management decision making, the Pacific Disaster Center (PDC) provides disaster management information integration and sharing throughout the Asia Pacific Region. The PDC has developed an integrated decision support system for disaster management and humanitarian assistance. The system supplies access to many disaster-related databases, including emergency services, public facilities, utilities, transportation communications, political boundaries, demographics, hazard, image data, elevation, hydrograph, climate, weather, landforms, and land use. Importantly, the user chooses what and how to display the data (PDC, 2005). Another effort in the Asian region, the Asian Disaster Reduction Center (2005) has worked to establish an Internet mapping site to disseminate base data along with hazard information to the 22 member countries.

At the international level, mapping has increasingly become important at the United Nations (UN). The UN's Project of Risk Evaluation, Vulnerability, Information, and Early Warning is an online, interactive mapping project that gives users the capability to decide what to display, giving them access to tremendous amounts of global information on hazards and vulnerability (UNEP, 2005). The Humanitarian Early Warning Service (IASC, 2005) is a more extensive illustration of integrating data from a variety of sources to support UN and non-UN humanitarian programs in coordinating humanitarian assistance efforts.

All of these Internet-based projects illustrate the importance of integrating new and emerging information technologies, observation systems, and communications for disaster management. The further development of tools such as these will provide new and enhanced capabilities for decision makers about disaster management.

Vulnerability Mapping

Vulnerability science is a relatively recent research area needing much attention with few explicit guidelines for how a comprehensive, multihazard vulnerability assessment should be conducted at the local level (Cutter, 2003a). Cutter's Vulnerability of Place Model (1996) and Tobin and Montz's Hazard Dimensions Model (1997) are two models that offer a framework for geographic analysis, both utilizing GIS. Geographic approaches bring many unique insights to vulnerability assessment, including extensive knowledge about scale, spatial analysis, cognition of geographic information, and the systematic study of physical and human processes. Cutter, Mitchell, and Scott (2000) combined physical and social risk variables in Georgetown County, South Carolina, illustrating one approach for incorporating all-hazards risk along with social variables into a single depiction.

In an effort to integrate social data with hazard risk modeling, FEMA's HazUS/MH (Hazards U.S. Multihazards) estimates potential losses from earthquakes, floods, and hurricane winds and approximates loss to the built environment, populations, and critical infrastructure from these models (FEMA, 2005b). National datasets and models for the hazard events are included. However, it is not truly multihazard in the sense that the models cannot be run in a single session. Further, with the emphasis on loss estimation, the role of social vulnerability is not prominent. In fact, many aspects of social vulnerability are not easily incorporated onto a map (Morrow, 1999), but still GISs also offer many opportunities that should be further investigated and developed.

Technological Hazards and Security

The potential for applying a disaster SDSS to technological hazards and security is immense. In fact, natural and technological hazards are frequently so closely tied that an SDSS incorporating both would be necessary for disaster management. Chemical releases are commonly modeled for assessing the impacts on health. In the case of chemical accidents, the Computer-Aided Management of Emergency Operations (CAMEO) was developed by the U.S. Environmental Protection Agency (USEPA) and NOAA to assist emergency managers and first responders with necessary information about the dispersion of the chemical along with response recommendations (USEPA, 2005). Results are directly linked to mapping capabilities.

Two examples of SDSS applied to shipping illustrate their use for emergency response and for security planning. Pourvakhshouri and Mansor (2003) implemented a multicriteria SDSS for oil spill incidents. The aim was to determine priorities in emergency response conditions through detecting coastal area sensitivity and advising decision makers so they could choose the most reasonable method to control spills and consider cleanup alternatives. Tzannatos (2003) combined threat assessment, vulnerability assessment, and consequence assessment in a decision support system environment to support the development and implementation of shipboard and seaport security plans with maximum flexibility. The challenge for shipping is the time and place variability of threats.

The use of GIS after September 11, 2001 in New York City highlights some of the ways in which spatial technologies support decision making in the aftermath of a terrorist event (Thomas, Cutter, Hodgson, Gutekunst, & Jones, 2003). As with most natural and technological events, a multitude of maps and analyses were produced and developed to support the response efforts. The application of these technologies for the prevention of terrorism and potential for response to any future event is further explored by Cutter, Richardson, & Wilbanks (2003). In most respects, a fully functional disaster SDSS will perform equally well for natural and unintentional human-induced hazard events, as well intentional terrorist events in the response phase. One of the key differences for this particular application is surveillance activities employed to prevent a terrorist event. Instead of monitoring hazard events, tracking and monitoring people become the focus for security purposes.

TRENDS AND FUTURE NEEDS

The previous section emphasized examples of GIS use within the context of a disaster SDSS. Current work often centers on one particular hazard, rather than providing a truly multihazard approach. Further, examples are frequently aimed only at either response or mitigation, not both. Ideally, a disaster SDSS should encompass all of the elements of disaster management and incorporate all hazards. The technological and data needs of such a system are immense and the needed physical and social models vast. The ideal system has not yet been realized as a practical system. This section focuses on needs and considerations for the development of such a disaster SDSS, suggesting future directions for research. The first part concentrates on technical issues, while the second speaks to organizational and social concerns, with the last addressing issues of knowledge driving the technology.

Technical Implementation

The technical concerns surrounding the implementation of a disaster SDSS include such issues as spatial data acquisition and integration, interoperability, distributed computing, dynamic representation of physical and human processes, scale, spatial analysis and uncertainty, and system design (Cutter, 2003b; Radke et al., 2000). A disaster SDSS must allow the efficient and effective interchange of data between modules and modeling techniques, while at the same time must be easy to use. Interoperability ensures that data, algorithms, and models can be shared between various GIS systems that are housed in diverse agencies, departments, or organizations contributing to disaster management.

The development of a disaster SDSS requires that most of the functionality is not technically difficult for the end user. Keenan (1998) points out that the decision maker should not have to go through long sequences of commands. In other words, the system itself should be user friendly and should meet informational needs accessing appropriate data and running analytical process in the background (not actually seen by the user), representing physical and human processes in an understandable format. Thus, GIS software must be seamlessly integrated with other software.

Data concerns are mentioned by nearly everyone who writes on this subject and are one of the greatest challenges facing the development of effective and robust disaster SDSSs (NRC, 1999). Because these technologies are by definition data-driven, the lack of documentation about the information, lack of data standardization, lack of up-to-date information during the disaster (victims, rescue teams, damage), and lack of access to existing data and action plans all limit their usefulness. Further, recent studies surveying emergency managers revealed that real-time decision support mostly require *temporal* detail in combination with the mapped information (Zerger & Smith, 2003). For example, the general movement of people and vehicles is necessary for evacuation modeling, but also for understanding what population is at risk at a given time. Data on many vulnerable and special needs population, such as tourists, homeless people, or undocumented workers are not collected or maintained (Cutter, 2003b; Morrow, 1999). These groups remain entirely unrepresented in disaster GIS as a result. Daytime populations (e.g., work or school) and their socioeconomic composition are also not well understood (Thomas et al., 2003). In terms of real-time disaster response, mobile (field) data collection and processing efforts could be important for understanding response efforts and vulnerable populations if they integrate directly to a SDSS (Erharuyi & Fairbairn, 2003). Importantly, disaster management requires both geographic and nongeographic data, all of which must be incorporated into any disaster SDSS. Although efforts are underway, coordination of information and data is necessary to avoid interoperability issues as well as simple information overload with too much available in too many disparate locations.

Disaster managers and others involved in response and mitigation to disasters come mostly from fields that are far from geography or geographic technologies and thus they require technical GIS education and training. Further, they are frequently not aware of spatial analytical capabilities of GIS or the functionality and decision support role of SDSS. The general perception is that GIS provides cartographic capability rather than spatial modeling and analysis capabilities (Zerger & Smith, 2003). In short, not only do technical GIS staff and researchers need a better appreciation of the needs of disaster management, but practitioners and researchers in disaster management also should understand the ways in which these technologies support decision making.

Social and Organizational Needs

Because disaster SDSSs are used by people within a particular context, social and organizational considerations are fundamentally important; there are many concerns beyond strictly technical details. In other words, a disaster SDSS may be developed and run efficiently, but may never be utilized to the fullest capacity without taking social and organizational issues into account. This encompasses implementation and system development issues (coordination between organizations and user needs), as well as access to technologies.

Interoperability requires the cooperation of organizations for the transfer of data and models. Agreements must be in place and a plan for the flow of information and models must exist. An example of this type of data sharing agreement internationally is the International Charter, "Space and Major Disasters," which gives organizations in countries affected by major disasters access to necessary remote sensing data if they are an authorized user. In many instances, these types of agreements are not established before an event occurs. Further, lack of effective communication between different actors will ensure the failure of the disaster management process. Of course, this entails embedding the disaster SDSS into a broader organizational plan for disaster management. A system must also meet the needs of the organization as well as the end user/disaster manager.

There is a need to more completely understand how these geographic technologies are actually being used, both within and between organizations and by individuals (public, disaster managers, and policymakers). Dymon (1993) observed that the spatial data needs of emergency managers are simpler than expected in studying GIS use after Hurricane Andrew. Rather than requiring advanced spatial analysis, simple map products were viewed as essential. The reliance on paper maps rather than more advance digital approaches could be attributed to the early application of the technology, but more recent work has also found similar results. Zerger and Smith (2003) observed that the detail provided was not always used, access was often too slow, and paper maps could be used in the event of a power failure. While GIS is perfect for planning and preparation, people generally prefer to discuss emergency task on paper rather than a computer screen. Whether this emerges from a lack of awareness/training, that the current geographic technology does not meet the needs of disaster managers, or some combination, has not been established.

Clearly, providing adequate GIS/SDSS training to disaster managers and other end users is vital to their successful implementation. Otherwise, the maps and results could even hinder response and decision-making capabilities. Along with training, appropriate tools giving new insights into hazards that are useful to the end user, rather than just creating lovely pictures, must be developed. In designing systems, user need assessments should reveal how technology could support the decision-making process, which is a much more desirable approach than creating a SDSS without input from disaster managers.

If the goal is loss reduction, then individuals (public) as well as experts must have access to disaster decision-making information. Thus, various segments of society should also have access and have input to at least a portion of the developed system. One mechanism for accomplishing this is public participation GIS (PPGIS), which focuses on including all stakeholders, including residents in neighborhoods and local communities, in the GIS process (Elwood & Leitner, 1998). When used in a participatory fashion, database development and interpretation involves an exchange of information, not just communicating risk to a community, but also integrating information about hazards and assets from citizens (Talen, 1999).

In an era of digital geographic data, the very data that are utilized to support improved hazard mitigation and preparedness may, in fact, reveal too much detail about communities and individuals. Many challenges exist to maintaining privacy within this technological environment and the ways in which places are reconceptualized by GIS must be understood (Curry, 1997). The ethical issues surrounding data accessibility and security have not been adequately addressed to ensure geographic technologies actually contribute to reducing loss, while not infringing on individual or community rights.

Technology transfer, cost and data availability, and ethical issues extend to differences in utilization in various parts of the world. Software and hardware may not be as readily available in less developed countries, although there are exciting and interesting examples of GIS use in these settings. Data availability and accessibility may also be more problematic in some places, with data not even being collected or disseminated. Remote sensing and GPS can both offer alternatives to some of the deficiencies in data, but may not always be practical solutions, particularly with regard to challenges of depicting social vulnerability. The disasters themselves are frequently different in developing countries, such as famine or HIV/AIDS epidemics in Africa. As with other types of hazards, the use of GIS as a tool for managing these types humanitarian emergencies is increasing (Kaiser, Spiegel, Henderson, & Gerber, 2003). Importantly, disease outbreaks are not unique to developing nations and so special consideration should be given to how surveillance systems link with disaster SDSSs to better coordinate emergency response efforts.

SDSS Supporting Disaster Management Research and Practice

Beyond the technical, organizational, and social issues surrounding the creation of a disaster SDSS, the subject-based knowledge necessary for its creation is immense. The models and algorithms incorporated should be grounded in theory, as well as meeting the requirements of the user. This is a huge challenge and requires an interdisciplinary disaster management approach, bringing together the physical and social sciences, engineering, along with geographic information science. Both research in the theory and the development of robust methods is necessary.

A fully functional disaster SDSS should incorporate multihazard assessment combined with vulnerability science. Many options exist for retrieving data and maps for individual hazards and several of the Internet mapping sites described in the previous section even allow the display of multiple hazards and sometimes select socioeconomic data, but do not frequently combine them in meaningful ways. There is a need to expand, refine, and test vulnerability models, explicitly focusing on place and space, and GIS is a fundamental tool for accomplishing this (Radke et al., 2000). Appropriate methods for assessing vulnerability as an ill-structured problem should be explored. Rashed and Weeks (2003) illustrate one method for accomplishing this for urban vulnerability analysis using fuzzy logic and spatial multicriteria analysis, which are methodological approaches that could provide mechanisms for more advanced vulnerability models. Further, qualitative information along with quantitative data must be incorporated into the disaster SDSS, a methodological challenge requiring attention. Clearly, deriving social and physical indicators of risk and social vulnerability and developing models for combining the two will require working across disciplines and integrating an expanded set of methods with GIS into a disaster SDSS.

   Theory development and research are needed in the cognition of geographic information for disaster management and risk communication. So, knowing how people process and understand spatial data aids in the creation of appropriate and effective maps and other corresponding output from the SDSS. Related to this is developing theory-based mechanisms for conveying uncertainty that exists in all physical and social models as well as in the data itself. If disaster management will be successful, changing behavior and getting people to respond is cornerstone for reducing loss. But, in the face of information that is not 100% correct, disaster managers still must make costly decisions about evacuation or prioritizing mitigation measures. Individuals and communities are faced with the same dilemma. Through better risk communication and display mechanisms, all involved have the opportunity to improve decisions.

CONCLUSION

Technological solutions for the sake of technology are not particularly useful; it is cutting-edge approaches that support disaster decision making that will ultimately reduce loss. This will require continued research in many areas. The geographic information science and disaster research communities will need to explore the integration of improved modeling techniques with GIS for multihazard and vulnerability assessments. The potential for remote sensing and GPS must be more fully investigated, not only for environmental modeling, but also for assessing social vulnerability. Further, issues of spatial cognition and understanding the needs of the end user (whether the disaster manager, policymaker, or public) must be more fully understood, both in support of decision making and risk communication. Social and organizational issues surrounding the use of GIS should also be the focus of extensive research so that the ways in which the technology is applied and utilized are understood in order to develop improved tools. As their utilization increases, critical reviews of the technology should be undertaken, focusing on data privacy and confidentiality considerations. The design of an effective SDSS cannot occur without a thorough comprehension of all of these issues.

   Geographic technologies as part of disaster SDSS have great potential as a decision-support tool. If designed with proper considerations, the system should reduce information overload and assist all stakeholders in disaster management. Perhaps a disaster SDSS should not be entirely a single system, but should include systems that "talk" to one another. Ideally, these systems can link disaster management with environmental planning, development, and sustainable development to reduce duplication of efforts and integrate disaster management into these broader areas. Technology cannot take the place of people who make decisions about disaster management, but if designed and used properly, it can provide an extremely valuable tool.

ACKNOWLEDGMENT

The authors thank Rafael Moreno, Amanda Gierow, and the two anonymous readers who all made extremely valuable comments.

CHAPTER 6

Morbidity and Mortality Associated with Disasters[1]

LINDA B. BOURQUE, JUDITH M. SIEGEL, MEGUMI KANO, AND MICHELE M. WOOD

Disasters disrupt the natural, built, and social environments, affecting communities and the people within them. Disasters can be triggered by climatic, geophysical, technological, or human-initiated events, or a combination of these. Their impact on the health of a community can be immediate or delayed, and changes in health status may be attributable to the original event or result from events subsequent to the disaster. Deaths, injuries, and other health outcomes of a disaster are usually caused by the destruction of the built infrastructure. In the absence of people living in built communities, disasters do not occur.

The frequency and severity of disasters triggered by natural hazards have increased over the last 15 years, part of which is attributable to cyclic changes in climate patterns. Of even greater relevance, however, is the fact that population density in cities and in geophysically vulnerable areas has increased dramatically since 1950, both in developed and developing countries. The majority of the world's largest cities (17 of 20) are in developing countries, 80% of the world's population will be concentrated in developing countries by 2025, and half of the large cities in the developing world are vulnerable to natural disasters such as floods, severe storms, and earthquakes (Noji, 2005). Disaster-related health problems in developing countries are exacerbated by lower immunization rates and poor nutritional status relative to those in the United States and other developed countries, and greater vulnerability of the facilities that provide water and handle sewage.

Health effects vary across disaster types. For example, death by drowning rarely occurs during earthquakes, but is a major cause of death during hurricanes and floods. The extent to which infectious diseases occur is determined by the health of the affected community before the disaster, and the ability of the infrastructure to recover sufficiently to prevent, or at least control, the spread of infectious diseases. In general, increases in infectious disease rates following disasters are more common in developing than in developed countries.

---

[1] The authors thank Elizabeth Tornquist for her rapid editorial assistance. While Linda Bourque took the lead on this chapter, the four authors were equal partners in assembling the information and writing the manuscript.

It has often been stated that "vulnerable" populations, such as women, children, the elderly, nondocumented immigrants, underrepresented groups, and the poor, are differentially and negatively affected by disasters (e.g., Bolin, 1976; Bolin & Bolton, 1986; Bolin & Stanford, 1991; Drabek & Key, 1984; Kaniasty & Norris, 1994; Kilijanek & Drabek, 1979; Tierney, Lindell, & Perry, 2001). Research on physical morbidity and mortality associated with natural hazards and terrorist events generally does not support that perception, at least in the United States. In contrast, the literature on mental health morbidity shows that vulnerable persons are particularly prone to post-disaster stress, a topic addressed at the end of this chapter.

Age is the only characteristic that has been consistently reported to have a weak association with disaster-related morbidity and mortality. Following the Northridge earthquake, studies of hospital admissions and emergency room logs found that older persons were more likely to be hospitalized because of injuries suffered (Peek-Asa et al., 1998; Seligson & Shoaf, 2003) and were somewhat more likely to present at emergency rooms (Mahue-Giangreco, Mack, Seligson, & Bourque, 2001), but when residents were asked about injuries in community-based samples following three California earthquakes, women and younger persons were more likely to report being injured (Shoaf, Nguyen, Sareen, & Bourque, 1998). The elderly were also more likely to be killed in the Hanshin-Awaji earthquake in Kobe, Japan, but here the higher death rates for elderly are confounded by the fact that the elderly tended to sleep on the first floor of "bunka jutaku," two-story wooden houses with heavy tiled roofs and thin walls that were built after World War II (Kunii, Akagi, & Kita, 1995).

It is somewhat easier to conclude that *recovery* from disasters favors those with knowledge and money. In a series of analyses conducted at UCLA, we have demonstrated that persons with higher education and income are more likely to engage in preparedness and hazard mitigation activities before earthquakes, are more likely to take first aid courses, and know more about where to obtain assistance after disasters. Conversely, immigrants and persons who are linguistically isolated are less likely to have invested in preparedness and hazard mitigation, or to know where to go for assistance (e.g., Goltz, 2005; Kano, Siegel, & Bourque, 2005; Nguyen, Shen, Ershoff, Afifi, & Bourque, in press; Nguyen, Shoaf, Rottman, & Bourque, 1997; Russell, Goltz, & Bourque, 1995). Interestingly, however, during the Northridge earthquake, newer homes inhabited by middle-class whites were more likely to be damaged than older homes that were inhabited by groups more often considered vulnerable (Comerio, 1995; Shoaf & Bourque, 1999), but African-American residents more often *perceived* themselves to be victims of the earthquake than did other groups with more property damage.

The inability to demonstrate a relationship between traditional indicators of vulnerability and morbidity and mortality does not automatically mean that it does not exist. Rather it may reflect the generally weak methodology of most studies. Very few studies allow prevalence estimates and rates to be calculated for the morbidity and mortality associated with disasters (Bourque, Shoaf, & Nguyen, 1997; Dominici, Levy, & Louis, 2005; Ibrahim, 2005). Most studies describe those cases in a coroner or medical examiner's office, or at a hospital or emergency room, with no effort to describe the denominator population from which the cases are drawn. A study focused only on the dead, injured, and sick who present at a particular location provides no insight into how deaths and injuries are distributed across the population at risk, and whether certain groups are more vulnerable to death and injury. Increased use of cluster samples in rapid needs assessments after floods and hurricanes provides some ability to generalize to a larger population. Unfortunately, rapid assessment techniques do not work well following earthquakes where structural damage is less predictably distributed (Noji, 2005).

Other useful, but underutilized, methodologies include case-control designs, geographic information systems (GIS), comparative cohorts, and probability proportionate to size (PPS) surveys. All have the potential to provide information about whether morbidity and mortality are differentially distributed across populations. A case control design considering persons who died or were hospitalized as a result of the Northridge earthquake and sets of age-matched and geographically matched controls selected from a post-quake survey of Los Angeles County residents revealed that persons at elevated risk of death or hospitalization were females, elderly, close to the epicenter, in areas of high peak ground acceleration or high Modified Mercalli Intensity, or in buildings that were damaged or constructed after 1970 (Peek-Asa, Ramirez, Seligson, & Shoaf, 2003). Comparative cohorts were used by Semenza, McCullough, Flanders, McGeehin, and Lumpkin (1999) to examine excess hospital admissions during the July 1995 Chicago heat wave, and by Leor, Poole, and Kloner (1996) and Kloner, R. A., Leor, J. U., Poole, W. K., and Perritt, R. (1997) to examine deaths on the day of the Northridge earthquake. GIS could, for example, be used to "map" the addresses where the injured and dead lived or were at the time of impact (Peek-Asa, Ramirez, Shoaf, Seligson, & Kraus, 2000). This information could then be compared with census data about the populations who live in those areas, similar to what Klinenberg (2001) did after the 1995 Chicago heat wave. But these methodologies require substantial resources, which are not readily available to researchers. Similarly, ongoing surveillance systems in hospitals and emergency rooms would increase our ability to determine whether the number and pattern of presenting cases change in the aftermath of a disaster. Surveillance has long been advocated by the public health community, but has yet to be instituted widely in the United States.

Further complicating research is the lack of agreement on what constitutes a disaster-related death, injury, or disease. Twenty years ago, the Centers for Disease Control and Prevention (CDC) took the lead in attempting to develop a standardized definition of disaster-related deaths and injuries; more recently, Seligson, Shoaf, and colleagues have attempted to develop standardized procedures for identifying earthquake-related deaths and injuries (Seligson & Shoaf, 2003). In spite of these attempts, the majority of researchers continue to develop their own definitions of which injuries and deaths are counted, often with little regard for or even knowledge of past research and discussions. Disaster-related mortality is more accurately described than are injuries, where official numbers are often guesses compiled by a public health employee who contacts the Red Cross and hospitals within an affected area for estimates of the injured and sick seen in emergency rooms. The majority of injured do not utilize emergency rooms and the person representing the hospital usually does not know which patients are injured or sick because of the index disaster and which are not. Thus, the numbers reported simultaneously exaggerate and minimize actual counts. Careful review of emergency logs and admissions records is necessary to determine whether a condition is related to the event and, even with careful review, not all cases can be resolved.

The health effects of disasters can be categorized in many ways, but for purposes of this chapter we adopt the typology defined by Combs, Quenemoen, Parrish, and Davis (1999) and used by the CDC: "... disaster-attributed deaths [are] those caused by either the direct or indirect exposure to the disaster. Directly related deaths are those caused by the physical forces of the disaster. Indirectly related deaths are those caused by unsafe or unhealthy conditions that occur because of the anticipation, or actual occurrence, of the disaster" (p. 1125).

We concentrate on how natural hazards worldwide and terrorist events that occurred in the United States have affected the health of populations. These events are neither more important nor more lethal than events not described, but they are the centerpiece of this chapter because a greater quantity of methodologically rigorous research has focused on these disasters. This work provides insights into the types of morbidity and mortality that would be expected to occur when natural hazards and terrorism result in a "disastrous event." As highlighted in this chapter, definitions of what constitutes a death or injury *caused* by a disaster vary within a type of disaster, as well as across disasters. The CDC has attempted to develop a system that differentiates the time (relative to the disaster) when the death or injury occurs, and whether the event is directly or indirectly related to the disaster, but the protocol is difficult to apply. The most accurate estimates of morbidity and mortality are probably those reported in studies conducted after the Northridge earthquake in California (1994) and the Murrah Federal Building in Oklahoma (1995). Even there, as discussed in the section on earthquakes, the range of reported morbidity and mortality is wide. Estimates from events outside the United States, especially in areas that lack mechanisms for centralized data gathering, are expected to be even lower in accuracy. This chapter concludes with a note about the mental health effects of disasters.

HURRICANES

According to current estimates, hurricanes caused about 75,000 deaths during the 20th century (Nicholls, Mimura, & Topping, 1995; Rappaport & Fernandez-Partagas, 1997; Shultz, Russell, & Espinel, 2005). Most deaths occurred in developing nations, with 42% in Bangladesh and 27% in India.

Prior to the development of effective warning, evacuation, and shelter systems, most deaths were caused by drowning in storm surges (Shultz et al., 2005). Japan and the United States, two developed countries at high risk of hurricanes, cyclones, and typhoons, have experienced no storms that resulted in more than 1,000 deaths since 1959, while 50 high-fatality storms (with more than 1,000 deaths) occurred in developing nations of the Asia-Pacific region and 16 in the Caribbean and Central American area. At the time of this writing, the full consequences of Hurricane Katrina (November, 2005) are unknown.

Data available on deaths and injuries from Hurricanes Elena (1985), Gloria (1985), Hugo (1989), Andrew (1992), Marilyn (1995), Opal (1995), Georges (1998), Floyd (1999), and Isabel (2003) provide information about how and when deaths and injuries occur (Centers for Disease Control and Prevention [CDC], 1986b, 1989b, 1989d, 1989e, 1992a, 1992b, 1992c, 1993a, 1993c, 1996a, 1996c, 1998b, 1999, 2004d, 2005). A total of 208 deaths were attributed to these hurricanes. Of the 103 for which CDC assigned a time of death, 9 occurred before, 57 during, and 37 after the hurricane. Of the 142 individuals for whom a cause of death was clearly indicated, 62 drowned with 26 in motor vehicles and 20 in or when beaching boats. Others died when hit by falling trees, in fires, from carbon monoxide poisoning, by being crushed or asphyxiated in collapsing structures, by electrocution, by blunt or penetrating trauma, while using a chain saw, by falling in the absence of electricity, in motor vehicle crashes, and in cardiovascular events. Some information is available on injuries that occurred during these hurricanes. Although the numbers of pre- ($N = 198$) and post-hurricane ($N = 184$) injuries from Hurricane Opal were about equal, most of the injuries from Hurricane Andrew ($N = 321$) took place after the hurricane, with only 15 before and 70 during the hurricane. In all hurricanes, the majority of injuries, regardless of when they occur, are cuts, lacerations, sprains, and strains and fractures, generally in the upper or lower extremities. Both corneal abrasions and insect bites and stings have been found elevated after hurricanes. As many as 75% of the injured are male, a substantial number of whom had been injured while using chain saws during cleanup activities.

The 2004 hurricane season was one of the most destructive to the state of Florida in recent history, and hurricanes in 2005 exceeded those in 2004. Four hurricanes hit Florida, with Hurricane Charley resulting in 35 deaths, Hurricane Frances in 40, Hurricane Ivan in 29, and Hurricane Jeanne in 19 (Dahlburg, 2005). In Hurricane Charley, 17 of the 35 deaths, 10 on the day of impact, were due to trauma caused by falling trees, flying debris, and destroyed physical structures. Only one death was caused by drowning. Other causes of death, all after impact, included carbon monoxide poisoning, electrocution, suicide, exacerbation of a medical condition, and lack of necessary respiratory equipment (CDC, 2004c).

Surveys after the hurricanes found that the most prevalent risk factor for indirect morbidity and mortality was improper use of portable gas-powered generators. "A total of 167 persons had nonfatal CO poisoning diagnosed during the study period, representing a total of 51 exposure incidents. The number of cases and incidents peaked within three days after landfall of each hurricane" (CDC, 2005, p. 699). Environmental concerns considered most important by respondents included water quality (50.9%), sewage disposal (13.2%), and food protection (11.8%). Only 51.3% of respondents reported having an evacuation plan before the hurricanes.

TORNADOES

Although tornadoes occur in other parts of the world, information about morbidity and mortality associated with tornadoes comes exclusively from North America, primarily the United States. Reports generally provide information on Fujita scores or wind speed.[2] Data on deaths and injuries are available for the following tornadoes: Topeka, 1966; Omaha, 1975; Wichita Falls, Texas, F4, 1979; the Carolinas, 1984; Pennsylvania, 1985; Southern Ontario, 1985; Saragosa, Texas, F4, 1987; Illinois, F5, 1990; Kansas, F5, 1991; Alabama, F4, 1994; Arkansas, F4, 1997; Texas, three tornadoes at F3, F4 and F5, 1997; and Oklahoma, F5, 1999 (Bell, Kara, & Batterson, 1978; Carter, Millson, & Allen, 1989; CDC, 1984c, 1986c, 1988, 1991, 1992d, 1994c, 1997b, 1997c; Daley et al., 2005; Erickson, Drabek, Key, & Crowe, 1976; Glass et al., 1980; Pereau, 1991). Four hundred and sixty-one deaths and 5,882 injuries were attributed to these tornadoes.

Deaths were overwhelmingly instantaneous, occurring at the time of tornado impact, and resulting from head, chest, and body traumas: 89% (43/48) in Wichita Falls, 100% (12/12) in Ontario, 82% (23/28) in Illinois, 84.5% (22/26) in Arkansas, and 89.7% (26/29) in Texas in 1997. Victims died as a result of becoming airborne and being slammed into structures and objects, or from being crushed by structures. Some reports attributed deaths to brief, nonexistent, or insufficient warnings.

Although the majority of deaths occurred in buildings, persons in mobile homes, motor vehicles, and outdoors were at high risk of death. In Wichita Falls in 1979, 60% (26/43) of the deaths from multiple traumas occurred in motor vehicles, and 77% (20/26) had entered their vehicles expressly to outrun the tornado. Studies of Oklahoma victims, however, found that risk of death in motor vehicles was not elevated but that persons in mobile homes and persons outdoors were at high risk (Daley et al., 2005). The authors attributed this difference in findings to improved warnings about the expected path of tornadoes, which led residents to evacuate the predicted impact areas.

The most common injuries from tornadoes are contusions, lacerations, abrasions, strains/sprains/muscle spasms, fractures, penetrating wounds, and closed head injuries (CDC, 1984c, 1997b). What differentiates those hospitalized from those treated and released is the

---

[2] Tornadoes are graded on the Fujita Scale, which ranges from F-0 to F-12. Anything above F-5, or 319 mph, rarely occurs (Fujita, 1987).

a population-based sample of households, found that 8.1% of households reported an injury to at least one member of the household. Ten percent of those injured, or 0.81% of the total sample, sought treatment from some source, with a third of them (0.27% of the total sample) seeking treatment from a hospital. Thus, extrapolating to Los Angeles County from these studies, the death rate was 0.38/100,000 population; the hospitalization rate was 1.5/100,000 population; there were approximately 240,000 minor injuries, of which 6.6% sought out-of-hospital treatment; and 3.3% went to emergency departments (Seligson & Shoaf, 2003). These numbers are quite different from those that continue to appear on official Web sites.

Earthquakes in other areas of the world have resulted in many more casualties and other devastating health effects. The 2001 Gujarat, India earthquake resulted in 20,000 or more deaths, and the 2003 Bam, Iran earthquake resulted in 30,000 or more deaths (Earthquake Engineering Research Institute, 2005a). As in the United States, the primary cause of death and serious injury was structural collapse (De Brucycker, Greco, & Lechat, 1985; Glass et al., 1977; Noji et al., 1990), which occurs more often in areas with weak or nonexistent building codes (Ramirez & Peek-Asa, 2005).

VOLCANOES

Three active volcanoes have erupted in the United States in the last 25 years—Mount Saint Helens in Washington in 1980, Mauna Loa in Hawaii in 1984, and Kilauea, which has been continuously active in Hawaii since 1982. Thirty-one bodies were recovered from the Mt. St. Helens eruption and 32 persons were missing and presumed dead. Deaths were from asphyxiation by dense ash exposure (19/31), burns (7/31), falls (1/31), flying rocks (1/31), and falling trees (3/31) (Merchant et al., 1982). Hospital visits and admissions for respiratory illnesses, especially asthma, increased following the eruption. Repeated exposure to volcanic ash increases risk of pneumoconiosis, especially if particles are inhaled (CDC, 1986a), putting persons involved in post-disaster cleanup and those who work outdoors at elevated risk. The presence of free silicon increases future lung damage, but results of a longitudinal study of loggers exposed to Mt. St. Helens indicated that risks of chronic bronchitis or pneumoconiosis were negligible.

More insidious is the air pollution caused by sulfur dioxide gas when it combines with other gases emitted by volcanoes and interacts chemically in the atmosphere with oxygen, moisture, dust, and sunlight to create vog. This has been a constant problem since 1986 on the island of Hawaii, where the Kilauea volcano produces a nearly constant outflow of lava and gas. Vog, in turn, produces acid rain which damages crops and is thought to increase health problems, particularly asthma among children (Elias, Sutton, Stokes, & Casadevall, 1998; Sutton, Elias, Hendley, & Stauffer, 2000; United States Geological Survey, 2001).

TSUNAMIS

The tsunami in Papua, New Guinea, and the tsunami caused by the Sumatra-Andaman Islands earthquake are the first for which attempts were made to ascertain population-based rates of deaths and injuries. Deaths resulting from fifteen tsunamis occurring since 1946 have been estimated at 291,058,[3] with the vast majority (283,100) caused by the December 26, 2004,

---

[3] Number of dead were: 173, Hawaii (1946); 61, Hawaii after the Chilean earthquake (1960); 11, Crescent City, CA after the Alaska Earthquake (1964); 920, Mindenaio, Philippines (1976); 1,000, Flores Island, Indonesia (1992); 170,

tsunami associated with the Sumatra-Andaman Islands earthquake, and 4,966 caused by the 1998 Papua, New Guinea, tsunami. In Papua, New Guinea, although no pre-tsunami census data existed for the area, fatality rates were estimated at 18.8% (Dengler & Preuss, n.d.), 23.1% (International Tsunami Survey Team, 1998), and 28.9% (Office for the Coordination of Humanitarian Affairs, 1998). Death rates ranged from 2.3% in Sissano to 49.1% in Warupu.

Injury estimates were reported first for the 1964 tsunami in Crescent City, California, by Lander and colleagues, with 35 injuries, and the 1996 Chimbote, Peru tsunami, with 55, including one serious injury (Humboldt State University, Geology Department, n.d.; Petroff, Bourgeois, & Yeh, 1996). In Papua, New Guinea, 1,000 injuries were reported by the International Tsunami Information Center (2005, March 23), 668 major injuries were reported by the Office for the Coordination of Humanitarian Affairs (OCHA) (Office for the Coordination of Humanitarian Affairs, 1998), and 369 injuries in Warupu were reported by the International Tsunami Survey Team (1998). The most common injuries were fractures, abrasions, deep cuts, and broken limbs (Dengler & Preuss, n.d.). In some cases, delayed care (beyond 12 hours) led to the development of gangrene and amputations.

The tsunami caused by the Sumatra-Andaman Islands earthquake[4] destroyed miles of coastline in 12 countries with devastation, death, and injuries correlated with the number and height of waves, the amount of runup, and the extent of development. Adger, Hughes, Folke, Carpenter, and Rockström (2005) noted that coastline in Sri Lanka that remained covered with indigenous mangrove forests and that had not been degraded by mining of coral reefs fared better than areas that had undergone development. Preliminary data reported by the many affected areas on mortality, morbidity both from physical injury and other disease sequelae, and the impact on the health structure have been considerably more extensive than those from the more contained Papua, New Guinea tsunami. The most comprehensive data are available from Thailand, owing to the well-developed national health care system that was in place before the tsunami. Estimates of dead and missing presumed dead as posted on various Web sites in June 2005 averaged 283,100, with 125,000 reported injured. The latter figure is presumed to be a substantial underestimate, given the unreliability of most injury reports following natural disasters. In Sumatra, Indonesia, reported mortality rates ranged from 13.9% in Meulaboh to 22.2% in Banda Aceh (Doocy, Rofi, Robinson, Burnham, & Shanker, 2005, May); in Sri Lanka, from 4.2% in the Northern Province to 20.0% in the Southern Province (Pomonis, 2005); in Thailand, death rates were 25% for residents and 50% for tourists in Phang Nha, and 3% to 5% in Phuket (Pomonis, 2005; Wilkinson, 2005, April); and in India, 3.3% were dead and 13.7% were missing in the Nicobar Islands (Jain et al., 2006).

HEAT

Deaths directly caused by heat occur from hyperthermia, which is defined as a core body temperature of 105° Fahrenheit or 40.6° centigrade. When bodies are found in a hot, unventilated environment, with unknown core body temperature at the time of death, heat is frequently

---

Nicaragua (1992); 320, Okushiri Island, Japan Sea (1993); 250, East Java, Indonesia (1994); 62, Mindoro Island, Philippines (1994); 11, Kuril Islands, Russia (1994); 1, Alaska (1994); 1, Indonesia (1994); 12, Chimbote, Peru (1996); 4,966, Papua, New Guinea (1998); 283,100, Sumatra-Andaman Islands Earthquake (12/26/04).

[4] Nineteen countries were affected by the tsunami: Indonesia, Sri Lanka, India, Thailand, Somalia, Maldives, Malaysia, Myanmar, Tanzania, Seychelles, Bangladesh, Kenya, Singapore, Madagascar, Mauritius, South Africa, Mozambique, Australia, and Antarctica (Earthquake Engineering Research Institute, 2004).

listed on the death certificate as a contributing cause of death, and the death is considered heat related (CDC, 1994b).

A heat wave is defined by the U.S. National Weather Service as three or more consecutive days of temperatures 90° Fahrenheit (32.2° centigrade) or higher (CDC, 1995a). Between 1979 and 1997, an average of 371 deaths per year in the United States were attributed to "excessive heat exposure," which translates into a mean annual death rate of 1.5 per 1,000,000 persons (CDC, 2000a). Of the 8,015 heat-related deaths in the United States between 1979 and 1999, 48% were due to weather conditions, yielding an average of 182 deaths per year (CDC, 2003a).

The criteria used to determine which deaths are attributable to hot weather and heat-related illness vary by state and among individual medical examiners and coroners. In Dallas, for example, at least one of three criteria must be met for a death to be listed as heat-related: (1) a core body temperature of 105° Fahrenheit (40.6° centigrade) or higher at the time or immediately following death, (2) substantial environmental or circumstantial evidence of heat as a contributory cause of death, or (3) the decedent is found in a decomposed condition without evidence of other causes of death and the decedent was last seen alive during a heat wave (CDC, 1997a). In the absence of consistent definitions for defining a heat-related death, the number of deaths caused by heat may be substantially over- or underreported.

Heat-related deaths are higher for persons older than 60 years of age and children younger than 5. Generally, elderly women are at greater risk of death, in part because they live longer than men, but this trend was reversed in the 1995 Chicago heat wave, in which elderly men died at disproportionate rates (Klinenberg, 2001). African Americans are at greater risk of heat-related death, largely reflecting living conditions associated with lower socioeconomic status and residence in densely populated urban centers without air conditioning. Among adults younger than 65 years of age, men are at greater risk of heat-related death (CDC, 1984a, 1984b, 1989a, 1995b, 1996b, 2000a, 2001).

Semenza et al. (1999) examined the hospital admissions in 47 non-VA hospitals in Cook County in 1995 and compared them to admissions during the same period in 1994. The majority of excess admissions were because of dehydration, heat stroke, and heat exhaustion. Persons older than 65 years of age with the underlying medical conditions of cardiovascular diseases, diabetes, renal diseases, and nervous system disorders were at higher risk of being admitted.

ICE AND SNOW

The impact of blizzards, ice, and snow on morbidity and mortality has not been widely studied. In the 1978 New England Ice Storm, total mortality did not increase but a third ($N = 37$) of all deaths were classified as storm related (CDC, 1982). Eight persons stranded in cars died, with five dying from carbon monoxide poisoning. Mortality from ischemic heart disease increased significantly in Rhode Island, although the number of visits to emergency rooms declined by 64% in Rhode Island and 65% in Eastern Massachusetts during the blizzard. No disease outbreaks occurred and no water or sanitation hazards could be verified, although seven were reported in Eastern Massachusetts.

Ice storms during 1994 in the Washington, D.C., area resulted in 53 National Institute of Health (NIH) employees having acute musculoskeletal injuries (CDC, 1995c). Of these, 22 (42%) were bruises and contusions, 24 (45%) were strains or sprains, and 7 (13%) were fractures. Thirty-nine of the 53 injuries resulted from falls on ice on the NIH campuses, including all seven fractures, 63% of the strains/sprains, and 77% of the bruises and contusions.

Rain combined with freezing temperatures caused trees and utility poles to fall in Maine in January 1998, leading to loss of power (CDC, 1998a). An assessment found that presumptive carbon monoxide poisoning increased from 0 to 101 cases compared to the 1997 reference period. Visits to emergency rooms increased 47% over the reference period, and most types of injuries showed absolute increases, but proportional increases were found only for cold exposure and burns.

WILDFIRES

Historically, wildfires in the United States occurred in unpopulated areas and were allowed to burn out. Starting in the 1940s and escalating during the last 20 years, development has occurred in areas traditionally considered wildlands. Areas where residential structures and fire-prone wildlands intermix are referred to as urban–wildland interfaces. One of the first fires to receive widespread attention was the Oakland, California, fire of 1991, which resulted in 25 deaths and 150 injuries ("Charring cross bottleneck was big killer," 1991; East Bay Hills Fire Operations Review Group, 1992).

Subsequent fires in Malibu, Laguna Hills, and those that occurred throughout Southern California in October 2003, which resulted in 20 deaths and 121 injuries, have emphasized the increased importance of wildfires as a type of natural disaster (Greenberg, 2003). There have been no systematic studies of the deaths and injuries that occurred in these fires; most available information is contained in press reports and other informal sources. It is clear that deaths occur because persons are unable to evacuate the area of fire and either do not consider or are unable to initiate procedures that would allow them to shelter in place. Most deaths appear to be caused by smoke inhalation and burns. How injuries occur and whether they occur pre-impact, during impact, or post-impact is unknown.

TERRORISM

Since September 11, 2001, the disaster community has examined the extent to which terrorist incidents do or do not resemble the natural disasters that have been studied over the last 60 years. Bombs, planes, arson, gases (e.g., sarin), pathogenic microbes including *Bacillus anthracis* (anthrax), variola virus (smallpox), *Yersinia pestis* (plague), *Francisella tularensis* (tularemia), *Clostridium botulinum* (botulism), the hemorrhagic fever viruses (e.g., Ebola), and nuclear devices have been hypothesized to be or actually have been selected as the agent of choice by terrorists. Clearly, cause of death and the kinds of morbidity experienced after a terrorist attack differ with the agent used. Devices are frequently delivered by individuals who intentionally commit suicide as part of the delivery process. Between 1980 and 2001, the FBI reported 482 terrorist attacks in the United States, with 67.2% being bombings (Federal Bureau of Investigations, n.d.). This section examines the deaths, injuries, and disease potentials associated with the 1993 bombing of the World Trade Center, the 1995 bombing of the Murrah Federal Office Building in Oklahoma City, and the 2001 attacks on the World Trade Center and Pentagon.

The majority of deaths in such events are caused by instantaneous dismemberment, crushing by debris, burns, and smoke inhalation. Morbidity is primarily the result of physical injuries, but disease syndromes associated with inhalation or other kinds of exposure to toxic substances are also of concern. In contrast to earthquakes, which result in similar kinds of injuries, the lethality of bombs is increased by the force with which the blast transforms parts of structures and other materials into projectiles.

Six persons were killed and 1,042 were injured when a truck bomb exploded at the World Trade Center in February 1993 (Parachini, 2000). There is no available information about what exactly caused the deaths, how the number of injuries was determined, or the nature of the injuries.

When the Murrah Federal Building was bombed on April 19, 1995, the Oklahoma State Health Commissioner "... mandated that physical injuries and other health conditions associated with the bombing be reportable conditions for the purpose of special study" (Mallonee et al., 1996, p. 383). Of the 167 fatalities, 162 persons died at the scene. The probable cause of death included multiple injuries (73%), head trauma, chest trauma, head and neck trauma, traumatic shock, and fractured spine.

Mallonee et al. (1996) defined a case as " ... any person with a physical injury directly related to the bomb blast that resulted in death or treatment at a medical facility or physician's office between April 19 and April 25, 1995" (p. 383). Of the 769 persons injured, 167 died, 83 were hospitalized, and 509 were treated and released. Similar to injuries observed in earthquakes, soft tissue injuries (lacerations, abrasions, contusions, and puncture wounds) were most common followed by musculoskeletal, head, ocular injuries, and burns. The most common locations of injuries were the extremities (74%), head and neck (48%), face (45%), and chest (35%). Eighty-eight percent of the persons who were in the building at the time of the blast were injured. Persons killed were disproportionately located on the upper floors (4 to 9) in the collapsed part of the building (risk ratio = 16.3, 95% CI 8.9 to 29.8).

In a later study, 8% of 684 survivors sustained an ocular injury, with 12 having injuries to both eyes (Mines, Thach, Mallonee, Hildebrand, & Shariat, 2000). Seventy-one percent of these persons were within 300 feet of the point of detonation, and glass caused two thirds of the injuries, with persons who were facing windows at the time of the blast being most likely to have open globe injuries.

As of August 22, 2002, 2,819 persons were estimated to have died in the September 11 attack on the World Trade Center, and a total of 2,734 death certificates had been issued (CDC, 2002a). In the Pentagon attack, 125 occupants of the Pentagon and 64 occupants of the plane were killed, and 106 persons were treated for injuries in local hospitals (Jordan, Hollowed, Turner, Wang, & Jeng, 2005; Wang, Sava, Sample, & Jordan, 2005). Fifty-four patients were treated and released, 47 were admitted, and 7 were transferred to other sites. Injuries treated were primarily burns, respiratory problems (smoke inhalation), and orthopedic injuries.

It is more difficult to determine the number and type of injuries that occurred in New York. CDC reported in January 2002 that 790 survivors with injuries were treated within 48 hours at four hospitals and one burn center. Of the 790, 49% had inhalation injuries and 26% had ocular injuries, primarily attributable to smoke, dust, debris, or fumes. Of the 139 hospitalized, the distribution of injuries was as follows: 37% inhalation, 7% ocular, 18% lacerations, 12% sprain or strain, 21% contusions, 19% fractures, 19% burns, 6% closed head injuries, and 4% crush syndrome. Two hundred and thirty-nine rescue workers sought care, with the majority suffering from inhalation (42%) and ocular (39%) injuries (CDC, 2002f). Since the original studies reported by the CDC, more detailed reports about patients seen in a number of hospitals have been published (Cushman, Pachter, & Beaton, 2003; Kirschenbaum, Keene, O'Neill, & Astiz, 2005) but no single article has attempted to describe all of the injured who sought care.

In the years since 9/11, numerous articles have reported on attempts to monitor the long-term health effects of the World Trade Center attack on the population of New York City. The majority have reported efforts to monitor the impact of environmental contamination on health. Reports of asthma, respiratory symptoms, eye irritations, and rashes by persons who lived or worked in the immediate area increased after 9/11, but researchers have not been able to establish a link to the attack itself or to changes in ambient air in the months following the attack (CDC, 2002e, 2002g, 2003b; Trout, Nimgade, Mueller, Hall, & Earnest, 2002).

Fifteen months after the attack, firemen and other rescue and recovery workers exhibited lower-airway hyperresponsiveness which may be due to high levels of airborne contaminants from smoldering fires, dust resuspension, and diesel exhaust from heavy equipment. Respiratory medical leaves by firefighters increased fivefold during the 11 months after the attacks (CDC, 2002b, 2002c, 2004b; Prezant et al., 2002).

A NOTE ON PSYCHOLOGICAL MORBIDITY

This chapter has considered the impact of disasters on physical health. Not surprisingly, the type of disaster has a strong influence on the particular health outcomes that occur. In contrast, the impact of disasters on mental health is less differentiated by type of disaster and more strongly affected by the pre-disaster characteristics of the individual and the parameters (severity, suddenness, human intent) of the disaster event. This section provides an overview on the research concerned with the influence of disasters on mental health. The interested reader is referred to two excellent papers by Norris and colleagues (Norris, Friedman, & Watson, 2002; Norris, Friedman, Watson et al., 2002) for a more detailed review of this literature.

Despite considerable diversity in circumstances, methods, and outcome measures, some commonalities emerge from the research on the mental health impact of disasters, both in regard to characteristics of individuals and parameters of the disaster events. Persons surviving natural disasters generally do not meet criteria for psychiatric disorders. Posttraumatic stress disorder (PTSD) is by far the most common disorder studied, followed by depression, anxiety, and panic disorders (Norris, Friedman, Watson et al., 2002; Vlahov et al., 2002).

In a careful study of two communities (one affected by a tornado and the other by a flood), Steinglass and Gerrity (1990) found that symptoms of PTSD were a normative reaction to disaster exposure, yet few respondents reached the threshold for a diagnosable disorder. Following Hurricane Andrew, a majority of adolescents in a multiethnic sample reported symptoms of PTSD, yet only a small proportion met criteria for the disorder (Garrison et al., 1995). Likewise, very few respondents met criteria for PTSD after the Northridge earthquake, although scores were elevated on a measure of psychological distress (Siegel, 2000). Most studies reveal a significant drop in symptoms over time (Briere & Elliott, 2000; Norris, Friedman, Watson et al., 2002). For example, three successive surveys in New York City 1 month, 4 months, and 6 months after the 2001 terrorist attack yielded PTSD prevalence rates of 7.5%, 1.7%, and 0.6%, respectively (Galea et al., 2003). These and other findings have led some researchers (see McMillen, North, & Smith, 2000) to propose a subthreshold, or partial PTSD diagnostic entity that would apply to survivors who are impaired yet do not meet diagnostic criteria.

Human-initiated disasters tend to yield higher rates of mental impairment, with mass violence being the most disturbing of all (Norris, Friedman, Watson et al., 2002). Beyond the lack of prediction and control that is characteristic of all disasters, human-initiated events shatter fundamental beliefs about vulnerability, mortality, and human nature, leaving survivors with a sense that their lives have spun out of control (Difede, Apfeldorf, Cloitre, Spielman, & Perry, 1979; Ursano, Fullerton, & Norwood, 1995). These disasters also raise continuing uncertainty about the future (Ofman, Mastria, & Steinberg, 1995) and appear to result in episodes of impairment that are lengthier as well as more severe than those that arise from natural disasters (Kopala & Keitel, 1998).

Two studies of survivors of the Oklahoma City bombing reported PTSD rates of 34% (North et al., 1999) and 8% (Sprang, 1999), respectively. The study yielding the higher rate included only survivors who had been *directly* exposed to the blast, whereas the latter sample *excluded* respondents who were direct victims of the bombing or had experienced another traumatic event in the 5 years preceding data collection. A study of the rescue and recovery workers, including volunteers, from the 2001 attack on the World Trade Center indicated that 13% met criteria for PTSD, a rate about four times what would be expected in the population (CDC, 2004a). Stress-related illness increased 17-fold among FDNY rescue workers in the year following the attack (CDC, 2002d). Nonetheless, communities exposed to chronic threat of terrorism do appear to adapt. Sixty percent of a nationally representative sample in Israel felt that their lives were in danger, yet rates of PTSD were less than 10% (Bleich, Gelkopf, & Solomon, 2003).

Similar to research on other major stressors, the disaster literature shows that vulnerable persons are particularly prone to post-disaster stress, with vulnerability encompassing prior distress, social class, gender, and linguistic or social isolation. Disasters enhance socially structured inequalities already in place and generate new, secondary stressors that further tax coping capacity (Kaniasty & Norris, 1995; Norris, Friedman, Watson et al., 2002; Tierney, 2000), particularly among community members who experience chronic adversity (Richmond, 1993). Paramount among these secondary stressors is disruption of social networks. After a disaster, demand for support can exceed the network's capacity to provide support (Kaniasty & Norris, 1993; Norris, Friedman, Watson et al., 2002). In the face of disaster stressors, instrumental, as opposed to emotional, support is especially important (Haines, Hurlbert, & Beggs, 1999), yet potential support providers may not be in a position to provide instrumental support.

A national survey, fielded 5 days after the September 11 attacks, confirmed the greater vulnerability of certain groups, but also found significant distress among most of those surveyed, even respondents who lived far from the affected areas (Schuster et al., 2001). In other research on 9/11, women who were already experiencing chronic stress were most likely to respond with anxiety and increased alcohol use (Richman, Wislar, Flaherty, Fendrich, & Rospenda, 2004). Female survivors of the Oklahoma City bombing were twice as likely as men to meet criteria for PTSD, depression, and generalized anxiety (North et al., 1999). These findings are compatible with a meta-analysis of psychological impairment following disaster which showed that effect sizes were directly proportional to the number of females in the sample (Rubonis & Bickman, 1991).

Epidemiologic studies identify degree of involvement with the disaster as the most consistent predictor of individual response (Bromet & Dew, 1995; Burkle, 1996; McDonnell et al., 1995). Physical injury, witnessing death or injury, and property loss are the most robust predictors of mental health sequelae, and are more important in this regard than the type of disaster (Briere & Elliott, 2000). Following the Armenian earthquake, an especially severe natural disaster, two thirds of survivors met criteria for PTSD (Goenjian et al., 1994). Health and disaster services were inadequate, and death tolls in this earthquake approached 100,000. Among survivors of a severe earthquake in Western India, 59% met criteria for a psychiatric diagnosis, six times the usual rate in rural India (Sharan, Chaudhary, Kavathekar, & Saxena, 1996). Early reports from the December 2004 tsunami indicate that rates of disaster-related mental disorder are high relative to those following other natural disasters. After the September

11 attacks, several studies documented higher prevalence of PTSD among those with greater exposure (Galea et al., 2002; Schlenger et al., 2002). It is worth noting that research on psychological responses to the events of September 11, 2001, shows that one third of those with PTSD had *not* been directly exposed to the World Trade Center or Pentagon attack (Galea et al., 2003). The immediacy and extensive nature of the media coverage, coupled with the profound psychological impact of the event, appeared to have expanded the boundaries of disaster impact.

The available literature on post-disaster mental health interventions converges to suggest that resources should be devoted to facilitating a speedy return to normalcy in affected communities (Norris, Friedman, & Watson, 2002; Siegel, 2000). In instances of international aid, mental health workers may be most effective when they contribute to the local relief effort by providing information and reassurance, rather than attempting to adapt Western therapeutic techniques to other cultures (Barron, 2004). Survivors of disasters need concrete and timely information on how to find shelters and access other forms of assistance (Joh, 1997). Social support and social resources are also effective in ameliorating distress (Tyler & Hoyt, 2000), as social cohesion improves when other social structures return to their pre-disaster forms (Sweet, 1998). Family, friends, and religious institutions are especially important in light of data that relatively few disaster survivors utilize mental health services (Bourque, Siegel, & Shoaf, 2001; Sprang, 1999).

CONCLUSIONS

In most disasters, the majority of deaths occur because people drown, are crushed by collapsing buildings or other structures, are hit by moving objects, or are thrown against structures and objects. People drown in hurricanes, tsunamis, and floods, with death often occurring instantaneously. People die from crush and multiple traumatic injuries in tornadoes, earthquakes, hurricanes, tsunamis, and terrorist bombings. In hurricanes, floods, and tornadoes, people who are in motor vehicles, motor homes, and outdoors are at greater risk of injury or death; in earthquakes, people who are outdoors are at less risk of injury or death. Burns and asphyxiation are major causes of death and injury following volcanoes and in terrorist bombings, and probably in wildfires. Many of these deaths could be avoided if warnings and evacuation plans were better and more effectively disseminated.

Physical injuries are the primary cause of nonfatal casualties after all disasters, and the majority are soft tissue injuries and fractures, generally to the arms and legs. When electrical service is disrupted, the use of generators and other sources of light and heat lead to increased incidents of carbon monoxide poisoning and burns.

After every disaster, certain myths emerge about how disasters affect the health of populations. Prominent among them are the misconceptions that dead bodies cause disease, epidemics and plagues follow every disaster, local populations are in shock and unable to function, and outsiders are needed to search for bodies and bring supplies. In particular, our review did not find any evidence to support the popular belief about disasters and the occurrence of infectious disease outbreaks. Jean Luc Poncelet, Claude de Ville de Goyet, and Eric Noji have been among the most persistent in trying to address these misconceptions (e.g., de Ville de Goyet, 2004; Noji, 2005, September; Pan American Health Organization, n.d.; Poncelet, 2000), but the beliefs persist, nonetheless.

Despite the unpredictability of disasters, it is incumbent on researchers in this area to utilize strong research designs that are population based and incorporate pre-disaster measures, where feasible. Standardized methods of data collection are imperative, as is increased reliance on multivariate analytic strategies that can be replicated across time and events. Questions about who is at greatest risk of morbidity (physical and psychological) and mortality during and after a natural hazard or terrorist event can be adequately addressed only when researchers and practitioners agree on what constitutes an event-related health effect, and utilize research designs that allow for generalizations to the larger or denominator population.

CHAPTER 7

Race, Class, Ethnicity, and Disaster Vulnerability

Bob Bolin

Hurricane Katrina and the disaster that unfolded in its wake provided a stark example of the pervasiveness and perniciousness of race and class inequalities in the United States. The media images constructed an unambiguous story: tens of thousands of mostly low-income African Americans were left to fend for themselves as the city of New Orleans flooded from breached levees on Lake Pontchartrain. Their only refuge was a large sports arena unequipped to serve as an "evacuee center" and devoid of any resources to support the thousands of people who gathered, many arriving only after wading through the toxic flood waters gathering in the city. In a city with a poverty rate of more than 30%, where one in three persons does not own a car, no significant effort was made by government at any level to assist the most vulnerable people to escape the disaster (Alterman, 2005). While Hurricane Katrina momentarily and unavoidably called attention to issues of race and class vulnerabilities, hazards and disaster research has clearly shown that social inequalities are core conditions that shape both disasters and environmental inequalities on a global scale. My goal in this chapter is to discuss what five decades of hazards and disaster research have revealed about race, class, and ethnic inequalities.

My primary interest is the relationship between social inequalities and hazard vulnerability in disaster processes. In the United States, the imbrication of race and class is significant, a product of a long history of racist and exclusionary practices that have marginalized groups of people deemed inferior by those holding political and economic power. Such practices, both intentional acts of discrimination and more covert, diffuse, and persistent institutionalized racism, have produced deep and lasting social, political, and economic disadvantages for people in targeted racial categories (Winant, 2001). Those disadvantages have historically expressed themselves in class position, primarily through their effects on employment, educational, and residential opportunities denied to those in marked racial categories. Given that racial and ethnic minorities will form the majority of the U.S. population by 2050 (Wilson, 2005), this is an area, as I will argue, that warrants increasing research attention in the hazards community. While people's vulnerability to environmental threats is shaped by a concatenation of sociospatial and biophysical factors, race/ethnicity and class have proven central in understanding social processes during hazard events (e.g., Duffield, 1996; Wisner, Blaikie, Cannon, & Davis, 2004). (Gender, also a significant factor in class processes and hazard vulnerability, is discussed elsewhere in this handbook and is not considered here.)

My goal here is to discuss theoretical and methodological issues in research on race and class in hazard vulnerability and disaster. This is not intended to be a detailed review of the disaster literature, as such reviews are available elsewhere (e.g., Fothergill, Maestas, & Darlington, 1999; Wisner et al., 2004). Nor will I be discussing human acts of collective violence, including war, genocide, or terrorism, as these raise complex and contested political issues beyond the scope of this chapter. (For recent discussions of terrorism from hazards geography and vulnerability perspectives see: Cutter, Richardson, & Wilbanks, 2003; Mustafa, 2005). Lastly, my comments about disaster research are made only in reference to research on race and class factors.

This discussion is divided into four sections. In the first I provide a review of some recent theoretical discussions of four key concepts: vulnerability, race, class, and ethnicity. I use this section to illustrate some of the theoretical issues invoked by the terms and to provide a context for discussing hazard and disaster research on these topics. Next I provide a chronological sketch of U.S. studies that discuss race and class, beginning with disaster research from the 1950s and continuing to the present. The third section reviews studies that utilize what has been referred to as a "vulnerability approach." Because vulnerability research is situated within a political ecological rather than a sociological framework (cf. Quarantelli, 1994; Robbins, 2004), I treat it as a separate body of literature. Notably, it differs from earlier approaches to disaster in that it considers a broad range of political economic, historical, and sociospatial factors in the genesis of disasters. In the concluding section, I briefly consider a body of hazards research that I suggest is a rich source of insight on race, class, and environmental hazards: the environmental justice literature (e.g., Bullard, 1993, 1994; Szasz & Meuser, 1997). My goal in the last section is to review elements of the environmental justice literature to illustrate race and class issues in the allocation of environmental risks, a focus largely missing in U.S. disaster research (e.g., Cutter, 1995b; Wisner et al., 2004).

THEORIZING INEQUALITIES

For my purposes, race, class, and ethnicity are key markers of a person's potential vulnerability to environmental hazards of all types. In the hazards and disaster literature a "vulnerability approach," with its focus on an ensemble of sociospatial and political economic conditions that shape disasters, is a two-decade-old research approach grounded in political ecology (Hewitt, 1997; Wisner & Walker, 2005). Vulnerability analysis, or vulnerability science as it has been recently labeled (Cutter, 2003b), is currently formulated as a broad theoretical approach for investigating hazards, environmental inequalities, and questions of sustainability (Kasperson, Kasperson, & Dow, 2001). Beginning with the publication of Hewitt's foundational volume, *Interpretations of Calamity from the Perspective of Human Ecology,* in 1983, vulnerability analysis has attempted to shift the analysis of disasters away from the physical hazard agent and a temporally limited view of disasters as "unique" events separate from the ongoing social order (Hewitt, 1983a, 1983b). Vulnerability researchers have for some time argued that environmental calamities are shaped by the already existing social, political, environmental, and economic conditions and thus should not be considered as "natural" occurrences (e.g., Cannon, 1994; Maskrey, 1993). Indeed, as Quarantelli notes (1990, p. 18) in this vein, "... there can never be a natural disaster; at most there is a conjuncture of certain physical happenings and certain social happenings."

Wisner et al. (2004, p. 11), in the most systematic statement of hazard vulnerability research to date, define vulnerability as "... *the characteristics of a person or group and their situation that influence their capacity to anticipate, cope with, resist, and recover from the impact of a natural hazard"* (Italics in original). They go on to note that vulnerability is determined by a variety of factors, variable across space and time, that differentially put people and places at risk of loss from environmental hazards. Wisner et al. (2004, p. 11) suggest that among these factors are class, caste, ethnicity, gender, and immigration status. Vulnerabilities are variable by hazard type, contingent on a variety of circumstances, and unevenly distributed across individuals, households, communities, and regions (Bankoff, Frerks, & Hilhorst, 2003; Morrow, 1999). Hazard vulnerability has been consistently linked to people's class locations and the effects of race/ethnicity on the ensemble of social advantages and disadvantages they routinely experience (Wisner et al., 2004). While a very large social science literature has been built around each of these concepts, space allows me to focus only on a few key ideas to suggest their theoretical complexity.

RACE AND ETHNICITY

Omi and Winant (1994) contend that postwar U.S. sociology has attempted to apply a white ethnic immigrant framework to *racialized* minorities, including African Americans, Latinos, American Indians, and Asians. This strategy obscures the complex class and cultural differences among people so labeled, and it directs attention away from the structural ways in which such groups are "racially constructed" in the United States (Omi & Winant, 1994, p. 23). For example, in the United States one can stop being ethnically Irish or Italian in ways that would not allow to stop being labeled black or Asian, however much one is assimilated into dominant cultural forms. Race (and racism) exists at the level of social structure in the sense that one cannot opt out of the effects of racial categories.

The challenge for researchers is to approach race (and ethnicity) as complex and contested social constructs that form the axes of a variety of historical and contemporary social struggles across a range of scales (Smith & Feagin, 1995). In using race to explain observed individual differences in social research, Omi and Winant (1994, p. 54) claim that scholars too often treat "race as an *essence*, as something fixed, concrete, and objective." Against such essentialism, they contend that race should be understood as "an unstable and 'decentered' complex of social meanings constantly being transformed by political struggle ...: *race is a concept which signifies and symbolizes social conflicts and interests by referring to different types of human bodies"* (Omi & Winant, 1994, p. 55, Italics in original). What types of bodies are included in what racial categories reflect place-specific historical processes that produce distinct patterns of advantage and disadvantage based on such classifications (e.g., Hoelscher, 2003; Pulido, 2000). These accumulated advantages and disadvantage can have distinct relevance for hazard vulnerability. Racialized groups, for example, may be spatially segregated and forced to occupy unsafe and hazard-prone spaces that privileged groups can avoid occupying (Wisner et al., 2004). Such racially marginalized groups can also be denied access to necessary resources to recover from disasters, deepening their vulnerability to future hazard events (Bolin & Stanford, 1999).

The changing categories of races and ethnicities in the U.S. Census are an example of an arbitrary and shifting discursive terrain. In recent decades, Japanese Americans have moved from being considered "nonwhite" to Oriental to Asian, and Hispanics, a term dating to the 1980 census, may be "white" (or another race), and all are ostensibly ethnically different from "non-Hispanic whites" in unspecified ways. And though Hispanics and Asians have different national origins (Korean, Chinese, Cuban, Mexican, etc.) in the census, whites appear as ethnically monolithic. The unstable and changing census categories and attached cultural representations that "move" people in or out of racial and/or ethnic categories over the decades hints at the ambiguities and fluxes of such identity markers. Regardless, these categorical shifts should not obscure the fact that both Japanese and Latinos have faced intense discrimination and dispossession as racially defined minorities at various times and places in U.S. history (e.g., Smith & Feagin, 1995; Winant, 2001). Hazard and disaster studies that rely solely on census classifications leave unexplored the meaningfulness of the labels for affected people in particular localities and the cultural, class, and gender diversity these terms may obscure. For a deeper understanding of race in disaster, it is necessary to investigate the complex historical, social, and geographic processes in which racial identities are socially constructed and given significance in systems of domination and subordination in specific places.

Omi and Winant (1994) offer two key theoretical formulations useful for understanding the ways that race and racism relate to hazard vulnerability: racial formation and racial project. Racial formation refers to the historical process "by which racial categories are created, inhabited, transformed, and destroyed" (Omi & Winant, 1994, p. 55). Such formations incorporate specific "racial projects" that represent and organize human bodies and social practices across space and time, privileging certain categories of people over others (Pulido, 2000). Thus, racial formations are historically produced, hierarchical, and hegemonic, and are expressed materially, spatially, and in discourse (Hoelscher, 2003; Omi & Winant, 1994). Grounding understanding of systems of racial inequality in specific sociohistorical processes marks a theoretical and methodological advance over treating race and ethnicity as demographic givens that are fixed, measurable, and unproblematic. For hazards research, understanding racialized social processes requires a historically informed understanding of the particularities of racial formations in specific places and times and how those shape the environmental risks to which people are exposed (e.g., Bolin, Grineski, & Collins, 2005; Pellow, 2000). It also avoids the essentialist treatment of race found in quantitative studies, wherein racial/ethnic categories are treated as concrete attributes with ensembles of presumed, but unmeasured, social characteristics.

According to Omi and Winant (1994), ethnicity is frequently either used as a substitute for or conflated with race in sociological literature, although it too is an unstable concept that escapes easy definition. And as with race, relying on shifting census categories elides any consideration of the instability of labels or the political struggles over cultural identities they incorporate. Anthropology, beginning at least with Barth's classical statement on ethnic groups (Barth, 1969), has produced an extensive literature on ethnicity and ethnic groups as *the* key subject of contemporary cultural anthropology. At its (deceptively) simplest, ethnicity implies an ensemble of cultural characteristics and interaction patterns that distinguish one group from another. Ethnicity shapes individual identities and group characteristics while at the same time drawing boundaries with others who ostensibly do not share a set of cultural characteristics. Thus, ethnicity involves both identities and cultural practices by which one set of people can distinguish themselves from another, and are likewise recognizable by "outside groups" (Eriksen, 1991). However, the cultural features and practices that either unify or divide groups are frequently difficult to identify, particularly in complex postcolonial and multicultural social formations (Gupta & Ferguson, 1997). Further, anthropologists are well aware that knowledgeable lay people often disagree with social science descriptions of their cultural or "ethnic" characteristics (Eriksen, 1991).

There are other confounding issues as well. Individual members of ethnic groups are also class situated and certain "cultural features" attributed to ethnicity may be more directly concerned with class position and practices (Williams, 1989). Further, the disadvantages that accrue to women in a variety of cultural or ethnic contexts can be severe, pointing to the need to always consider gender at its intersection with ethnicity and attached cultural practices. The literature on famine, for example, provides numerous examples of the vulnerability of women as a consequence of their marginal and subordinate status within specific ethnic, tribal, and religious groups (Oliver-Smith, 1996; Watts, 1991).

As illustrated below, the historical and cultural complexities of race and ethnicity are typically not investigated in any real depth in the disaster literature (see Fothergill et al., 1999). Perhaps because of the exigencies of disaster research, there is an tendency to rely on commonsensical treatments of racial and ethnic categories rather using in-depth sociohistorical and ethnographic analyses of local racial and ethnic projects (e.g., Aptekar, 1994; Bolin & Bolton, 1986). Given the typical applied, pragmatic, policy focus of disaster research, it is not surprising that researchers do not engage extended theoretical discussions and qualitative unpacking of their key terms. However, to provide an empirically richer, more contextualized understanding of race and ethnicity requires explicit theorization of key concepts, as some researchers have begun to undertake (e.g., Peacock, Morrow, & Gladwin, 2001). The complex mechanisms by which certain ethnic (and racial, gendered, and classed) categories of people are disadvantaged in relation to hazardous environments will remain invisible as long as researchers are concerned with statistical *differences* between groups rather than the pervasive social *inequalities* that produce measured difference to begin with (Holifield, 2001).

CLASS AND POLITICAL ECONOMIC TRANSFORMATIONS

While an in-depth understanding of ethnicity may be more the domain of social anthropologists than sociologists (Oliver-Smith, 1996), the opposite holds for social class. Indeed, social class cuts across and is imbricated with all other demographic factors, as one is always class situated, whatever other determinants of social positionality may be simultaneously at work. Class theory, particularly in its Marxist and poststructuralist forms, is both complex and at the center of a variety of new theoretical developments (Gibson-Graham, Resnick, & Wolff, 2001). While there are a number of competing Marxist and Weberian approaches to class and economic positionality in capitalist political economies, here I use class as a trope for aspects of an agent's dynamic position in processes of economic and social production and reproduction. In Marxist terms, classes are elements of the social relationships of production, which include not only people's primary productive activities, but also patterns of ownership, the appropriation and distribution of surplus value, and the legal and cultural systems and practices that justify and reinforce existing class inequalities (Harvey, 1996a; Peet, 1998). In this sense, classes are processes that extend beyond the "economic" in any narrow and essentialist reading. As Glassman (2003, p. 685) writes, "... classes are always already constituted as economic, political, cultural, and ideological entities—including being gendered and racialized in specific ways ... "

It is common in the social sciences for people to be assigned class position based on a variety of indicators, including income, their position in the extraction of surplus value, occupation and education, ownership of means of production, and labor market position (Arvidson, 1999, p. 138). However, different meanings of class may produce different conclusions about class processes, pointing to the need to theoretically distinguish different class and nonclass indicators used in the course of research. Class processes are connected to a complex range of issues, from political and economic power and job security to modes of consumption, identity formation, subjectivities, legal rights, and sociospatial processes (Bourdieu, 1984; Harvey, 1990). The latter include a range of issues from economic segregation to land uses and the distribution of hazards.

As with the other concepts discussed here, class processes and class compositions should be understood as historically constructed, overdetermined, contingent, and dynamic (Glassman, 2003). In the case of class, change can be pronounced as dominant regimes of accumulation shift with political economic crises and as localized class struggles crystallize over specific issues (Merrifield, 2000; Peet, 1998). It bears noting that in the United States class and race are often coupled, a historical effect of racially exclusionary practices in sectoral employment and the formation of industrial working classes in the United States. The exclusion of blacks from early labor unions (other than the International Workers of the World) helped establish a racialized (and gendered) labor hierarchy in which well paying skilled industrial jobs were reserved for whites while low paying service work was the province of blacks and Latinos. The pervasive effects of this segmentation and inequality remain today (McIntyre, 2002).

The structural instability of class position in the context of a crisis-prone capitalist system is perhaps most visible with the economic restructuring in the United States beginning in the 1970s. This restructuring led to the deindustrialization of the Midwest and Northeast beginning with post-Vietnam War economic crises and the subsequent emergence of an ascendant and hegemonic neoliberalism in the 1980s (Soja, 2000). This restructuring produced the "deproletarianization" of significant fractions of the industrial working class as jobs and factories were moved toward nonunion, low-wage sectors of the United States and to the global South (Harvey, 1996a, 1996b; Soja, 1989). Economic restructuring has been simultaneously accompanied by the growth of insecure low-wage, service sector employment, geographic shifts in employment opportunities, weakened trade unions, reshaped industrial and residential landscapes, and reduced real incomes for significant fractions of the working class (Davis, 1992; Harvey, 1990, 2001; Yates, 2005). These changes led to the decline of class-based social movements and the advent of "new social movements" focused on "fragmented group identities that have filled the class void in increasingly polarized urban spaces" (Arvidson, 1999, p. 136). The shift toward flexible accumulation strategies in the United States, coupled with "lean and mean" corporate restructuring, has likewise begun a historically unprecedented job and wage squeeze on the middle and working classes over the last two decades (Soja, 2000). And these pressures are disproportionately impacting people of color, where today in the United States more than 30% of black workers and 39% of Latino workers earn poverty wages or below (Yates, 2005).

With neoliberal economic policy being imposed on indebted Third World countries through the World Bank and the World Trade Organization, social inequalities and processes of marginalization are being intensified in the global South as well (Peet & Watts, 2004). The imposition of "free market discipline" through structural adjustment programs has a variety of impacts including growing income inequalities, increasing production for export rather than domestic consumption, reduced social welfare services, privatization of common property resources, the dispossession of peasants, and increased ecological disruptions (Klein, 2005; Robbins, 2004). It is also argued that these transformations increase vulnerability to hazards through environmental degradation, magnify losses from disasters, and increase recovery difficulties in the post-disaster period (Bankoff et al., 2003; Oliver-Smith, 1996). Class and the larger political economic relationships that shape class processes are a key, if neglected, part of understanding disaster. Class positionality connects closely with the types of resources people can use in crises and the types of social protections granted or denied, and it has a strong spatial dimension linked to occupation of hazardous areas (Arvidson, 1999; Wisner & Walker, 2005).

In sum, race, class, and ethnicity are theoretically complex signifiers of social processes that involve struggles over legal and political rights, access to resources and livelihoods, and the constitution of identities (e.g., Peluso & Watts, 2001). The combined effects of these factors are linked to sociospatial processes in disasters as shown in the research literature (Fothergill et al., 1999; Wisner et al., 2004). In the following sections, I provide an overview of how these concepts have been utilized in disaster and vulnerability research.

DISASTER RESEARCH FOCUSING ON RACE
AND CLASS

Disaster research as an academic specialization was first developed in the United States in the aftermath of World War II. Its roots can be traced to the Strategic Bombing Surveys of World War II, conducted to understand the "morale" of civilian populations subjected to sustained military attacks (including the U.S. nuclear attacks on Japan) (Mitchell, 1990). This general interest carried over into the Cold War, during which research, funded by the military, was conducted on civilian disasters. A "sociological perspective" on disaster emerged in a series of studies funded by the Army Chemical Center and conducted by the National Opinion Research Center (NORC) at the University of Chicago (Drabek, 1986; Quarantelli, 1987a). After the NORC studies concluded in 1954, federal funding of disaster research continued through the Office of Civil Defense and ultimately led to the establishment of the Disaster Research Center (DRC) at Ohio State University in 1963 by sociologists Quarantelli and Dynes (Dynes & Drabek, 1994). The DRC (now at the University of Delaware) was the first of several disaster research centers in the United States, establishing the country as an early leader in disaster and hazards studies (Quarantelli, 1991a).

In keeping with dominant approaches in U.S. sociology in this period, disaster research in the 1950s and early 1960s paid minimal attention to victim diversity or social inequalities by race or class. Instead, studies focused on event characteristics and overall effects on a given community (e.g., Drabek, 1986; Form & Nosow, 1958). Although social inequalities were not directly investigated by any major studies in the 1950s, because of opportunistic nature of disaster research, some initial findings found their way into the published literature. An exemplar of this is Moore's *Tornadoes Over Texas* (1958), which includes findings on a limited number of blacks and Mexican Americans who turned up in his sample. Moore, for example, found that blacks had disproportionate losses from a tornado and consequently had greater need for external assistance to recover (as did the elderly in his sample). He also found that blacks had a higher injury rate than whites, a finding echoed in Bates, Fogleman, Parenton, Pittman, and Tracy (1963) that found that mortality was significantly higher among blacks than among whites after Hurricane Audrey. These are among the earliest findings suggesting that being black and poor in the United States was associated with disproportionate environmental risk, although such conclusions were not highlighted in the studies. Moore also observed some differences in the use of public shelters, noting that people at the "lower end of the socio-economic scale" were more likely to use public shelters than white-collar individuals (Mileti, Drabek, & Haas, 1975).

Clifford's (1956) study of two Texas–Mexico border towns evacuated for flooding offered some early observations about "ethnic" differences in evacuation behavior. According to Dynes (1972, pp. 236–237) Clifford's research "found that in the Mexican community, there was a greater dependence on the kin groups as sources of advice and help. There was a greater reluctance to accept 'official' warnings and aid." A study of a 1965 Denver, Colorado flood

(Drabek & Boggs, 1968, p. 447) found that "Spanish-American [sic] families will evacuate to the homes of relatives more frequently than Anglos." In neither case was there any direct consideration of the how social class and related political economic factors might account for these ostensible "ethnic" or cultural differences (cf. Yelvington, 1997). The interest in demographic differences in warning, emergency response, and evacuation behavior was strong in early disaster research (see Drabek, 1986 for a review), as was the impulse to generalize and systematize findings irrespective of their fragmentary nature (e.g., Barton, 1970).

It was not until the 1970s that the first studies on reconstruction and recovery were conducted, driven by new interest in demographic differences in disaster response. The expansion and theoretical elaboration of disaster research were abetted by the publication of the first major assessment of hazards and disaster research in the United States in the early 1970s, a work that brought together much of the sociological and geographical research available to that time (White & Haas, 1975). This work, under the leadership of the hazards geographer Gilbert White, helped establish an agenda for new hazards and disaster research that would appear over the next two decades (Mileti, 1999; White & Haas, 1975).

Part of the new agenda for hazards research of the 1970s included studies focusing on racial, ethnic, and socioeconomic differences in disaster response. However, a recent review notes ". . . existing studies on racial and ethnic differences cover such a wide spectrum of time, disaster event, place and racial group, that it is difficult to identify patterns and draw conclusions" (Fothergill et al., 1999, p. 157). Considerable variation in theoretical sophistication, diverse research methodologies, and study designs, as well as disciplinary differences, contribute to this lack of patterning. Since class, race, and ethnicity are concepts attempting to capture dynamic constantly changing phenomena, it should not be surprising that a variety of studies covering more than 30 years produce findings that are difficult to generalize from. Certainly studies since the 1970s offer a variety of practical insights into racial and ethnic differences in various aspects of disaster processes (e.g., Oliver-Smith & Hoffman, 1999; Peacock, Morrow, & Gladwin, 1997). Far less attention has been given to class and theorizing class-related phenomena in published disaster research. Most quantitative studies in the United States have not gone beyond measuring socioeconomic differences, usually restricted to income, in disaster responses, failing to explore class structures in the context of local political economies and the structuring of urban space (see Peacock et al., 1997 for an important exception).

Disaster recovery studies in the 1970s began to examine race, class, and ethnic differentials, marking a new direction in the research (Haas, Kates, & Bowden, 1977). Some of the first explicit discussions of class issues (concerned mostly with poverty) and race come in discussions of a catastrophic flood in South Dakota as part of the Haas et al. reconstruction study. Class (as socioeconomic status) and racial differences in access to assistance, victim experiences in temporary housing, and general recovery processes were discussed (Haas et al., 1977). A historical analysis of the 1906 San Francisco disaster, as part of the reconstruction research, highlighted the changing pattern of ethnic and racial segregation in the city as it was rebuilt, marking an important early example of historical geographic disaster research concerned with race and ethnicity. Coming out of this reconstruction research was a study comparing household recovery in Nicaragua and the United States that emphasized important class/socioeconomic and cultural/ethnic dimensions in accounting for different household recovery strategies (Bolin & Trainer, 1978).

In the 1980s new studies comparing ethnic/racial groups in disasters were undertaken by Perry and Mushkatel (1986) and by Turner, Nigg, and Paz (1980; see also Perry, 1987). Both studies found various statistical differences among Anglos, blacks, and Mexican Americans regarding risk perception, disaster preparedness, and warning responses, differences attributed to ethnic characteristics of the subjects investigated. Perry and Mushkatel (1986) found ethnic minorities were less likely to evacuate in the face of warnings than their Anglo comparison group. This quantitative study did introduce statistical controls on income to discern direct or indirect "class" effects on reported ethnic/racial differences in response. Income measures are often the extent of class analysis in disaster studies of this period, leaving class-related factors largely untheorized and uninvestigated as a structuring factor in disaster response.

Another study at this time also explored racial and ethnic differences, focusing on long-term household recovery. Bolin and Bolton (1986) discussed race, ethnic, and class differences at disaster sites in Hawaii, California, and Texas, comparing across different hazard agents and racial and class mixes. Consistent with other more recent studies, they found that blacks were more likely to live in mobile homes provided as temporary housing by the federal government than were whites (in Texas). African Americans were also less likely to obtain adequate aid for their recovery needs from both house insurance and from the federal government (see also Bolin, 1986). Such observations reflect class differences which, in this setting, were tightly coupled with race. Bolin and Bolton also reported that at their California earthquake site, Latinos were less likely to receive adequate recovery assistance than Anglos and more likely to rely on kin groups for aid in coping. The Hawaiian site provided comparisons of Japanese, Filipino, and white victims. However, differences in ethnic groups appeared related to differences in initial damages rather than other factors. The authors did recognize the confounding effects that class inequalities had on assumed ethnic differences, noting the significance of poverty in disaster vulnerability and in inhibiting long-term recovery (Bolin & Bolton, 1986). These findings and others from 1980s studies would receive more in-depth investigation and elaboration in 1990s studies that provided more in-depth analysis of race and class processes in disaster.

It bears noting that many of these 1980s studies were explicitly quantitative and statistical, and included, for the time, relatively sophisticated attempts at statistical modeling. The primary limitation of cross-sectional survey research of this sort is that while race, class, and ethnic differences can be measured and their independent statistical effects can be controlled for, why those differentials exist, how they came about, and how they manifest themselves over time cannot be addressed. As discussed extensively in environmental justice studies, the focus on the relative statistical effects of race versus class obscures any understanding of the concrete ways that race and class are bound together and embodied in human subjects, structuring people's everyday lives, including where and how they live, and their particular ensembles of capacities and vulnerabilities (Downey, 1998; Holifield, 2001; Pulido, 1996; Szasz & Meuser, 1997).

More recent U.S. disaster literature focusing on race and class has been shaped by studies on California earthquakes and Hurricane Andrew in Florida. The 1987 Whittier Narrows earthquake and the 1989 Loma Prieta earthquake each became the focus of research on race/ethnic and class differences in various aspects of response. Bolton, Liebow, and Olson (1993), using detailed ethnographic research, provided an examination of how low-income Latinos, most housed in unstable unreinforced masonry buildings, coped with housing damage and displacement after the Whittier Narrows earthquake (in a suburb of Los Angeles.) That study detailed linguistic barriers Latinos experienced in trying to obtain housing information and in attempting to work through the federal aid system (see also Bolin, 1993a). While lacking the scope of earlier quantitative race studies (e.g., Perry & Mushkatel, 1986), Bolton and colleagues' ethnographic research provides a good example of a study providing numerous insights into how particular people (embodying race, class, age, and gender differences) experience and cope with disasters in specific contexts and settings.

The issue of language and other cultural and class barriers is an important theme in several 1990s disaster studies (e.g., Phillips, 1993). As with Whittier Narrows, the 1989 Loma Prieta earthquake in Northern California provided opportunities for researchers to examine specific race, class, and ethnic issues. Several Loma Prieta studies approached their research ethnographically, providing detailed descriptions of how vulnerable and marginalized groups coped with the aftermath of a destructive earthquake (Bolin & Stanford, 1991; Laird, 1991; Phillips, 1993; Schulte, 1991). Each of these studies investigated processes of political, social, and cultural marginalization that systematically disadvantaged African Americans and Mexican Americans in a variety of ways, from housing assistance to political representation. These studies documented how federal assistance programs consistently failed to meet the needs of the homeless, Latino farm workers, and low-income African Americans.

Several studies also discussed political mobilizations by Latino farm workers challenging the Anglo power structure in Watsonville in the wake of the earthquake (Bolin & Stanford, 1991). Class and race-based mobilizations and the protracted conflict that ensued catalyzed Latinos politically, leading to new class and ethnic coalitions opposing a historic Anglo hegemony in Watsonville, and prompting the development of new earthquake assistance programs (Bolin, 1994; Schulte, 1991). This research highlighted the importance of grass-roots movements working with community-based organizations (CBOs) to address local disaster needs (see Laird, 1991; Phillips, 1993). In reference to the earlier theoretical discussion, these studies illustrated the specific ways that class, race, and ethnicity articulate in specific ways in actual disaster processes, something that conventional quantitative survey studies generally do not.

What I take as a leading example of recent research on race and class, providing both quantitative scope and ethnographic depth, focused on Hurricane Andrew (1992) in the Miami, Florida metro region. This research provided a theoretically informed discussion of race, class, gender, and poverty dynamics, explored in a series of case studies (Peacock et al., 1997). Consistent with vulnerability studies described later, Grenier and Morrow (1997) offered a historical overview of the development of the Miami urban region to show how processes of political and economic marginalization were creating at-risk people and communities, especially between Caribbean immigrant groups and African Americans (see also Peacock et al., 2001). Although not using the explicit language of racial formations and racial projects, the Hurricane Andrew volume stands as one of a few U.S. disaster studies that has examined racial projects in the context of vulnerability and disaster.

Throughout the Hurricane Andrew case studies, the authors highlight how race, ethnicity, and class inequalities shaped people's experiences, from impact related losses to access to assistance, inequities in insurance settlements, the effects of pre- and post-disaster racial segregation, and the calamitous effects of disaster on an already marginalized and impoverished black community (Dash, Morrow, & Peacock, 1997; Girard & Peacock, 1997; Peacock & Girard, 1997; Yelvington, 1997). Each of these studies documents how already existing social conditions in greater Miami shaped the contours of disaster and the ways that marginalized populations variously endured continuing or increased disadvantages in the recovery process (see Dash et al., 1997). However, the research also demonstrates that race or ethnicity by itself is not an adequate explanatory element: What matters is how these factors (and immigration status, gender, and age) intersect in spatially specific ways to shape a person's class locations and his or her access to social and economic resources (e.g., Yelvington, 1997). That is, race, ethnicity, and other "identity" factors are intertwined with class processes and the privileges or disadvantages that flow from these converge to shape a person's vulnerability to hazard events.

Overall, race and ethnicity have received more attention in the U.S. literature than have social class processes in disaster. Apart from the Hurricane Andrew research, there is little in the U.S. literature that provides a detailed spatially and historically informed analysis of race and class in disaster. This is an area in the disaster literature where there is clearly a need for more place-specific, historically informed case studies. Until the 1990s, quantitative differences among ethnic or racial groups were the primary interest in the literature on race and ethnicity, the not inequalities or the discriminatory practices that produce those inequalities. There is a need in disaster studies to go beyond the too often superficial discussion of race as a mere nominal variable, and to examine it as a pervasive structuring feature linked to a wide variety of sociospatial processes (e.g., Peacock et al., 1997). Class factors also require greater attention and more adequate theoretical work to move beyond reducing them to a relative income measure. The question of poverty has received more attention than other aspects of class in the research, but it appears almost exclusively as an issue of inadequate income, not a condition actively structured by multiscalar political economic processes (see Arvidson, 1999). Historically and spatially informed research such as Peacock and colleagues' (1997) work should serve as a model for studies that combine qualitative and quantitative techniques to examine the ways that class, race, and ethnicity shape vulnerability and disaster.

RACE, CLASS, AND VULNERABILITY

While the work of Peacock et al. (1997) is, by self-description, situated within a "sociology of disaster" framework, it is also one of the few U.S. studies that addresses issues central to vulnerability analysis (see also Kroll-Smith & Couch, 1991). Peacock and his colleagues explicitly situate the disaster in the context of historical, spatial, and political economic processes in urban space, and focus on the particular ways social inequalities develop and shape people's vulnerabilities to disaster. While vulnerability analysis is treated as separate body of research here, I emphasize that the research on Hurricane Andrew marks a potential convergence between prevailing U.S. approaches and those explicated by Hewitt (1983a, 1983b, 1997) and more recently Wisner et al. (2004). Until recently, the majority of vulnerability studies have focused on disasters in the global South (see Blaikie et al., 1994 and Wisner et al., 2004 for reviews). Generally, this research has adopted a critical, sometimes Marxist, analysis of Third World development projects in generating hazard vulnerabilities and environmental degradation. This general approach draws off political ecology (Robbins, 2004) rather than sociology, as many of the U.S. studies cited in the preceding text do.

Vulnerability analysis, dating to its classic statement by Hewitt and others in 1983, distanced itself from the "dominant approach" to disaster and has engaged in an extended critique of conventional disaster research and management (e.g., Hewitt, 1997; Susman, O'Keefe, & Wisner, 1983a; Watts, 1983). That critique and a series of critical exchanges since have produced a lively, if not always productive, debate among disaster researchers of different theoretical and political positions (e.g., Hewitt, 1997; Quarantelli, 1995c; Wisner et al., 2004). Recent vulnerability analysis is discussed in *At Risk* (Wisner et al., 2004), which offers an extensive hazard-specific review of research. In general terms, the research examines political economic and spatial processes of marginalization that not only produce or intensify poverty, but that also, in given instances, constrain certain portions of a given population (often by class, race, caste, or ethnicity) to occupy hazardous areas and hazardous structures. Prime examples can be seen in the proliferation of unsafe, unplanned, and impoverished squatter settlements in many of the world's major urban centers (Davis, 2005).

Wisner et al. (2004) provide a detailed discussion of vulnerabilities across a range of hazards under a variety of specific spatiotemporal conditions. At the core of their analysis is a process model of vulnerability accumulation and the production of differential environmental risks. Specifically, hazard vulnerability is understood as a process comprising three linked elements: root causes, dynamic pressures, and unsafe conditions. The underlying causes refer to the general historical, political, economic, environmental, and demographic factors that produce unequal distributions of resources among people, by a variety of positional factors, including race and class. These processes produce environmental vulnerability through specific social processes, including, for example, rapid urbanization, environmental degradation, economic crises, political conflict, and poorly planned and executed development programs (Peet & Watts, 2004). These processes generate unequal exposure to environmental risk by creating "unsafe conditions" in which people live and work. Unsafe conditions may involve both spatial location and characteristics of the built environment, but they also include fragile livelihoods, inadequate incomes, legal and political inequities (often by race, ethnicity, and gender), and a lack of social protections offered by the state (Bolin & Stanford, 1999; Cannon, 1994).

The anthropologist Oliver-Smith has been an important contributor to this literature, offering historically and ecologically informed, ethnographical research on Latin American disasters (e.g., Oliver-Smith, 1986; Oliver-Smith & Hoffman, 1999). Recent anthropological research examines vulnerability and disaster in the context of colonialism, underdevelopment, and increasingly severe environmental degradation (Johnston, 1994; Oliver-Smith, 1996, 1999a; Peluso & Watts, 2001). Much of Oliver-Smith's work has involved detailed analysis of a devastating earthquake and mudslides in Peru in 1970, generally considered to be the worst disaster in the Western hemisphere (Oliver-Smith, 1986). In his political ecology of disaster, he considers the Peruvian disaster to be five centuries in the making, a combined effect of colonially imposed building and settlement patterns and economic policies that marginalized Indians and peasants, engendering a chronic rural poverty that survived and expanded into the postcolonial period. Oliver-Smith (1994) shows that it was not simply bad judgment or "bounded rationality" that led people to occupy unsafe ground and pursue marginal livelihoods (cf. Burton, Kates, & White, 1993). Rather, he argues that the cumulative and constraining effects of underdevelopment, chronic poverty, and racial/ethnic marginalization, all part of a legacy of colonialism and antidemocratic development programs, were determining factors in people's vulnerability to earthquakes (Oliver-Smith, 1999b).

The geographer Maskrey's (1994) account of the 1990 Alto Mayo earthquake in Peru provides a second example of vulnerability research that considers class and cultural/ethnic marginalization, set in a broad historical geography of a farming district in the interior. He shows how a moderate earthquake produced a broad-scale disaster, occurring as it did in a region going through protracted political, ecological, and economic crises—products of short-sighted development programs—and an ascendant neoliberal economic policy. Peru's crushing international debt, hyperinflation, and deteriorating infrastructure ensured the failure of its new export agricultural economy, producing in turn a deepening economic crisis in the interior region of Alto Mayo in the 1980s. The pauperization of small-scale farmers as result of failed export programs led them to shift to coca production in order to survive, which in turn accelerated environmental degradation through deforestation (Maskrey, 1994). With growing poverty, increasing marginalization of peasants, and a lack of state support, the region was in the midst of a protracted economic and ecological crisis when a moderate earthquake hit, destroying fragile adobe homes, displacing people, and intensifying the ongoing crises. Maskrey offers a critical assessment of the top-down, technocratic approach to disaster response and reconstruction by the state and international NGOs in the temblor's aftermath. He notes the many failures of programs initiated by NGOs and the state can be attributed to inadequate incorporation of local knowledge and the lack of democratic participation in recovery. Maskrey's focus on processes of marginalization, particularly of low-income farmers in the region, shows how failed development programs, under the guise of "modernization," produced poverty and increasing hazard vulnerability (see Peet & Watts, 2004; Robbins, 2004).

Historically and geographically informed disaster research of the type just described is relatively rare in U.S. disaster research (cf. Fothergill et al., 1999; Mileti, 1999). At the risk of calling attention to my own research, a colleague and I developed a vulnerability analysis of the 1994 Northridge earthquake. That study was specifically developed from Blaikie, Cannon, Davis, and Wisner's (1994) vulnerability approach (see Bolin with Stanford, 1998; Bolin & Stanford, 1999). In that research, we reviewed century-long processes of sociospatial marginalization by race, ethnicity, and class in the Los Angeles urban region. We adapted a vulnerability approach to conditions encountered in an urbanized and ostensibly wealthy area of the United States. We noted, in contrast to Third World studies, that populations marginalized by class and race in the United States were not necessarily driven to live in areas with the most natural hazards, however much they were otherwise spatially segregated along class and race lines. Rather Bolin and Stanford (1999) argued that vulnerability in the United States related most closely to people's capacities to either avoid or cope with hazard losses, capacities influenced by access to recovery assistance and other social protections linked to class privilege.

The research draws a distinction between availability of and access to assistance, the latter often determined by class, race, legal, and cultural factors. While a broad range of federal resources were made available after Northridge, those most in need of assistance often could not access those resources because of qualification requirements (Bolin & Stanford, 1998a). Federal housing assistance programs were criticized for their class biases. Programs provided far less (or no) assistance to renters, the unemployed, and the homeless while they provided the most generous aid to middle-class employed homeowners (Bolin & Stanford, 1998). These critiques were developed through a series of case studies of impacted communities near Los Angeles, to show in each instance how hazard vulnerability accumulated between certain class fractions and racial groups based on specific historical and sociospatial processes. Those vulnerabilities were often highlighted by inadequate post-earthquake recovery programs that only intensified existing inequalities (Bolin & Stanford, 1999; see also Peacock et al., 2001). The Northridge research also highlighted the importance of political vulnerabilities in the United States, specifically as they related to the question of "illegal" immigrants and their access to post-disaster resources. Our study found that, with the threat of deportation a constant feature of daily life, undocumented low-income Mexicans faced the challenges of recovery without assistance while living under the political risks of discovery and deportation (Bolin & Stanford, 1998). One element in the Northridge work examined the historical and current class, racial, and ethnic conflict involving Mexican American farm workers in Ventura County pitted against an entrenched Anglo power structure. These conflicts were expressed in a series of contestations over whether new affordable housing would be built to accommodate the area's large low-income Latino population (Bolin & Stanford, 1999). It was argued that these class and ethnic conflicts could not be understood without also understanding the history and political ecology of farming and farm workers in the U.S. Southwest (Bolin & Stanford, 1999).

While Latino farm workers were characterized as a chronically vulnerable population, we also noted that situational vulnerability may affect class fractions not "normally" considered vulnerable in the literature (Bolin with Stanford, 1998). An example of this involved small numbers of middle-class homeowners in Los Angeles, recently unemployed as a result of retrenchment in the aerospace industry. Unemployed middle-class homeowners, with large mortgages on houses that had slipped in resale value, found themselves in an uncharacteristic position of severe economic insecurity following losses incurred in the earthquake. These earthquake victims were unable to qualify for Small Business Administration disaster housing loans because of their unemployment, while simultaneously also needing to pay mortgages on homes with negative equity (Bolin with Stanford, 1998: see also Tierney, 1997). Bankruptcies followed and houses were repossessed. While such cases were few in number in Northridge, it points to caution necessary in making blanket assertions about risk and vulnerability by race and class.

In sum, vulnerability research emphasizes political economic inequalities and processes of racial and ethnic marginalization in relation to risks from environmental hazards. It also stresses the importance of historical political economic factors in the production of inequalities and their links to land use patterns (Oliver-Smith, 1996). It contrasts with mainstream disaster research that has developed a view of disasters as acute events, concentrated in space and time, that engender "unique" social processes different from those found in the pre-disaster setting (Kreps, 1995). The evidence from vulnerability studies is that disasters are produced and shaped by normal operations and material expressions of politics and economics in a place and thus have to be understood in that context. The central focus of the approach on the dynamics of race, ethnicity, and class/economic inequalities has an affinity with approaches used in the environmental justice literature, and I turn to that topic in the conclusion.

RACE, CLASS, AND ENVIRONMENTAL JUSTICE

There is a notable lack of connection between the sociological literature on disasters and burgeoning sociological and geographic research on environmental equity or environmental justice (Fothergill et al., 1999). In this concluding section, I highlight some salient features of the environmental justice literature to suggest ways in which its general approach could be used to strengthen disaster research in the area of race, class, and ethnic inequalities.

The environmental justice literature examines inequalities by race and class in the exposure to technological hazards across a range of spatial and temporal scales. The environmental justice literature, by the very nature of its subject matter, places the subjects of this chapter—race, class, and ethnicity—at the center of its theoretical and empirical concerns (e.g., Boone & Modarres, 1999; Hurley, 1995; Pellow, 2000; Pulido, 1996, 2000). This focus is consonant with political ecological theory and the core of vulnerability analysis, providing important conceptual and research linkages (e.g., Robbins, 2004; Wisner & Walker, 2005). I contend that disaster sociology, in particular, could be broadened and enhanced by more fully engaging environmental justice theoretical and methodological issues. While U.S. disaster sociology clearly can stand alone as a well developed and self-contained specialty, it is not well connected to other realms of socioenvironmental research. The fact that disaster research receives scant mention in recent environmental sociology or political ecology texts can be read as a sign of its lack of recognition or integration in socioenvironmental studies (e.g., Bell, 2004; King & McCarthy, 2005; Robbins, 2004).

While disaster research, almost by definition, has used a temporally bracketed "extreme event" focus (e.g., Quarantelli, 1994), environmental justice research examines the hazards of everyday life at a variety of spatiotemporal scales (e.g., Cutter, 1995b; Tiefenbacher & Hagelman, 1999). At the core of environmental justice is a concern with distributions of hazards and other unwanted land uses, the race and class composition of proximate and distal populations, and the processes that produce landscapes of differential risk. This contrasts with the problematic of disaster research, which with a few important exceptions, seldom targets race and class inequalities in disaster processes. Environmental justice research has devoted significant attention to the question of environmental racism, a discussion that has provided detailed, historically informed analyses of class and race in the production of urban spaces (see Bullard, 1994; Pellow, Weinberg, & Schnaiberg, 2005).

Research on race, class, and environmental risk dates back to what are now considered canonical studies in environmental justice, Bullard's *Dumping in Dixie* (1990) and the United Church of Christ's (UCC's) 1987 report on race and hazardous waste sites in the United States (UCC, 1987). Both studies put class and racially defined minorities at the center of research on environmental risk inequities, focusing on the disproportionate exposure of people of color and the poor to hazardous waste sites. In revealing race-based environmental discrimination, these studies invoked civil rights and social justice issues, and highlighted the pervasiveness of environmental injustices. The UCC studies have since been followed by a large number of sociospatial studies on technological hazards in relation to demographically diverse populations. These studies have developed both in theoretical and methodological sophistication, now drawing off the latest in Geographic Information Systems (GIS) technologies as well as employing innovative methods to assess risks and spatially determine their distributions in relation to vulnerable populations (Cutter, Hodgson, & Dow, 2001).

While a variety of methodologies are employed in this literature that could be adapted to disaster research to understand pre-disaster vulnerabilities and post-disaster processes, I briefly discuss historical environmental justice research as a case in point. Historical equity studies provide in-depth, spatially attuned studies of how racial and class inequalities in hazard exposure develop as an intrinsic part of processes of urbanization and industrialization (e.g., Boone & Modarres, 1999; Hurley, 1995; Szasz & Meuser, 2000). In these historic geographic studies, race and class are dealt with not simply as demographic categories, but as structuring factors in the production of urban space and land uses. These studies probe the historical sources of environmental discrimination through processes of marginalization linked to political–economic processes and other exclusionary practices (Holifield, 2001). Marginalization takes a variety of sociospatially specific forms documented in the research. These may include a wide range of phenomena such as residential sequestration in dilapidated housing and tenements, living in environmentally degraded and hazardous regions, having limited income earning and educational opportunities, persistent discriminatory land use practices, and the penetration of industrial land uses in residential areas (e.g., Pellow, 2000; Szasz & Meuser, 2000). The consequences of these processes are inequalities in access to opportunities and in exposure to hazards, phenomena also at the core of vulnerability analysis of disasters (Varley, 1994a).

Pulido's discussion of the development of environmental injustice in Los Angeles provides an exemplar of a historical geography of race, class, and the production of an urban hazardscape (Pulido, 2000; Pulido, Sidawi, & Vos, 1996). In explaining how landscapes of environmental injustice developed over the course of a century, Pulido (2000, p. 15) advances the concept of "white privilege." In her usage, white privilege denotes a hegemonic form of racism, deeply embedded in ideologies, institutions, and practices, that produces an ensemble of social, political, and economic advantages for Anglos across time and space. In the Pulido research, it manifests itself in whites' abilities to historically control the locations of hazardous industries and waste sites, while being able to avoid the most hazardous and polluted areas of Los Angeles. A variety of mechanisms have been used over the course of a century to construct such inequities, from race-based residential segregation to zoning decisions, bank redlining, and disinvestment in low-income minority neighbors (Pulido, 2000; see also Davis, 1992). Conceptually, it calls attention to the persistence of unequal power relationships of different racial groupings in urban space and the ways that "whiteness" has conferred economic and social benefits to those so identified.

Applied to hazards research in general, historical environmental justice studies illustrate the value of tracing the development of urban hazardscapes and comparative analyses of populations facing the greatest risks with those who are able to avoid them through residential, employment, and land-use decisions. It entails a detailed examination of the political economic mechanisms by which specific environmental inequalities develop and change over time (Szasz & Meuser, 2000). Thus, the growth of white suburbia can be understood as a spatial expression of white privilege, one that has inexorably shifted both environmental and economic burdens onto those who remain in decaying central cities (Bolin, Grineski, & Collins, forthcoming; Bullard, Johnson, & Torres, 2000). Historical environmental justice research directly investigates the development of specific racial projects (Omi & Winant, 1994) by examining how racial categories are instantiated in and shape political economies and urban spaces over time.

I have called attention to both vulnerability analysis and environmental justice research in this chapter to highlight areas where I would judge disaster research to be weak. Much of the disaster literature reviewed in the preceding text fails to provide information on the historical development of the places where disasters occur, likely a by-product of a temporally limited event focus. It also tends to neglect theoretical issues of race or class formation or their specific spatial expressions. As a consequence, few available U.S. studies examine the ways that historical inequalities may affect the unfolding of disasters in particular places (see Kroll-Smith & Couch, 1991 and Peacock et al., 2001 for exceptions).

LOOKING FORWARD

To enrich future disaster research, a better grounding in the historical geographic development of class and race relations in particular places is necessary. This should be combined with more attention given to theoretical issues regarding race and class processes and to spatial analysis of patterns of segregation. Environmental justice research and vulnerability studies both provide models for such analyses that could be incorporated into the ensemble of methodologies already deployed by disaster sociologists (e.g., Morrow, 1999). The regional catastrophe that emerged in the aftermath of 2005's Hurricane Katrina provides researchers with a mandate to attend to the complex historical and political ecological factors that have shaped race and class relations and produced the landscapes of risk so clearly and tragically revealed in the disaster.

With disasters growing in number and severity, often combined with long-term environmental degradation, technological failures, anthropogenic climate change, racial and ethnic conflicts, and growing class inequalities, the shared interests of disaster research, vulnerability studies, and environmental justice research appear clear (Oliver-Smith & Hoffman, 1999; Robbins, 2004). The increased use of political–ecological theory, spatial analysis, and studies of racial formation and class inequalities would strengthen disaster research by providing a spatially and historically informed understanding of the conditions that shape the severity and consequences of disaster. It would also help connect disaster research with a larger intellectual community in environmental sociology, environmental justice studies, and political ecology.

Enhanced understandings of race and class in disasters require more attention to social theory and to a research approach that situates disasters in the context of historical geography and political economy of places and regions. In-depth, interdisciplinary case studies spanning disaster sociology, political ecology and environmental justice research would provide the necessary theoretical and methodological tools to investigate the intersections of social inequalities, hazards, and the production of space. Lastly, new research will require a willingness to critically investigate social inequalities and the social and environmental policies that put people and places at risk.

CHAPTER 8

Gender and Disaster: Foundations and Directions

ELAINE ENARSON, ALICE FOTHERGILL, AND LORI PEEK

Gendered disaster social science rests on the social fact of gender as a primary organizing principle of societies and the conviction that gender must be addressed if we are to claim knowledge about all people living in risky environments. Theoretically, researchers in the area are moving toward a more nuanced, international, and comparative approach that examines gender relations in the context of other categories of social difference and power such as race, ethnicity, nationality, and social class. At a practical level, researchers seek to bring to the art and science of disaster risk reduction a richer appreciation of inequalities and differences based on sex and gender. As the world learns from each fresh tragedy, gender relations are part of the human experience of disasters and may under some conditions lead to the denial of the fundamental human rights of women and girls in crisis.

We begin by briefly discussing the dominant theoretical frameworks that have guided gender disaster research to date and seem likely to develop further. We then organize and review the extant literature around seven interrelated themes. The literature review is designed to highlight published research conducted on human behavior and social consequences in primarily natural disasters and thus does not include, for example, armed conflict and displacement, HIV/AIDS, and other related literatures. The third section of the chapter examines international perspectives in the gender and disaster field. Finally, we point out knowledge gaps and some new directions we hope will guide the endeavors of those who produce and use knowledge about disasters.

THEORETICAL APPROACHES

No single theoretical lens frames disaster research on gender. Indeed, most researchers use insights freely borrowed from all angles of vision, though most begin with a social vulnerability approach (Blaikie, Cannon, Davis, & Wisner, 2004; Bolin, Jackson, & Crist, 1998; Hewitt, 1997). This way of thinking assumes that disasters are fundamentally human constructs that reflect the global distribution of power and human uses of our natural and built environments. Disaster risk is socially distributed in ways that reflect the social divisions that already exist in society. Not a question of "special" populations or a quality of the individual, social vulnerability to disaster is a social dynamic rooted in gender, class, race, culture, nationality, age, and other power relationships. Situational and contextual dimensions cut across these lines, for example, physical (dis)abilities and health concerns, household size and composition, functional literacy, citizenship status, political experience with uniformed state authorities, different degrees of ease on the street at night, and so forth. Used uncritically, this approach can lead to overgeneralizations about women as a social category and overemphasize women's dependency and need (see Fordham, 2004). However, it also inspires many researchers to investigate specific structural sources of vulnerability related to sex and gender, from reproductive health and gender violence to land rights and poverty (Enarson & Morrow, 1998).

The sociopolitical ecology perspective, most clearly used by Peacock, Morrow, and Gladwin (1997) in their edited book on Hurricane Andrew, also calls for a broad ecological and political approach and focuses on interactions—not solely the interaction of human systems and the physical environment, but of all social systems. This way of thinking about hazards and disasters is concerned with conflict, competition, and inequality, rejecting the notion that a community is a single, autonomous social system and conceptualizing community instead as an ecological network of interacting social systems (Peacock & Ragsdale, 1997). From this perspective, social systems are no more gender neutral than they are race neutral (Enarson & Morrow, 1997; Morrow, 1997; Yelvington, 1997).

Feminist political ecology integrates many of these ideas, examining gender relations in specific environmental contexts with an emphasis on women's practical environmental knowledge and the nexus of gender inequalities, environmental degradation, and disaster vulnerability (Rocheleau, Thomas-Slayter, & Wangarai, 1996). Women's roles as primary resource users and managers, their dependence on natural resource based livelihoods, and the responsibilities they have to dependents in the household and community are central concerns. Women are therefore viewed as especially sensitive to hazardous conditions that put their families, homes, and neighborhoods at risk of mudslides, toxic spills, forest fires, gas explosions, and other environmental and technological hazards (among others, see Cutter, 1995b; Cutter, Tiefenbacher, & Soleci, 1992; Steady, 1993). Without accepting the essentialist identification of women and nature embedded in popular eco-feminism, disaster sociologists can and do draw on feminist political ecology to link gender relations to specific environmental contexts. Empirically, feminist political ecologists have analyzed gendered environmental knowledge and survival strategies in drought-prone regions and female leadership in grassroots movements against the destruction of forest resources and toxic waste disposal, among other topics.

Gender and disaster researchers also draw explicitly on feminist theory. Enarson and Phillips (forthcoming) argue that disaster sociology and feminist theories work well together and should forge an even closer relationship as they use similar concepts (e.g., social power, privilege, domination, vulnerability, empowerment, political economy, and social change) and equally embrace global, interdisciplinary, and practice-oriented inquiry with libratory intent. When disaster scholars posit that disasters disrupt "the social system," feminist theory poses the question "whose social system?"

While there are theoretical openings for understanding disaster risk in socialist feminism, postmodern feminism, multiracial feminism, and eco-feminism, most researchers draw either on liberal feminism or gender and development theory. Based on ideas from the western Enlightenment, liberal feminist theory posits that gender differences are for the most part socially created, and that women as much as men have inalienable human rights. They attribute social inequality to unfair barriers to education and achievement, focus on the cultural devaluation of women as well as the gendered division of labor, gender violence, and limitations on reproductive choice (Lorber, 1998). Disaster researchers use these ideas to explain why some women and girls may not have access to equal resources and information in a disaster situation or face discrimination in the aftermath. This approach also leads researchers to investigate how gender stereotypes affect disaster services and emergency operations; the careers of women in the field; and gender bias in the design, funding, implementation, monitoring, and evaluation of emergency shelters, water and sanitation, health care, and other post-disaster initiatives. While liberal feminist thought potentially leads to an equal focus on gender as a factor in men's disaster experiences, this avenue of research has not been developed (but see Alway, Belgrave, & Smith, 1998; Klinenberg, 2002; Scanlon, 1998c, 1999b).

Most of the international research in the field is grounded in gender and development theory (e.g., Fernando & Fernando, 1997; Tinker, 1990). From this perspective, disaster vulnerability cannot be understood outside patriarchy and the historical dynamics of global capitalism and colonialism still shaping the developing world today. Free trade policies that undermine local markets and increase pressures on men to migrate for wage work, for example, leave more women and children impoverished in unsustainable rural environments or displaced to risky urban settlements. Like liberal feminists, gender and development theorists view inadequate maternal and child health care and lack of education for girls as important factors in gendered disaster vulnerability. But gender and development theorists also emphasize the possibilities for women's agency and self-protective action in risky environments based on their reproductive, productive, and community work. This perspective is moving the field from a beneficiary or victim model to one based on barriers to the realization of women's and girls' fundamental human rights in disasters (Acar & Ege, 2001; Enarson & Fordham, 2004). It also invites attention to women's coping strategies in risky environments and brings into view such marginalized groups as female migrants and refugees, women agriculturalists, street vendors, home-based workers, single mothers, widows, and impoverished and low-caste women.

There is ample room for development in every set of ideas that is currently guiding the work of researches and practitioners concerned about gender. As noted by Quarantelli (1998), the focus on gender relations in disaster contexts is one of the contemporary forces for change in thinking and theorizing about hazards and disasters.

KEY EMPIRICAL FINDINGS

While some early disaster research included sex as a survey variable, no careful, thorough, explicit, and purposeful examination of gender in disasters was undertaken until the 1990s. In a key review of the literature to date, Fothergill (1996) summarized a wide range of work documenting significant empirical findings on gender differences and inequalities across the disaster cycle. In the intervening decade, the field has grown considerably and has become increasingly international (see the special issues in the book edited by Morrow & Phillips, 1999 and Phillips & Morrow, forthcoming). Catastrophic events such as the Indian Ocean tsunami and Hurricane Katrina will certainly inspire more gender-focused research in the future. In the following sections we highlight some of the major work to date and draw conclusions in seven interrelated areas.

Class and Gender

Though in-depth class analysis is still relatively rare in gender-focused disaster research, studies that have been done in this area show that class status is an important difference in women's disaster experiences (Finlay, 1998; Fordham, 1999). Indeed, when a disaster does occur, it is clear that those already living in poverty are impacted in different and significant ways compared to other members of society, as Fothergill and Peek (2004) concluded in their major review of the disaster and social class literature. Feminist theorists have long argued that women's experiences and social locations are not universal but are shaped by critical differences grounded in class, caste, age, sexuality, race, ethnicity, religion, nationality, and other factors.

Disaster vulnerability is not synonymous with poverty, however, as the rich can and do buy their way into harm's way. While affluent women are certainly more resilient to economic loss, they do not escape the emotional impacts of evacuation and losing their homes and belongings, the stress of rebuilding, and the anxiety over health and safety in general (Enarson & Fordham, 2004; Fothergill, 2004; Hoffman, 1998). Yet it is clear that economically insecure, low-income, and poor people are most often exposed to environmental harm and have less social choice, more practical constraints, and fewer recovery resources. Because women are generally the poorest of the poor, this is most true for women; disasters frequently leave poor women even more impoverished (Bradshaw, 2001a; Enarson, 2000a, 2001a; Kafi, 1992).

Poor women have a more difficult time recovering from a disaster, as they are often living in crisis before a disaster strikes (Fordham & Ketteridge, 1998). When hunger prevails, women's and girls' food insecurity and their lower caloric intake relative to that of male relatives in some societies makes them physically weaker in the crisis of the moment and less able to survive injuries and deprivations in the aftermath of disaster (Rivers, 1982). Poor women are also more likely than other women to depend on community-based services such as public transportation and health care, including crisis counseling and shelter from violence; when these resources and services are destroyed or undermined by disaster events, poor women's health and safety are affected (Enarson & Fordham, 2001). Low-income women also tend to live in housing that exposes them to harm, living more often than low-income men in poorly maintained public housing, manufactured homes, shelters, and rental properties, and more often than men as low-income single heads of households (Enarson, 1999a). After Hurricane Andrew, poor women of color were observed to be those most in need of housing several years after the disaster (Morrow & Enarson, 1996).

The impacts of disasters on women's paid and unpaid work are well documented, and livelihood protection is the main focus of gender and disaster projects on the ground in the world's poorest nations. In the 1985 Mexico City earthquake, poor single women with children were the hardest hit by the disaster and many of them lost their homes, which were also the site of their livelihoods, as they prepared food at home to sell on the street (Dufka, 1988). Poor women do not have the economic resources (i.e., insurance, land, access to labor, tools) needed to reconstitute their lives and homes following a catastrophe. Low-income women are also unlikely to receive the mental health care that would advance their recovery, though most researchers find that gender relations put women more than men at risk of reports of posttraumatic stress (Ollenburger & Tobin, 1998; Van Willigen, 2001).

Women's long-term economic status following disasters has not been sufficiently studied to arrive at conclusions, but the work of Bradshaw (2001a), Buvinić (1999), and Delaney and Shrader (2000) from Latin America suggests that household structure and ethnicity must also be taken into account. The International Labour Organisation working paper on gender, work, and disaster (Enarson, 2000a) observed that working-class women dependent on social protection, secure employment, public services, and/or home- and homestead-based livelihoods were severely impacted by disasters.

Race/Ethnicity and Gender

Researchers have found that people marginalized by race and/or ethnicity in the United States face barriers stemming from language, culture, experience, stereotypes, discrimination, segregation, and social isolation in the aftermath of disasters (Fothergill, Maestas, & Darlington, 1999). However, race-sensitive gender research conducted on the disaster experiences of race-specific groups of women or men is lacking. For example, while risk communication researchers are sensitive to population diversity, we are aware of no studies that directly address these interactive effects. One early study did find that gender as well as ethnicity, measured and analyzed separately, were important factors in effective communication about earthquake preparedness in southern California (Blanchard-Boehm, 1997).

As might be expected, the intersection of poverty and race/ethnicity may combine to disadvantage women. Researchers from the United States, while rarely focused explicitly on these links, report in qualitative studies that women in subordinated ethnic and racial groups face housing-related difficulties coupled in some cases with discrimination in relief systems. Enarson and Fordham (2001) reported that after the 1997 Grand Forks flood in North Dakota, flood relief was geared away from migrant workers, hurting primarily Hispanic single mothers. Morrow and Enarson (1996), in their research on Hurricane Andrew in Florida, interviewed immigrant and migrant women from Haiti, Cuba, Mexico, and Central America, African-American single mothers and grandmothers, and others. They found that these women faced numerous obstacles, including lack of affordable housing, especially for Latinas and others with large households, slow repair of their residences in public housing units (damaged when managers failed to protect windows), interpersonal violence in the temporary trailer camps in which minority women disproportionately resided, increased "kin work" as ethnic families combined resources, and unnecessarily complex aid applications. Researchers also report that women already marginalized by racial/ethnic bias or economic exclusion are less likely than more privileged women in dominant racial groups to take an active part in long-term recovery efforts. For example, the neglect of issues specifically affecting women of color was one of the reasons for the cross-cultural coalition of women in Miami that arose in the wake of Hurricane Andrew (Enarson & Morrow, 1998). Lacking a sense of political efficacy, Latina migrant workers interviewed after the 1997 Grand Forks flood (Enarson, 2001b) reported feeling excluded from formal political power and informal community rebuilding initiatives, and some expressed interest sparked by the flood in organizing a political presence for Latinas who had worked and lived for many years in the Grand Forks region.

Systematic cross-cultural investigations with emphasis both on gender and culture or ethnicity are also rare. Enarson & Fordham (2001) reported on the "lines that divide" in their comparative discussion of how race, class, and gender affected women before, during, and after major floods in the United States and Scotland. As noted later in this chapter, gender and disaster researchers writing from low-income nations and regions often focus on poor women who are also marginalized by caste or religion, rarely addressing gender in the abstract but as a social construct embedded in a rich cultural context (Ahmed, 2004; Bhatt, 1998; Lovekamp, forthcoming; Rozario, 1997; Shroeder, 1987).

Gender Violence

It is well documented by humanitarian relief agencies and other responders that the risk to girls and women of emotional abuse and physical violence increases in the aftermath of disasters in low-income countries. In their influential report for the United Nations Development Programme (UNDP), Wiest, Mocellin, and Motsisi (1994) state that girls are vulnerable to sexual abuse and exploitation following disasters, and displaced girls especially. More recent studies also find that violence against girls and women is a post-disaster issue for survivors. For example, Nicaraguan families hit by Hurricane Mitch faced many problems including increased family conflict and abuse that may be explained in part as the unintended consequence of the practice of many external relief agencies of targeting women in relief programs (Bradshaw, 2001a). In Cambodia, women worried about the risks of rape and sexual abuse of their daughters who were forced to migrate to find work after floods as a debt repayment strategy (CARE International, 2002). Following the 2004 Indian Ocean tsunami, there were numerous media accounts of violence against women and sexual exploitation of girls. Fisher (2005) corroborated these accounts through interviews with women's advocacy organizations and local experts able to gain the confidence of tsunami-affected women.

Measured by increased requests for service and documented in qualitative interviews with survivors and with the staff of antiviolence agencies responding to them, studies from North America also find that violence against women, especially intimate partner violence, tends to increase in disaster periods (Dobson, 1994; Enarson, 1999b; Honeycombe, 1994; Morrow, 1997; Morrow & Enarson, 1996; Palinkas, Downs, Petterson, & Russel, 1993; Williams, 1994). In North Dakota after the 1997 flood, there was an increased demand for services from the local battered women's shelter, such as counseling and protection orders from abusers, in the immediate and more extended aftermath of the disaster (Fothergill, 2004). Researchers reported that in that same event, some women apparently returned to their abusers if they were desperate for their help or had no housing alternatives (Enarson & Fordham, 2001; Fothergill, 2004). It is also possible that these events afford women the opportunity to leave abusers as a result of relief money and perhaps increased self-confidence (Fothergill, 2004; Morrow & Enarson, 1996).

In her comparison of the preparedness of antiviolence shelters and the impacts of recent earthquakes, floods, hurricanes, ice storms, and landslides on these refuges, Enarson (1999b) found more commonalities than difference between the United States and Canada. For example, more reports of increased violence surfaced in the 12 months after a given disaster event than in the emergency period, owing either to decreased levels of violence, obstacles to reporting and assistance, or some combination of these factors. Following extreme events such as earthquakes and floods, there is a decrease in police protection as social control norms change and laws regarding domestic disputes are often not enforced (Wenger, 1972). In addition, how organizational personnel perceive domestic violence issues before a disaster strongly influences the perceptions and handling of domestic violence issues after a disaster (Wilson, Phillips, & Neal, 1998).

The Gendered Division of Labor

Building on their knowledge of women's multifaceted work roles involving productive, reproductive, and community labor, gender scholars of disaster have analyzed how the division of labor at home, particularly regarding caregiving roles and responsibilities, may increase women's pre-disaster vulnerability and place additional burdens on women during recovery. Women's labor often helps their families to prepare for and cope with disastrous events, and some researchers posit that it is women who have held their families together after a disaster (Dann & Wilson, 1993; Fothergill, 1999; Millican, 1993; Morrow & Enarson, 1996). Disaster work takes on added significance as part of the "second shift" of household labor documented by sociologists (Hochschild, 1989). In most societies, the everyday and immediate responsibilities of parenting and caring for dependents are women's work. In the event of evacuation, it falls to women to create and re-create a sense of security for children in what is often a series of makeshift shelters or temporary houses; for women on the other end, hosting evacuees or displaced relatives and friends, the emotion work of disaster reconstruction can take a large toll (Enarson & Scanlon, 1999). Women's and men's ideas about their appropriate family and household responsibilities have major consequences for their risk perception (Major, 1999), preparedness (O'Brien & Atchison, 1998), and evacuation (Bateman & Edwards, 2002), all of which have documented gender differences. Generally, women often appear to find risk warnings more credible and act on this knowledge by taking protective actions for themselves and their family members (Fothergill, 1996).

In a disaster, mothering becomes more difficult and complicated as conditions become unsafe and as surviving children need more attention during and after the crisis. Slow-onset disasters often degrade water quality and quantity, which puts women's and children's health at risk and greatly expands the demands on mothers to keep children well (Halvorson, 2004; Sultana, forthcoming). A study in Cambodia discovered that women, as the health and child care providers in the family, were under great stress as they felt compelled to keep a vigilant eye on young children while also carrying out other critical work responsibilities in flood disasters (CARE International, 2002). In the aftermath of a disaster, caretaking also becomes much more difficult for women who care for disabled family members, or are disabled themselves (Fothergill, 2004). In the United States, lack of child care was a major barrier to women's return to work and hence to business recovery after the Red River flood that destroyed child care centers and home-based child care facilities (Enarson, 2001b; Fothergill, 2004).

At the most fundamental level, Ikeda (1995), Miyano, Jian, and Mochizuki (1991), Rivers (1982), and others note that caregiving responsibilities put women more at risk of injury and death as they strive to save their children. Gender differences in fatalities can in large part be attributed to the daily patterns of life that put women and men, respectively, at higher risk depending on the time of day and gender-differentiated working patterns.

While female headship is not synonymous with disaster vulnerability, Wiest et al. (1994) argued that women are particularly vulnerable in the developing world because of the large number of women-headed households and the difficult conditions of household management in poor communities in the best of times. The increase in households maintained entirely by women is a well-documented effect of recent disasters. After Hurricane Mitch, women's domestic labor expanded greatly as a result of male desertion and/or the imperative of economic migration (Delaney & Shrader, 2000). Wiest (1998) also documented the "flight of men" in the case of Bangladesh floods with the result that women were forced into wage labor for local landowners.

Field researchers internationally find that, except where cultural norms limit women's contacts outside the home, securing relief assistance and the immediate necessities of life falls largely to women. Both women and men in the United States and elsewhere resist the stigma and shame of receiving public assistance after a disaster event, but it is women who ultimately stand in the lines, negotiate the bureaucratic paperwork, and seek long-term help for family members (Enarson & Fordham, 2004; Fothergill, 2003). Regarding the gendered division of labor in agricultural work, Paolisso, Ritchie, and Ramirez (2002) reported on women's and men's substantially different views of economic impacts on their coffee crops in post-Hurricane Mitch Honduras, suggesting the practical need for gender-specific data and gender-aware impact assessments, especially of economic recovery programs affecting primarily low-income families.

Relief Services and Recovery Efforts

Research shows that gender is relevant in understanding who is assisting with disaster relief services and recovery efforts. For example, women's groups are often actively involved in the crisis period, delivering food and other supplies. Occasionally these are newly formed groups, but more often they are preexisting women's community groups that expand their work to disaster relief operations. Women generally step into relief from established leadership roles at the neighborhood level (Serrat Viñas, 1998) and it is not uncommon for some to move on to progressively more responsible relief and recovery positions (Barnecut, 1998). Both women and men work voluntarily for the most part, sometimes in a sex-segregated fashion, as Cox (1998) demonstrated in her account of a rural Australian community coping with wildfire, and sometimes in more gender-integrated ways, such as in sandbag lines during floods in the United States (Fothergill, 2004).

Overall, however, despite women's considerable work in relief and recovery, most research finds that women are not in positions of authority. A survey on women's roles in disaster management in the Caribbean demonstrated that women were involved in the implementation of relief activities, but not in the decision-making and planning process (Noel, 1998). This was also found in Bangladesh, where women were excluded from disaster response decision-making activities (Khondker, 1996), given fewer relief supplies, and not trusted with response tasks (Begum, 1993). An early Red Cross survey documented organizational barriers to the occupations and rankings of women (Gibbs, 1990), a finding echoed by more current investigations from emergency management organizations in the United States (Wilson, 1999). Women were found to represent only 5% of those trained in emergency management in Australia (Wraith, 1997). Phillips's (1990) groundbreaking study of gender bias in emergency management reported that women were underrepresented in the emergency management field and easily excluded from the organizational "old boys' network." However, the study also found that women contribute positively to the profession and often bring a heightened sensitivity to the socioemotional needs of survivors.

Regarding access to help, women's short-term needs and long-term interests are often neglected. Social class, race, and ethnicity were found to be powerful determinants of aid in qualitative profiles from the aftermath of Hurricane Andrew (Enarson & Morrow, 1997; Morrow, 1997; Yelvington, 1997). Poor women did not always receive the assistance to which they were entitled as relief was based on a single "head of household" model that tended to privilege men (Morrow & Enarson, 1996). Childers (1999) found that low-income elderly women were disproportionately in need of economic assistance but less likely to receive it. Women were also at a disadvantage in federal disaster relief programs for small businesses (Nigg & Tierney, 1990), and women-owned businesses had disproportionately high failure rates in one flooded mid-western community (Staples & Stubbings, 1998). Women are less often employed in housing construction roles than men but do find work in human service jobs created after a disaster; hard-hit women lacking college degrees or professional experience often benefit the least from these new jobs (Enarson, 2001a).

Limited political rights and lack of information about existing legal rights compound the barriers to women's recovery created by gender relations, as illustrated in the accounts from

is, researchers in different regions have many common concerns about gender but distinct empirical and theoretical foundations.

Writing from affluent societies in North America and Europe, researchers tend to examine gender (read: women) as a stand-alone category, explore discrete disaster events, address response and relief issues and the social vulnerabilities of gender, undertake studies at the individual and household levels, and are especially interested in women as caregivers and professional emergency managers. The contrast is striking when compared to the work of researchers studying cyclones, floods, earthquakes, and drought in the poorest countries of the world. Here researchers tend to work with gender in cultural context as one among other dimensions of social life; study communities from the inside-out, often utilizing participatory research methods; and take a much stronger interest in risk management through vulnerability reduction, hazard mitigation, capacity building, and sustainable development and reconstruction. Researchers focus more on collective than on individual impacts and responses and on the transformative potential of disasters for empowerment. Women's livelihoods and earning potential and women as grassroots community leaders in risk reduction are major concerns. A disastrous cyclone or landslide is understood as the manifestation of a process with deep historical, cultural, political, economic, and environmental roots. Indeed, women may be more visible to disaster theorists from lesser-developed countries because what is under investigation is not the crisis, but the conditions leading up to the crisis. Some of these differences in theoretical perspectives are explained by environmental context, stage of development, and research inspired by high-profile disasters in which gender differences and inequalities were difficult to miss on the ground or theoretically. Other factors are the research agendas of international women's organizations and movements and the particular development of disaster sociology in the United States. It may be that some of the effects of globalization will foster a convergence of what now appear to be distinct lines of analysis and research. At a minimum, extremes of wealth and poverty arising through increased globalization mitigate against simplistic analysis of "gender relations" or "women" as unitary concepts.

We argue that the best theoretical work with the most urgently needed practical dimension is written from the world's most dangerous places and about women and men who must learn to live with risk. Practitioners, policymakers, community leaders, emergency managers, activists, and scholars concerned about gender equity and open to gender analysis have much to learn from those writing at the turn of the century from the world's most fragile places.

KNOWLEDGE GAPS AND FUTURE RESEARCH

Once conspicuous by its absence, a gender perspective is embraced today by an international community of scholars who see gender as an intersecting dimension of human life and hence of disaster risk management. Since 1990, researchers, policy makers, community members, and disaster practitioners have gathered seven times for major conferences in Costa Rica, Australia, Pakistan, Canada, the United States, and Turkey. United Nations agencies focused on gender and on disasters, respectively, have made the experiences of women and children salient, for example, through the 1995 United Nations International Decade for Natural Disaster Reduction (UN/IDNDR) campaign on "women and children as keys to prevention" and, more recently, the 2001 United Nations Division for the Advancement of Women Expert Working Group on Gender, Environmental Management, and Disaster Risk. In the wake of the 2004 Indian Ocean tsunami, the World Health Organization (WHO), the United Nations Development Fund for

Women (UNIFEM), the International Labour Organization (ILO), and other international governmental organizations (IGOs) and international nongovernmental organizations (INGOs) took a strong interest in the survival needs of women and children. The United Nations International Strategy for Disaster Reduction (UN/ISDR, 2003) continues to strongly promote gender equality and disaster risk reduction (see Briceño, 2002). It is noteworthy that the electronic Gender and Disaster Network (2005) now includes more than 300 women and men in its membership database. While this is a rich and productive field, there are many areas in need of further study. In the following section, we briefly present nine specific knowledge gaps where we believe more research is warranted. We present these using the imperative verb form, but with appreciation for researchers already working in these areas.

Think More About Bodies and Sexuality

It is important that scholars and practitioners recognize that in real emergencies there are no disembodied "emergency managers," "volunteers," or "parents" and no degendered "disabled," "poor," or "seniors." All people are embodied social actors with multiple and fluid identities and interests. Our bodies imply differences that matter in disaster contexts. Aging populations are female dominated, so planning with and for elders means attending to gender issues germane to older women. Imbalanced sex ratios in disasters hitting women or men disproportionately matter in assessments of community vulnerability generally and gendered vulnerability specifically; these warrant much more attention. Sexual difference demands more analysis of women's and men's reproductive health needs and maternal health in particular. Gender violence is a fact of life for legions of girls and women and must be investigated as a factor reducing individual, household, and community resilience. Among "the disabled" are women living with cognitive and/or physical disabilities, HIV or AIDS, and chronic illness— and with disproportionately high rates of gender violence, poverty rates, and responsibilities for others.

Sexual orientation is a vastly understudied dimension of human experience in crisis. In the aftermath of the September 11 attacks, gay and lesbian communities were among those not well served by disaster assistance organizations (Eads, 2002). Gay and lesbian advocacy organizations are rare in all countries and hard pressed to meet even the most fundamental needs of gay, lesbian, bisexual, and trans-gender persons after disasters. How can emergency managers plan to help without even rudimentary knowledge of their living conditions, capacities, and vulnerabilities in a social crisis?

Focus on Girls and Women

Gender scholars are often charged, correctly, with focusing mainly on women. While in the following paragraphs we call for more gender analysis of men in disasters, here we argue for more research on gender inequalities—and that means women and girls first. We say this not because gender norms do not matter as much to men, but because there is already evidence that girls and women are endangered in times of crisis by sexual and domestic violence, cultural constraints on their mobility, poverty, language and literacy barriers, insecure housing, limited or nonexistent land and inheritance rights, barriers to their fair access to new information technologies and to "old" media such as radios, and overt and covert constraints on their public presence and voice. In the 2004 Indian Ocean tsunami, the everyday facts of life for women and girls cost tens of thousands their lives—simply because they did not know how to swim or wore restrictive clothing or, more often, because of the gendered division of labor, the cultural imperative to protect their children, lack of autonomy to move freely in a world of men, and the urgent need of poor women to protect the dowry jewelry and other assets that represent their daughters' futures (Oxfam International, 2005). Having said this, it is also vital that we de-link "women and children" analytically and ask: Which women? Which children? Girls and boys? In what context? The lives of children in risky environments cannot be fully understood without gender analysis but, too often, we are quick to assume a common interest rather than empirically investigating when or whether the needs and interests of women and their sons and daughters are the same.

Acknowledge Capacities and Strengths

While it is important that we understand the ways in which women and girls may be vulnerable in disasters, it is just as critical that we understand their capacities and strengths in disaster situations. Gender scholars have been concerned that females are portrayed in the media and in scholarship as helpless victims who need rescuing in a disaster, and that by focusing solely on that image we have lost sight of the ways in which women are capable, strong, and resilient. Therefore, in future research we must investigate gender-based resources and strengths with the same enthusiasm we bring to the study of gendered vulnerability. Gender researchers across the disciplines have shown that the life experiences of women and men often lead them to different kinds of social bonds, community knowledge, information networks, power and influence, technical and administrative skills, family care experience, livelihood assets, environmental knowledge, and activist traditions. These experiences are relevant to our central research questions and must be considered in order to develop a more complex and comprehensive understanding of women's and men's lives.

Look Inside the Household

In any society the household is a distributive system in which different actors bring different resources to bear as they prepare for disasters and strive to recover from their effects. Gender analysis helps answer: Who has access to and/or control over property, time, information, labor, and relief goods and services? Gender is also a key factor in decision-making in intimate relationships, for example, regarding household preparedness, evacuation, or relocation. With this knowledge, preparedness campaigns and early warning systems can be fine tuned and perhaps gender targeted; without it, initiatives may fail. We must also consider constraints on women's autonomy, asking in any community under study which women, if any, are free to speak publicly, attend community meetings, act outside the household, access shelters, and otherwise act independently of men. Gender violence against women and girls in their homes—from intimate partner abuse and "honor" killings to forced early marriage and marital rape—makes fear an everyday reality for millions of women around the world. Their risk of trafficking to sex work and other forms of coerced labor may also increase after disasters. It is important to consider how community members and risk managers can best use this knowledge.

In addition, interior living spaces and the homestead area are typically workplaces for girls and women. Here they earn income or otherwise support themselves and their families through direct care for dependents (paid and/or unpaid), food preparation (for consumption and/or sale), and home-based production and service work of all kinds. A gender lens is needed when we study residences as workplaces in our work on economic and social vulnerability, preparedness, impact, and short- and long-term recovery.

Think Globally

To understand disaster vulnerability and gender relations, we must examine the root causes of social changes—including the global political economy, religious fundamentalism, and social movements for and against the liberation of women. This means we need to think globally. For example, we need not only document the numbers of women now heading households alone in the aftermath of an earthquake, but also analyze the gendered dimensions of international labor migration and of armed conflict that may have made them heads of households long before the disaster. Global trends impacting women can be seen as "early warning signs" of reduced capacity to anticipate, survive, and recover from the effects of disasters of all kinds. For example, women need to be included in economic recovery after a disaster in order to realize full family and community recovery. Increasing economic gaps between women in high- and low-income nations can be analyzed in light of cross-national movements for risk reduction. We note with optimism the impetus to gendering climate change research and policy and call for more context-specific research addressing gender relations as a factor in mitigation, impact, and adaptation. Action research partnerships crossing the borders of the nation-state are also essential if we are to understand and address the gendered effects of globalization on hazards and disaster risk.

Engage Gender Politics

The construction of knowledge is always a social process, so there is always a gender politic to our work as students of disaster. In our view, scholars must link women's human rights to disaster risk theoretically, in research, practice, and political work. We must ask: How do increasing social inequalities within and between nations and regions impact the fundamental human rights of men and women in crisis? How do land-use decisions affect the housing, employment, and transportation options of women and men, respectively?

What kinds of gender relations, political–economic and military contexts, and environmental pressures increase women's risk in disasters of death, injury, or disempowerment? Conversely, what configuration of gender relations enhances disaster risk reduction? As communities with more egalitarian relations between women and men seem better able to reduce and cope with the effects of disasters, we must develop this line of research.

Explore Difference

Close examination of gender power as a social fact affecting all dimensions of risk management can and must be integral to our analysis of ethnicity and race, caste and class, age, sexual orientation, mental and physical (dis)abilities, citizenship, religion, and other categories of power—and the inverse is no less true. Gender cannot be understood in isolation. We find gender and disaster scholarship generally more nuanced and intersectional than the norm but there is much room for improvement. Understanding differences among women based on race and ethnicity, caste and class, nationality and culture, sexuality, religion, life stage, and physicality is vital. Indeed, it can be life saving. Like differences among women based on employment, marital status, and household size and structure, these must be more carefully explored in support of gender-aware disaster risk management. We call specifically for more direct attention to gender and race/ethnicity and to gender and cultural difference more broadly.

Work with Men as Well as with Women

Unless the theoretical questions at hand relate exclusively or predominantly to men or to women, the "gold standard" of our research must be interrelationships between women and men, girls and boys. Without asking, how will we know whether or to what extent hazards and risks are constructed and experienced differently by women and men in different social, cultural, and geographic locations? How, whether, or to what extent masculine norms impinge on men and boys, for example to disempower or empower them, or make them more or less safe? Sex differences in mental and physical health should be investigated as a disaster public health concern as well as boys' exposure to gender violence and male-on-male interpersonal violence generally. Sex-based differences in vulnerability to human-induced pandemics will surely be a topic of interest to future researchers. We await more research on the gender-related experiences of South Asian men widowed by the 2004 Indian Ocean tsunami in such large numbers and now stepping into unanticipated domestic and caregiving roles in villages and towns across the region.

Collaborate with Women's Groups

Grassroots women's groups may have first-hand knowledge about environmental and population pressures, local political dynamics, and leadership structures in high-risk neighborhoods. They may have insight for researchers into those most "hidden in plain view" among the socially invisible (e.g., old women in substandard housing, women with newborns, and those caring at home for the terminally ill), stigmatized groups (e.g., women and girls living with HIV/AIDS or profound cognitive disabilities), persecuted groups (e.g., trafficked women, undocumented women doing migrant labor), and transient, homeless, and displaced women. Participatory action research is needed with women's professional, civic, educational, and faith-based organizations, and also with women working "under the radar" against environmental racism and for the rights of sexual minorities, against unsustainable local development, and for school, neighborhood, and workplace safety. More insight is needed, too, about how the actions of local activists—to name a few, those organizing locally around land-use and transportation challenges, community health, affordable housing, land rights, immigrant rights, indigenous land rights, children's rights, and disability rights—relate to disaster resilience. Their expertise and local knowledge is as valuable as the insights of professional women in disaster response and emergency management roles.

GENDERING RESEARCH AND ACTION TO REDUCE DISASTER RISK

Many lessons can be learned from gender and disaster researchers but only with concerted effort to synthesize the applications and exchange insights and concerns about gender with practitioners. There is a long way to go. In most training courses or college classes, gender is addressed sparingly in "special populations" courses or texts. Few teaching resources are available and much of the best work has not yet been translated, especially from Spanish to English. This work must be shared and mined for use in ways that reduce avoidable suffering and mitigate the human impacts of disastrous events. The 2004 Indian Ocean tsunami is a case in point. In the weeks and months following the tsunami, NGOs, IGOs, and INGOs posted repeated e-mail requests for "checklists and guidelines" for assisting women and children. The research community readily responded with reference to existing guidelines and bibliographies, and women's groups in Sri Lanka and elsewhere articulated emerging gender threats and needs. But the large gap between survivors, policymakers, funders, practitioners, and academics was hard to miss and is more likely than not to recur.

Within the research community, moving from knowledge to action is a familiar challenge, but what accounts for the resistance to a more gender-sensitive approach? Among the answers are lack of enthusiasm for the critique of gender power, a misreading of gender analysis as an artifact of Western feminism, and the power of funding agencies, governments, and mainstream NGOs to drive the research and action agenda in every region. In the developing world, the urgent need to connect gender, development, and disaster risk reduction is clear and scholarship in these regions reflects this. But this writing is too little known or used. Internationally, we note barriers of language, technology, secure employment, technical support, travel funds, Internet access, and a host of other material resources that keep the strong gender analysis of researchers and field workers in low-income nations out of the mainstream even of gender and disaster scholarship.

What is needed? Appropriate levels of public- and private-sector support can help researchers with a new or established interest in gender undertake more gender-sensitive and theoretically informed research on a host of critical questions across regions and disciplines. Then we can teach what we learn by revising and developing courses and educational resources, and use what we learn by bringing science-based knowledge about all people to the management of risk in our increasingly risky world. Assessments are needed of how and where the gender literature is taught and what teaching techniques and resources are most effective. International teaching exchanges, paper competitions, and mentoring programs are needed for young professionals interested in gender and disaster, and material support for gender researchers from low-income countries and regions. Certainly, teaching about gender and disasters through training modules and distance education would advance the field. It is also necessary to encourage and fund scholarship that bridges the North–South divide, promote the use of gender experts on international research teams, plan special journal issues on international perspectives of gender and disasters, and support gender-sensitive multidisciplinary workshops, roundtables, consultations, and policy-oriented networks. These are among the many useful strategies that researchers in this field can advocate to see their work put to use.

CONCLUSIONS

Disaster social science is at a critical juncture, challenged by new definitions of "homeland security," the urgency of climate change, the threat of new pandemics, increasing global militarization, extreme development pressures on people, places, and resources, and entrenched social inequalities in an increasingly divided world. We are optimistic that gendering disaster theory and research will help us connect with the energies, passions, and knowledge of a larger community of activist scholars equally concerned about people, place, and risk. Expanding the field of disaster social science in this way would be a major contribution of the gender and disaster paradigm.

ACKNOWLEDGMENTS

The authors thank the editors of the *Handbook of Disaster Research* for their support and feedback. Portions of this chapter were delivered by Elaine Enarson at the 2004 conference sponsored by the University of Delaware Disaster Research Center on "Disaster Research and the Social Sciences: Lessons Learned and Future Trajectories."

CHAPTER 9

Globalization and Localization: An Economic Approach

J.M. ALBALA-BERTRAND

The aim of this chapter is to assess, from an economic perspective, ways in which actual globalization is likely to affect disaster vulnerability. We approach the issue by putting forward an economic concept of disaster localization. It is first shown that a localized disaster is unlikely to affect the macroeconomy in any significant way. In addition, development tends to make all disasters localized as an incidental consequence of its endogenous and exogenous processes. The people and activities directly affected by a disaster may still undergo severe difficulties, but these are likely to be less intense and more rapidly counteracted in countries with higher levels of integration, diversification, and general development. That is, as economic resilience and economic disaster confinement increase, disaster vulnerability is bound to decrease. However, the effect of current globalization on vulnerability seems to be double edged. On the one hand, globalization is likely to speed up the downgrading of vulnerability at the national level by helping to upgrade localization. On the other, however, at least in the short and medium terms, globalization may increase vulnerability at the local level by disenfranchising communities and individuals as well as adding new sources of economic instability. Does globalization help the process of disaster localization? Is current globalization beneficial for the people and activities that can be directly affected by a potential disaster? In other words, we look at the ways in which the main economic features of actual globalization might affect disaster vulnerability, at national and local levels.[1]

GLOBALIZATION, THE BUSINESS CYCLE, AND VULNERABILITY

Globalization, the business cycle, and vulnerability are three interacting processes of economic life, which we use as a basic framework for an analysis of economic localization and resilience.

---

[1] Given restriction of space, there is no attempt at detailing some propositions and statements, but to refer them to reliable sources where they have been treated appropriately. The thesis proposed in the present chapter is novel and derives from my own approach and work, as referred to here.

As in themselves they are not the focus of our analysis, it is necessary to define them consistently so as to set up their boundaries to help our ensuing analysis.

Globalization

Globalization is a societal process that widens and deepens the interactions between each country and the rest of the world. In general, these interconnections refer to the institutions associated with the flows of goods, services, people, information, and cultural traits in a worldwide context. In particular, economic globalization refers to the institutions associated with the flows of traded goods and services, financial and direct capital, migrant labor and tourism, and economic information and ideas, within a global arena of cultural institutions and traits. All this will tend to make global administrative and communication structures more flexible and expedited, while transport and means of exchanging and distributing information become cheaper. The most forceful advocates of economic globalization, normally associated with the so-called "Washington Consensus," claim that as more countries join their preferred and currently dominant policy package, economic and social benefits for everybody will come over time. The detractors normally agree that higher levels of global integration could be economically and socially beneficial, but have serious doubts about the type of economic policies that are currently pursued for this purpose. The main reason for their misgivings is that a rapid, unregulated, and socially unaccommodating transition to higher stages of globalization has often produced deleterious consequences for the economy in general and for the most vulnerable people in particular. The transition length toward the supposedly equitable benefits of a higher stage of globalization remains so far undefined (for a good collection on the issues above, see *Oxford Review of Economic Policy* 2004, Vol. 20, No. 1).

In short, the "Washington Consensus" represents a package of neoliberal policies agreed to mainly by U.S. officials, the International Monetary Fund (IMF), and the World Bank in the mid-1980s, in connection with the required stabilization and structural adjustment of the countries affected by the 1980s debt crisis (Stiglitz, 1998). This later became the policy package behind the dominant model of current globalization. Its main components are free foreign trade, specialization via static comparative advantages, liberalization of capital flows, the "flexibilization" of the labor market, balanced budgets and privatization, a minimal and subsidiary role for the state, and the deregulation of most if not all price signals (Fischer, 2003; Williamson, 1990). The main alternative, and seemingly more successful, model of globalization is the Asian Model, which is the one followed by Taiwan and South Korea, based on the economic experience of Japan after World War II. Here the state has an important role to play, as free markets are not considered as self-adjusting toward the best socioeconomic outcome, as regards industrial policy, employment, growth rates, technological sophistication, income distribution, and poverty. These Asian countries demonstrate the greatest success in all these areas among most countries, let alone developing countries (Chang, 1996; Chang & Grabel, 2004).

In a social vacuum, we can theoretically describe economic globalization as a continuum from autarky (a fully closed economy) to a fully liberal (fully free-market) world, just as if the world were to become a single unrestricted economy. In practice, however, the fully liberal ideal appears as economically farfetched and socially undesirable even within a country (Ibid.). In addition, there are increasing problems associated with the deepening and enhancing of economic globalization via the currently dominant policies, which have been widely studied in the real world. First, there appears to be normally a short- to medium-term increase of vulnerability, especially of the poorest sections of society, increasing poverty, and inequality. The latter appears unchecked even in countries that the "Washington Consensus" would consider as prime example of success, such as Chile, which has the ninth worse income distribution in the world (Human Development Report, 2004; Pizarro, 1996). Second, a good deal of economic instability and economic destruction has also been associated with unregulated financial flows (Weisbrot & Baker, 2001; Weller, 2001). Third, this has also carried serious political instability and social victimization, such as in Argentina 2001 (Damill, Frenkel, & Maurizio, 2003; Frenkel, 2003). Finally, there appears to be a clear asymmetry in the compliance with current globalization precepts between the developed and developing countries (Guadagni & Kaufmann, 2004)· In fact, no serious economist would argue about the existence of such actual problems, but about their interpretation and solutions, and not least about their socially acceptable time-length persistence. This may have not unimportant consequences for the globalization project as a whole, but it also shows that current globalization, in its purist "Washington Consensus" guise, may have significantly become a political ideology (Stiglitz, 2002; Wade, 1996; Weiss, 2002).

The main visible aspect of current globalization is the strength and speed of capital flows and secondarily the integration of domestic production into the world market. Restrictions on labor mobility, however, appear as an uneasy countertrend. Free-trade integration has already created serious transition cost associated with the fast, uncoordinated, and inequitable domestic structural change that seems required to fit into the global economy (Rudra, 2002). Free unregulated capital flows, in turn, have rendered economies even more unstable and less policy independent than before (Eichengreen, 2001; Grabel, 2002). Therefore, at least in the medium term, these processes are likely to render significant numbers of people more differentially at risk and hence more vulnerable than before. There are, however, proposals for other ways of inserting into the global economy, which do not require enduring the worse social and economic costs of this enterprise (Chang & Grabel, 2004; Mansoob, 2002; Nayyar, 2002, Stiglitz, 2002; Wade, 1990; World Bank, 2001).

The Business Cycle

Another point to consider is that globalization policies and effects occur in interaction with the business cycle, which means that some negative aspects of disaster vulnerability may be amplified in recessions. The business cycle is a sequence of sustained upturns and downturns of gross domestic product (GDP) and employment, associated with economic shocks and/or agents' decisions, affecting aggregate demand (investment, consumption, trade, public expenditure), which are in turn mediated by a collection of societal factors and expectations of economic and political nature. The mediating aspects are not well understood and, therefore, policy attempts at preventing, rather than correcting, the cycle may not normally be forthcoming or successful (Bergtrom, 1995). Up until recently, the seeming absence of a synchronic cycle in the developed countries grouped in the Organization for Economic Cooperation and Development (OECD) contributed to smoothen and soften the world cycle. That is, when Japan was in a downturn phase, the United States and Germany (or the EU) would be in an upturn phase, and vice versa. Lately, it seems that the domestic cycles of OECD countries have become both more synchronic and more dependent on the phase of the U.S. economy than before, China being both a dependent and modifying factor of the U.S. cycle. However, the business cycle of open developing economies, especially small ones, has always been very much synchronic with that of the main OECD trading partner. But there has also been the possibility of diversifying trading partners over time, so as to reduce their vulnerability to single-partner economic cycles. This is something that globalization could foster, but such a diversifying strategy may be tampered with in the presence of a business cycle that appears to be more synchronic with the U.S. world locomotive than before. Globalization itself seems to be behind this hegemonic tendency. If the cycle becomes more synchronic and more people are rendered increasingly vulnerable by virtue of the current dominant type of globalization, then the timing of a major disaster in the developing world may have more serious consequences than currently, as is shown later.

Vulnerability

A disaster impact is normally the result of a physically or societally uncompensated tension, which translates into death, damage, destruction, and the disarticulation of societal frameworks. In the case of natural disasters, the uncompensated tension is due to the physical weakness of structures and societal processes that fail to compensate for extreme natural events, such as earthquakes, hurricanes, floods, and the like. As such, even if the natural event were fully exogenous to society, the physical resistance to geophysical phenomena would not be. It depends on both disaster-proof technology and sociopolitical access to it, which is mostly an endogenous societal process. This is also true in the case of technological disasters, but here the inducing phenomenon is also fully endogenous, associated with the institutional failure to put a check on the production, containment, and the use of risky technology. This is then a societal process fully in-built in construction regulations and technology handling as well as technology monitoring and disciplining, control systems and warning, and a range of compensatory actions. In turn, a socially/politically induced disaster impact, such as riots, civil wars, wars, and the like (i.e., "complex humanitarian emergencies") is normally the result of a societal/institutional weakness that fails to accommodate competing identity groups. This is a fully endogenous phenomenon, in-built in social structure and dynamics (Albala-Bertrand, 2000a). In this chapter, however, we concentrate on natural hazards only, as the other disaster types have characteristics of their own, which are beyond the scope of this chapter. This takes us to the issue of vulnerability.

We generically define vulnerability as the exposure of both physical and societal frameworks to violent events. The latter refers to the exposure of institutions and organized people to violent or extreme events. The degree of exposure is in turn associated to the risk of failure (or dislocation) of an item (or framework) to a potential event of a given magnitude. This gives rise to two not independent types of vulnerability: physical and societal. Society's physical arrangements are paramount in explaining disaster damage. But these are the result of societal processes that confine people and activities to a physically vulnerable built-up environment (and unsafe technology) or to societal processes that increasingly weaken the physical environment where people live and work, or both. These societal processes are the result of prevailing institutions, and in turn institutional arrangements are also paramount in explaining resilience and recovery from a disaster impact.

The main processes behind physical vulnerability to both natural and technological hazards are unsafe living quarters (building quality and location) and unsafe economic activities (engineering quality and location of structures and risky processes). In turn the main societal factors, which may increase the proneness and destructiveness of disasters, are entitlement erosion (economic and political possessions, access, and rights) and environmental degradation (pollution, deforestation, overcrowding, and the like). These four factors are the result of society's processes of production and reproduction, which may differentially affect some individuals and groups as well as increase overall risk in unpredictable ways. Hence, whatever the potential unleashing event (geophysical, technological, or political), the proneness of the social/physical system and its increased vulnerability to such events are largely part and parcel of society's ongoing structure and dynamics. It is therefore society itself that, by creating and modifying institutions, may increase or reduce its proneness and vulnerability to geophysical and socially made events (see Albala-Bertrand, 1993, 2000a, 2000b).

Lack of political influence, lack of economic alternatives, poverty, and overall societal disenfranchising may be at the foundation of vulnerability. A good deal of increased vulnerability and disaster risk can be attributed to the wholesale policy rearrangements demanded and imposed by a socially unconcerned globalization. Notice also that rural disenfranchising, associated with multinational cash-crop agriculture, with its enclosures, evictions, and capital-intensive technology, pushes masses of impoverished people to unsafe locations and buildings in both rural and urban areas (ravines, shanty towns, overcrowded inner city), increasing their vulnerability. In addition, some cash crops, which may be efficient to produce hard currency, might not constitute food to live on, like peanuts. So when a world recession comes, some communities may find themselves with less food available than before, with both countryside and cities affected (Albala-Bertrand, 1993).

This is translated into a policy inconsistency, in which institutional rearrangements are imposed with a pace and extent that are significantly faster, deeper, and wider than the ability of the most vulnerable people and activities to adapt and accommodate within a minimum of stability. This often puts people and activities in both a precarious livelihood condition and a safety vacuum, which could be aggravated by a synchronic business cycle. That is, some features of unfettered globalization might largely explain safety negligence, entitlement erosion, and environmental degradation.

DISASTER LOCALIZATION

Overall economic vulnerability to disasters, from a macroeconomic viewpoint, can be traced back to a weak, undiversified, and unresponsive economy. If after a disaster, the economy of a country holds, then there would potentially be more domestic capacity to respond both endogenously and exogenously to it. In addition, a more responsive economy would require less foreign aid, while aid and loans would be more forthcoming. In which circumstances would an economy then be more likely to hold in the face of a natural hazard? Are these circumstances favored by globalization? These questions can be answered by using an appropriate concept of localization.

In most studies, the word localization is used often, and usually refers to the geographic extent of either the event or the disaster impact itself in a rather ubiquitous manner. Given that this type of extent does not appear to mean much in the absence of the type of economy that is within the affected area, we proposed a combined concept in another work (Ibid.). That is, a disaster is localized if it affects a confined geographic area and/or a confined area of economic activity. This implies that a geographically widespread disaster can be economically localized (e.g., a drought in a diversified country) or widespread (e.g., a drought in an agriculturally

TABLE 9.1. The Issue of Localization[a]

		Economic Viewpoint	
		Localized	Widespread

G
E
O
G
R
A
P
H
I
C
	L
	O
	C
	A
	L
	I
	Z
	E
	D
		(11)
		
		Most disasters
		
		e.g., <u>Malawi</u> and <u>Bangladesh</u>
		  (both in later years)
			(12)
			
			Some disasters
			
			i.e., Capital city or key industry
			  (e.g., <u>Ecuador</u> 1987 earthquake)
			e.g., <u>Bangladesh</u> (in earlier years)

V
I
E
W
P
O
I
N
T
	W
	I
	D
	E
	S
	P
	R
	E
	A
	D
		(21)
		
		Diversified economy
		
		e.g., drought in Uruguay or hurricane
		  in <u>Ecuador</u>
		
		e.g., <u>Dominica</u> (in later years)
			(22)
			
			Undiversified agricultural economy
			
			e.g., <u>Malawi</u> (in earlier years) and
			  Sahelian countries
			
			Small islands (with diversification.
			
			e.g., <u>Dominica</u> (earlier years) and
			  Monserrat's volcano

[a]This classification refers only to direct disaster effects (stock effects). Notice also that some countries are underlined when they appear in two different cells at different times. This is to show how similar disasters are likely to become more localized over time, as countries both generally develop and specifically protect against hazards.

undiversified least developed country, like a Sahelian country). Hence, our early conclusion is that as most disasters are economically localized, they are unlikely to have serious macroeconomic effects, especially on GDP (Ibid.). This assertion can be presented and analyzed by means of a double entry table and some useful examples, especially from Benson and Clay (2004), so that the concept of localization can be unambiguously defined for later usage (see Table 9.1).

Our concept of localization corresponds to the first column of Table 9.1: cells (11) and (21), that is, economic localization. As a corollary, the second column shows that a disaster can be economically widespread, whether it is geographically widespread or not. Cell (11) shows the most common case, as it is likely that the majority of geographically localized disasters are also economically localized. As examples, we can focus on Bangladesh (especially floods and cyclones) and Malawi (droughts). Since the 1990s these countries underwent geographically localized disasters, which had severe impact in the affected areas, but did not translate into significant losses for the economy as a whole. The initial impacts were short lived and more than compensated within a year or so. Cell (12) shows that some geographically localized disasters can also be economically widespread if they strike a key industry (normally an exporting one, like oil, bananas, etc) or a main industrial/political city (normally the capital city). For example, in 1987, an earthquake in Ecuador damaged the main oil pipe for this export. This is, however, a rare event, as even when major earthquakes struck a capital city (e.g., Managua 1972, Guatemala City 1976, Mexico City 1985) they do not translate into widespread economic effects, so this is more possibility than necessity. Another example would be the cyclone and floods in Bangladesh (then East Pakistan) contributing to the separatist momentum and civil war of independence in early 1970s. The disasters appear to have acted as triggers of a growing institutional conflict with West Pakistan (Albala-Bertrand, 1993). But the above disasters were geographically localized, which in normal times would unlikely create significant widespread effects on the macroeconomy, as was shown in the previous point.

Cell (21) shows that geographically widespread disasters can also be economically localized. This is the case when a geographically widespread disaster strikes a diversified economy, mainly affecting one economic sector, normally the agricultural sector (e.g., droughts in Latin America or even widespread hurricanes in diversified islands like Dominica since the 1980s). It would be unusual that this unleashes important macroeconomic effects, unless the affected sector was pivotal for the rest of the economy, which is unlikely in diversified open economies. Notice also that even when one sector or industry undergoes the brunt of damage from a sudden disaster, such as a flood or an earthquake, this would unlikely be fully impaired, as disaster impact effects are never homogeneous. Finally, cell (22) represents the case of geographically widespread disasters that also have an economically widespread impact. This normally refers to a geographically widespread disaster that strikes an undiversified agricultural economy (e.g., droughts in Sahelian countries) or a small semidiversified island (e.g., hurricanes in small Caribbean islands, such as St. Lucia and Dominica in the late 1970s—fishing, agriculture, and tourism might suffer considerably). It also includes rare events such as the Monserrat's volcano in 1995. The latter would have been widespread however economically diversified the country was at the time, as all sectors would have suffered total or partial impairment, which might be expected to cause structural change (Benson & Clay, 2004). In most cases of widespread disaster, however, the persistence of the macroeconomic effects would be confined to around 2 to 3years after the disaster impact, except in slowly developing disaster such as droughts (Albala-Bertrand, 1993; Benson & Clay, 2004).

If we look again at the table above, we can see that some disaster-prone countries, which were located in cells (12) and (22) in early years, reappear in cell (11) or (21) in later years, that is, the countries undergo more localized disasters from similar natural events over time. For example, Malawi moves from (22) to (11), while Dominica does from (22) to (21), and Bangladesh from (12) to (21). This is an indication that for disaster-prone countries, as a rule, development can be conceived as a process that transforms all types of disaster into economically localized ones, that is, toward cells (11) and (21). This appears to have been the case of the three countries mentioned above (Benson & Clay, 2004). This is then also an indication that development and reduced macroeconomic vulnerability to disasters might go hand in hand. This process would be reinforced and sped up by disaster policies that explicitly seek such an outcome, but such policies are more likely to come up in the aftermath of large natural disasters than in normal times. In what follows, the term "disaster zone" is used for any stock affected by the initial impact, whether this is located within a given geographic area or not.

From this and other studies (Albala-Bertrand, 1993, 2004; Benson & Clay, 2004; Charveriat, 2000) it can be see that indirect (flow) effects on the economy do not appear to be highly significant or long lasting, but they are bound to become even less important as localization increases and therefore vulnerability decreases. This does not mean that directly affected people and activities are necessarily less vulnerable to disaster. This would depend on general institutions and disaster-specific ones. But it does mean that as development progresses disasters may have less intense and less widespread impact effects than otherwise it would have been. It does also mean that the affected economy would have more scope and resources for a rapid recovery, even in the absence of concessional foreign support.

ISOLATION AND INSULATION

An isolated, autarkic, local economy cannot by definition have spreading effects toward the national economy. If it were affected by a disaster, however large its direct or stock effects, the indirect effects would be contained within its boundaries, which may make the total local effects more intense. Without outside aid and endogenous macro integrative reactions the recovery would likely be more trying, as it would have to be met with resources and reactions within the local economy alone. From the viewpoint of the macroeconomy, the disaster would be localized and nonintrusive. In contrast, if the local economy is integrated to the national economy via mutual demands and supplies of factors, goods, and finance, then the disaster can remain local only insofar as the indirect spreading effects can be contained within the disaster (economic or geographic) zone boundary. From a national standpoint, the disaster would be localized if the macroeconomy could insulate itself from the indirect effects that originate in the disaster zone. For this to happen, the national economy has to create compensations via in-built economic and community reactions, which in addition are likely to be reinforced by exogenous domestic and foreign responses. This would initially insulate the disaster, and later help recover the disaster zone itself. The basic containment of wider indirect effects would normally occur rapidly via relief and local physical rehabilitation, at the time when the macroeconomic organism was already taking care of itself.

We then expect that a more developed country will be more economically diversified and more internally and externally articulated. This will make both its interindustrial and income linkages more all embracing and dynamic, less dependent on given domestic sources, and not least its people will more likely be institutionally integrated to a more responsive center of allegiance or state. This means that a disaster might have the possibility of spreading via linkages to the wider economy, through indirect or flow effects, which would not happen from an autarkic location. But at the same time the interlinked system is likely to generate market endogenous reactions via buffer stocks, substitutions, and new supply/demand opportunities that would dampen down negative effects. In addition, other in-built or institutional mechanisms, plus the standard exogenous ones, would also respond in the same direction (Albala-Bertrand, 1993). That is why, in this conception, both indirect effects and long-term effects from localized disasters are likely to be unimportant for the macroeconomy. In autarky they would be irrelevant and in diversified societies they would be rapidly compensated and outweighed, even in the disaster zone itself. So the direct disaster stock loss, which is associated with residential, infrastructure, social, business, and inventory capital, plus current production and labor, might represent almost all of the total loss. In sudden, localized, disasters this is unlikely to have major effects on the macroeconomy even in the short term, especially after relief and rehabilitation are well under way, as shown below (Ibid.). Globalization via trade, financial development, and speedy communications is bound to support and foster the general requirements for localization, despite its current shortcomings.

A MACROECONOMIC ARGUMENT

In the above context, even if the capital stock lost to the disaster were not completely replaced, it would be unlikely that the economy be affected in the short and medium terms, let alone in the long term. This can be shown by means of a macroeconomic argument. Setting aside the normally large overestimation of disaster losses, the argument can be based on well-supported facts about both localized disasters and developing economies. Among them are the facts that capital losses to disaster are both not homogeneous and normally lopsided toward the less productive capital, that most losses are to the capital stock rather than to income and that reconstruction investment is likely to be of better quality than that of the capital lost. In addition, it is well known that the growth of output does not depend on the contribution of the capital stock alone, but also on labor, technology, and other societal requirements. Likewise, it is accepted that new investment opportunities are normally taken up when their risk is low, especially when private investment is publicly supported and protected. And it is also accepted that public investment in infrastructure normally complements or "crowds in" private investment (Albala & Mamatzakis, 2004; Aschauer, 1988; Taylor, 1983). Further, developing countries exhibit large levels of unused or underused productive factors, in terms of idle capacity, underemployed labor, and other resources, which may be one of the reasons why inflation is either not significant or very short lived after disasters. Idle capacity is mostly due to narrow domestic markets and single primary exports, lack of domestic credits and savings, lack foreign exchange and expertise, and not least lack of information about investment opportunities and know-how (Thirlwall, 2003).

In the context of a disaster situation, which includes the impact, the response, and derived societal interference, an economy would normally generate endogenous reactions from within and from outside the disaster area. For example, market reactions that follow opportunities, either by filling profitable gaps left by the disaster losses or by complementing new (disaster) public investment, or both. There will also be economic counteractions via the use of buffer stocks, like savings and inventories plus fast imported inputs, to partly make up for the initial losses to both final and intermediate goods. Buffer stocks in a disaster aftermath will contribute to contain both negative multiplying effects on the economic machinery and the spreading effects from the disaster zone to the rest of the country (Albala-Bertrand, 1993). The more diversified and openly integrated the economy was, the more important would these reactions be. In other words, the disaster itself endogenously creates domestic and foreign economic incentives and reactions, which are reinforced via public, private, and foreign exogenous responses. New concessional foreign exchange could even relax a complementary foreign-exchange constraint if this was present before the disaster, as can be shown via a two-gap model (Taylor, 1994, 2004), increasing investment and hence growth. The stimuli from disaster-induced incentives may also unlock and create economic opportunities, inducing a reconstruction investment multiplier larger than the disaster loss multiplier, making the recovery less costly to undertake and more rapidly to succeed than it would otherwise have been. But the main argument about localization would actually hold even if there were no multiplying effect from the disaster response, when the multiplier was equal to unity.

A MODEL FOR A LOCALIZED DISASTER

Within this framework, an economic model to assess the output effects of a localized disaster can be articulated as follows (for the full mathematical version, see Albala-Bertrand, 2004/1993). One unit of capital loss will always have a lower impact on future output than one unit of capital replaced via new investment. This is because the value of the productivity of capital is always smaller than the value of the investment multiplier, even if the latter were equal to unity. The average productivity of capital represents a fraction of the value of the capital stock, normally around 40% of it, that is, the ratio total output-to-total capital is around 0.4. That is, 2.5 units of average capital normally produce around 1 unit of average output. Given that disasters affect more the less productive capital types, like residential and infrastructure capital, then the average productivity foregone to the disaster will be lower than normal, say half of it. That is, five units of capital loss would represent one unit of foregone output. And given that the less productive capital is the more affected within any capital type, say half of it again, then 10 units of average capital loss would represent only around 1 unit of average foregone output. That is, the capital–output ratio for the disaster loss will be equal to 10. If we also allow for noncapital contributions, then the impact of capital losses on future output will be even smaller, but to make our point we can stick to the moderate capital–output ratio above.

In turn, one unit of reconstruction investment will represent at least one unit of future income, and significantly more via the multiplier, say conservatively two units. This means that a unit of reconstruction investment would have 20 times more impact on income and output than one unit of capital loss. In other words, to recover the possible negative effect of disaster loss on future output, reconstruction investment can be only one-twentieth of total capital loss, in the first aftermath year. That is, if capital loss represented 10% of GDP, then the required ratio of investment to GDP would have to be only 0.5 percentage points more than otherwise it would have been. As this investment ratio is normally around 15% of GDP, after the disaster it requires to be around 15.5% of GDP, which is not an onerous additional effort. Most countries do fulfill such a requirement within a year or so. That is why only rarely a localized disaster has a negative impact on GDP even in the first accounting year. If anything, because of the new disaster-associated opportunities, related directly to reconstruction or otherwise, and the unlocking of potentials due to public expenditure, domestic finance and foreign exchange, it is likely that there will be a significant acceleration of growth. This will normally be confined to the first 2 or 3 post-disaster years, especially but not only in the case of earthquake disasters (Albala-Bertrand, 1993; Charveriat, 2000). It can also be shown that, after the first post-disaster year, the required investment ratio can be even more moderate than in the first year to keep GDP unaffected. Lastly, and not less important, this is partly the reason why it is unpersuasive that a localized disaster can have important indirect, let alone longer-term, effects on the economy. And it is also partly the reason why the assertions about the existence of harmful cumulative disaster effects on the economy are little convincing.[2]

An application of this model (Albala-Bertrand, 2004/1993) appears to confirm the patterns above. For example, the large Guatemalan earthquake in 1976, which reported a loss-to-GDP ratio of 17%, required a total expenditure ratio (including both investment expenditure and other expenditure) of 1.2 percentage points more than otherwise it would have been in the first post-disaster year, and significantly less afterwards. In turn, the Honduran Hurricane of 1974, which reported a loss ratio of 45%, required a total expenditure ratio of 8.7 percentage points more than otherwise it would have been in the first post-disaster year, which is huge.

---

[2] As indirect, long-term, and cumulative effects of disasters are intractable to direct observation, most disaster "experts" and other observers, like relief operators and journalists, normally get away with noncheckable and nonfalsifiable statements about their importance, which then feed back and are repeated by everybody else as a buzzword. In turn, some studies via abstract modeling also attempt to establish their importance. The latter are interesting but normally fail in their realism. For example, a study by Freeman, Martin, Mechler & Warner (2002), for some regions prone to floods and other localized disasters in some Latin American countries, relies heavily on fixed coefficients, an actuarial concept of losses, and an inert conception of society. Fixed coefficients would normally be a problem for any projection beyond 3 to 5 years, but more so in the case of a serious upheaval resulting from a disaster. The actuarial concept might be useful for isolated items, but certainly not for social processes. And associated with the latter, the inert approach to society is simply untenable. Society, including the economy, is not a collection of inert items or a static cake, which can be wound up as a toy or cut to size, but a living organism that generates societally endogenous reactions. These are bound to produce adaptations, substitutions, economic shifts, migration, diversification, and other in-built societal traits, altering somehow the dynamics and structure of the affected location and country (see Albala-Bertrand, 1993).

The difference is mostly due to the different proportions of current output lost to the disaster, that is, 2% and 18% of the total loss, respectively. However, Honduras current output loss is likely to have been grossly overestimated by the Economic Commission for Latin America and the Caribbean (Cepal) at the time (Albala-Bertrand, 1993). It can be shown that the ensuing GDP losses in the first two aftermath years were also due to the fact that the hurricane did seriously affect the key economic sector of banana plantation. In this sense, the disaster was significantly less localized than the one in Guatemala, that is, closer to cell (12) in Table 9.1. However, there was here also an economic conflict with the banana multinationals who were boycotting production as a reaction to a higher tax. Not surprisingly, as soon as a more pliable dictatorship dropped the tax, banana production and the GDP jumped up to unprecedented levels (Ibid.). Whatever it is, in all the cases in this study, the required investment ratio was generally fulfilled, making potential growth losses more than compensated either in the year of the disaster or within the first two post-disaster years. That is, even in the worse cases, the negative disaster effects on the economy were short lived and more than compensated afterwards.[3]

Therefore, reactivity via domestic and foreign linkages in a diversified economic environment is paramount to explain why disasters might not have the dramatic negative economic effects that are so commonly portrayed in the mass media and other sources. That is, market behavior and information, economic diversification and integration, public institutions and expenditure, and domestic and foreign interactions will all endogenously and exogenously help counteract, if not outweigh, actual and potential disaster effects. These processes are likely to be enhanced by globalization.

VULNERABILITY IN THE CONTEXT OF GLOBALIZATION

One conclusion so far is that globalization does appear to help the process of localization in general by endogenously enhancing economic diversity and synergy via all-embracing economic networking. These enhanced interlinkages are bound to increase the resilience of an open national economy, making it more able to insulate from general local failures. But does globalization also contribute to reduce vulnerability to natural disasters in particular? This can be analyzed in the context of a disaster situation by looking at the characteristics of a potential impact and a potential response, within their likely societal interfering effects.

Societal Interference

Societal interference is the result of the impact and its effects as well as the responses and their effects, which are bound to have some variable degree of intromission in normal society and economy, making the prevailing resources undergo some rationalization and redirection. Some societal interference effects are normally called "secondary effects" in the literature, but they are normally confined to a few economic accounting results, such as inflation and the public deficit. This is incomplete, as they do not appear to come from societal channels

---

[3] A disaster with similar geophysical or hydrological characteristics, striking the same places today, would highly likely have significantly less negative economic consequences on GDP than then. This result would come from the upgrading of the enonomic conditions for localization that development itself brings. Not surprisingly, as a rule, disasters in developed countries are always economically localized.

that have been affected by both the impact and the response, but mostly by an overall disaster claim on finance. In addition, they appear too confined to visible financial traits, ignoring endogenous societal processes. Societal interference can be expressed in short-term changes in the public and trade deficits, in inflation and relative prices, in capital flows and remittances. But it can also be seen in terms of institutional changes, which can translate into fragmentation and politicization, technological changes and migration, corruption and speculation, and in less common long-term changes in economic and political structures. In the case of natural disasters, this interference is for the most part an incidental effect of the impact and the response to a disaster situation. But there could also be some interference that intentionally seeks to reduce societal vulnerability to future disasters via preventive policies, which may in addition have a developmental component (Ibid.).

The emergency and especially reconstruction may be highly invasive, but they are likely to have different degrees of potential interference. In natural disasters, emergency response is likely to have a high degree of incidental interference, derived from general institutional stress. But it may also stimulate some deliberate political interference, derived both from the fragmentation of the state apparatus and the ensuing inward activities of identity groups (Albala-Bertrand, 1993; Chakrabarty, 1978; Geipel, 1882). This interference is unlikely to be dramatic and is usually the incidental effect of physical, rather than institutional, demands. In some cases, however, like the Sahelian drought/famine of 1974, the emergency response itself became the problem for long-term recovery, as it created a strong foreign-assistance dependency, weakening the domestic capacity for autonomous social and economic recovery as well as further general development (Lateef, 1982).

Disaster Impact Effects

Once a disaster impact has occurred, two main types of effects ensue: direct or stock effects and indirect or flow effects. Direct effects have an impact on the quality and levels of human populations (injury and deaths) as well as on the quality and levels of physical and animal stocks (damage and destruction). In turn, indirect effects derive from the former, affecting the interrelationships between physical structures and between people. These two types of effects cause losses to society's stocks and flows. For example, for the economic system, direct effects represent losses to the capital stock and labor, whereas indirect effects represent losses to functioning flows, in terms of foregone production and income, savings and investment, productivity and efficiency, and the like. For socially made disasters, like complex emergencies or technological hazards, there is also an institutional effect, as the triggering event, the proneness, and vulnerability to breakdowns are themselves both institutionally based and due to institutional failure.

Indirect effects can be usefully decomposed into four disarticulations of societal frameworks, which are not independent from each other. Two disarticulations, while secondarily affecting the social system, primarily affect people's basic needs and welfare. These represent the effects that can potentially come from the disarticulation of both household conditions (i.e., homelessness, services shortages, displacement, and livelihood erosion) and the states of health and nutrition of the population (i.e., environmental degradation, hygiene problems, increase in disease and food scarcity). The other two disarticulations, while secondarily affecting people, primarily affect the social system, and represent the potential effects from the disarticulations of both the economic circuit (i.e., effects on intermediates markets, final markets, policy and expectations) and public activities (i.e., overburden, discontinuities, fragmentation, and politicization). With some qualifications, these potential disarticulations and potential effects are common to all types of disaster.

Indirect effects, however, appear to be more remarkable for the effects they do not have than for those they do. There is little evidence that the consequences of the disarticulation of household conditions are long lasting, even when the direct effects can dramatically affect some vulnerable social strata. The case is similar with the disarticulation of health and nutrition frameworks, where its potential consequences normally appear to be small, containable, or nonexistent. The economic circuit may be initially disrupted, especially in the directly affected zone, but there is no much evidence that a localized disaster would have significant macroeconomic repercussions, even in the short term, as was shown above. Lastly, the disarticulation of public activities might have more serious consequences than the other ones, especially if an administrative center or a capital city is directly affected, but it normally does not. Fragmentation of institutions and politicization of the response activities are common traits of disasters, but only rarely do they translate into a major structural change or are they significant beyond the emergency activities. Notice these two traits also represent endogenous mechanisms to counteract disaster effects. Disaster-induced structural change appears to depend more on the affected society's prevailing structure and dynamics than on the disaster effects themselves. But only an effective emergency response may guarantee that the potential disarticulations and their effects are not only short-lived, but also the emergency itself is not wasteful (Albala-Bertrand, 1993).

Direct Impact Effects

It is well known that the most affected capital stocks by the direct effects from natural disasters are normally both residential capital and infrastructures, usually representing more than half of the total loss, private housing and roads being the most affected. The former would impinge on household conditions directly, while the latter would initially disarticulate utilities and the transport system, potentially affecting economic flows within the disaster area and between this area and the rest of the economy. This would indirectly rebound on households and the local economy. It is also known that business capital, especially the fixed assets of the secondary (manufacturing) and tertiary (service) sectors, normally undergo a small share of direct losses, between negligible losses (floods) to around 10% of them (earthquakes and hurricanes). Primary sectors can bear an important share of the total capital loss in sudden hydrometeorological disasters, mainly in terms of agriculture and cattle loses, but it can also be shown that this is often macroeconomically compensated in the short run (Ibid.). At any rate, the less productive capital and labor are normally the more affected, which also means that the required investment to compensate for potential growth losses is smaller than otherwise it would have been, as was shown in the previous section (Albala-Bertrand, 2004/1993). Can globalization alter favorably the above patterns?

GLOBALIZATION AND IMPACT PREVENTION

Prevention is also part of the anticipatory response to disasters, as discussed below, but here we concentrate on prevention of the impact itself, that is, the interface between a geophysical event and a social system. How could globalization modify the intensity of the direct effects of a disaster impact? This would depend on factors that could modify either the strength of the geophysical event or the physical resistance of a disaster-prone community. As regards the event, there is little that globalization can do directly, as it would mostly depend on highly sophisticated technology to alter the strength of earthquakes, hurricanes, floods, and volcanoes at source, which is hardly available (Kunreuther & Rose, Vol. I, Part V, 2004).

Economic globalization, however, does appear to be damaging to the environment and also to some sections of society. For example, vulnerability of both the people and the environment can increase when cash crop agriculture evicts and pushes already vulnerable people to marginal lands, also when the rain forest succumbs to trade, or when carbon dioxide pollutes the environment, or when urban areas undergo accelerated overcrowding. Some of these factors may increase the frequency and magnitude of floods and other natural events. Carbon dioxide emissions, arguably associated with global warming, might intensify desertification, erosion, hurricanes, flooding, and tsunamis (Albala-Bertrand, 1993; Haas, 2003). This is a current debate that has captured the public imagination and can be exemplified by the Kyoto Protocol to control emissions. But for as long as the United States does not appear willing to participate there will be little changes, as this economy is still the largest polluter. As a countertrend, however, the global community has become closer by virtue of globalization, so it has also become easier to point the finger against violators of world well-being, and press more effectively for positive changes. Hence, debate about economic, political, and legal aspects of environmental and human protection have also become more expedient. The likes of the Kyoto Protocol would not have been approved only a decade ago (Faure, Gupta, & Nentjes, 2003; Hanley & Owen, 2004).

As regards the community's exposure and resistance to disasters, a first contribution from globalization would be the setting up of early warning systems associated with preparedness for appropriate responses to them. This is likely to modify the intensity of direct impact effects on people, via organized evacuation toward less exposed areas and buildings (Mileti & Sorensen, 1988; Tsuchiya & Shuto, 1995). It is likely that the massive death toll from the 2004 Asian tsunami would have been largely avoided had early warning systems been in place in that area of the world. Globalization can create more awareness about the need for concerted regional safety systems and can also pool the costs of such systems more easily (e.g., http://tsunami.report.ru/).

As regards the strength of the physical built-up environment, the main mechanisms to reduce the disaster impact vulnerability are regulations of buildings and structures, such as construction codes, land use licenses, and regulations about land location and the handling of risky technology. Globalization, via dissemination of information about best practices, may contribute positively to a better understanding of design and use of structures as well as their monitoring and legal enforcing. In addition, insurance can also play a role at this juncture, by disciplining construction and land use, as conditions to qualify for insurance cover. Also, the requirement to introduce disaster-risk factors in both cost–benefit analysis and private investment projects, as a condition for international and domestic loans, can also work toward this aim (Mechler, 2003). Globalization also assumes an increasingly more open and transparent society, which may favor the observance and application of legislation, and at the same time that also contribute to reduce traditionally unchecked corruptive practices.

This is not unimportant, but its effective implementation depends more on the type of society than on globalization itself. So the role of the state, as a necessary complement or substitute for private markets, should not be overlooked. Current globalization, however, does not primarily favor this role in any significant way, which is another insufficiency to address. In addition, it can be shown that the current dominant, but increasingly criticized strain of globalization, the Washington Consensus, even when successful at the macroeconomic level, generates and perpetuates large income inequalities and disparities in purchasing power, at least in the short and medium terms. It can also be shown that this type of globalization does not count with many unqualified successful cases, even at the macroeconomic level (Rodrick, 2004; Taylor, 2000). This means that if current trends remain unchecked and unmodified, more people in more countries are likely to be rendered more vulnerable than currently are. There are, however, alternative roads to a more all-embracing type of globalization, like the Asian model, but Washington and its followers have so far resisted such alternatives on arguably ideological grounds (Chang & Grabel, 2004; Wade, 1996). But if the disaster impact itself cannot be fully prevented, how would globalization fare in the area of actual disaster responses?

DISASTER RESPONSE

Disaster response can be defined as a wide array of endogenous and exogenous reactions, measures, and policies that are aimed at mitigating, counteracting, and preventing disaster impacts and effects. The response side of a disaster situation can be articulated as follows: once a disaster impact has arisen, the impact effects themselves stimulate both the unfolding of systemically incorporated mechanisms of response and the creation of especially designed response measures. These two sets of responses aim at compensation via emergency activities that temporarily counteract functioning flow losses (i.e., emergency relief and emergency rehabilitation) and at reconstruction activities that permanently redress the consequences of stock losses and institutional insufficiencies. The impact effects and the derived compensatory responses also stimulate an anticipatory response aimed at prevention and mitigation of future potential disasters. This then generates three not independent main areas of attention, which make up the response side of a disaster situation: response mechanisms, compensatory response, and anticipatory response (Albala-Bertrand, 1993). In addition, as a disaster situation always generates varying degrees of societal interference, then the disaster response should also be contextualized in terms of response-induced interfering effects, as described earlier.

RESPONSE MECHANISMS

Response mechanisms refer to endogenous and exogenous processes of response. Endogenous response mechanisms are those channeled through society's in-built institutional processes. These processes represent a series of formal and informal feedback mechanisms, which are part of the existing self-regulatory social organism, for example, the family, informal finance, the informal sector, formal markets, political and administrative frameworks, cultural norms and customs, psychological attitudes and habits, and so on. These involve a wide array of activities that range from highly automatic to nonautomatic in-built responses. For example, extended family solidarity represents a highly automatic endogenous reaction, while the use of the hazard reserve item of the public budget is mostly a nonautomatic in-built response. Likewise, market reactions and emergent coalitions appear to lie somewhere in between. A good deal of these processes may act as an informal insurance mechanism, associated with social cooperation and solidarity as well as individual reciprocity and altruism, both societally founded processes, which can be resorted to in times of distress (Albala-Bertrand, 1993; Hirschleifer, 1975).

Exogenous mechanisms, in turn, are those channeled via ad hoc, irregular, processes that are not patterned or guaranteed. These are expressed in action, measures and policies that may formally fill gaps left by in-built responses, by-pass endogenous channels, shift initiatives away from regular actors, or superimpose alternative structures. This normally implies private and public interventions that go beyond in-built actions, and international assistance and aid that go beyond existing guarantees. In the long run, however, these two response types might not be necessarily independent. This is because the endogenization of societally useful exogenous initiatives and behaviors, via education and other social institutions, is the normal way in which society strengthens and develops (see Albala-Bertrand, 1993; Barton, 1970; Cuny, 1983; Davis, 1978; Dynes, 1970; Prince, 1920; Quarantelli, 1978; Sorokin, 1942; White, 1974).

Some of these response mechanisms might be helped by globalization. One of the main planks of globalization is the deepening and enhancing of international trade. Foreign trade benefits a country by unlinking the domestic structure of production from that of demand. Domestic production then can also satisfy a foreign structure of demand via exports, while domestic demand can also be satisfied via imports of final and intermediate goods. This diversifies the sources and markets of inputs and outputs. In addition, in countries with small markets, it allows using capacity at a higher level than otherwise it would have been. This is bound to increase the localization of a disaster, as the output and capital losses as well as the ensuing demand losses in the disaster zone can now be more easily made up with alternative domestic and foreign markets. This may not only reduce even more effectively the potential for widespread effects on the macroeconomy, but also change the structure of supplies and demands toward more stable markets. Although this may promptly shelter and compensate the macroeconomy from unwanted indirect flow effects, it may also put out of business a number of affected economic activities in the disaster zone. That is, even if foreign-free trade may contribute to confine and isolate the potential for widespread indirect effects, it might not necessarily contribute directly to the recovery of activities and people in the affected zone. This may make the disaster even more economically localized than before, but it might also worsen the plight of affected communities by passing them over. But if the macroeconomy is not affected, then it should be more expedite and less onerous for the affected country to counter the effects in the disaster zone both exogenously or otherwise. So again the main focus of exogenous disaster response should be people and activities directly affected in the disaster zone, as an open macroeconomy is highly unlikely to be affected in any significant way by localized disasters, even in the absence of important exogenous public and foreign responses.

A wide opening to international trade, however, has also a number of downsides for developing countries. Among other problems, first, there will be an initial destruction of indigenous uncompetitive firms and a probably long-lasting confinement to the production of primary products (Weiss, 2002), increasing general and disaster vulnerability in passing. This is the consequence of the elimination of tariff and other trade protections, which is demanded by the WTO for foreign trade agreements (FTAs), not always readily observed by OECD countries. Second, it may also make the economy more vulnerable to international fluctuations, again weakening domestic response in the event of disaster. Third, it may also stifle domestic technological sophistication and the economic efficiency of domestic intermediate inputs, which may in the long run make an economy less flexible to adapt to sudden changes. Hence the positive aspects of free trade have to be balanced against the negative ones when analyzing it, let alone when designing policy for the real world and current generations (Albala-Bertrand, 1999; Andersen, 2003; Chang, 1996; Chang & Grabel, 2004; Stiglitz, 2002). Both exogenous and endogenous responses may become strengthened via enhanced communications, regional free-trade agreements, or by attracting foreign tourism. This may increase international solidarity and concessional aid to deal with emergency relief and emergency rehabilitation. But on the downside, free trade may affect standard endogenous social mechanisms of response in negative ways by disenfranchising traditional economic activities via foreign competition. This translates both in losses of traditional livelihood and lack of alternative livelihood in the short to medium terms. It also translates in increases in inequalities and instability of especially the most vulnerable sections of society, which normally represent the overwhelming majority in developing countries. Both the extended family and community support are bound to be weakened by this kind of societal disenfranchising. This means that the well-known endogenous reactions in the disaster zone, which are paramount to deal with the early relief and rehabilitation, are bound to be impaired, requiring faster and larger exogenous and endogenous responses from outside the disaster zone than otherwise it would have been.

It is, however, not enough that an open macroeconomy has available resources to deal with an actual disaster, as countries with acceptable GDP per capita and good growth rates can and do carry unacceptable levels of inequalities and poverty, that is, the so-called "trickle down" does not appear to work. Therefore, a policy balance between positive and negative aspects of free-foreign trade should actively consider the formalization of well-funded and well-managed public and private mechanisms of response to potential disasters (Benson & Clay, 2004).

COMPENSATORY AND ANTICIPATORY RESPONSE

If the disaster impact cannot be prevented, we then should look for ways to reduce and effectively absorb and counteract its effects as they occur. Emergency relief and emergency rehabilitation are likely to be enhanced by globalization via macro insulation, local integration, buffer reactions, and general exogenous resources vis-à-vis the said impairments to endogenous reactions. Once the emergency response has contained the spread and the deepening of indirect effects, the basis for starting to reverse the direct effects would be feasible. This would come in the shape of physical reconstruction plans, which is partly an exogenous type of activity, but financing from insurance, market reactions, and other in-built systems would also be involved. These responses do require public involvement out of public finance via contingency funds, new grants and subsidies, tax and bills write-offs, and the like. But it would also require foreign aid and credits, including material, technical, and labor assistance. These responses are therefore bound to interfere with standard activities that compete for the same resources, but it may create or unlock new resources that were not available before the disaster (Albala-Bertrand, 1993). These responses can also be made less intrusive and therefore more effective by resorting to in-built financial mechanisms that transfer risk and that increase the available funding for reconstruction, that is, the use of financial anticipatory mechanisms either as a specific disaster aim or as an incidental by-product of financial deepening.

This takes us to the second main plank of globalization, the development of domestic financial markets and its integration with a global financial market, in terms of bank loans, portfolio investment, and foreign direct investment. These are meant to increase greatly in coverage and depth, via the development and creation of financial instruments and products. Setting aside, for the moment, the serious problem of domestic regulation of foreign financial flows, a more extensively developed financial market would include some mechanisms to fund, spread, transfer, and reduce risk and vulnerability. Instruments such as disaster insurance and reinsurance, catastrophe bonds and weather derivatives, hedge funds and disaster credit, reserve funds and remittances, are all part of the current need to establish a financial architecture aimed at disaster vulnerability reduction (Andersen, 2003; Doherty, 2000; Keipel & Tyson, 2002; Kunreuther, 1996).

If this was the case, then the impact of a natural or technological disaster might be at least partly absorbed, via improved access to the above instruments and better information about risk vis-à-vis materials and design. But for as long as the collateral requirements were not readily available, loans and other forms of financial protection might not reach the people who need it most in the wake of a disaster. Insurance premiums might be an unaffordable cost for precisely the people and activities more likely to be directly affected by a disaster impact. Still, the easier availability of these products for firms and employers, by virtue of globalization, might reduce the livelihood vulnerability of employees, even if the latter cannot afford insurance of their own. But, even if the domestic and international financial market for insurance were easily available, voluntary insurance and other risk-transfer instruments, as a norm, are poorly demanded (Albala-Bertrand, 1993; Cochrane, 1975; Dacy & Kunreuther, 1969; Giarini, 1984; IDB, 2003; Kunreuther, 1997). These anticipatory actions would also involve the monitoring of markets, migrations, and general people's reactions, so that response effectiveness can be maximized, while antisocial and speculative behaviors can be minimized. Most of these responses may have strong societal implications as they aim to modify people's behavior and institutions. State involvement, as a guiding drive, becomes of paramount importance. These include the setting up of land-use regulations and building codes, with their associated legal enforcement. It also includes the supervising of financial transfer mechanisms and people's participation in prediction/warning, preparedness, and self-help systems, including microfinance. All this requires government intervention at all levels for effective reactions to potential and actual impact effects (Albala-Bertrand, 1993; Dreze & Sen, 1990/91; Godschack, Beatley, Berke, Brower, & Kaiser, 1998; Mileti & Sorensen, 1988).

DISASTER VULNERABILITY AND GLOBALIZATION

We have seen above that globalization is likely to help the process of localization, hence helping insulate the macroeconomy from disaster effects. We also saw that trade and financial resources can act in favor of reducing disaster vulnerability by increasing disaster-specific absorption capabilities and the resilience of those who can afford it. But lower macroeconomic vulnerability is perfectly compatible with higher social vulnerability at a local level, especially that of those directly affected by a disaster.

Globalization and Social Exclusion

Community, defined as a stable array of institutions that set patterned societal interaction and hierarchies, within and between particular identity groups, like family, neighborhood, workplace, formal and informal working relationships, might be the first casualty of fast and unfettered globalization (Chang & Grabel, 2004; Stiglitz, 2002). As indicated earlier, there is plenty of evidence that the fast opening of trade is bound to make small and financially precarious firms especially uncompetitive, and therefore unviable. These would affect formal firms and their workers as well as informal economic activity that depends on these firms, which may represent the overwhelming majority of economic activity in some developing countries (Thirlwall, 2003; Thomas, 1992). In addition, the current globalization push for privatization, deregulation of labor markets and general restructuring of firms, which seek fast efficiency and productivity improvements, does not generally pay much attention to the ensuing social costs. This is bound to make matters even worse for the precarious social fabric of many communities and people. If there were no alternative means of livelihood, nor was there any public protection on these affected people, and the transition to higher employment and stability was slow, then both informal and formal endogenous mechanisms might well be badly impaired at the time of a disaster impact.

The hope is that this will only be a short-term passage to a stronger economy and society. But as it happens, this transition is slow to deliver better general conditions and access. And even when things might be improving, the trickle down to poorer social strata would either be too slow or not forthcoming. In addition, the liberalization of especially short-term capital flows is now well known to create negative economic shocks and instability associated with lack of regulation and controls, which is bound to further impair the stability and strength of endogenous response mechanisms. Therefore, globalization, as it has been carried so far, may significantly weaken useful local endogenous response mechanisms at the time of disaster, thus demanding a stronger exogenous presence of domestic and foreign sources when a disaster strikes. There might then be the requirement of international concerted efforts to improve the soundness and safety of globalization policies as an aim in itself, so that the masses of vulnerable people and activities get a better deal than currently, especially in the face of natural hazards.

Synchronization of the Business Cycle

If globalization makes the cycle synchronic, and there is a recession in the US locomotive, then the downturn will become global, affecting globalizing economies in a number of ways. First, it would reinforce the negative effects coming from unfettered globalization, as described earlier. This would also affect informal financial markets, which might become less agile and effective in the wake of fast globalization, again impairing recovery. Further, people's remittances from abroad would be strongly hindered. As this is usually a very important type of informal financial response at the family and local level, recovery of household and individual livelihood conditions would likely be additionally impaired. Second, as export demand, commodity prices, and capital flows decline, then both less domestic financial resources will be available and the already depressed communities would be further impaired, which would further weaken endogenous response mechanisms. Third, in a similar vein, both bilateral and multilateral sources of foreign finance might become strongly procyclical, reducing significantly their role in recessions. Fourth, nongovernmental organizations (NGOs) depend on donations from a variety of people, which might dry up with a synchronic recession, curtailing their functions. Finally, international private sources might, however, be undergoing excess liquidity, which can contribute to easy, but risky, lending.

A country in recession may, however, have more idle capital resources to put in the service of rehabilitation and reconstruction, which may be stimulated via appropriate domestic demand policies in the aftermath of disaster. This would be expected to engage other domestic activities not directly related to disaster response, and so affecting the whole economy positively. But globalization itself may make this useful expansionary policy less effective than otherwise it would have been, as most capital is not malleable and therefore cannot be switched to alternative types of production in the short and medium terms. So if the economy were significantly open, then most types of output would have already been geared for exports. A recession then will have both the export sector and its backward domestic linkages operating with significant idle capacity. Domestic demand can normally be satisfied with only a small fraction of these exportable goods. This would make disaster-induced expenditure less effective as a mechanism to compensate the economy and stimulate other sectors than in a closer economy. On the other hand, if the world economy is in an upturn, then the situation for foreign aid and resources would likely be relaxed and forthcoming, but also domestic financial resources would be more readily available. This can contribute to speed recovery from disaster, although it could affect the economy somehow via inflation, uncoordinated sectoral shifts, labor shortages, and other bottlenecks.

CONCLUSIONS

Our main conclusions are as follows. First, disasters may impose large residential, infrastructure, and agricultural losses as well as large death tolls and injuries within the disaster zone, but it is highly likely that these losses and problems will be economically localized. Second, economically localized losses of capital and activities, death tolls, and injuries are unlikely to affect negatively the macroeconomy in the short term, let alone in the longer term. Third, it is unlikely that this general pattern would significantly change by virtue of the negative features of globalization; if anything, the positive features of globalization may help make a disaster even more economically localized than otherwise it would have been. Fourth, development itself appears to be a process whereby all disasters become more economically localized. That is, "disasters are primarily a problem *of* development, but essentially not a problem *for* development" (Albala-Bertrand, 1993, p. 202). Fifth, the negative features of current globalization may, however, make a significant difference for increased direct local victimization, as the local endogenous mechanisms of response may be seriously impaired by both the structural changes associated with international trade competition and the potentially recessionary effects of unmanageable capital flows. But successful globalization itself may also provide the resources for speedy local recovery if there was political will. Sixth, given that globalization appears to make the world business cycle synchronic and dependent on the U.S. economy, a U.S. recession would also become a global situation. Hence, financing disaster response might become procyclical, affecting a disaster-struck country more adversely than it would otherwise have been. The jury is still out about the issue of synchronization, so time will tell how relevant it is. Seventh, globalization can provide new opportunities for both improving physical prevention and diversifying risk, via information about best practices, access to appropriate technology, disaster insurance, equity mechanisms, international cooperation, and the like. But the useful incorporation of these opportunities into the economy and polity would depend not only on domestic society and its ruling regime, but also on globalization policies and their social concern. A good deal of work is being carried out by academics and international institutions, but it would always be useful to entertain a further diversity of positions and studies.

As a main suggestion for disaster research, it would be useful to enhance the duality thesis proposed here by explicitly assessing disaster events within this framework in a systemic manner. First, it would be useful that future studies start classifying disaster impacts according to some meaningful concept of economic localization, within the general definition proposed here. This may allow establishing some useful patterns at more focused levels (regional, demographic, political, and the like). Second, many studies have unintentionally shown that localized disasters do not have significant effects on the national economy, but shy away from making this connection explicit. The framework proposed here might help overcome such reluctance and encourage making such connection both systematically and in the appropriate institutional context. Given that different institutional frameworks are likely to unleash different response patterns, knowing more about them may contribute to recovery, reducing victimization and costs. Third, as regards development, it would be useful to look at the particular development factors and policies that can incidentally make a contribution to enhance disaster localization, therefore reducing vulnerability in both given countries and in general.

Therefore, I would suggest that approaching the study of disaster vulnerability via a framework of economic localization vis-à-vis the actual globalization experience of disaster-prone countries could produce useful understanding and policy rewards.

Finally, given that a macroeconomy would unlikely be affected by an economically localized disaster, communities and activities directly affected should be the main target of response policies, rather than the unwarranted belief that the economy as a whole would be impaired. In addition, apart from early warning, disaster preparedness and general resource management in the case of hazards, the design of more inclusive and stable approaches to globalization should be a fundamental way to reduce the natural hazard vulnerability of most people in developing countries.

CHAPTER 10

Local Emergency Management Organizations

David A. McEntire

Two days after Hurricane Andrew struck the southeastern coast of Florida, the emergency manager of Dade County asked in desperation, "Where the hell is the cavalry on this one?" Pleas for help are common in most widespread disasters as municipal and county governments may not have sufficient material and human resources to deal with the devastation and disruption they leave behind. Mass emergencies and major calamities are therefore characterized by the need for outside assistance, and state and federal assets are sent to the affected area to assess damages, explain national relief programs, and provide financial assistance, among other things. For instance, when the World Trade Center towers collapsed after being struck by hijacked aircraft, hundreds of government agencies and departments converged in New York. Among these individuals and organizations from the public sector were search and rescue teams, law enforcement personnel, environmental enforcement officials, intelligence agents, congressional representatives, the National Guard, interstate mutual aid partners, and the Federal Emergency Management Agency (FEMA). Emergent groups, religious organizations, businesses, and nonprofit agencies also arrived at the scene from distant locations to provide various kinds of disaster assistance. Nonetheless, the bulk of responsibility in disasters typically falls on local jurisdictions. The burden of dealing with a disaster is never felt more intensely than at the community level. For this reason, it is imperative to understand local emergency management organizations.

This chapter reviews what is known about official and unofficial participants in emergency management at the community in the United States and around the world. It first provides the context of emergency management and identifies the organizational arrangements in which emergency managers operate. A history of emergency management is provided and the functions of this profession are discussed. The chapter then illustrates that the emergency manager is heavily dependent on other departments, preparedness councils, mutual aid partners, regional consortiums, and emergent groups. Attention subsequently turns to the nature of emergency management organizations in other nations, although this portion of the chapter is somewhat limited owing to a continued lack of comparative research. An assessment of current challenges and future opportunities facing local emergency managers and related stakeholders in the public sector then takes place. Research needs pertaining to emergency management organizations are also identified. One of the major conclusions to be drawn from this exposition is that the emergency manager is only one of many actors interested and involved in disaster issues at the local level, and that increased effort needs to be given to networking and improved intergovernmental relations. Another finding is that local emergency managers may want to become more proactive by pursuing integrative policies based on the popular concepts that scholars and practitioners consider to be imperative for the reduction of future disasters.

EMERGENCY MANAGEMENT AND ITS CONTEXT IN THE UNITED STATES

Emergency management is "the discipline and profession of applying science, technology, planning and management to deal with extreme events that can injure or kill large numbers of people, do extensive damage to property, and disrupt community life" (Hoetmer, 1991, p. xvii). In conjunction with this definition, emergency managers may therefore be regarded as public servants who employ knowledge, techniques, strategies, tools, organizational networks, and other community and external resources to reduce the occurrence of disasters and successfully deal with their impacts in order to protect people, property, and the environment. Because the mayor is the designated emergency manager under most city ordinances, emergency managers are often referred to as emergency management coordinators or disaster planners. For the purpose of this chapter, however, these coordinators and planners are referred to as emergency managers.

These preliminary comments bring up several interesting points about the nature of the field and they also invite further commentary about this area of study and emerging profession. First, it is necessary to recognize that there are several problems with the term "emergency management" (McEntire, 2004a). In spite of its name, emergency management is generally more concerned about disasters than emergencies because first responders are fully capable of addressing most needs in routine incidents. When a disaster occurs, however, police, fire, and emergency medical service (EMS) personnel cannot always cope with the resulting widespread impacts unless an emergency manager and numerous others are available to acquire resources for first responders and take care of broader response and recovery needs in the community (e.g., warning, sheltering, debris management, donations management, rebuilding, etc.). The concept of emergency management is similarly questionable in that emergency managers may have less control over the unfolding of extreme events than they would like to admit. Because of the unique, complex, and dynamic features of disasters, the activities of emergency managers may be significantly influenced by these disruptive occurrences rather than the other way around. Emergency management might likewise be a reactive name for a profession that should give more attention to a reduction of both the quantity and quality of disasters. From an epistemological standpoint, the term emergency management seems to suggest that we can only react after a disaster rather than take steps to reduce our vulnerability before the event occurs. These weaknesses aside, awareness of emergency management appears to be on the rise. Media coverage of major disasters in recent years has certainly spread recognition of this important field.

These observations should not be taken to imply that emergency management is as widely recognized a discipline as English or History, however. From an academic standpoint, emergency management is still in its youth or adolescent stage, and there is even debate as to whether the field constitutes "a discipline or a multi-disciplinary endeavor" (Phillips, 2003). Nonetheless, the fact that there are now more bachelor's, master's, and doctorate programs in this area should begin to discredit questions of legitimacy (see FEMA's Higher Education Program list at http://training.fema.gov/EMIWeb/edu/collegelist/_ for examples). A growing number of students are pursuing emergency management as a career of first choice and many educators report expanding enrollments at FEMA's annual Higher Education Conference. In addition, the content of these academic programs in emergency management is changing slowly but surely. Students in the field now have a greater exposure to the physical and social sciences as well as other disciplines related to disaster (Falkiner, 2005; McEntire, 2004a; Neal, 2000). Today's emergency management students also spend more time than their predecessors did considering how disasters can be prevented and how post-disaster operations can be made more effective in the future. Besides focusing on ways to protect life and limit the disruption disasters cause, these students are increasingly concerned about politics, law, social and economic relations, technological impacts, environmental protection, and multiorganizational coordination. Knowledge, skills, and abilities regarding the administration of emergency management programs in the public sector are now more commonplace as well (although much improvement remains to be seen).

The evolving educational opportunities are also leading to more respect for the position of local emergency manager. According to many job postings, a degree in emergency management is now preferred and is often required. More and more jurisdictions are unwilling to hire individuals without the necessary background and credentials. To be certain, emergency managers are undoubtedly not yet comparable to the medical, legal, or engineering professions, and several strategies must be pursued if emergency management is to achieve similar status in the future (Oyola-Yemaiel & Wilson, 2005). Regardless, many cities currently employ at least one emergency manager and others will hire one or more as time passes. The U.S. Department of Labor (2005) reports that the demand for emergency management positions is projected to rise by more than 28% by 2012.

The existence of an emergency manager is not uniform across all jurisdictions, however (Kreps, 1991b). Small, rural towns may not have sufficient resources to hire a full-time disaster specialist. If this is the case, the job remains vacant or someone may voluntarily fill this function. At other times, the emergency manager may work on a part-time basis, or the fire chief, police chief, public works director, city manager, or mayor fills this role. Certain municipalities may not get involved in emergency management as the county takes a more active stance regarding disasters. Most large cities do recognize the need for and value of emergency management, however, but the size of such offices varies dramatically. Omaha, Nebraska has two emergency managers while the City of Fort Worth, Texas has five. Major metropolitan areas have even more sizable emergency management staff. There are 13 on the payroll in Los Angeles, California, and New York City has 125 employees. This does not include, of course, individuals in other departments who perform related emergency management functions.

The emergency management position may also be included in one of many common organizational arrangements (Kreps, 1991). Most fall under another department such as fire, police, or public works. Some may be independent, lacking direct ties to other peer entities. Others may report to a city manager or even the mayor directly, and movement toward this trend is gaining momentum. Regardless of the location, there are advantages and disadvantages to each of these positions in the city's organization. Those integrated in separate departments may theoretically have access to large budgets and their host departments may be closely associated with emergency managers (e.g., fire departments are involved in emergencies on a daily basis). Nonetheless, the needs of emergency managers could be downplayed because of the general goals of the organization, and programmatic objectives of emergency management could be dismissed as a result of the final say of other department heads. Emergency managers who are isolated from other organizations may be free to build a program with minimal outside control, but they may consequently lack financial resources or the buy-in of other departments. Being placed under city leadership would most likely provide adequate political and monetary support, although this may engender hostile attitudes on the part of different departments. Policies pertaining to emergency management could also vary dramatically among elected administrations, leading to dramatic fluctuations in the direction of such programs. Despite the divergent organizational situations, emergency managers must use political acumen to promote their programs and overcome interpersonal or interorganizational conflict. In other words, the art of the profession is just as important as the science of emergency management.

Finally, it should be noted that the name of the emergency management department also varies dramatically in different cities. In Portland, Oregon, it is known as the Office of Emergency Management. Indianapolis, Indiana, labels it as the Emergency Management Agency in the Department of Public Safety. Some organizations reflect the past traditions of Civil Defense, as in Shakopee, Minnesota, while others now reflect the current terrorist threat, as is the case with the Homeland Security Department in McKinney, Texas. This complexity results not only from the federalist and decentralized system of government in the United States (Drabek, 1985), but also from the dynamic nature of emergency management in general.

THE HISTORY AND FUNCTIONS
OF EMERGENCY MANAGEMENT

Emergency management—whether at the federal, state, or local level— has been influenced significantly by world events and the occurrence of disasters (Quarantelli, 1987a). The impetus behind emergency management was initially World War II and subsequent Cold War hostilities (Waugh, 2000a, p. 13). Many European countries were bombed during this drawn-out conflict, leading to civil defense initiatives for advanced warning and related evacuation and sheltering. When allied forces pushed back Hitler's army, disagreements about the future of Europe began to appear between the United States and the Soviet Union. Communist leaders feared the expansion of U.S. capitalism and they viewed the use of the atomic bomb in Japan as a potential threat to their security. A nuclear arms race ensued between these two superpowers, producing a potential of mutually assured destruction (MAD). Governments in both countries gave impressive attention to war planning and civil defense wardens helped prepare cities by developing siren systems, stockpiling nuclear bunkers with supplies, and planning how to move citizens to untargeted areas. Little attention (comparatively speaking) was given to other types of disasters by local governments during the 1950s and early 1960s.

After witnessing the devastation caused by natural events including Hurricane Betsy, Hurricane Camille, and the Alaskan earthquake, federal officials began to see civil defense as a dual-use activity (i.e., for nuclear strikes and natural disasters) (Drabek, 1991a, p. 18). This consequently altered the goals and scope of civil defense, and emergency management offices were created in cities around the nation. When technological disasters began to occur with increased frequency as a result of ongoing industrialization, emergency management began to focus on hazardous materials releases. Effort was given to track dangerous chemicals in manufacturing plants and build local capabilities to deal with such disasters (Lindell, 1994). This shift to man-made disasters was dampened when Hurricane Andrew, the Midwest flooding, and the Northridge Earthquake occurred in the early 1990s. Under the direction of FEMA director James Lee Witt, local emergency managers began to stress hazard and vulnerability assessments in addition to mitigation through land-use planning, improved engineering, and public/private partnerships. The Witt revolution helped the profession become more proactive by attempting to reduce risk and expedite the recovery process (Haddow & Bullock, 2003, p. 10). Even though emergency managers gave attention to the possibility of computer-related disasters (e.g., Y2K), priority was still directed at natural disasters during the first few months of the new millennium.

With the 9/11 terrorist attacks, emergency management has again changed course by taking on the homeland security perspective. Local officials, recognizing the challenges of the response to the World Trade Center attacks and the use of anthrax in Washington, D.C. and in Florida, began to stress law enforcement, interoperable communications, and public health concerns (Fischer, 1999; McEntire, Robinson, & Weber, 2003; Perry, 2003; Waugh, 2001). Emergency management has in some ways come full circle (Alexander, 2002), although homeland security is certainly more complex than civil defense. Attention is now given to intelligence gathering, border control, and preparation for a possible attack involving weapons of mass destruction (nuclear, biological, and chemical agents) (Bullock et al., 2005). Federal grants enable cities to prepare for possible terrorist attacks, but tension has resulted because of the apparent downplaying of natural hazards (Waugh, 2004c). The four hurricanes and one tropical storm that struck Florida in fall, 2004, the devastating Tsunami in the Indian Ocean, and the dislocation of thousands of people after Hurricane Katrina were vivid reminders that natural disasters cannot be overlooked. It is unclear to what extent these events have influenced or will alter federal policies and local emergency management activities, however.

Although policies and funding stress counterterrorism activities, local emergency managers still undertake a variety of steps within what is known as the comprehensive emergency management framework (Godschalk, 1991). Mitigation includes efforts to prevent disasters or minimize impact through hazard and vulnerability assessments, improved construction practices, and better land-use decisions. Preparedness activities attempt to enhance post-disaster operations through planning, training, exercises, and community education. Response operations entail warning, evacuation, search and rescue, emergency medical care, fire suppression, and other methods to care for disaster victims and minimize disruptions. Recovery implies efforts to return the community to normal or improved conditions after disaster strikes, and often involves damage assessment, debris removal, disaster assistance, and rebuilding measures. Since disasters are fairly rare occurrences, most of the emergency manager's time is spent attending meetings, promoting more stringent disaster policies, educating the public, creating plans, updating resource lists, and conducting exercises (Daines, 1991; Pickett & Block, 1991; Scanlon, 1991). In recent years, emergency managers have become heavily involved in managing numerous grants including the Nunn-Lugar-Domenici Domestic Preparedness Equipment Program, the Urban Area Security Initiative, the Citizen Corps and Citizen Emergency Response Team (CERT) Programs, and the Homeland Security Grant Program. This has added a significant work load to what is typically an already overburdened and limited staff. It is apparent that emergency managers cannot be considered the only participants in emergency management.

INVOLVEMENT WITH OFFICIAL PARTNERS

Emergency managers do not (or should not) act in isolation from others. To the contrary, the success of emergency managers is largely determined by the extent to which they involve other departments, planning committees, mutual aid parties, and regional networks in pre- and post-disaster activities. In other words, because emergency managers cannot possibly perform every function in emergency management alone, they must attempt to ensure that someone is completing each vital activity pertaining to the reduction and management of disasters (Hoetmer, 1991, p. xx).

For their part, local government departments often fail to recognize their important role in a disaster. Since there is a designated emergency manager in many cities, and since the jurisdictional domains for disasters are spread across so many organizations, most individuals and institutions do not perceive themselves as being responsible for emergency management (Auf der Heide, 1989, p. 8). However, natural and technological incidents may adversely impact economic development as well as schools, public utilities, and transportation systems. Terrorist events could have similar impact on those concerned with infrastructure, the environment, and public health. Flood plain managers and the planning department are heavily involved in land management and development while engineering is relied on to enforce building codes. The engineering department will also be needed for damage assessment, and public works and possibly parks and recreation will be used to remove debris. The police department is utilized for traffic control, the fire department has responsibility for fire suppression as well as search and rescue operations, and the public information officer must deal with media requests. To facilitate recovery, the city will work with the chamber of commerce to point out business needs whereas the budget or finance department will process federal funding for reconstruction projects. Permits will likewise be needed for rebuilding (thus requiring the engineering department again), and city managers and political leaders will coordinate efforts and oversee progress of the entire emergency management program. Every local government organization has some relation to disasters and emergency management operations. Emergency managers must therefore educate city leaders about disasters, and involve them as much as is possible in prevention and preparedness processes.

Besides the public officials and departments mentioned above, emergency managers create several types of planning advisory boards and involve other organizations in their activities (Gordon, 2002). The most common example is a local emergency planning committee (LEPC). LEPCs were instituted in the late 1980s in response to the Emergency Planning and Community Right to Know Act (SARA Title III) to prepare communities for industrial accidents such as explosions or hazardous materials releases. There is no standard list of constituting agencies, but typical members include the emergency manager(s) and representatives from fire departments, hospitals, environmental protection agencies, and petrochemical facilities. Lindell has studied these advisory councils extensively and concludes that they have a positive impact on disaster preparedness as they reject the isolated planning undertaken by former Civil Defense Directors (1994, p. 103). The facilitation of preparedness is especially evident when the committee is well funded, organized, committed, and capable of assessing risks, acquiring resources, developing HazMat teams, and identifying evacuation routes. LEPCs are not the only type of planning council, however. Cities may utilize several committees to monitor development, enforce building codes, establish warning systems, enhance bioterrorism preparedness, plan drills, carry out exercises, foresee land acquisition needs during recovery, promote public health and emergency medical care, manage grants, and protect critical infrastructure.

Emergency managers also work with neighboring jurisdictions to ready themselves for disasters. One way of increasing preparedness is through a mutual aid agreement, which is a "pact between local governments whereby each pledges to assist the other in time of need" (Poulin, 2005, p. 1). Mutual aid agreements prove useful because internal resources are often insufficient during response and recovery operations. Disasters typically outstrip emergency personnel because a fire has spiraled out of control, or because there are too many victims who need medical treatment, too many roads to be cleared of debris, and too many volunteers to be managed. Material resources, in terms of generators, heavy equipment, or WMD diagnostic tools, may be inadequate as well. Such shortages are not automatic, however. Research illustrates that too many people or supplies may sent to the scene of a disaster, thereby complicating response and recovery operations (Lowe & Fothergill, 2003; Neal, 1994). Emergency managers should consequently establish mutual aid agreements, considering there is no way to know or predict exactly what each disaster may bring. The mutual aid agreement should address the conditions under which it will be implemented, exclusion clauses, financial responsibility, repayment issues, and death or victim benefits (McEntire & Myers, 2004). Most importantly, the mutual aid agreement must be approved by the legal counsel for each local jurisdiction to avoid liability.

Emergency managers are also actively involved in regional planning consortiums. Cities work with other jurisdictions to save resources and increase the effectiveness of emergency management. The Department of Homeland Security, the Office of Domestic Preparedness, FEMA and many states now require a regional approach if certain grants are to be distributed. The logic is that funds will be conserved under this organizational arrangement. For instance, instead of funding a hazardous materials team and a mobile command vehicle for each community, a regional strategy dictates that each of these items are given to different cities with an expectation that they are to be shared with all jurisdictions in that particular area. A vivid example of this approach is seen in the efforts of the Emergency Preparedness Department of North Central Texas Council of Governments (NCTCOG) (see http://www.nctcog.org/ep/index.asp). The NCTCOG includes 16 counties and 230 member governments, and the staff and city personnel involved disaster planning work together to promote advocacy, information sharing, and collaboration. The Emergency Preparedness Department is especially active with the major cities in the Dallas-Fort Worth Metroplex area (Collin, Denton, Dallas, and Tarrant counties) to promote Citizen Corps, homeland security initiatives, and the regional coordination plan. Such efforts require an extreme amount of cooperation, which may be complicated because of different community priorities and interjurisdictional politics. However, regional approaches are becoming more common and are gaining in importance as all types of government stakeholders see a further need to collaborate to address complex disaster problems.

PARTICIPATION OF EMERGENT GROUPS

Although local governments are undoubtedly major players in emergency management, it is necessary to recognize that they are not the only actors involved in disasters. Because earthquakes, hurricanes, industrial explosions, terrorist attacks, and other types of disasters create large numbers of victims, disable transportation systems, and place excessive demands on first responders, many important and urgent post-disaster needs cannot be addressed quickly or adequately. For these reasons, people do not simply wait for fire fighters, police officers, or the American Red Cross to show up at the incident scene. Bystanders and victims instead take initiative to care for themselves and for others.

Research has consistently shown that citizens engage in emergency response after a disaster (Drabek & McEntire, 2002). For instance, a great deal of research emanated in the 1950s from the National Opinion Research Center (NORC) detailing the convergence of people and organizations to provide humanitarian assistance in disasters (Fritz & Marx, 1954; Fritz & Mathewson, 1957). Scholars have since added to these findings, illustrating that the human desire to help those in need is nearly an irrefutable fact in virtually every type of disaster, perhaps even regardless of location (Aguirre, Wenger, Glass, Diaz-Murillo, & Vigo, 1995; Bardo, 1978;

Comfort, 1996; Drabek, 1986; Dynes, 1970; Wenger & James, 1990; Wilson & Oyola-Yemaiel, 1998). Such was the case in New York after the 9/11 terrorist attacks; volunteers came from all across the United States to assist those affected by this world-changing event (Lowe & Fothergill, 2003). These altruistic endeavors are known as "emergent behavior" and the people involved in disaster responses are labeled as "emergent groups."

Emergent behavior may be loosely defined as a form of collective activity (being distinct from prior behavior resulting from a consensus on new norms) which creates a unique social order that has not yet become institutionalized (see Killian, 1994, p. 278). In the context of disaster, this means that individuals see needs that are not being met and therefore attempt to address them in an informal manner. People join together to complete tasks that often include, but are not limited to, search and rescue, emergency medical care, donations management, and debris removal. Those who participate in these atypical disaster functions are considered emergent groups—citizens and others who come together in an informal manner to address the new tasks that are made evident by the disaster (Stallings & Quarantelli, 1985, p. 94).

Emergent groups are therefore different than other types of organizations (Dynes, 1970). For instance, emergent groups (e.g., unaffiliated volunteers) undertake activities that were previously foreign to them and develop a social structure that lacks formalization, tradition, and endurance (Stallings & Quarantelli, 1985, p. 94). In contrast, an established organization (e.g., a fire department) performs routine functions in a disaster and maintains its traditional organizational relationship with the chief and the subordinates. An extending organization (e.g., the American Red Cross) completes routine functions in a disaster but creates new relationships as workers from around the country converge to the scene of a disaster. Finally, an expanding organization (e.g., a church that gets involved in disasters) tackles new tasks but maintains traditional relationships among the pastor and the members.

While emergent behavior and groups are most evident during times of emergency, this should not be taken to imply that such phenomena are nonexistent in other phases of emergency management. One study of 50 emergent groups reveals that emergent groups have become involved in a variety of issues and activities:

- educating a community about earthquakes,
- opposing the location of a hazardous chemical waste site,
- preventing further development in a flood plain,
- informing citizens about the dangers of a nuclear power plant,
- protecting a creek from being polluted,
- developing an emergency operations plan,
- proposing a flash flood warning system,
- training neighbors on disaster response,
- obtaining funding for homes damaged by landslides,
- replanting trees destroyed by a tornado, and
- protesting decisions regarding post-disaster housing (Stallings & Quarantelli, 1985, p. 95).

As can be seen, emergent groups may provide numerous benefits for a wide-range of emergency management activities. The emergency manager should be aware that emergent organizations do at times present challenges for those involved in this profession, however. In one disaster, one telephone call to a religious organization generated more than 6000 volunteers to help sand bag in a little more than an hour (Armstrong & Rosen, 1986, p. 23). Situations like this typically generate logistical difficulties in that volunteers need to be checked in, given equipment and directions, and monitored to ensure they are performing the job correctly.

In other cases, well-intentioned citizens may unintentionally hurt the trapped victims they are trying to rescue, and the donations sent to a disaster area may require sorting, storage, distribution, or disposal. The major implication for local emergency managers is that emergent groups are inevitable (Stallings & Quarantelli, 1985, p. 98) and they are major participants in emergency management.

EMERGENCY MANAGEMENT ORGANIZATIONS IN OTHER NATIONS

There have been repeated calls for studies about emergency management and emergence in other nations (Drabek, 1986; Dynes, 1988; Peacock, 1997). However, much of the research is still conducted in developed countries such as the United States. A number of studies have examined international responses to disasters (Cuny, 1983; Green, 1977; Kent, 1987; McEntire, 1997). Scholars have also investigated the causes and consequences of earthquakes, famines, hurricanes, technological disasters, complex emergencies (Cuny & Hill, 1999; McEntire, 2003; Minear & Weiss, 1995; Oliver-Smith, 1994; Perrow, 1999) and a host of other disasters (Farazmand, 2001), subject areas (Mitchell, 1999), and processes (Porfiriev, 1999a). There are far fewer studies about official and unofficial disaster organizations around the world, but there are some notable exceptions including the informative chapter about the Philippines, Japan, and New Zealand in this text by Neil Britton.

One of the first comparative studies of official emergency management organizations was completed by Bejamin McLuckie, a Ph.D. student at the renowned Disaster Research Center. McLuckie explored the management of disasters in Italy, Japan, and the United States (1970). He discovered that each nation decentralized authority in time of disasters, although the former two countries were more centralized than the latter. His research reveals that organizational arrangement can have a dramatic impact on the effectiveness of disaster institutions. Other in-depth studies have been conducted about Russia (Porfiriev, 1999b), Australia (Britton & Clark, 2000), and the United Kingdom (O'Brien & Read, 2005). These illustrate that hazards, historical circumstances, culture, political objectives, and current events influence the organizational arrangements for emergency management. They also reveal that many actors are involved in disaster planning and management, although this varies by country. Less is known about disaster organizations in developing nations, where governments tend to be highly centralized and the military is more heavily involved in emergency management functions. While comparative research has undoubtedly increased over the years, Quarantelli's admonition (1989c, p. 6) for more studies remains justified.

In comparison to the above studies regarding official organizations in other countries, there has probably been more research on emergent behavior in foreign disasters. Of course, anyone with an interest in disaster behavior is aware of Prince's description of human collective action after the Halifax, Nova Scotia shipping explosion and the impact that this has had on scholarship in the area (Scanlon, 1988). Similar studies on post-disaster behavior have been conducted around the world. Among the first truly cross-national projects was Clifford's research (1956) on the response to the Rio Grande River that flooded Eagle Pass, Texas and Piedras Negras, Mexico. He wanted to know how cultural values would affect the response, and found that family and informal organizations were more important in Mexico than in the United States where victims relied more heavily on government institutions. This line of research has been continued by Aguirre and his colleagues (1995), illustrating that routine social patterns are often witnessed after a disaster. Dynes' work (2003) also reiterates social continuities after disasters.

One of the most universal findings in many different disaster contexts around the world is that people generally come together to meet disaster demands. However, at least one study has revealed that political unrest may emerge after major disasters (Olson & Drury, 1997). There are also some differences in terms of the degree of convergence, therapeutic activity, and nature and extent of emergent groups in Mexico, the United States, Russia, and Japan (Comfort, 1996; Drabek, 1987a; Porfiriev, 1996; Quarantelli, 1989c; Scawthorn & Wenger, 1990; Vigo & Wenger, 1994). Reports of antisocial behavior (e.g., looting) may also be more common in certain types of disasters (Drabek, 1986, p. 231), although we lack sufficient evidence to make such statements across countries. It is thus problematic to generalize at times about emergent behavior in other nations.

CURRENT CHALLENGES AND FUTURE OPPORTUNITIES

This assessment of local emergency management organizations would be incomplete if it did not provide a discussion about future expectations. This final section therefore outlines some of the problems facing the profession in addition to various measures that should be taken to improve performance. First, there can be little doubt that emergency managers must increase their awareness of the trends pertaining to disaster occurrence and impacts, and accordingly do a better job of sharing such information with decision makers and citizens in their communities. Quarantelli's research (1992b) indicates that industrialization and urbanization are among several factors that augment the frequency and severity of disasters. Rising losses have also been reiterated and projected in the most recent assessments of the field (Mileti, 1999). Therefore, emergency managers must do a better job of educating themselves and others to counter prevailing apathetic attitudes about disasters.

In conjunction with this step, emergency managers must also develop improved communication skills and master the art of persuasion (to increase the possibility of buy-in among politicians, department leaders, and other organizational stakeholders). In spite of the current educational opportunities, professionalization is still desperately needed among the rank and file of those working in the field. Future emergency managers must also possess expanded knowledge of different academic disciplines, distinct practical functional areas, and key partners in the public, private, and nonprofit sectors. Today's complex and dynamic disasters require knowledgeable professionals who understand effective management principles and are able to make good decisions based on unique disaster contexts.

To assist them with the difficult choices they often face, emergency managers should become more versed in modern technological tools. Geographic information systems (GIS), computers, remote sensing, personal digital assistants (PDAs), and other equipment may help the emergency manager understand what has occurred and how the disaster may unfold, along with projected needs and what to do about them (Dash, 1997; Fischer, 1998b; Gruntfest & Weber, 1998; Stephensen & Anderson, 1997; Sutphen & Waugh, 1998; Waugh, 1995). For instance, GIS may help emergency managers identify the number of people affected by a hurricane while decision support software such as E-Team and Cameo/Aloha can track human and material resources or the plume of a hazardous materials release. A reliance on technology should always be coupled with a realization of its potential drawbacks and limitations, however (Quarantelli, 1997a). Technological approaches cannot resolve all of the social problems inherent in disasters (e.g., miscommunication).

Local emergency managers and related organizations should also be weary of an overemphasis on homeland security. It is true that the threat of terrorism is both real and menacing in our current era, and the consequences of attacks involving WMD could kill thousands, hundreds of thousands, or even millions. However, it is also the case that terrorist attacks have historically been less likely than natural and technological disasters, and the effects of these latter incidents can be equally devastating as the Indian Ocean Tsunami and Hurricane Katrina revealed. Emergency managers should accordingly consider all types of hazards, and ensure that they do not neglect the range of potentialities and disaster needs. New programs espoused by the Department of Homeland Security should be integrated into emergency management organizations, but they should not discount the value of traditional approaches for floods, fires, industrial explosions, and the like.

The emphasis on homeland security does present a great prospect for further funding for emergency management however. A great deal of political support has been given to the terrorism threat, and funding for professionals in the field may be at historically high levels. Some of these grant programs may be specific to terrorism (e.g., Urban Area Security Initiative) but others may have broad application to all types of events (e.g., first responder equipment initiatives). Understanding what grants are available and how to obtain them are likely to be coveted skills in the future. If these grants are funded, emergency managers will then need to administer them according to federal rules and regulations. This will require a larger emergency management staff in most communities, which brings up an additional recommendation for the future.

Emergency managers have traditionally been underfunded and overworked in most jurisdictions. New terrorism preparedness initiatives and grant programs discussed above have only exacerbated the already thinly stretched human resources. Politicians and communities must therefore hire additional personnel in emergency management, and emergency managers should take advantage of the current context to promote their programs and departments. Increased responsibilities cannot be adequately addressed by a limited number of emergency managers.

Fortunately, there are many stakeholders to whom the load can be distributed. Emergency managers should therefore spend more time and energy interacting with others. Therefore, networking is a vital activity for everyone involved in the field. Mileti has provided useful recommendations for those establishing and participating in such networks. He asserts that these networks must be inclusive, function in a democratic manner, promote continuous learning, adapt to changing circumstances, and work for the benefit of all parties involved (Mileti, 1999, p. 270).

As emergency managers network and prepare with other departments, planning committees, mutual aid parties, and regional consortiums, it will be imperative that interoperability be developed. This implies not only that all organizations successfully communicate with others, but that they also understand their own roles in times of disasters and how others fit into the overall system of emergency management. Organizational barriers in terms of culture and politics will have to be overcome, and the equipment and language needed to coordinate must become more standardized. The National Incident Management System promoted by FEMA and the Department of Homeland Security will be extended to all jurisdictions in the country in order to foster increased collaboration, and states may desire to emulate California's exemplary Standard Emergency Management System. Everyone needs to have the same strategy (i.e., to reduce the impact of disasters through coordination), even if the individual organizational responsibilities vary in dramatic ways. The overarching goal should be to reduce fragmentation and integrate activities both vertically among levels of government and horizontally across departments. This is especially crucial as disasters span geographic space and distinct authority domains.

Local emergency management organizations must also recognize that unofficial players will continue to respond to disasters of all types. Emergent behavior is to be expected when extreme situations occur, and this poses advantages and disadvantages for the emergency manager. Consequently, emergent groups must be taken into consideration during the planning process; emergency managers cannot afford to ignore emergence as was done in prior years (Dynes, 1994a). Care must be therefore be given to integrate emergent groups into the response in such a way as to harness their potential contributions in disasters while also minimizing the challenges they present to emergency managers. The current Citizen Corps and CERT programs may help local emergency management organizations reach these goals (Simpson, 2001).

Another possible way to improve emergency management is to learn from other nations. Although hazards might vary by country, the lessons regarding mitigation, preparedness, response, and recovery might have application beyond national borders. As comparative research expands in the future, emergency managers should stay on top of the literature. Furthermore, emergency managers should stay in tune with current disasters around the world and consider the implications of those events for their own jurisdictions. Emergency managers should therefore be continuous students, seeking to apply best practices for the benefit of the community in which they reside.

Finally, and most importantly, local emergency management organizations must become more proactive in their efforts to prevent disasters and prepare to more effectively deal with their adverse impacts. For too long, emergency managers have seen themselves as an extension of first responders who react after an event occurs. Although it will certainly be impossible to eliminate all disasters because of powerful natural hazards, human fallibility regarding the use of technology and seemingly endless social conflicts, there is no reason why more cannot be done to reduce their frequency of occurrence and intensity of impact through more holistic policies (Mileti, 1999; Quarantelli, 1992b).

Unfortunately, local emergency managers have been faced with continuous changes in federal programs. Not only has the nation focused more heavily on one hazard than another at any given time in history, but there has also been an introduction of one policy proposal to be followed by a completely different programmatic objective. As an example, the nation shifted in the 1990s from the comprehensive emergency management concept to a risk-based approach that attempts to build disaster-resistant communities (FEMA, 1997). After the 9/11 terrorist attacks occurred, the federal government again changed priorities—this time to homeland security. Such fluctuations create a serious challenge for small emergency management programs in that momentum built up in one area is repeatedly lost through continuous alterations in policy directions.

Scholars have also proposed additional concepts for emergency managers to consider, and they have brought recognition to variables that have heretofore been neglected. The social vulnerability school asserts that we must take into account people's susceptibility owing to the political and economic structures (Wisner, Blaikie, Cannon, & Davis, 2004, p. 11). Mileti (1999) has encouraged practitioners to consider the utility of the sustainable hazards mitigation concept in that development must be linked to disasters. Others espouse the notion of resilience to disasters to improve institutional capacity (Buckle, Mars, & Smale, 2000; Paton, Smith, & Violanti, 2000). But these and other viewpoints have perhaps inadvertently added to the ongoing confusion.

What is needed is a policy guide that considers the advantages and disadvantages of each of the prior perspectives. For example, comprehensive emergency management attempted to be an inclusive policy, but it was much too reactive (Britton, 1999, p. 23). A risk-based approach is proactive, but it is generally associated with a technocratic approach to disasters (Wisner et al., 2004, p. 4). Implementing the disaster resistance policy will help to limit losses, but it is a restraining concept in that it may ignore social variables (Mileti, 1999, p. 264). The current focus on homeland security takes into account a real and menacing threat, but it appears to ignore the all-hazards approach that has guided the field for several years (Waugh, 2004c). Those who focus on susceptibility bring to light important social variables although they may inadvertently downplay hazardous locations and dangerous construction practices (Wisner et al., 2004, p. 15). Sustainable hazards mitigation brings to light the value of environmental protection, but it appears to neglect certain phases and actors in emergency management and possibly even actual disasters themselves (Aguirre, 2002b, p. 121; Berke, 1995a, p. 14–15; Mitchell, 1999, p. 505). Resilience is definitely a laudable goal, but it deals less with mitigation and preparedness functions and more with response and recovery operations (Geis, 2000, p. 41; Kendra & Wachtendorft, 2003, p. 41). All of these issues raise the question as to how local emergency management organizations are to operate effectively under what might be termed as a condition of conceptual or policy anarchy.

One possible method to overcome the individual weaknesses of these concepts but retain and integrate their divergent strengths is through the principles of liability reduction and capacity building (which can be regarded as a broad form of disaster vulnerability management) (McEntire, 2000, 2004b; McEntire, Fuller, Johnson, & Weber, 2002).). This suggests that local emergency managers, community stakeholders, and all citizens should strive to reduce liabilities by limiting each of the factors that contribute to disasters (i.e., risk from the physical, biological, built and technological environments, and susceptibility from the social, political, cultural, economic, and institutional realms). Emergency managers should also build capacity through mitigation measures and preparedness steps to reduce impact and advance coping abilities (i.e., resistance and resilience). Such principles are therefore based on—but go much further than—FEMA's prior policy of integrated emergency management (IEM), which never met its goal of reducing risks and focused on the development of response capabilities alone (see Table 10.1).

Interestingly, the literature from diverse scholars—when considered collectively and not individually—may add support for this model of emergency management. For instance, it has been illustrated that culture, exposure to hazards, social structure, root causes, dynamic processes, and unsafe conditions (i.e., liabilities) augment vulnerability (Bogard, 1989; Dow & Downing, 1995; Watts & Bohle, 1993; Wisner et al., 2004). Scholars also imply that capability or capacity has a direct relation to vulnerability (Anderson & Woodrow, 1998; Bohle, Downing, & Watts, 1994; Dow, 1992; Kates, 1985; Pijawka & Radwan, 1985; Timmerman, 1981; Watts & Bohle, 1993).

In their article about risk and resilience, Britton and Clark (2000) acknowledge that both physical variables and social and demographic patterns increase the possibility of disaster, and they state that engineers, emergency planners, and a host of others may implement actions to minimize impact. Don Geis (2000), a major proponent of the resistance paradigm, illustrates how land-use planning, construction materials and techniques, and environmental protection can reduce the risk of disaster. He also accepts the possibility of social proneness as a result of quality of life issues, and discusses how resilience relates to resistance

TABLE 10.1. Comparison of Two Emergency Management Models

Integrated Emergency Management	Disaster Vulnerability Management
1. Assess risks	1. Assess risks and susceptibilities
2. Assess capabilities	2. Assess resistance and resilience
3. Close the gap between them	3. Reduce liabilities/raise capabilities

(Geis, 2000). Scholarship in the area of homeland security continues these themes as well. Falkenrath, Newman, and Thayer (1998) point out how to reduce the probability or risk of a terrorist attack involving WMD. Webb (2002a) asks if certain individuals or groups are less likely to recover because of their susceptibility to disasters. Warn, Berman, Whittaker, and Bruneau (2003) seek to understand how the structures and infrastructure targeted by terrorists may be constructed in such as way as to promote resistance. Kendra and Wachtendorf (2003) explore the resilience of New York after 9/11, specifically focusing on creativity and improvisation. Although the social vulnerability camp downplays physical variables at times, Wisner et al., do assert at times that risk and susceptibility are products of environmental factors such as land use and construction (2004, p. 4). Wisner et al., also illustrate how the degree of resistance (2004, p. 4) and resilience (2004, p. 54) relate to the social forces that affect individuals and communities. Thomas and Mileti, who support the sustainable hazards mitigation concept, declare that professionals in emergency management should "acquire a basic understanding of risk, susceptibility, resilience, [and] resistance" (2003, p. 7). *Disasters by Design*, arguably the most important book in the field, discusses the risk, susceptibility, resistance, and resilience concepts in various portions of the text (1999, see pp. 106, 125, 174, 264).

Many scholars likewise stress the centrality of vulnerability and request a shift in emphasis to this paradigm (Alexander, 2002c; Britton, 1986b; Comfort et al., 1999; Hewitt, 1983b; O'Keefe, Westgate, & Wisner, 1976; Peacock, Morrow, & Gladwin, 1997; Salter, 1997/98; Wisner et al., 2004). One possible explanation for this shift is that we are recognizing that policy tends to reflect the most recent or most devastating type of hazards, and not the commonalities in all disasters. In addition, we cannot always control hazards themselves, but our vulnerability to the hazards (Cannon, 1993). Interestingly, Weichselgartner's review (2001) of numerous definitions of the vulnerability concept stresses liabilities in an indirect manner and capabilities in a direct manner. His research also notes a close relation of risk, susceptibility, resistance, and resilience to many scholars' definitions of vulnerability.

Even practitioners appear to emphasize vulnerability, risk, susceptibility, resistance, and resilience. Those designing policy for the International Decade for Natural Disaster Reduction, the Yokohama Strategy, and the International Strategy for Disaster Reduction clearly use these terms repeatedly in their respective documents. Reviews of the recent World Conference on Disaster Reduction likewise stress capacity, risk, resilience, and root causes (e.g. liabilities) (Jigyasu 2005; La Trobe, 2005; Pelling, 2005; Rodriguez, 2005; Wisner, 2005). Commenting on this gathering, Villagran Da Leon observes that "the initial risk model based on hazards and vulnerabilities now encompasses issues such as coping capacities, resilience, susceptibility and [other] new terms" (2005, p. 145). Scholarship therefore appears to be converging on several important concepts, and a consensus about policy priorities may be occurring (Britton, 1999b, p. 227; Cole & Buckle, 2004; Weichselgartner, 2001). Local emergency management organizations might therefore want to consider liability reduction and capacity building as ideals to be pursued in order to minimize their community's vulnerability to future disasters (McEntire, 2004a).

RESEARCH NEEDS

The evolving nature of emergency management as well as current challenges and opportunities open up several research avenues for scholars. A few of them will be mentioned here. First, more studies need to be conducted on emergency management organizational arrangements, and the pros and cons of independent emergency management offices and those integrated into other departments. Not enough is known about the optimal location for local emergency managers. An updated and thorough assessment of all types of emergency management organizations would increase understanding of roles and responsibilities, and thereby facilitate improved coordination. There are many actors and agencies involved in disasters, and there is a dearth of literature on the contributions each one makes. Another research opportunity pertains to the skills needed to be developed by local emergency managers. There are very few studies about how to successfully promote and administer emergency management programs at the local level. Scholars may also desire to reexamine the value of planning councils, the importance of and difficulties associated with mutual aid arrangements, and the strategies for regional integration of emergency management programs. Information about intergovernmental relations is scarce, particularly as it pertains to local interaction with state and federal emergency management agencies. There is a lack of investigations about emergency management organizations in foreign nations, and research on emergence in other countries could be revisited. This would help generate additional lessons for emergency managers in the United States and around the world. In light of the current emphasis on terrorism, there is insufficient information about technology to detect and deal effectively with WMD, grants administration, and the impact of NIMS and the Department of Homeland Security on emergency management organizations. The advantages and disadvantages of current homeland security policy on emergency management deserve significant attention—especially when one considers the less than desirable response to Hurricane Katrina. Finally, a serious assessment of alternative policies for emergency management is warranted. A specific recommendation is to consider the utility of the concept of vulnerability and its relation to other popular terms being discussed today among scholars and practitioners (McEntire, 2004b).

CONCLUSION

Emergency management is a crucial and complex profession that has changed dramatically over time. Emergency management organizations vary dramatically in terms of their name, size, and position in municipal government, although each organization increasingly strives to reduce disasters through mitigation, preparedness, response and recovery activities. Because there is no way local emergency managers can fulfill all of these responsibilities alone, they frequently call upon and work with other departments, planning committees, mutual aid parties, regional consortiums, and even emergent groups. In the future, progress will be seen in numerous areas of emergency management, especially in relation to awareness of disasters, the art of administration, and the use of technology. Effective emergency managers should maintain a balanced approach to the hazards that confront their communities, seek grants and additional personnel for their organizations, network with other agencies, improve intergovernmental and multiorganizational relations, and learn from disasters and emergency management institutions in other countries. Of paramount importance is the need to integrate proactive concepts and holistic policies in order reduce vulnerability and minimize the adverse impacts disasters produce. Scholars also play an important role in understanding emergency management, and several areas of investigation deserve additional academic attention. As professionals and researchers give further attention to these issues, emergency management organizations will be better able to address the major challenges that disasters will certainly present in the future.

CHAPTER 11

Community Processes: Warning and Evacuation

John H. Sorensen and Barbara Vogt Sorensen

Almost every day people evacuate from their homes, businesses or other sites, and even ships in response to actual or predicted threats or hazards. Evacuation is the primary protective action utilized in large-scale disasters such as hurricanes, floods, tsunamis, volcanic eruptions, releases of hazardous or nuclear materials, and high-rise building fires and explosions. Although often precautionary, protecting human lives by withdrawing populations during times of threat remains a major emergency management strategy. There have been some instances in which removal of property and livestock to safer places has been a major evacuation activity for some businesses such as automobile or boat dealers or specialty farm managers, but these evacuation activities lack systematic validation. Although there is some excellent research on evacuation behavior in other countries, such as the Holland floods in the early 1950s, the focus of this chapter is on evacuation behavior in the United States.

The term "evacuation" is used to describe the withdrawal actions of persons from a specific area because of a real or anticipated threat or hazard. The time period for the span of withdrawal is elastic in that the evacuation may last for any amount of time, and may occur more than once or sequentially should there be secondary hazards or a reoccurrence or escalation of the original threat. For example, while the primary hazards form hurricanes are wind and storm surge flooding, secondary threats could include inland riverine flooding that might necessitate a second evacuation effort. Further, the evacuation experience can include events when a return to the original site is not feasible or forbidden, as when the federal government buys out or relocates communities prone to recurring floods or when a state or federal agency quarantines a contaminated area. In this sense, the definition of evacuation used here deviates from that of some other researchers, such as Quarantelli (1980a), who have suggested that evacuation be considered a round-trip event. Given such events as Hurricanes Andrew and Katrina, Chernobyl, drought and civil wars in South Africa, and sites made uninhabitable by persistent chemical hazards, the decision to include long-term resettlement or relocation as part of the evacuation continuum appears appropriate. Long-term relocation of populations and the issues associated with extended evacuation periods such as after hurricanes or terrorist events may signal a trend affecting evacuation research agendas in the future.

As an alternative to evacuation, people may take protective shelter inside structures to prevent harm during severe weather that includes lightning, tornados, and hail as well as exposure to harmful substances in the air, or to quarantine during an infectious outbreak. "Vertical evacuation" in hurricanes in which people move to the upper floor of a modern high-rise building is also a form of sheltering and should not be termed evacuation. In some incidents, officials have advised both sheltering and evacuating either simultaneously for selected groups or sequentially for fast moving hazards. For example, when a toxic chemical cloud is moving rapidly over an area, people may be told to shelter and then evacuate their shelters once the major threat has passed the structure. This is because the build-up of contaminated air inside the structure will likely be higher than that of outside air once the cloud has passed. In comparison to evacuation, sheltering behavior is less understood with only a few social science studies having been conducted in the past 25 years, including Three Mile Island (Cutter & Barnes, 1982) and a hazardous material release from an explosion in Arkansas (Vogt & Sorensen, 1999).

In the last two decades there has been a greater focus on the varieties of subgroups that require special attention, such as assisted care individuals or high-rise building occupants, and on the timing of warnings to alert and notify residents of the potential threat. The attention to occupant evacuation behavior after the 2001 World Trade Center (WTC) disaster has been the most crucial in changing the evacuation and engineering paradigms for high-rise buildings that are likely to be felt worldwide as the findings are disseminated (Natural Hazard Research and Applications Information Center, 2003). These trends have led to better typologies and planning models and more critical attention to factors affecting protective actions in planning and response. Real-time transportation models developed over the past decade also allow transportation engineers to better direct egress routes but the models require more sophisticated computer modeling that many communities, especially the more rural or those with a number of absentee owners, may not have resources to incorporate into their emergency plans.

Although evacuation behavior has been closely associated with officials issuing warnings, people often spontaneously evacuate (evacuate without an official order) or refuse to comply with an evacuation order for a variety of reasons (Lindell & Perry, 2004). Evacuations work best if a community plans, organizes, develops, installs, and maintains a warning system (Lindell & Perry, 1992; Mileti & Sorensen, 1990). Developing the warning system is both an engineering process and an organizational process. Warning systems are more than technology—involving human communication, management, and decision-making. As was solidly demonstrated by the experiences on September 11, 2001, disaster in the WTC high-rise buildings, warning systems also extend far beyond "official systems" as most of the evacuees in WTC 2, the second building to be hit, initiated their evacuation before they were warned to evacuate by the building's public address system, which occurred 1 minute prior to impact (Averill et al., 2005).

In this chapter we first briefly discuss the social construction of evacuation and the changing social and technological context of evacuation. Next we examine the extent of systematic studies conducted by disaster researchers on warnings that lead to protective actions. Four major research themes are then examined:

- warning and warning response,
- societal characteristics,
- organizational response, and
- behavior in evacuations.

EVACUATION AS A COMMUNITY PROCESS

Although evacuations occur daily in the United States, it is difficult to typify a generic model because evacuations lack both definition and consensus on specific parameters. Drabek and Stephenson (1971) defined four types of evacuation: by invitation, choice, default, or compromise. Evacuation by invitation occurs when someone outside the area at risk provides the means or impetus to leave. Evacuation by decision or choice involves individuals processing warning information, deciding to leave, and then taking action. Evacuation by default involves behavior dictated by actions other than seeking safety from the hazard (such as not being allowed by officials to enter an evacuated zone or structure upon one's return). Evacuation by compromise is characterized by people following orders even though they do not want to or feel it necessary to leave (Sorensen, Vogt, & Mileti, 1987). By cross-classifying two dimensions of evacuations—timing and period of evacuation—Perry, Lindell, and Greene (1981) distinguished four types of evacuations: preventative (pre-impact, short-term), protective (pre-impact, long-term), rescue (post-impact, short-term), and reconstructive (post-impact, long-term).

Occurring across various time periods and affecting various numbers of people or groups, evacuations can also impose significant psychological and physical impacts on those involved or who are close to evacuees. Evidence from the 2004 hurricanes in Florida suggests that those impacts may be delayed as well as have effects at significant distances from the hazard source. For example, after the 2004 hurricanes many low-income elderly evacuees found it impossible to rebuild their damaged residences and as a result were forced to move to other states to live with family members. Evacuees from Floyd traveled to destinations across several counties and even into other states seeking refuge (Hazards Management Group, no date). Public outcry over congested highways used for evacuation routes for Hurricane Floyd also forced states to consider coordinating with other state's departments of transportation on traffic planning (Wolshon et al., 2005).

Evacuation is rarely an individual process. Even in single-person households, the first response to the initial evacuation warning is to seek further information on the validity of the threat or to consult with a friend, co-worker, neighbor, family member, or relative. Evacuations usually take place in a group context (Drabek & Stephenson, 1971). Families will try to reunite, if possible, to evacuate as a group, but not necessarily in a single vehicle if two or more vehicles are owned. In business settings, co-workers typically evacuate in groups (Aguirre, Wenger, & Vigo, 1998), and may be expected to regroup once evacuated.

Events that necessitate evacuation vary widely from natural or technological disasters to deliberate terrorist events. Aside from the fundamental issue of intent in terrorist-induced disasters, there are some commonalties in evacuations from deliberate and nondeliberate disasters, particularly relating to response and recovery. For example, response parallels exist between wildfires and arson, accidental explosions and bombs, airplane accidents and aviation terrorism, floods and dam sabotage, chemical releases and chemical attacks, and epidemics and biological terrorism (Demuth, 2002).

THE CHANGING TECHNOLOGICAL AND SOCIAL CONTEXT OF WARNINGS

Warning processes have traditionally been linear communication systems. In a linear process, governmental organizations identify the presence of a hazard through validated monitoring and detection systems. The data are then assessed and analyzed and could lead to the prediction of an extreme event. Such predictions typically included a forecast of the estimated lead time until impact, general location to be affected, estimated magnitude of the event, the probability of occurrence, and the likely consequences for residents. The organizations making these predictions communicate the information to public emergency officials, who in turn interpret the information, decide whether to warn, determine the content of the warning, decide the method to disseminate the message, and then issue the warning to citizens. Again, such a system is linear, going from one actor to the next. The warning that eventually gets to citizens at risk is official. People at risk are expected to respond to these official warnings. This warning process has served our nation for over a half a century, and may still be of use in rural areas with widely dispersed population and few resources.

Significant changes in American society have occurred since this linear warning process was developed. Both cultural and technological shifts in the last decade have altered our view of the public warning process and require a different approach to planning and issuing warnings. These changes include:

- new warning technologies (cell phones, Internet, pagers, palm pilots)
- private warning subscription providers,
- nationalization of news coverage,
- increased availability of visual images and information, and
- increased use of a Global Positioning System (GPS) for alert and notification.

In addition to technological changes, societal changes have impacted the warning process. Today the public does not rely on a single official source of warning information. Instead, people access or are forced to listen to multiple sources of information, some of which may be unreliable or not supported by valid models or detection systems. Increasing transmission of warning messages now compete for an individual's attention creating problems especially for fast-moving events with no communication cues. Media coverage of high-consequence/low-probability events draws attention from more common occurring risks for which warnings generally protect people. To further compound the problems America's increasing ethnic diversity with a multiplicity of languages has created more barriers to communication with minority groups at the same time that the number of such groups has grown tremendously.

Demographic changes have also affected warning communications. Increases in single-person, single-parent, and elderly households have affected people's abilities to respond to warnings, or even to respond at all. Added to these problems is the increase in residential and institutional development in vulnerable areas (especially coastal surge zones) that has led to greater number of special populations at risk. Placing nursing homes and assisted living facilities on exposed barrier islands further saps scarce resources for communities that must also plan for evacuating large seasonal tourist populations who may never have experienced an evacuation.

THE RESEARCH RECORD

The empirical study of public evacuation and response to emergency warnings has proceeded for more than 40 years (Baker, 1979; Drabek & Stephenson, 1971; Lachman, Tatsuoka, & Bonk, 1961; Leik, Carter, Clark, Kondall, Gifford and Ekker, 1981; Mileti & Beck, 1975; Perry & Mushkatel, 1986, 1984; Quarantelli, 1980a). These studies, when viewed collectively, have compiled an impressive record about how and why public behavior occurs in the presence of impending disaster or threat. For example, it is well documented that emergency warnings are most effective at eliciting public protective actions such as evacuation when those warnings are frequently repeated (Mileti & Beck, 1975), confirmatory in character (Drabek & Stephenson, 1971) and perceived by the public as credible (Perry et al., 1981). Excellent summaries of

TABLE 11.1. Behavioral Surveys on Evacuation Behavior of Residential Population in the United States

Event	Source
Rio Grande flood	Clifford, 1956
Hilo Tsunami	Lachman et al., 1961
Hurricane Carla	Moore et al., 1964
Hurricane Camille	Wilkinson & Ross, 1970
Denver flood	Drabek & Stephenson, 1971
Rapid City flood	Mileti & Beck, 1975
Big Thompson flood	Gruntfest, 1977
Hurricane Eloise	Windham et al., 1977
Hurricane Eloise	Baker, 1979
Three Mile Island nuclear accident	Cutter & Barnes, 1982; Flynn, 1979
Mississauga chemical accident	Burton, 1981
Sumner flood	Perry et al., 1981
Valley flood	Perry et al., 1981
Fillmore flood	Perry et al., 1981
Snoqualmie flood	Perry et al., 1981
Clarksburg flood	Leik et al., 1981
Rochester flood	Leik et al., 1981
Hurricane David	Leik et al., 1981
Hurricane Frederick	Leik et al., 1981
Mt. St. Helens volcano	Perry & Greene, 1983
Mt. St. Helens ash	Dillman et al., 1983
Abilene flood	Perry & Mushkatel, 1984
Mt. Vernon chemical accident	Perry & Mushkatel, 1984
Denver chemical accident	Perry & Mushkatel, 1986
Hurricane Elena	Baker, 1987, Nelson et al., 1989
Hurricane Kate	Baker, 1987
Confluence PA chemical spill	Rogers & Sorensen, 1989
Nanticote chemical accident	Duclos et al., 1989
Pittsburg PA chemical spill	Rogers & Sorensen, 1989
Hurricane Andrew	Gladwin & Peacock, 1997
Hurricane Bertha	Dow & Cutter, 1998
Hurricane Fran	Dow & Cutter, 1998
Hurricane Georges	Dash & Morrow, 2001; Howell, 1998
Helena AR chemical accident	Vogt & Sorensen, 1999
Hurricane Brett	Prater et al., 2000
Hurricane Bonnie	Whitehead et al., 2000
Hurricane Floyd	Dow & Cutter, 2002; HMG, no date
Hurricane Ivan	Howell & Bonner, 2005

this research currently exist (Drabek, 1986; Lindell & Perry, 2004; Mileti & Sorensen, 1988; Tierney, Lindell, & Perry, 2001). Studies and summaries like these have done much to further social scientific understanding of how people process and respond to risk communications in emergencies; they have also served to inform practical emergency preparedness efforts in this nation and abroad.

The empirical research record on public behavior in evacuations is listed in Table 11.1. These studies represent major post-disaster surveys of the public that resided in areas for which a warning of an impending disaster was issued. The warning or warnings that were officially issued for these events included an order or advisory for the public to evacuate. Each study represents the following common characteristics:

- a discrete event took place,
- a clear threat to the population was present,
- an official warning was issued, and
- a more or less random sample of the population at risk served as the basis for the survey on which the researcher(s) compiled data on public evacuation behavior.

Disaster researchers have also studied evacuation behavior for discrete populations or in specific settings. Drabek (1996) studied tourist and transient behavior in Hurricanes Bob, Andrew, and Iniki and in the Big Bear Lake and Northridge earthquakes. Vogt (1990, 1991) examined evacuation of institutionalized facilities including hospitals, nursing homes, and schools. Drabek (1999) studied the evacuation behavior of employees in 118 businesses in seven disaster events around the country. Aguirre and colleagues (1998) and Fahy (1995) examined evacuation behavior of building occupants following the 1993 bombing at the WTC. More recently an extensive study about evacuation of the WTC on September 11 was conducted (Averill et al., 2005). Kendra, Wachtendorf, and Quarantelli (2002) examined the evacuation of Manhattan by water transport. Heath, Kass, Beck, and Glickman (2001a, 2001b) studied the evacuation of families with pets in a hazardous material accident and in a flood.

MAJOR RESEARCH FINDINGS

Warnings and Warning Response

These research questions focus on the information dissemination process, the quality of the information, and the timing of the message delivery and compliance with the warnings. Hurricanes and riverine floods typically have long warning periods during which both information on the physical characteristics of the event and recommendations on protective actions are widely distributed, often over national media outlets. Other incidents have a very short time span between detection and impact and require rapid warnings. For a radiological emergency at a nuclear power plant or a chemical release, emergency personnel may elect to shelter-in-place populations at potential risk instead of recommending evacuation. Some communities, with many large industrial facilities, recommend that residents initially shelter-in-place when sirens sound and then listen for further instructions to evacuate or not (Sorensen, Vogt, & Shumpert, 2004). Some research (Three Mile Island, the West Helena explosion) indicates that residents will often defy official recommendations and evacuate even when told to shelter or advised that no protective action is needed. Among the important topics that disaster researchers have studied with respect to warning and response are:

- community adoption of warning systems,
- the timing of warning receipt and warning diffusion, and
- factors influencing household decisions to respond to warnings.

Adoption of Warning Systems

Only a few researchers have investigated the community adoption of warning systems at the community level. Most research concerning adoption has focused on mitigation at either at the community (Berke, Beatley, & Wilhite, 1989) or household (Lindell, 1997) level. A study reviewing community emergency evacuations (Hushon, Kelly, & Rubin, 1989) found the methods most often used for notification and warning were door-to-door warnings coupled with emergency vehicle public address systems and TV and radio announcements. A survey of 18 early warning systems in the United States developed to protect communities against flash floods and dam failures revealed problems of unanticipated maintenance and malfunction costs of the warning systems' components, varying levels of local commitment to maintenance, and an underemphasis on response capacity (Gruntfest & Huber, 1989).

One of the few national studies of community preparedness for chemical hazards conducted by EPA looked at the types of warning systems used by communities with hazardous materials industries (Sorensen & Rogers, 1988). Warning systems were classified into three basic types: enhanced systems, siren-based systems, and ad hoc systems. Enhanced systems use sirens and some form of specialized alerting such as tone alerts. Siren-based systems rely on sirens for alert with use of media-based notification (if the siren has no voice capability to broadcast a warning message). Ad hoc systems generally rely on media reports, an Emergency Alert System (EAS), and on door-to-door or route alert. The study found that the predominant means to warn people in close proximity of the chemical facilities was usually by an ad hoc method (45%). Sixteen percent relied on route alert or door-to-door notification. Another 29% relied on EAS or media warnings. Siren-based systems were utilized in 33% of the communities. Only 12% had access to an advanced system involving both sirens and tone-alert radios for notification.

Timing of Warning Receipt

Overall we have good insight into timing of warning dissemination. Much of this knowledge has been derived by contentions over warning systems for nuclear power plants, primarily as a result of Atomic Safety Licensing Board (ASLB) rulings. The most significant debate on what constitutes a state-of-the-art alert/notification system came in an ASLB proceeding on the Shearon Harris Nuclear Power Plant in which disaster researchers served as expert witnesses. In their final decision the ASLB defined what constitutes "essentially 100% notification within 15 minutes in the first 5 miles of the Harris Emergency Planning Zone (EPZ)" (NRC, 1986). In this matter, the board required the utility to prove that more than 95% of the people within 5 miles of the facility would receive a warning in 15 minutes in summer nighttime conditions, one of the most difficult warning times. The utility could not do so by relying solely on a siren system. To exceed the 95% requirement, commercial tone alert radios were proposed for all households within the 5-mile radius. The ASLB accepted this plan as exceeding 95% notification.

Researchers have modeled the timing of warning dissemination for specific events with multiple sources (Lindell & Perry, 2004) or for different warning technologies (Rogers & Sorensen, 1988). Often warning time is broken down into the decision time (time for officials to reach a decision to issue a warning) and dissemination time (the time it takes for the message to reach the public) (Lindell & Perry, 1992; Rogers, 1994). Once the warning is given, a mobilization time or preparation time (referring to the time taken to prepare to implement the protective action) is modeled. Implementation time is defined as when the protective action is undertaken. Mobilization times are highly variable and seem to depend on the time to impact and the level of urgency to respond (Lindell & Perry, 1992).

Survey data collected on the Nanticoke, Pennsylvania, evacuation due to a metal processing plant fire enabled the construction of empirically derived diffusion curves for different

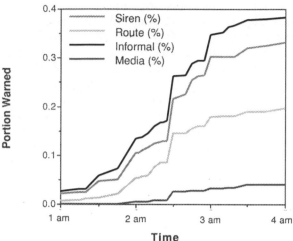

FIGURE 11.1. Source of first warning by warning technology.

warning technologies (Sorensen, 1992). The curves show the cumulative percent of the population receiving the first warning over time by the four major methods of warning. These are shown in Figure 11.1. The timing of the diffusion is very similar for siren, route, and informal alerting. Some of the early reporting of sirens and route alerts were likely made by people who heard emergency vehicles responding to the fire. The curves show a steep increase in notification when the official warning activity ensued. Data indicate that by 15 minutes into the official warning, about 65% of the public had been notified. About 22% of the public had received a siren warning at this point. The remainder had received an informal warning, from route alert or from the media.

Little research has been conducted on explaining individual variations in the timing of response (Sorensen, 1992). For example, what differentiates early or rapid responders from those who delay their response?

Factors Influencing Household Decision to Evacuate

A robust understanding of factors influencing evacuation compliance has been developed by social science researchers. The focus of the research has been on whether or not people evacuate when advised to do so (see Anderson, 1969; Baker, 1979; Cutter & Barnes, 1982; Dow & Cutter, 1998; Drabek, 1969, 1983; Drabek & Boggs, 1968; Drabek & Stephenson, 1971; Lachman et al., 1961; Leik et al., 1981; Lindell & Perry, 2004; Mileti, 1975; Mileti & Sorensen, 1988; Perry, 1979; Perry & Greene, 1982, 1983; Perry & Mushkatel, 1984, 1986; Perry et al., 1981, 1982; Quarantelli, 1980b, 1984a; Stallings, 1984; Williams, 1964; Withey, 1962).

Warning response involves a sequence of cognitive and behavioral steps. Perry and Lindell (1992, 2004a) characterize warning response as a four-stage process:

- Risk identification: Does the threat exist?
- Risk assessment: Is protection needed?
- Risk reduction: Is protection feasible? and, finally
- Protective response: What action to take?

Mileti and Sorensen (1988) characterize the process as sequential:

- *Hearing* the warning;
- *Understanding* the contents of the warning message;
- *Believing* the warning is credible and accurate;
- *Personalizing* the warning to oneself;
- *Confirming* that the warning is true and others are taking heed; and
- *Responding* by taking protective action.

Social scientists have identified both general and specific factors that affect the warning response process which include sender and receiver factors, situational factors, and social contact. The specific factors are summarized in Table 11.2 (Sorensen, 2000). Only a few of these factors can be manipulated as part of the warning process. The chief way warning response can

TABLE 11.2. **Major Factors Covarying with Evacuation Compliance**

Factor	Direction: As factor increases likelihood of evacuation ...	Level of Empirical Support
Physical cues	Increases	High
Social cues	Increases	High
Perceived risk	Increases	Moderate
Knowledge of hazard	Increases	High
Experience with hazard	Mixed	High
Education	Increases	High
Family planning	Increases	Low
Fatalistic beliefs	Decreases	Low
Resource level	Increases	Moderate
Family united	Increases	High
Family size	Increases	Moderate
Kin relations (number)	Increases	High
Community involvement	Increases	High
Ethnic group member	Decreases	Moderate
Age	Mixed	High
Socioeconomic status	Increases	High
Being female vs. male	Increases	Moderate
Having children	Increases	Moderate
Pet ownership	Decreases	Low
Channel: Electronic	Mixed	Low
Channel: Media	Mixed	Low
Channel: Siren	Decreases	Low
Personal warning vs. impersonal	Increases	High
Proximity to threat	Increases	Low
Message specificity	Increases	High
Number of channels	Increases	Low
Frequency	Increases	High
Message consistency	Increases	High
Message certainty	Increases	High
Source credibility	Increases	High
Fear of looting	Decreases	Moderate
Time to impact	Decreases	Moderate
Source familiarity	Increases	High

Source: Modified from Sorensen, 2000.

be affected by the emergency planner is in the design of the warning system including the channel of communication, public education, and specific wording of the emergency message. In addition, incentives can be offered to increase response, including information hotlines, transportation assistance, mass care facilities, and security and property protection for evacuated areas (Lindell & Perry, 1992).

One frequent response to a warning is to confirm the original message received (Drabek, 1969). Confirmation increases with longer lead-time to impacts (Perry et al., 1981), for warnings received from the media (Dillman, Schwalbe, & Short, 1983; Sorensen, 1992), and for alerts received by sirens (Sorensen, 1992). Confirmation levels decrease with the specificity of information in the first warning received (Cutter & Barnes, 1982) and when the initial warning is heard from police and fire personnel going door to door or using loudspeakers (Sorensen, 1992).

SOCIETAL CHARACTERISTICS

This research centers on the pre-emergency population attributes, including psychological, demographic, and social characteristics of those at risk. How a threat or potential risk is perceived and how (or if) people respond, especially in a rapid onset event, are often determined by existing conditions, including individual vulnerability. Some researchers have found that existing problems among population groups, such as domestic violence, escalates during disasters, especially if they include evacuation to a shelter or loss of residence (Enarson, 1998). Among the topics that disaster researchers have studied with respect to social issues are:

- how experience affects evacuation decisions,
- depersonalization and denial of risk,
- impact of preparedness effort on evacuation, and
- the relationship between culture, ethnicity, vulnerability, and evacuation.

How Experience Affects Evacuation Decision

Experiencing a disaster or a close call with an event often shapes people's response to future events; however, it does not do so in a predictable or systematic way. Direct hazard experience does not effect interpretation of warning information, decision processes, behavior, or information seeking (Lindell & Perry, 2004). Hurricane Kate led to an evacuation of the Tampa Bay area about 4 months after Hurricane Elena had prompted an unnecessary evacuation of the same area. Baker (1987) found that evacuation rates in the Tampa Bay area for Hurricane Kate were similar to that for Elena, despite the earlier false alarm. Others have suggested that long-term residents of coastal areas, who experienced minor hurricanes without severe damages, become complacent, and are less likely to evacuate in subsequent events (Windham, Posey, Ross, & Spencer, 1977). Others have suggested previous experience has had a positive effect on warning response (Lindell & Perry, 2004).

Personality, Depersonalization, and Denial of Risk

There has been a fairly widespread belief that personality factors such as locus of control (it is in the hands of others) or fatalism (what will happen will happen regardless of what I do) affect evacuation behavior. This is mainly supported by anecdotal information or newspaper coverage of people who refuse to evacuate and not by extensive empirical research. Good anecdotal examples are Harry Truman, who refused to leave his cabin near Mt. St. Helens volcano when warned because he felt his fate was in the hands of a higher authority (he died during the eruption) or people having hurricane parties. Several studies have concluded fatalism diminishes warning response for earthquakes (Turner, Nigg & Paz, 1986) and for tornados (Sims & Baumann, 1972). When faced with a warning to evacuate people often are initially in disbelief—it's not really happening to me (Drabek, 1999). Usually such perceptions are rapidly replaced by the reality of the situation.

Impact of Preparedness Efforts on Evacuation

There is no conclusive evidence regarding whether or not preparedness programs, public education, or information programs actually make a significant difference in increasing human response to warnings. The most reasonable interpretation of the evidence, when considering the empirical, anecdotal, and practical is that a good pre-emergency information program will increase response although the amount cannot be estimated (Sorensen & Mileti, 1991). Conversely, a poor program will not likely make a great overall difference. In addition, while providing information may lead to increased knowledge and preparedness, the effects drop off over time (Waterstone, 1978).

The Relationship Between Ethnicity, Culture, Vulnerability, and Evacuation

Some researchers argue that membership in a minority group typically isolates a person from information and decreases the likelihood of responding to a warning (Gladwin & Peacock, 1997; Perry et al., 1981). Other studies demonstrate that ethnicity has no significant effect on evacuation when perceived risk has the greatest influence (Perry, 1987). Language—the inability to understand the warning message—may also be a factor explaining why culturally isolated groups fail to understand a warning. The high number of deaths of Hispanics in the Saragosa, Texas tornado was attributed to a failure to provide a good translation of the warning into Spanish (Aguirre, Anderson, Balandran, Peters, & White, 1991).

In general, the literature suggests that members of minority ethnic groups are less likely to evacuate in an emergency (Mileti & Sorensen, 1988). Perry (1987) offers evidence that suggests that there appears that no ethnic differential exist with regard to the evacuation behavior when the relationships between warning belief and personal risk are controlled for. Perry (1987) also suggests from his research that some minority group members perceive authority figures—particularly uniformed "government" representatives—differently from majority group members. The higher the credibility of the warning source, the more likely the development of high levels of warning belief and the assessed personal risk, and consequently the more likely the recipient will engage in a protective action. Thus emergency managers should understand the authority figures that are regarded as credible by various population groups and have them issue warnings to achieve maximum warning compliance.

Wisner et al. (2004) offers a definition of vulnerability as it relates to hazards by suggesting vulnerability is defined by a combination of factors that influence people's ability to anticipate, cope with, resist, and recover from an identifiable event in nature or society. There is a time dimension to the definition as well, as Wisner et al. (2004) notes that vulnerability cannot be measured in immediate damages but takes into account damages to future livelihoods due to a person's (or group's) lack of resources and capacity to rebound. Although not directly related to poverty, though clearly related to socioeconomic status, Wisner's work relates to technological and terrorist events as well, and could be used for any threat that places people at risk relative to evacuation issues.

We currently know little about the social aspects of vulnerability. Social vulnerabilities, such as loss of community, are largely ignored, mainly because of the difficulty in quantifying them, which also explains why social losses are normally absent in after-disaster cost/loss estimation reports. The social mediation of vulnerability is also often overlooked (Cutter, Hodgson, Dow, 2001). Instead, social vulnerability is most often described using the individual characteristics of people (age, race, health, income, type of dwelling unit, employment). Socially mediated vulnerability is partially the product of social inequalities—those social factors that influence or shape the susceptibility of various groups to harm and that also govern their ability to respond. However, it also includes place inequalities—those characteristics of communities and the built environment, such as the level of urbanization, growth rates, and economic vitality, that contribute to the social vulnerability of places. To date, there has been little research effort focused on identifying socially constructed vulnerabilities or on comparing the social vulnerability of one place to another.

ORGANIZATIONAL RESPONSE

Typically this research has focused on the behavior of emergency preparedness and response organizations and their capacity to scale up to their response and resources if the event expands or secondary hazards occur. Among the topics that disaster researchers have studied with respect to organization are:

- the relationship between planning and response effectiveness;
- improving behavioral assumptions in planning; and
- reentry into evacuated areas, especially if decontamination effectiveness is problematical.

The Relationship Between Planning and Response Effectiveness

Evacuation warnings given without forethought or planning and without input from partners can be disastrous to both sender and receiver. It is important to plan for warning credibility, the warning message, the method of dissemination, rumor control, protective action recommendations, and incentives to response (Lindell and Perry, 2004; Mileti & Sorensen, 1990). Moreover, a warning may not be heeded by the public when the information is in direct contrast to what is being observed. To be most effective, a warning message should be planned with the concerted efforts to tell people where, when, how, and why the hazard has occurred (or is predicted to occur) and what people can do to avoid harm (Lindell & Perry, 2004). Plans should include the lead partner who will issue warnings for specific events.

Flexibility is also an essential element in planning and disseminating warnings (Mileti & Sorensen, 1990). A particular issue is how the hazard is defined, and therefore who is in charge. If an event is considered a potential crime scene, the emergency agencies responding may not be the ones who issue follow-up messages about the hazard. The key is to develop procedures to avoid conflicts in information in warning messages, recognizing that partnerships will fluctuate as the event unfolds.

Improving Behavioral Assumptions in Planning

Many emergency planning processes now involve the use of simulation models. All models concerning disaster management contain assumptions about human beings, be it an engineer's cognitive model of an equipment failure mode or a psychologist's model of how people respond to a stimulus. Few efforts have been made to identify and document behavioral assumption in models developed for and used in disaster management. It is essential that critical assumptions used in models be validated. For example, Lindell and Perry (1992) noted that the assumptions about warning and preparation times used in evacuation time estimates are based on engineering assumptions and not on behavioral data.

More work is need to develop robust models of human behavior in emergencies, including models of decision making, communication, interaction, warning systems, and protective action behaviors. For example, some dose assessment models assume people are passive receptors of an agent or are located in the same place during daytime as well as nighttime hours. Models based on these assumptions might not apply when people are fleeing or taking precautions in place. Santos and Aguirre (2004) argue that simulation models for emergency planning and intervention need to be linked to fieldwork and empirical investigations of emergency evacuations in order to provide modelers with the appropriate parameters for human behavior.

Reentry Into Evacuated Areas

Planning for reentry remains an issue that is often not addressed in plans. What is known on reentry procedures is not always implemented in practice. We know residents want to return as soon as possible to evacuated homes, that they do not travel far from home, and that considerable antagonism results if they are forced to remain away from their homes (Dash & Morrow, 2001). Research from Hurricane Elena evacuees indicated that approximately 75% of evacuees sought refuge in their home counties and reentry to designated evacuated areas became a significant issue (Nelson, Crumley, Fritsche, & Adcock,1989).

Guidelines for reentry into an area following a chemical release are practically nonexistent as are protocols and equipment for environmental monitoring in areas evacuated (Vogt & Sorensen, 2002). In the Miamisburg, Ohio, white phosphorus accident, citizens returned to their homes after being evacuated only to be forced to evacuate again as the situation worsened (Menker & Floren, 1986).

Managing traffic during reentry can be more problematic than during the evacuation. Witzig and Shillenn's (1987) study of traffic accidents in more than 300 evacuations traffic jams showed they were more likely during reentry than in the movement out.

BEHAVIOR IN EVACUATIONS

This category of research focuses on actual behavior in evacuations (and sheltering-in-place). Among the major research topics are:

- evacuation compliance,
- evacuation of special populations,
- evacuation of pets, and
- evacuation destinations.

Compliance with Evacuation Recommendations

Disaster researchers have studied issues associated with compliance with official orders to evacuate or not to evacuate. Such issues concern "shadow" evacuation, defined as people evacuating from outside the official evacuation zone, "early" or "spontaneous" evacuation, defined as people evacuating before an official warning is issued, evacuation rates in different risk zones, and "cry-wolf" effects. "Cry wolf" effects are defined as the noncompliance with warnings behavior that might be expected from residents who have responded to too many "false alarm" warning messages. "Warning fatigue" and the design of warning messages for special populations with limited sight or hearing have also been discussed in the literature but not in the same depth as the subjects previously mentioned (Mayhorn, 2004).

Evacuation rates vary by event, depending on the timing, perceived severity, constraints, susceptibility, and cost (Drabek, 1986). When warned properly, significant proportions of the threatened population respond in a reasonable manner (Drabek, 1986). In most evacuations, not everyone at risk or in areas in which evacuations are ordered or recommended, participate in the evacuation. Reasons for noncompliance include not having access to transportation, being mobility impaired, not being able to afford to evacuate, needing to work, needing to provide care, and thinking one's location is safe. Evacuation rates vary for different hazard types, for different events, and for different level of risk (as defined geographically). Evacuation rates are very high for most hazardous material accidents, where compliance may be in the high 90% range. Evacuation rates are typically low for slow onset events such as riverine floods. Evacuation rates vary in hurricanes depending on the strength of the storm and location. In high-hazard storm surge area evacuation rates may be as high as 90% in major storms. Evacuation rates are much lower for smaller hurricanes and in lower risk zones.

"Shadow evacuation" was well documented for Hurricane Floyd. The Hazards Management Group of Tallahassee, Florida (2000) studied the public's response to Hurricane Floyd in 1999 through 6900 structured telephone interviews with North Carolina, South Carolina, Georgia, and Florida residents in surge and nonsurge areas, as well as residents in noncoastal areas. Results revealed some of the highest participation rates ever experienced in an evacuation in the high-risk surge zone. Most evacuees cited evacuating because of notices from public officials and what they heard on the Weather Channel and local weather stations. A large percentage of respondents sought refuge out-of-county and out-of-state, with very few seeking refuge in official shelters. The data indicate that "shadow evacuation" in low-risk areas not told by officials to evacuate was high in almost every location. For example, evacuation rates in noncoastal counties, the lowest risk zone, ranged from 12% to 49%, with an average of 26%.

The concept of "spontaneous" evacuation grew out of analyses of the evacuation at Three Mile Island, when many more people evacuated than were advised to leave (Cutter & Barnes, 1982). In fact, spontaneous evacuation occurs in most evacuation events. People leave coastal areas when a hurricane seems eminent before officials order or recommend evacuation. In hazardous material accidents plant workers or first responders contact friends and relatives thought to be at potential risk before an official evacuation order (Vogt & Sorensen, 1999).

The effectiveness of people's responses to warnings is not always diminished by what has been labeled the "cry-wolf" syndrome. Two issues regarding false alarms are significant. The first concerns a false alarm that leads to the public taking a protective action such as evacuating. In this case, if the bases for the warning and reasons for the "miss" are told to the public in question and understood by them, the integrity of the warning system will be preserved. Data from hurricane evacuation studies indicate that false alarms do not prevent people from evacuating in the future if they know the basis for the uncertainty and the false alarm (Baker, 1987).

The second issue related to the "cry wolf" syndrome concerns repeated activation of the alert mechanisms. If such false alarms occur and no attempt is made to explain why they were false alarms, there could be a negative effect on subsequent public response to warning of a subsequent event (Breznitz, 1984). This is particularly true of inadvertent sounding of sirens if such malfunctions are frequent and not explained. It may also occur in populations around industrial facilities that use sirens to signal work shift changes.

Animals in Evacuations

Most disaster relief shelters or commercial lodging facilities do not allow people to bring in pets or other animals unless they are designated as certified companion animals for persons with disabilities. The Federal Emergency Management Agency (FEMA), however, recommends people evacuate with pets. An issue receiving increasing attention is what evacuees do with pets or other animals such as livestock when they leave their homes and whether having pets or animals impacts their decision to evacuate. Nelson et al. (1989) found that in Hurricane Elena, 25% of evacuees left their pets at home while they were gone. Most evacuees took their pets to either a friend or relative. The 11% of evacuees who took their pets to shelters left the animals in vehicles for the duration of the stay. Heath (2001b) found that in a flood evacuation, half of the pet owners evacuated with their pets and the other half did not.

For a protracted evacuation or one in which toxic fumes were involved, leaving pets behind could be a significant problem as premature reentry by evacuees could place residents at further risk. Cann (1990) found that during the 10-day Haggersfield evacuation from an area where burning tires created toxic fumes, residents routinely returned to their homes to care for livestock. Heath (2001a) found that in a chemical accident, 60% of the evacuees had dogs and cats. Of those, 49% evacuated with their pets, 41% initially left them home but later attempted to rescue them, and only 10% left them home without a rescue attempt. Buck (1987) notes that in certain situations evacuating livestock may be the only measure offering protection to animals. How that is best accomplished under various time frames remains problematic. Nelson et al. (1989) found that in Hurricane Elena people who had pets at the time of the hurricane were less likely to evacuate. Similar results were found in a study of evacuation behavior in Hurricane Bonnie (Whitehead et al., 2000).

Evacuation of Special Populations

Special populations are those groups of people who because of their special situations or needs require planning strategies different from those of general evacuation planning (Vogt, 1990, 1991). The term "special population" is somewhat misleading in that populations of institutions or special facilities are frequently considered homogeneous when in reality they exhibit many characteristics that differ by physical or geographic constraints (Lindell et al., 1985). While some populations may be concentrated in institutions such as schools, prisons, or hospitals, other will be widely dispersed. Among the dispersed individuals who make up such groups are the hearing or visually impaired, the non-English-speaking, transients such as motorists passing through the area, tourists or other temporary visitors such as day workers, and nonambulatory individuals confined to residences either temporarily or permanently.

The reason why these groups may fail to respond to warnings to take protective actions is that some groups may require special transportation while others require different types of warnings or technologies to receive a warning. Some groups must rely on caregivers (such as schools and daycare centers) to hear the warning and respond. Populations of nursing homes or assisted care facilities may combine various aspects related to mobility and mental competence that makes evacuation the last resort in protective action planning. Lack of mobility may not be voluntary, as in the case of prisons where continued constraints must be imposed during the evacuation process.

Destinations of Evacuees

Despite efforts by public officials to provide public shelters to house evacuees, most people evacuate to relatives, friends, or hotels. The use of public shelters is variable, ranging from less than 1% for the Three Mile Island evacuation to more than 40% in the Nanticoke hazardous materials evacuation. On average, shelter use is about 13%. It appears to be higher when the evacuating population is of low income and older and lower when the population is more affluent and young (Mileti, Sorensen, & O'Brien, 1992).

CONCLUSIONS

With the exception of hurricanes, very little research has been conducted in the past 10 years on warning and evacuation. Most of our understanding of human response to warnings is based on older research that has been based primarily on theories of persuasive communication. This linear model assumes a top-down flow of "official" warning information to the public. We suspect that this communication model, not without merit, needs to be revised. Social and technological changes have opened gaps in our knowledge about responses to warnings that requires research that will refine or replace extant theories.

We do not know the degree to which we can use past history to understand and predict how people will respond to events not yet experienced in our society, such assuicide bombings, a release of a biological agent, an attack with a radiological dispersion device, or a release of a chemical warfare agent. We will learn more about consistency and change in disaster response as we systematically study human response in new types of disasters. Preliminary findings from the large number of post-9/11 investigations suggest that some types of behaviors are similar to those exhibited in other large-scale disasters (such as the general absence of panic and considerable altruistic behavior). Other types of post-9/11 behavior, such as avoidance and economic spending, were unique. We must continue todocument differences and consistencies in disaster responses and learn what variables systematically shape them. This might require not just retrospective research but also rapid response teams of social scientists who, without interfering with emergency operations, can document behavior as it is occurring or very soon thereafter in a systematic and scientific manner.

Hurricanes Katrina and Rita caused large-scale evacuations of coastal areas in Mississippi, Louisiana, and Texas. Future research on these two events will likely provide opportunities to examine evacuation problems and strategies for large urban areas when a great level of infrastructure is destroyed. Such research will also add to the existing knowledge base on sequential hazards. The flooding of New Orleans from levee failure was a secondary event while wind and storm surge was the cause of destructive flooding for others along the Gulf coast affected by the same hurricane.

CHAPTER 12

Search and Rescue Activities in Disasters

Margarita Poteyeva, Megan Denver, Lauren E. Barsky, and Benigno E. Aguirre

The objective of this chapter is to review what is known about search and rescue activities in disasters, including heavy urban search and rescue teams. The accumulation of scientific knowledge about search and rescue (SAR), which is, as reflected in this chapter, disproportionately centered on disasters in the United States, allows us to identify certain recurrent patterns that should be considered in the development of an effective plan for national emergency response. The following sections present what is known about SAR, factors affecting survival, the behavior of victims, the impact of social and cultural arrangements, and ecological aspects of SAR in constrained and unconstrained spaces. This is followed by brief discussions of the search and recovery activities in the Columbia Shuttle Accident as well as by examinations of the World Trade Center (WTC) and Pentagon 9/11 SAR operations. The chapter concludes with an acknowledgment of the remaining research gaps in our understanding of SAR and with a summary of what needs to be done to improve SAR operations worldwide.

INTRODUCTION

There is widespread consensus among specialists that: (1) SAR is social, collective behavior of volunteers who share a culture and act as socialized human beings and are members of a human community; (2) Preexisting and emergent organizations, social statuses and social identities, such as neighborhood and work place relationships and family and neighborhood social identities, serve as a basis for the emergence of new SAR groups and constitute the fundamental concepts and categories that are needed to understand and improve SAR activities; (3) SAR activities do not emerge from a vacuum; as an example of the principle of continuity advocated by Quarantelli and Dynes (1977), there are always elements of the traditional social structure embedded within collective behavior entities, and their emergent division of labor, role structure, and activities are also dependent on prior social relationships and forms of social organization in the community or region; (4) "Breakdown" models of social organizational patterns in disaster are not useful to understand SAR. Television reports and misinformed reporters often misinterpret throngs of people moving seemingly at random at the sites destroyed by various hazards, and assume that the people were disoriented immediately after impact and had lost their ability to enact social roles. Despite these reports, scientific research shows the absence of widespread confusion, lack of coordination, and "panic" (Aguirre, 2005). The seeming disorganization and aimless movement of people is the result of their individual and collective acts as they try to accomplish multiple individual and collective goals under severe time constraints (c.f. Fritz & Mathewson, 1957). Creative problem-solving and rationality is a more accurate way of understanding their actions (Aroni & Durkin, n.d., p. 30); and (5) Advances in our understanding of SAR depends on multidisciplinary scientific collaboration involving, among others, structural engineers, emergency medical personnel, and social scientists. We next provide some of the reasons for these conclusions by reviewing what is known about search and rescue in the scientific literature.

WHAT IS KNOWN ABOUT SEARCH
AND RESCUE

Search and rescue (SAR) activities are part of a complex emergency system that emerges to respond to disasters, what has been termed "helpful behavior in emergencies" (Dynes & Quarantelli, 1980). During more than 40 years, disaster researchers (for information on SAR during the Kobe, Japan earthquake of 1995 see Kunii, Akagi, & Kita, 1995; for the Kocaeli Turkey earthquake of August of 1999 see Mitchell, 1999; for the Bam, Iran earthquake of December 2003 see Editorial, 2004; near-exhaustive literature reviews are available in Poteyeva, 2005; Prater et al., 1993) have endeavored to understand what accounts for the relative success of SAR activities in disasters, to include factors such as the nature of structural and nonstructural damage to the built environment (Anagnostopoulos & Whitman, 1977; Culver, Lew, Hart, & Pinkham, 1975; Hart, 1976; Hasselman, Equchi, & Wiggins, 1980; Lechat, 1989; Stubbs, Sikorsky, Lipnick, & Lombard, 1989; Tiedemann, 1989), the epidemiology of SAR events (De Bruycker, Greco, & Lechat, 1985; Glass et al., 1977; Glass, O'Hare, & Conrad, 1979; Lechat, 1976), and the effectiveness of medical services (Quarantelli, 1983a). Aguirre, Wenger, Glass, Diaz-Murillo, and Vigo (1995) have also argued for the importance of social organization in SAR in disasters.

The most extensive study of SAR activity was undertaken during the late 1970s by Drabek, Tamminga, Kilijanek, and Adams (1981), who conceptually recast the study of search and rescue into an emergent, interorganizational, systemic approach. While reaffirming a number of the previous observations made in the literature up to that time, their study highlighted the interorganizational managerial difficulties inherent in SAR. They found four common operational problems: (1) difficulties in interagency communications, (2) ambiguity of authority, (3) poor utilization of special resources, and (4) unplanned media relations. Quarantelli (1983a) analyzed the problem of locating victims and managing their entrance into the emergency medical system. Glass et al. (1977, 1979) provided epidemiological evidence on the etiology of injuries and deaths that had obvious implications for SAR behavior.

To restate the disciplinary consensus (see an earlier summary by Wenger 1990 and literature cited therein):

1. Volunteer and emergent group response is of critical importance.
2. The initial SAR activity is accomplished by volunteers and emergent groups.

3. Since most survivors are rescued within the first 2 days, this emergent and volunteer activity is critically important to the rescue effort, especially because buried and entrapped victims are likely to suffer from injuries that require rapid life-sustaining intervention including compromised access to air, severe loss of blood and body fluid, crushing injury, and internal damage to essential organ systems.

4. Despite the massive attention they usually receive from the mass media (Quarantelli, 1991c), most of the time urban search and heavy rescue (US&R) teams arrive too late to rescue anyone; instead, they undertake highly specialized recovery activities requiring sophisticated skills and equipment. This is due in large part to the particular nature of the sociogeography of disasters in which US&R teams are hampered by problems of timely access.

5. The integration of volunteer and established organizational activities is seldom efficiently achieved; many official responding organizations, particularly those from national governments, usually do not appreciate the work of the volunteers in SAR operations since they are often perceived as lacking sufficient credentialing, specialized training, and tools. In turn, the absence of disaster planning about how to use volunteers creates problems of its own as large number of volunteers converge on disaster sites (Quarantelli, 1996c). Problems of management of rescue activities are serious and include difficulties in coordinating activities across independent, autonomous organizations, disagreement over rescue strategy, and ambiguous authority relationships.

SOCIAL ACTORS

Dynes and Quarantelli (1980) identified four types of disaster volunteers, whom they term organizational volunteers, group volunteers, volunteers in expanded roles, and volunteers in new roles. As Dynes (1970) had theorized earlier, in the typical SAR site these types of volunteers become part of the process of organizational emergence involving extending, expanding, and emergent organizations, the last one often playing key roles in SAR activities (Quarantelli, 1999a). Preexisting networks of human relationships are used to alleviate novel and unexpected collective problems that demand immediate attention. People expand their sense of responsibility toward each other, and often do so by becoming members of new emergent groups that carry out SAR activities. Afterwards, there may be the institutionalization of these groups.

SAR activities are part of the mass assault phase of disaster. As such, multiple individual and collective actors participate in it. Many trapped victims are rescued by the uninjured bystanders and surviving local emergency responders (Aguirre et al., 1995; Auf der Heide, 2004; Durkin, Coulson, Hijar, Kraus, & Ohashi, 1987; Durkin & Murakami, 1988; Kunkle, 1989; Noji, 2003; see other literature in Poteyeva, 2005; Prater et al., 1993). For example, in southern Italy, in 1980, 90% of the survived trapped victims were extricated by untrained, uninjured survivors who used their bare hands and simple tools such as shovels and axes (Noji, 2003). Following the 1976 Tangshan earthquake, about 200,000 to 300,000 entrapped people crawled out of the debris and went on to rescue others (Noji, 2003). These volunteers became the backbone of the rescue teams. Durkin and colleagues (1987, 1988) specified that the primary rescue technique used by the SAR teams and volunteers was a human voice—the victims reacted to the rescuers calling out, and cried for help or made noise with available objects themselves.

The aforementioned institutionalization process can be observed in the thousands of local volunteer organizations that carry out SAR activities throughout the United States. The majority of these volunteer organizations came about soon after there was a mass emergency, a disaster, or there were cases of missing persons in their communities for which there was no organization in the communities to assist in the response. In a recent ongoing attempt to quantify this activity, we found that the earliest team in our nonrepresentative sample of teams (sampling frame included only those with Web sites during August 2004 to September 1, 2005) was the Hood River Crag Rats Mountain SAR, from Hood River, Oregon founded in 1926. We have identified more than 1000 SAR voluntary organizations in all 50 states, with more than 50 organizations in some states. Initially, most of these organizations were involved in mountain and wilderness search and rescue activities, although nowadays they engage in water rescue as well as a host of other response activities in the aftermath of mass emergencies and disasters. The most frequent team capabilities are: K-9 teams—31% of the teams had them; water rescue—26%; technical rescue— 22%; wilderness—21%; mine rescue—17%. Seventy-one percent of the organizations are supported by public donations, fund raising, and membership support; the breakdown for main sources of support mentioned by our respondents is: donations—56% of the teams mentioned it; sponsors—41%; fundraising—21%; member support—13%; private grants—8%; city, county, state governments—15%; others—6%. They compose a nascent industry in which, despite the recent effort by the Federal Emergency Management Agency (FEMA) to create a National Mutual Aid and Resource Management Initiative, there are at present no uniformed training standards or certification. Instead, these organizations follow various professional standards such as those of the National Association of Search and Rescue (NASAR) and FEMA, although many are not certified by these national organizations; most have developed their own regulations: 6% of the teams in our sample train to NASAR standards and 2% to FEMA standards. NASAR estimates more than 50,000 SAR missions annually—more than 90% carried out by unpaid professionals—missions that, while not all associated with mass emergencies and disasters, still give a sense of the importance of these voluntary organizations.

In contrast, another type of social actor, the urban search and rescue taskforces, has received a great deal of financial support and public attention. In the United States, the Urban Search and Rescue System (US&R) is a collection of multidisciplinary taskforces created from local emergency responders organized under a federal framework for response in the aftermath of structural collapses. These task forces arrive at the site complete with the necessary tools, equipment, specialized training, and skills. They were created to be deployed by FEMA at times of catastrophic structural collapse to engage in such varied activities as structural shoring, canine searches, complex rope systems, confined space entry, and technically assisted void search procedures, although for a number of reasons explored elsewhere (Trainor & Aguirre, 2005) they are now being used to do many other things not initially contemplated when the system was formed. In parallel, other taskforces are being formed by state governments in the United States and by national governments.

FEMA's US&R System is of fairly recent origin, with the first US&R taskforce certi-fied in 1991. The development of heavy rescue search capability was initiated in California, particularly after the 1971 San Fernando Earthquake (Naum, 1993). In 1990, FEMA, fresh from the problems created by Hurricane Hugo and the Loma Prieta Earthquake, organized a week-long meeting in Seattle, Washington where more than 90 specialists representing various constituencies met and developed the outlines of the program. They set up a system of local US&R taskforces that would be made up of personnel from local agencies and who would be federalized and deployed nationwide at the request of FEMA. State emergency manage-ment agencies were only marginally involved in the organization, which instead instituted an organizational link between the taskforces and FEMA. The taskforces have structural engineers to assess risks created by the configuration of collapsed structures, medical and hazardous material personnel, canine units, and very extensive cache of sophisticated tools and equipment for use in heavy rescue environments. When fully implemented each has more than 200 people. Today there are 28 US&R taskforces.

One of the great paradoxes of the present system is that U.S. federal and state funding is directed to these taskforces even though they too often arrive too late to save anyone, and that this is done to the near exclusion of the thousands of voluntary SAR organizations that do most of the rescuing and savings of lives in the United States.

The effectiveness of local SAR voluntary organizations and formal organizations such as fire departments in locating and rescuing victims is in part a result of the interaction of ecological characteristics of the site of the disaster with other factors such as the (1) the social, cultural, and behavioral patterns and social relationships between victims and responders; (2) behavior of victims during entrapment; and (3) nature of the buildings and other structures and their collapse configuration. The morbidity and mortality patterns associated with disasters depend on these other matters, to which we now turn.

CULTURAL AND SOCIAL ARRANGEMENTS

Cultural and social arrangements are often of primary importance (Pomonis, Sakai, Coburn, & Spence, 1991). Reflecting cultural practices, occupancy of buildings by time of day and season is significant in determining occupant exposure to specific hazards (Durkin et al., 1987; Tiedemann, 1989). Kuwata and Takada (2002), in their study of the 2000 Western Tottori earthquake noted the low occupancy of buildings at the time of the disaster as a major reason for the low number of dead and injured; the earthquake occurred at 1:30 P.M. on a weekday, meaning that the inhabitants of the building were awake and at once perceived the dangers of the earthquake. In addition, the most important factor was that the majority of people were not at home—the inhabitant occupancy was estimated at 27%. Knowing the time of the disaster helped Michael Durkin (Durkin et al., 1987) to reconstruct the location of his study's subjects during the 1985 Mexico earthquake: the impact had occurred at 7:17 A.M., when most of the medical students were in their dorm rooms preparing for the day, or on their way to the cafeteria for breakfast. Those who had morning shifts were already at work when the hospital collapsed.

Another issue directly related to community's culture and social relationships is the increased vulnerability to disasters of minority group members and residents of low-income households. These categories of people have lower ability to protect themselves from disaster. Income is positively related to access to better and safer housing and location. Older, unreinforced masonry buildings and mobile homes, which are highly susceptible to collapse in earthquakes, constitute an important source of affordable housing for lower-income residents in earthquake-prone cities such as San Francisco and Los Angeles.

Religious and ethnic minorities are often impacted by a number of erroneous assumptions about the management of the dead in the aftermath of major disasters which are often used to guide SAR activities. In Nicaragua, in 1998, because of an avalanche at the Casitas Volcano brought about by heavy rains from Hurricane Mitch, more than 2000 people died. Acting under the erroneous belief that human bodies are public health risks, and violating the rights of victims and their relatives to a burial in accordance to religious beliefs and local cultural practices governing the handling of the dead, the army incinerated more than 1000 victims;

the rest were buried. None were identified. To this day they are listed as "persons that are missing," an ambiguous status that creates legal and other difficulties for their surviving kin (Pan American Health Organization, 2004, pp. 163–170).

SURVIVAL

Several studies examine the relationship between changes in response time and the saving of trapped victims (Coburn & Hughes, 1987; Kunkle, 1989; Pomonis et al., 1991; Quon & Laube, 1991). Kunkle claims that 80% to 90% of entrapped victims who survive are recovered in the first 48 hours after the disaster impact, and that many more entrapped victims could survive with timely delivery of appropriate medical care. Comfort (1996, p. 134) reports that in the 1995 Kobe, Japan earthquake the percentage of those rescued who survived was 80.5% for the first day after the earthquake, 28.5% for the second day, 21.8% for the third, 5.9% for the fourth, and 5.8% for the fifth day. Quon and Laube developed a predictive model that suggests that a 10% to 20% reduction in response time would yield a 1% to 2.5% reduction in fatalities. In the 1988 Armenia earthquake, 89% of those rescued alive from collapsed buildings were extricated during the first 24 hours. Noji et al. (1990; see also Olson & Olson, 1987) documented that most lives are saved and victims rescued during this immediate post-impact period. The probability of being extricated alive from the debris declined sharply over time, with no rescues after day 6. Noji (1991) points out that people have been rescued alive after 5, 10, and even 14 days of entrapment, but these constitute rare events.

Pomonis et al. (1991) stress the importance of a victim's health condition inside a collapsed building at any given time; surviving entrapment can be expressed as a function of time and the injury level sustained at the moment of entrapment. Other factors need to be accounted for as well, such as exposure; dehydration or starvation after a long period of time; weather conditions and the amount of air voids that are created within the rubble; the weight of the rubble above the victim; and the victim's preentrapment health condition. Pomonis et al.'s study provides a number of empirical illustrations of the potential interplay among the mentioned factors. Thus, the collapse of the Juarez Hospital (a reinforced concrete frame building) in the 1985 Mexico earthquake trapped 740 people within the building. SAR operations lasted more than 10 days, but only 179 persons were extricated alive; 76% died. On day 1 the survival rate was 70% and this level was maintained until day 5. After that it dropped to 20% by day 9. The implication is that 30% of trapped victims were killed instantly or injured too seriously to survive more than one day while the rest of the victims suffered relatively slight injury and survived for a while but began to die after day 5 because of bleeding, exposure, compression, or some other reason.

Entrapment is the single most important factor associated with death or injury (Durkin & Murakami, 1988). As Noji (2003) states, in the 1988 Armenia earthquake, death rates were 67 times higher and injury rates more than 11 times higher for people who were trapped than for those who were not. Certain age groups are more vulnerable and have an increased risk for death and injury in disasters and others. People older than 60 years of age have a death rate that can be five times higher than that of the rest of the population during earthquakes. Children between 5 and 9 years of age, women, and the chronically ill also have an elevated risk for injury and death (Glass et al., 1977). As Noji (2003) points out, limited mobility to flee from collapsing structures, inability to withstand trauma, and exacerbation of underlying disease are factors that may contribute to the vulnerability of these groups. He also stressed the effect that certain social attitudes and habits of different communities may have on mortality distribution by age. For example, in some societies young children sleep close to their mothers and may be more easily protected by them.

BEHAVIOR OF VICTIMS

Scientific studies of the behavior of victims in disasters are infrequent (see Bourque et al., in this volume). While in need of replication, the few studies that have examined issues ranging from general behavioral patterns of communities during disasters to what building occupants did during the actual period of a disaster and experiences of trapped victims during SAR operations show that the much-feared social disorganization during the disaster periods is extremely rare (Aguirre, 2005; Durkin, 1989; Dynes, 1970), although conditions under which panic does occur have been identified in the literature (Dynes, 1970; Johnson, 1988). An atmosphere of human solidarity and cooperation characterizes the behavioral processes during and in the aftermath of a disaster. Residents of disaster-stricken areas are proactive and willing to assist one another. Research findings show that volunteer activity increases at the time of disaster impact and remains widespread during the emergency period (Dynes, Quarantelli, & Wenger, 1990). In the Guadalajara Gas explosion community residents who were not trapped or freed themselves from entrapment went to great lengths to search for their kin and neighbors (Aguirre et al., 1995). There were instances when individuals would call attention to other victims who were trapped nearby and could not free themselves; they would also speculate about the possible location of other victims, provided rescuers with information about the inner settings of the house, and reconstructed the architectural topography of the streets turned to rubble. Sometimes the victims, when trapped, were able to hear what was going on above or next door and thus maintained social ties with the world around them. They also engaged in imaginary interaction with significant others and saints, seeking spiritual and psychological support, which is so important for survival. More recently, Scanlon's recent observations (2005) of the London Underground's July 7th 2005 terrorist explosion also shows that victims helped fellow victims, that staff operating the trains helped the passengers, and that the first responders were not emergency personnel but people nearby, among them medical doctors who worked at the British Medical Association as well as workers from other commercial establishments.

Studies have paid particular attention to the importance of family as an institution during mass emergencies and disasters (Form & Nosow, 1958; see also Aguirre et al., 1995; Alexander, 1990; Quarantelli, 1988d). Family is a very powerful unifying factor for disaster victims, and, as Alexander points out, its influence could immediately dissolve other groupings such as friends. Family members are the first to be rescued by their kin. As soon as the nuclear family is reunited they concern themselves with other relatives. Second in importance is the concern for immediate neighbors and other nearby residents, and then other people farther removed from the spheres of everyday interactions (Aguirre et al., 1995). While in need of replication, a research finding is that the chances of people surviving the Guadalajara explosion were directly proportional to the presence among the searchers of a person or persons who cared for the victim and who knew the victim's possible location at the time of the explosion. Another important related pattern is that significant others acted as proxies for the victims, reminding the searchers that the family member was missing, and supplying information about their possible location.

Preliminary results from studies of occupant actions during disasters and trapped victims' behavior suggest that victims behave actively and assume responsibility over their rescue to the extent that they can do so. Thus victims trapped as a result of the Guadalajara gas explosion moved their bodies ever so slowly to create more room in the rubble; others called attention to themselves by screaming and making noise on the nearby debris (Aguirre et al., 1995). Seven of the eighteen victims trapped in the dormitory after the 1985 Mexico earthquake attempted to escape (Durkin et al., 1987).

Prior training and expectations play a significant role in the way that people respond to disasters (Durkin et al., 1987), but these beliefs and expectations have to be reevaluated depending on the physical setting of each particular case, for they may prove to be dangerous. Many beliefs about appropriate response can endanger rather then protect building occupants (Durkin & Murakami, 1988; Kunii et al, 1995). Thus, a significant number of respondents in Durkin's 1985 Mexico earthquake study reported that they chose to "stay where they were" once the shaking began, because they believed it was the right thing to do. As a result they were trapped in individual dorm rooms rather than trying to escape the building. A different example involves a person who moved into the doorway as the shaking began (as she was advised to do during earthquakes), and was hurt by the door being slammed shut. Another person was hurt trying to hide under a desk. Damage done to the General Hospital building by the 1985 Mexico City earthquake made the drills and bomb-threat evacuation routes inoperative, and the nursing staff had to find alternate ways out, demonstrating the ad hoc resourcefulness of disaster victims.

Traditionally criteria for evaluating structural safety have been tied to the structure itself (Stubbs & Sichorsky, 1987). However, nonstructural failures such as collapsing of cladding or partitions, ceilings, windows, equipment, fixtures, piping, ducts, and roof tile can also cause substantial harm. They should be physically connected to the structure (Cole, 1991; Jones, Noji, Smith, & Krimgold, 1990). Study of the Loma Prieta earthquake (Cole, 1991) documented many instances of overturned files and bookshelves that were not properly braced and anchored. These building contents caused a large number of injuries, with the ratio of injuries from building contents to those from structural elements being 3 to 1. People were hurt mostly by moving desks, filing cabinets, and furniture situated in the immediate vicinity of where those people were located. Therefore, building elements and contents play a clear role in endangering occupants' lives (Durkin & Murakami, 1988) when they are not appropriately braced and secured to the walls and floors of buildings. The 1979 El Centro, California earthquake study (Durkin, 1985) showed that 36% of office workers in the Imperial county services building that sustained considerable nonstructural damage, reported getting under their desks. The sort of evasive action that will prove effective depends not only on the nature of building collapse and the nonstructural failures associated with it, but also on whether the contents of the building are secured to the structure of the building. At the present time, knowledge of building collapse configurations is insufficient to provide valid answers to these matters (see below).

ECOLOGICAL FACTORS

Timely arrival of rescuers, proper behavior of victims, and propitious cultural and social arrangements impact the effectiveness of SAR operations in saving lives. Yet, it is also the case that the environment as it is impacted by human adaptation, what we call the ecological factor, is important as well. The next section reviews what is known about SAR in buildings and other enclosed structures. It is followed by the examination of the Columbia Shuttle Accident, in which SAR took place in a rural environment that presented very different challenges to responders.

SAR in Buildings

A number of studies explore structural vulnerability of buildings to earthquakes, taking into account a multitude of factors—for example, the variety of construction types, material and quality, the geology of the area, and the distribution of shaking intensity. It is possible to only briefly outline the characteristics of various building structures, associated modes of failure, and the consequences of building collapse for search and rescue. The type of building and the collapse patterns are important determinants for morbidity (Glass et al., 1977; Meli, 1989; Noji et al., 1990). Data on earthquakes and other disasters suggest that a relatively small number of damaged structures are the source of the vast majority of the serious casualties (Coburn, Spence, & Pomonis, 1992). For example, 50 of 62 deaths in the Loma Prieta earthquake occurred at the Cypress freeway structure in Oakland and 40 of 64 deaths in the 1971 San Fernando earthquake occurred as a result of a collapse of a Veterans Hospital (Noji, 2003). There is also information on the vulnerability of particular building structures. Noji (2003) states that by far the greatest proportion of earthquake victims have died in the collapse of unreinforced masonry buildings or unreinforced fired-brick and concrete-block masonry buildings that can collapse even at low intensities of ground shaking and will collapse very rapidly at high intensities. Other studies also support this conclusion (Sparks, 1985). Un-reinforced masonry buildings are from one to six stories in high and may be residential, commercial, and industrial. Their primary weakness is in the lateral strength of the walls and the connections between the walls and the floor or roof assemblies. Collapses are usually partial and are caused by the heavy, weakened walls falling away from the floors. Falling hazards are very widespread at these buildings because of the amount of small, loose masonry components that results from the collapse. At the same time large angular voids form, because large sections of floor or roof often stay together as a plane. Adobe structures have performed very poorly in many highly seismic parts of the world—for example, eastern Turkey, Iran, Pakistan, Latin America (see Ceciliano, Pretto, Watoh, Angus, & Abrams, 1993; Noji, 2003). These buildings not only have collapse-prone walls but also very heavy roofs that prove to be deadly to people when they collapse. On the other end of the spectrum of building vulnerability are wood-frame buildings, which usually comprise residential housing. They are one of the safest structures during an earthquake, because, despite their weakness to resist lateral forces and consequent collapse, they are constructed of light wood elements, and their potential to cause injury is much less serious than that of unresistant old stone buildings (Noji, 2003). A study of the 1995 Hanshin-Awaji earthquake in Nishinomia City (Hengjian et al., 2000) has concluded that most casualties occurred in relatively old two-story wooden buildings in which the ground floor collapsed completely without survival space. More than 84 percent of casualties occurred in buildings that collapsed without survival space.

Concrete-framed houses are generally safer in terms of their resistance to collapse, but they are also significantly more lethal than masonry or wooden buildings. Reinforced concrete requires sophisticated construction techniques; however, it is often used in communities around the world where either technical competence is insufficient or inspection and control are inadequate (Noji, 2003). Catastrophic failures of modern reinforced, concrete-slab buildings have been described in Mexico City (1985), El Salvador (1986), and Armenia (1988) (Bommer & Ledbetter, 1987; Wyllie & Lew, 1989). The principal weakness of concrete frame building (heavy floor) is the poor column reinforcement and inadequate connections between floor slabs and columns. Collapse from the failure of these parts can be partial or complete. These structures often fall down on themselves, or they may fall laterally if the columns are strong enough. Meli (1989) states that the failure of vertical members is worse than the failure of horizontal components and that to avoid a catastrophic collapse it is necessary to preserve the "main vertical load-resisting elements." Whereas the debris of buildings of adobe, rubble masonry, and brick can be cleared with primitive tools, reinforced concrete represents serious problems for rescuers, and requires special equipment. Other types of buildings discussed are pre-cast concrete buildings, which fail because of the weakness of the connectors between building parts such as floors, walls and roof; and heavy wall tilt-up/reinforced masonry. The latter have received mixed reviews as to their resistance to earthquakes (Cole, 1991). Walls in these structures usually fall away from the roof or floor edge, but because they are very strong panels, the top of the wall will fall far away from the building.

Empirical studies have evaluated the comparative performance during disasters of buildings of older and newer construction (Cole, 1991; Hengjian et al., 2000). Thus, during the Loma Prieta earthquake relatively modern buildings performed much better than buildings of pre-1973 construction. Most of the significant structural damage suffered by modern residences was due to the collateral effects of earth movement, that is, land sliding and soil rupture, although this particular earthquake was not a good test of the buildings because of its moderate intensity. Cole speculates that buildings designed and constructed to current codes would have fared well during a stronger, longer duration earthquake. On the other hand, residential buildings of older "archaic" construction suffered extensive damage.

Tiedemann (1989) lists the factors that impact the behavior of buildings during earthquakes and, therefore, affect the number of casualties: resonance between predominant frequencies of the foundation material and of the building structure; quality, that is, predominantly hardness of the foundation material; shear strength of the building resulting from the combined strength of structural and nonstructural parts; compatibility of behavior of building materials and components under dynamic loads; regularity and symmetry as regards floor plans, elevations, shear strength, distribution of masses and damping; type and behavior of nonstructural elements—their design, quality arrangement, and fastening; hammering between buildings; orientation sensitivity; and liquefaction. These factors determine the vulnerability of buildings to collapse during disasters as well as provide clues as to where void spaces might occur, and thus where surviving victims might be found during SAR.

The types of collapse generate known patterns of void spaces in the rubble which are very important to search and rescuers. The SAR literature discusses several types of collapse voids. For example, the Manual for the International Fire Service Training Association (Murnane, 2003) outlines five types of collapses (paraphrasing): (1) Lean-to collapse occurs when one exterior wall collapses, leaving the floor supported at one end only; the victims are likely to be found in the lower portion of the lean-to or positioned on the floor below the unsupported lean-to. Removal of debris that is supporting the "base" of the lean-to collapse can cause the floor to slide, collapsing the void. In the case of a supported lean-to collapse, most likely the victims will be located at the bottom of the lean-to near the wall surrounded by rubble, or they could be on the floor below the collapsed floor under the large void created at the opposite end of the failed construction. Victim survival profile is low to medium. (2) V-shape collapse occurs when an interior supporting wall or column fails. Victims are typically found on the floor below. They usually have a higher survival rate because of the sheltering effect of the collapse floor (prevents rubble landing on them). Victims on the top of the collapsed floor usually are at the bottom or near the center of the V, or trapped in the debris in various places. Because of large amount of debris concentrated in one area, survival rate for victims in this area is low. (3) Pancake collapse occurs when all vertical supporting members fail and most of the floors collapse on top of one another. This is more probable in heavy-floor buildings. This kind of collapse might not move the victim horizontally but drop the victim straight down in the collapse pile, so that victims may be located on several floors anywhere in the debris. Victim survival rate is very low. (4) Yet another configuration is the cantilever collapse. This type of collapse is similar to the pancake pattern with the additional problem of some of the floor planes extending, unsupported, from the debris pile. Victims might be found under the floor as in the pancake condition. (5) Finally, in A-frame collapse, the highest survival rate is for victims located near the partition wall at the center of the collapse. Victims located on the floor above can be pinned in the debris near both exterior walls, which results in a lower survival rate.

The location of people in the building at the time of the disaster is an important determinant of morbidity (Noji, 2003). For example, occupants of upper floors of multi-story buildings have been observed to fare less well than ground-floor occupants. In Armenia, there was a significant increase in risk for injury associated with the floor people were on at the moment of the earthquake. People inside buildings with five or more floors were 3.65 times more likely to be injured compared to those inside buildings less than five floors in height (Armenian, Noji, & Oganessian, 1992), and in the 1990 Philippine earthquake, people inside buildings with seven or more floors were 34.7 times more likely to be injured (Roces, White, Dayrit, & Durkin, 1992). As Coburn et al. (1992) point out, in a high-rise building escape from upper floors is improbable before the building collapses, and if it collapses completely, nearly 70% of the building occupants are likely to be trapped inside. In a low-rise building that takes perhaps 20 or 30 seconds to collapse, more than three quarters of the building's occupants may be able to escape before the collapse. In general, however, as Kunii et al. (1995) point out, needed are studies of behavior of individuals in disasters that protects them. Furthermore, developing scientific knowledge about the circumstances of entrapment and location of voids will contribute to the development of effective SAR techniques and effective injury-prevention strategies.

Very different ecological settings operated in the Columbia Shuttle Accident and in the WTC and Pentagon terrorist attack of 9/11, a matter to which we now turn.

The Columbia Shuttle Accident

In contrast to SAR in well defined and circumscribed ecological areas, the search and recovery effort that took place in the aftermath of the Columbia Discovery space shuttle accident of February 1, 2003 involved the simultaneous presence of local search and recovery groups and US&R taskforces working over a very large geographic area in central Texas, a region estimated to be 160 miles long and 35 miles wide. The incident was a federalized activity but it could not be done without the assistance of agencies from local and state governments and voluntary firefighters and SAR teams and other types of volunteers who were coordinated using a grill pattern map and geographic information system (GIS) that was initiated by Texas Forest Service (TFS), FEMA, and the National Aeronautic and Space Administration (NASA). The response was a mass assault in which the coordination function emerged over time. During the first 13 days, a great deal of the work of recovery was done by neighbors of the towns of Kerens and Rice in Navarro County, Texas and other towns in which the debris fell and by other local and state organizations who worked to secure the pieces of debris until these could be removed by NASA; in Hemphill and other towns, the churches got together and fed the volunteers and responders who came into the community to participate in the search and recovery. There were many individual and organizational participants. Interagency coordination problems that were eventually alleviated once an interorganizational managing group was set up and an understanding of agencies' capabilities, division of labor, and decision making system were established among the participants.

In this instance of a very large scale response operation involving a mass assault in which SAR volunteers and US&R FEMA taskforces operated simultaneously over a large geographic area, the official disaster response system as it was set up on paper had limited use. While outside this official system, neighbors, SAR groups, other organizational volunteers, and community institutions such as churches became critical although largely unrecognized actors in the federal effort. The large extension of terrain meant that it was not possible to establish a perimeter or control over the site. Instead, the mass media and existing emergency management and police systems were used to alert the public and instruct it in the ways it could assist the efforts of the federal government in securing and recovering the parts. Rather than entire US&R taskforces, only elements of some of these taskforces such as canine specialists and hazardous material specialists participated in the operation, again, a marked departure from their common pattern of operation; there was no need for a good portion of their equipment and trained personnel. This case study reaffirms earlier findings in the social sciences of disasters. It shows that SAR operations are, to a significant degree, impacted by the ecological settings in which they take place. Most of what we know about SAR applies to what take place in buildings and other well delimited areas, which is unrepresentative of the diversity of ecological contexts in which SAR takes place and the various challenges these contexts create for responders. US&R taskforces and other SAR groups had to adjust to the needs of the other organizational partners in what became an emergent multiorganizational coordinating search and recovery effort.

WTC AND THE PENTAGON

The nature of the structural collapses that rescuers had to deal with at the World Trade Center (WTC) and the Pentagon were very different from collapses caused by natural disasters, and represented a serious challenge for the US&R Task Forces (Hearing before the Committee on Science, 2002; Titan Systems Corporation, 2002). Typically, in case of a structural collapse caused by an earthquake, large pieces of the structure create void spaces in which live victims may be found (Murnane et al., 2003). The bomb explosion outside of the Murrah building in Oklahoma City "essentially pulverized" the structure (Comeau, 1996) and made it very difficult to shore up and stabilize the building. The destruction and fires from the plane explosion within the WTC Towers weakened the infrastructure of the buildings, collapsing the upper floors and creating too heavy of a load for the lower floors to bear. Heavy concrete and steel structure and massive fires impeded the survival of any victims after the collapse (Hearing before the Committee on Science, 2002).

WTC

After the September 11 terrorist attack on the World Trade Center "the very first rescue and evacuation activities were initiated and performed to a great extent by civilians who worked in the World Trade Center" (Petrescu-Prahova & Butts, 2005). Thousands of volunteers formed several staging areas close to Ground Zero. Community and religious organizations, charitable agencies, local businesses, and concerned citizens established and helped operate ad hoc catering, rest, and comfort stations near the disaster sites. Many off-duty emergency medical service (EMS), police, and fire personnel reported directly to the collapse, often traveling hours to reach the site. This phenomena of self-dispatching, also present after the Oklahoma City bombing and the Pentagon attack, was later criticized as adding to the confusion and disarray of the response scene, complicating a coordinate response effort. Unfortunately, it does not address the problem of how to incorporate the helping behavior of volunteers in disaster response planning. By 9:57 P.M. on the day of the attack, New York City Mayor Rudolf Giuliani made an announcement that no more volunteers were needed to help with the WTC rescue efforts.

What makes SAR at the WTC so different from other events of its type is the paucity in reestablishing command and control at the site. While still a subject of research, every indication we have is that perimeter control and a workable division of labor and cooperation among various responding official agencies were not accomplished until after the first 5 or 7 days after the terrorist attack. This was in part due to the impact of the attack on key organizations in charge of disaster response for the city. The destruction of New York City's Office of Emergency Management and Interagency Preparedness, the tremendous losses in special operations and command structures of the Fire Department of New York (NYFD) and less so of the New York Police Department (NYPD) and the Port Authority Police Department meant that it would take time and innovation to reconstitute the official response capabilities in the area of impact.

It is not possible to underestimate the impact of these events on the NYFD, the lead local agency in charge of operations at the site. Experienced officers capable of establishing an effective response were lost to NYFD at the start of the operations, which meant that officers with less operational experience and knowledge were placed in positions of responsibility at the site. Furthermore, many established bureaucratic procedures had to be suspended and superseded during the response period, which brought about innovation and adaptation but also a degree of confusion. It is in this context that the US&R taskforces attempted to insert themselves into SAR operations.

Twenty FEMA US&R task forces were present at the collapse site at one point in time. Preliminary findings indicate that they had a very difficult time accessing the site of SAR operations. There were no standard operating procedures understood by all responding organizations providing guidance to this interorganizational effort. Instead, it was an ad hoc process in which US&R taskforces used personal contacts and other ad hoc measures to "negotiate" access to the site from very often suspicious and unwelcoming NYFD officials. There were many reasons for this general attitude, foremost among them ignorance by NYFD personnel operating at the site about who the US&R were and their technical capabilities, in a context in which the site was peopled by many volunteers who made false claims regarding their technical competence in US&R procedures. The result was that very often US&R taskforces would be left waiting for things to do at the Javitts Center during the critical first days of the response. Eventually, many of them were given fire suppression responsibilities elsewhere in the city to allow NYFD personnel to participate in the WTC operations, in effect acting as regular fire department units, a worthwhile function but not one that reflected the purpose of the taskforces.

WTC illustrates the effects on SAR operations of the relative sophistication and resources of local fire departments. Before 9/11, the NYFD, probably the largest and most technically sophisticated and admired fire department in the world, was not accustomed to receiving assistance from any organization. Instead, it gave assistance to others. Thus, with its special operations unit decimated, it lacked the personnel who had participated in the development of the US&R system and who could have acted as a link between it and the taskforces. It also lacked the tradition of interagency coordination that would have facilitated the integration of the various organizational actors. Thus, the effects of the disasters were multiplied by matters of organizational culture.

The Pentagon

The severity of attack on the Pentagon—the force of the plane crash, which penetrated the inner wall of the complex, and massive fires from the explosion— reduced the chances of survival. Victims who were able to escape did so within the first minutes after the impact (Titan Systems Corporation, 2002). Partly because of the Pentagon being a U.S. military facility under the direct control of the Secretary of Defense, the emergency response to the incident was more tightly controlled and better organized. The Arlington County Fire Department (ACFD) dominated the response from the first minutes after the impact (Collins, 2002).

There is official secrecy about what happened during the evacuation and SAR that took place inside the buildings of the Pentagon impacted by the airplane and about the use and relative effectiveness during the emergency of cameras and other electronic censors that are placed in the buildings for security purposes. There is some indication that the monitoring and visualization systems in the Pentagon facilities worked quite well in identifying the danger zone, establishing the extent of the hazard, and isolating it through pressurization and movable doors/gates that delayed fire progress. Still, a few people died of smoke inhalation. Unconfirmed information indicates that people evacuated in an orderly manner both to outside and to other parts of the buildings, and that some Navy personnel doused themselves with bottled water prior to attempting to reenter the facility to rescue people. Volunteers participated in rescue efforts and in searches, forming human chains to remove rubble to create egress pathways, and developing a rough division of labor while doing so; exhausted rescuers, typically at the top of the chain, would be replaced by rested ones in the back of the chain. There is also indication that construction workers at the site on the day of the attack were very helpful in the evacuation of the impacted area (Natasha Thomas, personal communication).

In comparison to WTC, the SAR procedures in the Pentagon were in many ways a textbook example of high interorganizational effectiveness and cooperation (Collins, 2002). The primary reasons are that they took place in a federal facility that had a very secure campus and a system of safeguards and military discipline. Most of the responding organizations were part of the federal government, which eliminated many jurisdictional problems that are often seen in this type of operation. It also took place in a region that had experienced an important transformation in its readiness posture. There had been a two decades-long regional tradition of preplanning and coordination among fire and rescue units of Arlington County, Fairfax County, Montgomery County, Alexandria, and the District of Columbia (ICDRM, 2002). The need for such levels of cooperation became apparent after the Air Florida Flight 90 crash of January 13, 1982.

This set of ongoing planning tools and the social relationships and trust they propitiated increased the resilience of the inter-organizational system for disaster response in the region and provides the background to what has become an example of how it should be done. In contrast, there was no similar interorganizational system operating in the NYC region that would have provided the capability to respond more effectively to the enormous destruction that took place in lower Manhattan. Instead, there was the NYFD, and when it was weakened by the WTC collapses there were no preestablished alternative arrangements and a tradition of interorganizational coordination in place. Comparing these SAR case studies provides some understanding of the capacities and limitations of the US&R taskforce system and of the importance of disaster planning.

REMAINING RESEARCH GAPS

The foregoing is intended to convey the range of topics that have been addressed in the SAR scientific literature. We are painfully aware of its shortcomings. The majority of the existing research results reviewed here are in need of replication and expansion, while other needed research has not been carried out. For example, while information on the circumstances of entrapment and location of voids can contribute to the development of effective SAR techniques and effective injury-prevention strategies as well as national programs of response, to this day there have been no efforts to construct simulation models of building collapse configurations, develop a typology of building collapse, and ascertain empirically where the voids are in fact located in these types of collapsed structures which would then enrich and perhaps correct the practical knowledge of the practitioner community reviewed earlier.[1]

Moreover, there is little information about survival rates in reinforced concrete and in steel frame buildings, which are common on the West Coast region of the United States and elsewhere in the world. While common steel frame buildings perform relatively well in an earthquake, it is not known how they will respond to explosions caused by terrorists and accidents. An area that is almost untouched by research is the impact of different national and regional building codes and building practices on SAR. For example, a great many of the houses in Mexico are made of concrete, which presents very different challenges to SAR than is the case of the typical construction used in the United States. Most of the research conclusions in this area of study stem from events that occurred in foreign countries, where the building codes differ from the U.S. codes of practice. These differences in building codes and practices might lead to substantially different failure modes and survival rates in the United States.

There is also conflicting information on what is in fact the best behavior pattern for victims to follow during the actual occurrence of earthquakes and floods as well as immediately afterwards. A number of important research questions are still unanswered related to the entrapment of victims in the aftermath of disasters. Some of the most obvious of these are: What are the factors responsible for the survival of building occupants? How do the location of the occupants, actions of the occupants, nonstructural elements and building contents, nature and time of entrapment, and method of rescue play a role in survival? Most of the SAR literature is related to seismic disasters, with relatively little information about other types of hazardous events such as floods and blasts or explosions. In light of the new international focus on terrorism, there appears to be a gap in knowledge in this area. Our impression is that despite its obvious importance as part of the emergency response phase of disasters, SAR as a topic of scientific research has experienced a lull in interest; most of the scientific contributions included in this chapter, few as they are, are more than a decade old. The dearth of scientific research in SAR is such that it is not possible to establish findings using an international, inter-cultural comparative frame of reference (Dynes, 1993). Most of what is known is based on the United States and research is needed to establish the cross-cultural validity of what is known. A comprehensive and systematic research agenda for SAR would involve a multi disciplinary

---

[1] A partial answer to some of these questions, involving computer simulation of building collapse and behavior of victims is now being done by Sherif El-Tawil and B. E. Aguirre with partial financial support from the National Science Foundation, Grant no. 0408363.

effort by structural engineers, epidemiologists, emergency medical personnel, social scientists, and emergency planners using an international, comparative scientific research design. This research agenda will include understanding the social and cultural factors that (1) facilitate the development of emergent SAR groups, (2) are implicated in their institutionalization, (3) facilitate the upgrading of technical capacities of these voluntary organizations, and (4) facilitate their operational coordination with local and state, formal SAR responders as well as with other state organizations. It would also involve research on the victim–rescuer relationship and on the ways that the presence or absence of social relationships between them and the social visibility of the victims impact SAR activities and chances of survival. Another research goal would be to develop scientific knowledge of ways to increase the effectiveness of the interphase between emergency medical services and SAR by emergent groups and other volunteers.

CONCLUSION

US&R doctrine assumes that the main players in response are the local emergency management authorities, usually the local fire departments, that the federal taskforces are mobilized to assist them, and that the site of operations has been cordoned off so that only the "right" people are allowed in it. These assumptions are contradicted by the evidence we have presented from the incidents in the WTC and the Columbia Shuttle accident. These operations were so complex that not only is SAR in them an activity dominated by local volunteers and organizations, but the recovery of bodies is also a multiorganizational effort in which US&R taskforces had to share the site with multiple social actors. Greater importance should be placed on the social complexity of these sites of massive disasters, and on what this complexity implies for the operation of US&R taskforces. More attention should be given to the implications of the Pentagon response. It was a success that can be used to rethink the operation of these taskforces, particularly the ways in which they can become part of state-level systems of disaster response that would be linked to regional level capabilities through mutual aid agreements. Such a state level system would help ameliorate if not solve two of the seemingly intractable problems they now face—lateness in arriving at disaster sites and lack of previous interaction and a tradition of training and coordination with local responders that is key to effective response operations. More broadly, there is a need to rethink the distribution of public moneys spent in SAR, since so many of the rescues are made by emergent groups, neighbors, and volunteers who do not receive much assistance at present.

Needed is an international program of public education on first aid and emergency medicine, and programs to teach people what to do if they are victims and the right ways to conduct search and rescue in various types of terrains and the many other technical matters that they would need to improve their safety and their chances of rescuing victims. Associated with it is the pressing need to create government programs to make readily available the appropriate hand tools such as metal buckets, hand gloves, ropes, hydraulic arms, jacks, and drills that are needed by volunteers to carry out SAR activities during the mass assault phase of disasters. There is also a pressing worldwide need to give more attention and support to the emerging social organizations that SAR volunteers create in the aftermath of disasters (Drabek, 1987a; Forrest, 1978). This mass assault phase of disaster, if properly channeled and understood, constitutes the most important societal resource available for response in the immediate aftermath of disasters. It should become a key aspect of disaster preparedness planning. Unfortunately, at present, perhaps with the exception of the Community Emergency Response Team (CERT)

Program in California (Borden, 1991) and a few other states in the United States (Franke & Simpson, 2004) they are not so recognized, and instead SAR emergent actors and volunteers are typically seen as appendages to the work of state agencies or as impediments to the work of these agencies. Under the emphasis of professional ideologies emphasizing technology and specialization, the emergent features of the mass assault go unrecognized as key resources in improving the effectiveness of disaster response and the safety of people throughout the world. Change in this inappropriate approach to SAR is perhaps the most important factor that is needed in improving the public administration of SAR as a disaster preparedness and response function.

CHAPTER 13

Community Processes: Coordination

THOMAS E. DRABEK

COMMUNITY PROCESSES: COORDINATION

In your mind's eye picture the pyramids of Egypt or Peru. For they, like the darker side of human activity—think of the thousands involved in Alexander's military movements—reflect the social process labeled *coordination*. And while your mind is soaring, picture those magnificent structures that defined the skyline of Manhattan prior to September 11, 2001. In contrast to the macro systems of finance, engineering, and architecture that were integrated to create those structures, think of the coordination among those few who brought them down. Then, even before the toxic dust settled, scores of additional professionals sought to coordinate their activities so as to limit the death, injury, and physical destruction beyond that which had occurred. These considerations establish the context, importance, and relevance of this chapter.

At the very core of the practice of emergency management is the concept of coordination. In this chapter, research relevant to this key concept is summarized. The analysis comprises six topics: (1) introduction, (2) problem identification: fragmentation, (3) objects of study, (4) basic principles, (5) key strategies, and (6) future research agendas.

INTRODUCTION

Based on a survey of state officials, Benini (1998) concluded that "getting organized" really paid off during several large-scale disasters in California, such as civil disturbance (1992), earthquake (1994), and floods (1996–1999). Similarly, Irvine (2004) documented that local government preparedness that was completed after Hurricane Andrew (1992) produced more humane treatment of pets following Hurricane Charley (2004) in Charlotte County, Florida. But as 2004 began, reporter after reporter expressed doubts regarding the extent of coordination that would occur as representatives of thousands of agencies responded to the destruction brought by the tsunami that impacted coastal areas of 26 nations bordering the Indian Ocean in

I wish to thank Ruth Ann Drabek for her work on this chapter.

Southeastern Asia (December 26, 2004, Boxing Day). This juxtaposition illustrates the public policy relevance and theoretical importance of a fundamental concept—coordination.

Structure versus Process

Like many other sociological concepts, coordination has been defined differently by scholars with diverse objectives (Drabek & McEntire, 2003, pp. 204–205). As such it parallels many other constructs such as decision making or conflict, which also have been defined differently. Some have found each of these concepts to best fit their purposes when they were conceptualized as *structural* characteristics of social systems. Hence, the degree of centralization (or decentralization) within an organization or community, for example, has been a powerful tool in understanding all sorts of human consequences (e.g., Hage & Aiken, 1970). But likewise, the *processes* whereby decisions have been made regarding critical organizational, community, or even societal policies have produced critical insights in our understanding (e.g., Dewey, 1938; Janis, 1982).

So it is with *coordination*. Some have conceptualized the concept as a quality of social structure (e.g., Hall, 1987). In so doing, various types of social systems can be compared. Consequences of the degree or level coordination can thereby be assessed as can both determinant or consequence factors. Similarly, the *processes* whereby system coordination might be enhanced or undermined may also be examined (e.g., Haas & Drabek, 1973). While structural interpretations, and research reflective of such, will be noted within this chapter, the primary focus is on process.

Definition

As a process, coordination has been defined by community analysts such as Warren, Rose, and Bergunder (1974) and organizational researchers such as Rogers, Whetten & Associates (1982). Earlier, Haas and Drabek (1973) had defined coordination as "... those sets of behaviors through which the complex network of interrelated events are maintained." (p. 103). Building on studies by Lawrence and Lorsch (1969), Simpson (1959), and others, they proposed that many business texts were oversimplified. That is, administrators should not be viewed as *the* organizational coordinator. Despite the ego enhancement that such advice might foster, organizational coordination processes are much more complex than such images conveyed, for example, horizontal communications enhanced coordination within many businesses far more than administrative edicts. Their perspective was reinforced over the years as other analysts documented the inherent shortcomings in perspectives rooted in the articulation of "coordination principles" such as "the unity of command principle" that specified "... that no organizational participants should receive orders from more than one superior ... " (Scott, 1981, p. 65) (see also Hall, 1987, pp. 66–70).

Building on such insights as these, Rogers and his colleagues (1982) synthesized a large number of studies and perspectives focused on alternative approaches to coordination among organizations. Hence, they defined coordination "... as a legitimating mechanism used by those involved to divide up the territory and mutually work to prevent the entry of competition, and to dampen costly innovation." (p. vii). While similar to the definitions offered by these and other scholars, the formulation created by Gillespie (1991) is most relevant to the focus of this chapter and disaster research generally.

Gillespie proposed that "... coordination is the cooperation of independent units for the purpose of eliminating fragmentation, gaps in service delivery, and unnecessary (as opposed to strategic) duplication of services." (Gillespie, 1991, p. 57). Unlike other alternatives, this definition is most relevant to human service systems and disaster responses in particular. Although it reflects a managerial perspective, both in purpose and desired outcome, it pushes the profession of emergency management into a framework, orientation, and vision that reflect the turbulence, diversity, and scope of the social systems that comprise disaster responses. Others, of course, using alternative theoretical perspectives, such as Benson's (1982) political economy framework or the "vulnerability approach" proposed by Enarson, Childers, Morrow, Thomas, and Wisner (2003), would approach disaster coordination issues quite differently.

Enter the Emergency Manager

As implied in Gillespie's definition, coordination relevant to disaster within U.S. communities is very different from that applicable to other settings in other times. American society has been characterized in many ways, but all analysts from de Tocqueville (1947) to Williams (1970) to Drabek (2003a), agree that it reflects high levels of vertical and horizontal differentiation. Indeed, as Waugh (2000a) emphasized: "The horizontal and vertical fragmentation of the federal system creates jurisdictional confusion and leads to coordination problems" (p. 52). And he was referring only to one sector, albeit important, of the total response system relevant to disaster. When the community and state layers of government are added to the mix along with the myriad of voluntary and private sector units, the scope of the managerial task becomes much clearer.

Increasingly, however, the profession of emergency management has staked out this processual turf as its niche (Drabek & Hoetmer, 1991; Simpson & Howard, 2001). As reflected in the studies completed at Iowa State University (1962–1975), the post-World War II environment brought a fundamental shift in civil defense policy and especially local government priorities. The concept of a "community coordinator" became core to agency mission (Klonglan, Beal, Bohlen, & Shaffer, 1964, pp. 221–243). Here, and in numerous other publications, the Iowa State teams documented perceptions of local publics and local government officials that indicated major shifts. For example, "... preparedness for nuclear attack is not salient for most coordinators. One clear implication for DCPA is that appeals made to local coordinators on the basis of things a coordinator should do or be able to do in terms of the all-hazards approach are likely to be more readily acted upon than others" (Mulford, Klonglan, & Kopachevsky, 1973, p. 2). Indeed, during this era, in addition to more widespread adoption of an all-hazard approach, local government officials spoke in terms of "the coordinator." Despite the transitory shifts in priorities during the Reagan years (1980–1988) when such programs as crisis relocation programs (CRP) gained notoriety (Perry, 1982), the thrust of the seminal work completed by staff of the National Governor's Association (1979) proved to be paradigm changing. The *necessity* of intergovernmental and interorganizational coordination became recognized explicitly, and emergency managers within local, state, and federal agencies increasingly gained *legitimacy* in the eyes of their counterparts. They were viewed as "the coordinator" and their occupational role became increasingly professionalized including internal certification procedures and requirements (e.g., see Drabek, 1991a; Petak, 1984; Wilson & Oyola-Yamaiel, 2000). This transformation, like the specific principles and strategies of coordination, provides the basis for understanding the failures in agency action following the 9/11 attacks and the research needs highlighted for the future. In turn, it defines the sequential steps in the logic of this chapter and its remaining components.

PROBLEM IDENTIFICATION: FRAGMENTATION

To understand how coordination gradually evolved as the key responsibility of emergency managers—defining the very core of the profession—it is necessary to explore three interrelated streams of literature: (1) organizational theory, (2) disaster response assessments, and (3) studies of local disaster preparedness directors.

Organizational Theory

Thompson and Hawkes (1962) explored the implications of disaster for administrative theory. Conceptualizing disaster as a type of social system stress, they observed that "... the contemporary American community normally relies on pluralistic processes for allocating resources among its parts and for attaining integration of those parts." (p. 274). Furthermore, "... disaster interrupts normal relationships among these units, requiring them to operate more autonomously than before." (p. 274). And finally, "... the system's processes of allocation and integration are *fragmented* ... " (p. 274) (italics in original).

Increases in unit autonomy, preexisting levels of fragmentation, and pluralism give rise to the emergence of *synthetic* organizations whereby interorganizational communications can be established and/or enhanced and the information bases on which executive decisions can be made become expanded. In his now classic work, *Organizations in Action*, Thompson (1967) elaborated on these processes and adapted them into a general theory of organizational behavior. Numerous other scholars (e.g., Dynes & Quarantelli, 1977; Quarantelli, 1984a, 1984b) picked up on these themes and specified with greater precision the processes whereby the environment created by disaster redefined the managerial challenges confronting local decision makers (Kreps, 1991b). Analyses of these shifts in task environments, and the managerial models most appropriate for them, paved the way for the articulation of the range of strategies and tactics that came to define "comprehensive emergency management" (Lindell & Perry, 1992). Others proceeded to amplify these conceptual foundations through a series of elaborations, for example, Denis, 1997; Drabek, 1987b; Dynes, Quarantelli, & Kreps, 1972; Dynes & Aguirre, 1979; Pennings, 1981; Sorensen, Mileti, & Copenhaver, 1985; Turner, 1994).

Disaster Response Assessments

As Scanlon (1988, 1997) has highlighted so effectively, the *first* empirical study of disaster documented system fragmentation, conflict, and poor coordination among responders. Thus, in his seminal study of the Halifax ship collision on December 6, 1917, Prince (1920) laid the first stone in the foundation. As Scanlon put it, Prince described "... emergent organization, both homegrown and imported" (p. 221). Quoting Prince (p. 84), Scanlon hammered the point home. "There was also lack of cooperation among official committees themselves. Friction and crises arose from time to time, which were only stopped short of scandal" (Scanlon, 1988, p. 222).

Years later, individual disaster case studies continued to display organizational personnel tripping over each other as they mobilized to reduce the trauma brought by floods (e.g., Clifford, 1956), tornadoes (e.g., Form & Nosow, 1958), and hurricanes (e.g., Moore, Bates, Layman, & Parenton, 1963). Studies such as these provided others with the materials required for the next level. Thus, Fritz (1961) demonstrated the power of multidisaster analyses whereby the detail of the specific could give way to the generalization based on the many. Reading between the lines of dozens of single-community disaster studies, Barton (1969) expanded on his earlier (1962) more limited analysis of "the emergency social system" and created elaborate networks of hypotheses that linked hundreds of variables into more unified wholes. One such cluster of 71 hypotheticals sought to define the rise of the post-disaster "altruistic community" wherein some would put the pain and experience of disaster into redefinitions of deprivation that might neutralize the hurt and reinforce their sense of self worth and individual autonomy (Barton, 1969, pp. 216–279).

In contrast, Dynes (1970) stuck to realities that, while less abstract than Barton's models, were more rooted in empirically based observations. He emphasized that the post-disaster problem of coordination was exacerbated by numerous factors such as the sequential interdependence of tasks. This, in turn, required ". . . some overall view of the tasks and their relative priority" (Dynes, 1970, p. 207). Lacking mechanisms to accomplish this, some proposed that the coordination task could best be accomplished by strong leaders who could implement the classic principles of bureaucracy (e.g., Weber, 1947). "This myth tends to be perpetuated by those who assume military analogies are applicable and who speak in terms of commanding and controlling a disaster situation." (p. 207). Paralleling Thompson's (1967) analysis, Dynes (1970) concluded that such "commanders" rarely were successful at accomplishing the coordination required to adequately cope with such fragmented responses. Rather, the search for and eventual supply of information gradually leads to an emergent coordinating body. "Such a group is usually composed of officials of legitimate organizations plus individuals with special competence and knowledge and individuals who participate in many different institutional segments of the community" (Dynes, 1970, p. 208).

Organized disaster responses were not limited to the core emergency organizational executives that had become the primary units of analysis focused on by Thompson or Barton. Rather Dynes demonstrated the full scope of the community response and illustrated its various forms. What came to be known as "the DRC Typology" had its roots in this and other reports of its day (e.g., Quarantelli, 1966). Thus, the fragmentation of response was best understood, as emergency managers later came to realize, through the identification of at least four very different types of systems. These reflected two dimensions, that is, tasks (regular or nonregular) and structure (old or new). Cross-tabulation identified the four types of systems that comprised community responses to disaster: type I (established, regular tasks accomplished through old structures); type II (expanding, regular, new); type III (extending, nonregular, old), and type IV (emergent, nonregular, new). It is this mix of systems, with very different life histories and cultures, that defines the coordination task of emergency managers.

Numerous scholars documented the importance and usefulness of the DRC typology. For example, Stallings (1978) developed an insightful series of hypotheses that helped define the post-disaster community dynamic, for example, "Expanding organizations undergo greatest stress because their structures and functions change simultaneously, their boundaries are vague and permeable, and their emergency role is frequently ill defined" (p. 91). Similarly, by focusing on type IV systems, Forrest (1978) laced together the wisdom from numerous case studies by shifting abstraction levels and formulating numerous propositions pertaining to the internal dynamics of these systems, for example, "Prior interaction patterns identify and recruit specific actors for emergent group participation" (p. 115). While other examples could be noted, the long-term program of research directed by Kreps (1989a) and his associates (e.g., Saunders & Kreps, 1987) provides the best work to date that has tried to unravel the post-disaster structures described by Dynes and others using the DRC typology (e.g., Kreps and Bosworth, 1994). After extensive analysis of hundreds of interviews conducted by DRC staff, Kreps and Bosworth (1994) concluded: "The DRC typology will continue to be a very efficient and effective analytical tool . . . in part because it " . . . specifies nicely a micro-macro link between the individual and social structure" (p. 191).

Finally, others have built on this foundation by proposing various types of modification. Starting with the insights of Weller and Quarantelli (1973) and those of Forrest (1978), Drabek (1987a), for example, proposed elaborations by nesting the DRC typology within a much more complex analytic scheme comprised of three additional variables—system permanence, structural complexity, and disasters phase (pp. 268–274). Coordination processes were thereby recast from just the emergency response phase to the full life cycle of disaster, including preparedness, recovery, and mitigation. Likewise, Quarantelli (1984a, 1996a) has offered several reexaminations of the typology and has proposed various elaborations that reflect the observations gleaned from more recent case studies (see also Quarantelli, 1996a).

Disaster response assessments have been synthesized by others who have highlighted the variety of insights into coordination processes, barriers to coordination, and factors that might facilitate, for example, Drabek (1986), Drabek and McEntire (2002). These syntheses, like more recent field studies, are summarized below as various specific topics are explored.

Studies of Local Disaster Preparedness Directors

The third stream of research that helped define the problem of fragmentation was assessments of local emergency manager activities and programs. As noted earlier, this stream of research had its origins in studies conducted at Iowa State University between 1962 and 1975, for example, Klonglan et al. (1964) and Mulford, Klonglan, and Tweed (1973). After identifying a series of strategies used by local civil defense directors to improve coordination, that is, reduce program fragmentation, within their communities, senior team members began to examine other human service agencies, for example, Mulford and Mulford (1977) and Mulford and Klonglan (1981). They documented that more effective civil defense coordinators more frequently used such strategies as cooptation and resource building. Educating the public and local organizations also improved agency legitimacy, that is, audience strategy, as did inviting key local leaders to serve as an advisory board, that is, elite representation strategy (Mulford et al., 1973, pp. 3–4). Clearly these studies provided a solid foundation for our understanding of the dynamics of interagency coordination processes.

As noted earlier, numerous studies of disaster response were conducted, and continue to be completed, by staff of the Disaster Research Center (DRC) since its creation in 1963. Most relevant to coordination processes and explication of the key problem of fragmentation, of course, was the creation of the DRC typology. Beyond this, however, are specific assessments of local civil defense offices and qualities related to their effectiveness which frequently was defined as their capacity to coordinate. For example, in several statements, Dynes (1983, 1994) has emphasized that local managers would be better served by implementing an "emergent human resources model (later referred to as a "problem solving model") than the prevailing "command and control" approach. His wise understanding of the importance of legitimacy echoed the earlier observations of Anderson (1969c), who had highlighted issues of authority and acceptance in interagency contacts. Later comparative assessments (e.g., Wenger, Quarantelli, & Dynes, 1987) documented a typology comprised of eight types of local emergency management agencies that reflected: (1) extensiveness of response activities; (2) extensiveness of planning activities; and (3) agency structure, that is, autonomous or integrated (p. 60). Hence, local offices were found to vary from type 1 (traditional) agencies, that reflected an autonomous structure used to accomplish a very narrowly defined set of planning and response activities, to type 8 (established, i.e., broad response and planning activities implemented within an integrated structure). These analyses documented the utility of definitions of coordination paralleling that noted above by Gillespie (1991). Thus, these studies, like those of others, for example, staff at the International City Management Association (ICMA) (Hoetmer, 1982) and United Research Services Incorporated (Caplow, Bahr, & Chadwick, 1984), documented that the task environment within which most U.S. emergency managers operate differed significantly from that encountered by military commanders or those directing slaves who were moving stones for future pyramids.

OBJECTS OF STUDY

Researchers have examined coordination processes, and failures, from a variety of vantage points. The scope of this diversity is best understood by clustering studies into a typology comprised of two dimensions: (1) system complexity and (2) disaster phase. Given the brevity of this chapter, however, illustrations for each analytic cell are not specified; rather, a simple twofold break is made, that is, system level and disaster phase.

System Level

At the community system level, Sorensen et al. (1985) identified key factors that promoted cohesion within systems both at the intra- and intersystem levels. This work paralleled the earlier assessment by Dynes (1978a). Using the tornadoes that struck Ft. Worth, Texas in March, 2000, McEntire (2001b) documented the major factors that facilitated coordination, for example, program acceptance, preparedness activities, networking, technology, etc. (see pp. 10–12) and those that reduced it, for example lack of information, blocked access, language barriers, and so forth (see pp. 9–10). Denis's (1995) detailed assessment of the response to a PCB fire in Quebec, Canada demonstrated that "... coordination is negotiated by those who must respond to a disaster" (p. 25). Her work was extended to other events, for example, a used-tire dump fire, to dissect the dynamics of the types of "mega-organizations" that parallel the processes first described by Barton (1969) and Dynes (1970) and later by Drabek, Tamminga, Kilijanek, and Adams (1981). All of this work underscored the imagery of emergent systems being the key structures that emergency managers must first conceptualize and then develop strategies for managing if they are to be effective (see also Denis, 1997).

Relatively few have examined state level emergency management agencies, although Drabek (1991b) did assess the adoption and implementation of microcomputers in several. As will explored later, these were but one of several technologies that managers have used to improve their capacity for coordination.

Federal system level analyses have been completed in the United States that are both of a generic nature, for example, Kreps (1990) or Schneider (1998) and event focused, for example, FEMA's response during Hurricane Andrew by Carley and Harrold (1997). Most recently, Sylves and Cumming (2004) have documented the adaptations required by FEMA staff as they have turned more attention to terrorist attacks, both actual and threatened. Hence the drift toward a homeland security perspective has brought new problems and new organizational culture contacts that require additional coordination strategies. In contrast, researchers such as Scanlon (1995) have provided insight into the Canadian federal system. Britton (1991) has provided a counterpoint with the Australian experience. As highlighted below, what the future requires is multinational comparative study.

Wachtendorf's (2000) analysis of the Red River flooding that crossed from Canada into the United States is reminiscent of Cliford's border study of flooding in Eagle Pass, Texas and the nearby Mexican town of Piedras Negras. Here, the cross-national issues of disaster highlight the coordination difficulties nation-states confront. These issues are magnified when international relief agencies are scrutinized by scholars such as Kent (1987). The next few years undoubtedly will yield reports by many who will lament that lessons from the past were not learned as thousands of helpers rushed to locations in Southeast Asia following the Boxing Day tsunami of 2004.

Finally, as Petak (1985) noted years ago regarding the intergovernmental "partner-ships" that lace federal, state, and local emergency agencies into a loose federation, such "... complexity often leads to lack of a coordinated response, distrust, and conflict" (p. 5). The dynamics of these boundary-spanning processes, which were so well dissected by May and Williams (1986), have been scrutinized further in studies such as those of Kory (1998) and Toulmin, Bivans, and Steel (1989). From Kory's assessment, we learn of the reality of multiple local governments in a community such as Miami-Dade County, Florida. Regional, as opposed to local, planning for hurricane evacuation and recovery is but one approach to seek improved coordination. Deficiencies of a different type were documented by Toulmin et al. (1989), who applied Sanford's (1967) portrait of "picket fence federalism" to disaster communications. Their theory of "intergovernmental distance" (pp. 120–130) highlighted structural sources for weak and highly problematic interagency communication under non-disaster conditions. Indeed such poor communication, and consequently weak coordination, "... is not occasional, anecdotal or unique to particular disasters, but is endemic to all the intergovernmental disaster responses" (p. 130). In view of the conclusions reached by the members of the 9/11 Commis-sion (NCOTAUTUS, 2004) regarding "the wall" that hindered the "connection of the dots" by intelligence analysts operating within multiple agencies (pp. 254–277, 424), the conclusion offered by Toulmin et al. (1989) has a chilling relevance. "The theory of intergovernmental distance points to the complexity and difficulty—and yet the necessity—of planning for 'the big one'" (p. 131). Unfortunately, their wisdom never was implemented, thereby leaving the nation at risk.

Disaster Phase

Since the idea of disaster life cycles was first introduced by Carr (1932), dozens of researchers have discovered its utility although critics such as Neal (1997) have underscored a variety of limitations (La Plante & Kroll-Smith, 1989). Like the generic, rather than the agent-specific, approach to disaster preparedness (e.g., Quarantelli, 1992a), use of disaster phases often pro-vides a coherence to an analysis that is not otherwise possible. Wolensky and Wolensky's (1990) literature review is a case in point. For example, they documented "local government performance across four disaster phases" (pp. 704–708) and thereby demonstrated that within each phase actions by local officials emerged as "problematic." After dissecting strains within the intergovernmental system (pp. 708–710), vertical and horizontal fragmentation (p. 711), they concluded that "... the historic development of power relationships within the American community has supported a custodially oriented, limited-resourced government sphere and an influential, well-resourced private sphere" (p. 714). And in turn, "... we expect that disas-ter management will remain a low priority within a generally under-resourced local govern-ment" (p. 717). Others who have focused a study within a single disaster phase have provided the specifics as to how and why system coordination processes have all too frequently been implemented to adequately overcome the consequences of structural fragmentation (Lindell, 1994; Lindell, Whitney, Futch, & Clause, 1996a, 1996b).

Presumably, interagency coordination can be enhanced through a series of disaster preparedness actions (Perry & Lindell, 2003, 2004; Rogers et al., 1989). Empirical assessment of such a claim, however, has revealed many challenges. For example, Gillespie and Streeter (1987) unveiled a host of methodological issues when they attacked the first piece of the puzzle, that is, measures of disaster preparedness. Later, Gillespie and Colignon (1993) reported on their efforts to carefully measure network shifts before and after a major table-top drill involving an earthquake scenario. Validating the research of the past, but this time with far more precision, they concluded that shifts in the task environments of responding disaster organizations were met with changes in interagency relationships that reflected both elaborations in structure and increases in concentration (p. 159). These and related assessments reflecting network coordination processes were documented in detail in their book length presentation (Gillespie, Colignon, Banerjee, Nurty, & Rogge, 1993). To date, their work remains the most rigorous measurement and quantitative exploration of disaster preparedness networks although others (e.g., Hooper, 1999) have conducted related analyses that have provided important insights. Regardless of the precision or sophistication of the measurements used, however, one theme is underscored by all who have examined such social networks: preparedness activities frequently enhance, but do not insure, subsequent interagency coordination levels and in turn, the effectiveness of community responses to most disasters.

Studies of disaster response frequently have concluded that the coordination processes used during routine emergencies do not fit the task environment created by disaster (Dynes, 1970; Dynes & Aguirre, 1979; Dynes et al., 1972; Granot, 1997; Perry, 1991; Quarantelli, 1996b; Vigo & Wenger, 1994). As Auf der Heide (1989) stated, "...the reasons disaster response is difficult to coordinate is because disasters are different from routine, daily emergencies" (p. 49). As summarized by Auf der Heide (1989), numerous studies, especially those completed by DRC staff members, have documented various reasons why disaster responses require, and frequently produce, alternative coordination mechanisms, for example, unfamiliar tasks, crossing of jurisdictional boundaries, effects on equipment and/or personnel, large number of responders and responding organizations, urgent nature of demands, and so forth (see Drabek, 2004; Drabek & McEntire, 2002).

These realities were dissected in detail as the 9/11 Commission took testimony from those who sought to coordinate rescue efforts. Despite the guidance provided in a July 2001 directive by Mayor Guiliani titled "Direction and Control of Emergencies in the City of New York," "...the response operations lacked the kind of integrated communications and unified command contemplated in the directive" (NCOTAUTUS, p. 319). There were many reasons why the behavioral reality of the response did not match the framework spelled out on paper. Aside from the unique and massive quantity of attack-generated demands, the Commission documented that "...the FDNY and NYPD each considered itself operationally autonomous. As of September 22, they were not prepared to comprehensively coordinate their efforts in responding to a major incident" (p. 285). Intrasystem coordination processes were lacking as well, for example, "...the FDNY as an institution proved incapable of coordinating the numbers of units dispatched to different points within the 16-acre complex" (p. 319). Further, "Information that was critical to informed decision making was not shared among agencies" (p. 321).

Further validating the importance of improvisation in most, if not all, disaster responses, Kendra and Wachtendorf (2003c) carefully documented three significant developments following the 9/11 attacks. These "creative" responses partially reflected the destruction of the

responses, for example, Carley and Harrold (1997), Quarantelli (1997b), Paton and Johnson (2001), and Perry (2003, 2004).

After careful review of the literature and drawing upon his own work, Gillespie (1991) succinctly identified five core factors that facilitate interagency coordination: (1) "shared goals or expectations about what the organizations will and will not do"; (2) "shared leaders or overlapping board memberships"; (3) "diversity of roles and interests"; (4) "similarity in technologies and resource needs"; and (5) "high rates of environmental change" (p. 61).

Numerous studies have documented a variety of factors that at times can be barriers to interagency coordination. For example, Drabek (1985) stressed that inadequate communication flows among the multiorganizational search and rescue networks he studied prevented adequate coordination. He (1968) had stressed this factor previously in his case study of the Indianapolis coliseum explosion. However, he stressed that other factors operated as well. Many of these have been documented further by others. These include interagency conflicts and jurisdictional ambiguity (e.g., Kouzmin, Jarman, & Rosenthal, 1995); lack of experience and/or knowledge among EOC personnel (e.g., Auf der Heide, 1989); and lack of consensus regarding the nature of and need for coordination (Quarantelli, 1984a, 1984b, 1988b).

As he did with facilitators, Gillespie (1991) created a succinct list of barriers to coordination: (1) "the tendency of organizations to seek autonomy"; (2) "staff commitment to professional ideologies and work autonomy"; (3) "differences in organizational technologies and resource needs"; (4) "fear that the identity of the group or organization will be lost"; (5) "concern about the redirection of scarce resources; (6) "the proliferation of organizations and interest groups across multiple political jurisdictions; and (7) "differences in costs of and benefits from participating in coordination" (p. 58). Each of these factors has been documented by case study writers and those conducting comparative cross-event assessments.

Managerial Orientations

In 1983, Dynes first delineated the contrasts between a command and control managerial orientation that had become the prevailing orientation among civil defense directors. Reflecting in many cases their prior military training, they sought to apply the principles of coordination that they had learned within these bureaucratic systems. Unfortunately, both in everyday activities with the diverse array of organizational cultures they confronted, and especially in the turbulent environments of disaster response, this orientation failed them. Hence, Dynes argued then and focused his analysis later (1994) by explicating why the bureaucratic model was inappropriate to the task environment of the emergency manager. Most recently he extended his assessment to the responses to the 9/11 attacks (2003).

Others, such as Drabek (1987a, 1987b), Neal and Phillips (1995), and Schneider (1992) have developed parallel analyses. Waugh (2000) has stated the position well in several of his texts for emergency managers. "Given that authority and responsibility are often ambiguous in a disaster operation, the trend is toward more coordinative roles" (p. 162). "... [M]anagement theory today is far less 'command and control' oriented. It is based on a more participative, consensus-building approach to decision making" (p. 165). In short, regardless of the label used to identify the orientation, for examplee, "human resources model" (Dynes, 1983), "problem solving model (1994); "participative model" (Waugh, 2000), the coordination function increasingly is implemented by emergency managers who have come to realize the limited usefulness, indeed outright inappropriateness, of older managerial paradigms rooted within the rhetoric and orientation of "command and control."

Role of Emergency Operations Centers (EOCs)

During the past two decades, one structural creation has emerged in many communities that, apart from disaster drills and simulations, has done more to improve the quality of interagency coordination than anything else. But while the EOC concept has been around much longer, today it is a living, functioning unit in more and more communities. In the past, the so-called EOC might house only the emergency manager and other agency staff during an emergency response. Others just did not show up, or if they did, they did not stay long. Numerous field studies (e.g., Drabek, 1987b, 2003; Scanlon, 1994, 2002a) have documented the widespread presence of these facilities and their centrality within the multiorganizational network.

Role of Information Technology

Drabek (1991b) prepared a social history of the initial adoption and implementation of microcomputers into state and local emergency management offices. While there were barriers, these technologies enhanced the information processing and mobilization of resources, thereby facilitating interagency coordination. Further, many types of decision making tools have been developed (e.g., Belardo, Karwan, & Wallace, 1984) as have geographic information systems (e.g., Gruntfest & Weber, 1998) that have increased the visibility, reputation, and legitimacy of local emergency management agencies. Stephenson and Anderson's (1997) analysis of additional technologies is most insightful and underscores the impacts of a variety of new technologies (e.g., digital libraries, ultra-broadband networks) on the evolving profession of emergency management. Each of these has enormous potential for enhancing coordination although there are important issues that wise scholars such as Quarantelli (1997a) have identified.

COORDINATION STRATEGIES

Wolensky and Miller (1981) documented important differences in the everyday, and opposed to the disaster response, role of emergency managers. Drabek (1987b) integrated this analysis with insights about managing environmental uncertainty from organizational theorists such as Thompson (1967) and Pennings (1981). Through detailed community case studies and a multidimensional stratified randomly selected telephone survey, he documented 15 strategies used by effective emergency managers to nurture interagency relationships and maintain agency integrity. Thus, he built upon and extended the earlier pioneering studies conducted at Iowa State, the DRC, and elsewhere. These 15 strategies (Drabek, 1990) have been integrated into courses and seminars for emergency managers in the United States and elsewhere, for example, Australia. These strategies are: (1) constituency support; (2) committees; (3) cooptation; (4) joint ventures; (5) coalitions; (6) agenda control; (7) entrepreneurial actions; (8) organizational intelligence; (9) mergers; (10) media relationships; (11) outside expert; (12) innovation; (13) product differentiation; (14) regulation; and (15) flow of personnel. Drabek's data documented that those emergency managers who implemented the largest number of these strategies also ranked highest on a variety of effectiveness measures.

The response function was assessed years later in a complementary project (Drabek, 2003a). In total, 62 local emergency managers were interviewed (10 within community case studies and 52 through a telephone survey). By adapting a typology formulated by Osborne and

Plastrik (1998), Drabek documented five broad types of coordination strategies that were used to varying degrees during disaster responses. Within these five categories, 26 more specific strategies were identified: (1) core strategies (domain clarification, jurisdictional negotiation, and resource familiarization); (2) consequence strategies (display of decisions; use of information technologies; and maintenance of a hospitable EOC social climate); (3) customer strategies (communication of citizen expectations and requests, facilitation of media relations; documentation of damage assessments; and documentation of disaster repairs and restoration); (4) control strategies (appeals to prior legitimacy; reference to planning documents; reference to prior experiences; decentralization of decision making; use of self-managed work teams; emergent collaborative planning; and emergent community–government partnerships; implementation of mutual aid agreements); and (5) cultural strategies (enhance awareness of cultural differences among responding agencies; enhance awareness of vulnerable populations; enhance awareness of community diversity; promote interagency cross-talking; build a shared vision; develop an in-house schoolhouse; celebrate success; and monitor stress symptoms).

Using an assessment of effectiveness criteria proposed by Quarantelli (1997b), Drabek discovered that both the implementation of the 15 managerial strategies (pre-disaster) and the 26 coordination strategies were important factors in a prediction model. That is, those emergency managers who scored highest on the effectiveness index also reported using more of both sets of strategies (see Drabek, 2003a, pp. 143–146). Of course, other social factors also constrained effectiveness. Drabek's multivariate model also comprised one event characteristic, that is, lengthy forewarning; certain agency qualities, namely participation in disaster training exercises; and higher levels of both domain consensus and prior agency contacts. Each of these, reflected, in turn, more extensive use of the strategies identified that helped to maintain agency integrity.

FUTURE AGENDA

While this survey of research points toward many future research needs, five are highlighted that are most crucial: (1) development of a theory of disaster response effectiveness; (2) development of a theory of emergency management; (3) cross-national studies of complex catastrophes; (4) impacts and limitations of information technologies; and (5) assessments of alternative managerial models.

Development of a Theory of Disaster Response Effectiveness

At the conclusion of his study of coordination strategies, Drabek (2003, pp. 147–150) proposed a preliminary theoretical model whereby comparative study of response effectiveness might be conducted. Thus, he placed coordination processes within the broader context of disaster responses and the network of social constraints they reflect ranging from community, nation-state, and worldwide social trends and emergency management policies. While the events and response networks he examined were limited to "natural," and in a few cases technological, agents, responses to terrorist attacks such as those that occurred on 9/11 specify logical next steps. Although the matrix of agencies that comprise such multiorganizational networks will differ significantly, the basic logic of the model may apply. Such explorations, however, must be guided by greater sensitivity to the fundamental epistemological question posed by Quarantelli on several occasions, that is, "What is a disaster?" (Quarantelli, 1998). Through such work, expanded and more predictive models could be derived and subjected to further empirical exploration. Also required are improved measures for the many variables that comprise any such models.

Development of a Theory of Emergency Management

All societies confront vulnerabilities and changing levels and distributions of risk. Using models of disaster response effectiveness, with coordination processes at the very core, work should be undertaken to expand into other phases of the disaster lifecycle. Thus, the networks—conceptualized as nonlinear, mutually inclusive activity sets—through which recovery, mitigation, and preparedness programs are implemented should be studied. As these are completed and multivariate predictive models are tested with cross-national data sets, a true theory of emergency management may evolve. Such a theory must take into account the observations of those working within a wide variety of theoretical orientations including sustainability (Mileti, 1999) and social vulnerability (e.g., Enarson et al., 2003). In contrast to normative prescriptions about how to "do" emergency management, this model, or models, should seek to be predictive of alternative forms of emergency management programs and activities that exist behaviorally in societies throughout the world. Such a vision will bring the study of emergency management and its core components into the broader realm of sociological theory and scholarship, thereby strengthening both the discipline of sociology and the emerging profession of emergency management.

Cross-National Studies of Complex Catastrophes

Like the 9/11 attacks, the Boxing Day tsunami in Southeast Asia presented emergency managers with unique coordination challenges. Fortunately, such events have remained rare, but every effort should be made to learn from these and those of the past. While historical records present unique methodological challenges, much has been learned by creative scholars such as Oliver-Smith and Hoffman (1999), whose pioneering anthropological research provides an important counterpoint to the quick response tradition. Regardless of the events selected, however, theoretical models of coordination processes for such complex events must occupy a critical sector of the future agenda.

Impacts and Limitations of Information Technologies

As Drabek's (1991b) work demonstrated, microcomputers provided local emergency managers with a powerful tool that could enhance interagency coordination. But they were just another episode in the increasingly rapid speed of technological innovation (Rogers, Sorensen, & Morell, 1991). As Stephenson and Anderson (1997), like Gruntfest and Weber (1998) and Dash (2002), demonstrate so clearly, additional technologies ranging from digital libraries to the Internet to multilayered geographic information systems are transforming the profession of emergency management. All of these tools have enormous potential for enhancing interagency coordination. But as the 9/11 Commission documented so well, the fundamental problem is *social, not technological,* in nature (e.g., see NCOTAUTUS, pp. 297–300). Indeed, just the single issue of interoperability among response agency radio systems requires systematic and continuing assessments as new hardware and procedures are implemented (e.g., see National Task Force on Interoperability, 2003). As with the repeater system in New York City, that never was activated during the 9/11 response, the expected benefits of many technologies are not always forthcoming (NCOTAUTUS 2004, pp. 297–298). As Randell (2004) stated: "the fact remains that interoperability needs to be actively managed to avoid the chaos of everybody talking to everyone on the same radio frequency … " (p. 29).

Assessments of Alternative Managerial Models

As noted earlier, a key failure during the 9/11 response was the lack of unity of command (NCOTAUTUS, 2004, p. 285). One managerial tool that has become increasingly popular is the "incident command system" (ICS) (for history and basic concepts see Auf der Heide, 1989, pp. 134–151; Bean, 2002; Emergency Management Institute, 1998). Recognizing the lack of unity of command of as a major failing, the Commission recommended that: "Emergency response agencies nationwide should adopt the Incident Command System (ICS). When multiple agencies or multiple jurisdictions are involved, they should adopt a unified command" (NCOTAUTUS, 2004, p. 397). This recommendation is consistent with recent FEMA policy guidance regarding the National Response Plan (NRP) and the National Incident Management System (NIMS). But administrative edict does not necessarily translate into immediate or complete compliance. Rarely does the law on the books equate to the law in action. As noted earlier, Dynes (1994) and others have seriously questioned the assumptions and procedures that underlie much of the "command and control" mentality when it comes to civilian agencies who comprise most of the resource base that actually participate in the myriad of activities that reflect the full life cycle of disaster. While the ICS is a useful managerial model for use at the tactical level by a few highly disciplined agencies—namely law enforcement, fire, and emergency medical—it is not a panacea (Fennell, 2002). It alone will not provide the most effective guidance for the full range of more complex coordination processes that comprise the responsibility of emergency managers. Research must be conducted that documents the implementation process of the ICS, NIMS, and other aspects of any "Federal Response Plan" both within and among local communities and nation-states. Cultural differences both within agencies and among peoples do not disappear just because of policy adoption.

Haddow and Bullock (2003) stated the case well when they described the adoption of the ICS among fire departments. While it assisted in defining lines of authority, a more flexible "coordination model" was more appropriate for emergency managers. "… [T]he coordinational model is becoming more popular than the traditional command and control structure (p. 88)…. the new breed of emergency manager is typically more of a recovery coordinator than a field general" (p. 88). "The coordination model is also often better for negotiating turf battles among agencies and nongovernmental organizations providing overlapping services" (p. 88).

These views are more consistent with Gillespie's (1991) definition of coordination that was presented at the outset of this chapter. They also are more consistent with the critiques of the bureaucratic managerial model—an assumption base implicit within the ICS—summarized by Dynes (1994), Neal and Phillips (1995), and Drabek (1990, 2003a). Hence, it is highly likely that future researchers studying post-disaster communities wherein ICS and NIMS were implemented by emergency managers—at least to some degree—will document the costs of inadequate interagency coordination. Efforts to implement managerial prescriptions that are inappropriate for the task environment created by disaster are destined to fail. In short, the very structures some are trying to impose on their community to enhance subsequent levels of coordination may severely constrain the effectiveness of a post-disaster response. Only through carefully designed and executed disaster research will the theoretical foundations of emergency management be developed.

The above agenda would be expanded by many and reprioritized by others. This is as it should be. Regardless of the shape and contour proposed, however, coordination processes should be at the top of research funding agency concerns and budgetary allocations. Assessments of training impacts must also be part of the future effort. For clearly, even with these processes, that is, coordination, far more is known than is being implemented on a daily basis throughout the United States and especially throughout the world.

CHAPTER 14

Sustainable Disaster Recovery: Operationalizing An Existing Agenda

GAVIN P. SMITH AND DENNIS WENGER

Disaster recovery represents the least understood aspect of emergency management, from the standpoint of both the research community and practitioners (Berke, Kartez, & Wenger, 1993; Rubin, 1991). When compared to the other widely recognized phases of emergency management, that is, preparedness, response, and mitigation, scholars have yet to address fundamental questions, while practitioners have failed to establish an integrated policy framework or utilize readily available tools to improve disaster recovery outcomes (Berke et al., 1993; May and Williams, 1986; Mileti, 1999). Since the 1990s the concept of sustainability has been adopted by hazards researchers and applied to mitigation (Berke, 1995a; Burby, 1998; Godschalk, et. al., 1999; Mileti, 1999), recovery (Becker, 1994a; Berke, Kartez, & Wenger, 1993; Eadie et al., 2001; Oliver-Smith, 1990; Smith, 2004; United States Department of Energy, 1998), and to a lesser extent preparedness and response (Tierney, Lindell, & Perry, 2001). While recognized as a meaningful paradigm among scholars and a limited number of practitioners, achieving sustainable recovery following disasters is not a widespread phenomenon in the United States, owing in large part to the current recovery model in practice today. It is therefore the intent of this chapter to describe an improved policy implementation framework focused on achieving sustainable recovery. Emphasis is placed on the analysis of the United States model of recovery and the development of specific recommendations to improve the process. Key issues and research questions are identified in order to advance this agenda, including the need to develop a theory of recovery that emphasizes specific factors that facilitate or hinder this approach. Next, a review of the literature highlights the fact that while past research has addressed several recognized dimensions of sustainable recovery, the research has not been linked to a unifying theory that helps to clarify our understanding of how sustainable recovery can be achieved.

REVIEW OF THE DISASTER RECOVERY
LITERATURE

Disaster recovery has been analyzed using a variety of perspectives including the role of power in decision making (Olson, 2000; Platt, 1999), the practice of urban planning (Ohlsen & Rubin, 1993; Schwab et al., 1998), the sociology of disaster (Nigg, 1995a; Peacock, Morrow, & Gladwin, 1997), policy implementation (May, 1985; May & Williams, 1986; Olson & Olson, 1993), and more recently the application of sustainable development principles (Becker, 1994a,1994b; Becker & Stauffer, 1994; Berke, Kartez, & Wenger, 1993; Berke & Wenger, 1991; Eadie et al., 2001; Smith, 2004). Yet there exist a surprisingly limited number of theories explaining recovery (Chang, 2005). The widely recognized tenets of sustainability provide a robust and meaningful framework to synthesize the majority of existing disaster recovery research perspectives, develop a new theory of recovery, and outline a future research agenda that is directly applicable to both practitioners and scholars. As Table 14.1 demonstrates, a number of recovery-based studies have been conducted that can be classified across key dimensions of sustainability. Most of the research cited was not intentionally framed in this manner when it was undertaken. Rather, it became apparent during the review of the literature that past research provides important insights into our current understanding of this topic; serving as the roots of sustainable recovery.

Prior to the 1970s, a limited amount of research had been conducted on disaster recovery (Barton, 1969). The current range of research perspectives, including the increasing use of multidisciplinary teams to address complex questions dealing with hazards, can be traced back to the book "Assessment of Research on Natural Hazards" (White & Haas, 1975). The authors sought to evaluate the accumulating knowledge gained by hazards researchers, identify a future research agenda, and provide suggested national policy objectives. While the text clearly demonstrated the need for and use of multidisciplinary research, it did not generate a new paradigm (Mileti, 1999 p. 21).

The use of comparative analysis dominated the research agenda in the late 1970s and early 1980s (Friesemam et al., 1979; Geipel, 1982; Haas, Kates, & Bowden, 1977; Rubin, 1982; Wright et al., 1979). Particular emphasis was placed on the use of case studies to describe the process of recovery at the local level (Haas, Kates, & Bowden, 1977; Rubin, 1985). The Disaster Recovery Project, which focused on 14 localities, studied how local planning and management expedited recovery, the degree to which mitigation techniques were adopted and incorporated into the recovery process, and the extent to which communities sought to improve local conditions (Rubin, 1982; Rubin, Saperstein, & Barbee, 1985). Similarly, Kates and Pijawka (1977) suggest that as part of their four-phased sequential description of the recovery process (emergency period; restoration period; replacement and reconstruction period; and commemorative, betterment, and developmental reconstruction period), the final phase is representative of an opportunity to improve pre-disaster conditions. Today, these findings are considered important components of sustainable recovery (Beatley, 1995, 1998; Mileti, 1999).

Geipel, in his study of recovery following the 1976 earthquake in northern Italy, discovered that disasters serve to highlight existing cultural, social, and economic conditions that shape the path to recovery. In this case, the earthquake exacerbated existing class inequalities among merchants (who gained financially) and the elderly, who struggled to return to their pre-disaster condition. In areas that were the site of ongoing economic activity and growth, post-disaster reconstruction was more prevalent. Areas facing economic decline fell further into disrepair. Conversely, Friesema et al. (1979) argued that disasters caused little long-term

TABLE 14.1. A Summary of Recovery Research Across Key Dimensions of Sustainability

Environmental	Quality of Life	Social	Economic	Disaster Resilience	Participation, Political Process, Power
Pilkey & Dixon, 1996	Bolin (1985)	Quarantelli, 1989, 1999	Comerio, 1998	Burby, 2001; Burby et al., 1998, 1999	Olson, 2000
Burton, Kates, and White, 1993	Geis, 2000	Nakagawa & Shaw, 2004	Kunreuther, 1973	Schwab et al., 1998	Birkland, 1997
Cutter, 2001		Bolin & Stanford, 1998	Geipel, 1982	Beatley, 1995, 1998	Platt, 1999
Rees, 1992	Kates & Pijawka, 1977	Bolin & Bolton, 1986		Olshansky & Kartez, 1998	May & Williams, 1986
Becker, 1994b	Comerio, 2005; Alesch, 2005	Drabek, 1986		Berke, 1995; Mileti, 1999	Rubin & Barbee, 1985; Shaw, Gupta & Sarma, 2003
Phillippi, 1994		Cutter, 1996	Johnson, 2005	Rubin, 1982; Rubin, Saperstein, & Barbee, 1985	Olson & Olson, 1993
Thieler & Bush, 1991		Bolin & Stanford, 1999	Kunreuther & Roth, 1998		Francaviglia, 1978
			Chang & Miles, 2004		Berke, Kartez, & Wenger, 1993
		Peacock, Morrow, & Gladwin, 1997			

impacts, a finding that has been widely challenged (Cutter, 2001; Wright et al., 1979). Geipel also found that citizens envisioned a "post-disaster plan" emphasizing a return to normalcy, which competed with administrators, planners, and other experts who proposed change. The lessons, such as those described by Haas, Kates, and Bowden (1977) and Rubin (1982), suggest early components of a sustainable recovery framework (e.g., public involvement, equity, and the role of pre-disaster planning) as well as conditions that hinder a sustainable recovery, such as differing levels of social vulnerability and power.

A second assessment of hazards research, titled "Disasters by Design: A Reassessment of Natural Hazards in the United States," focused on the principles of "sustainable hazards mitigation" and the utilization of systems theory linking the earth's physical system, human system, and the built environment (Mileti, 1999). Many of the primary objectives described in the text (e.g., build local networks, strive for increased capability and consensus, establish a holistic government framework, and provide comprehensive education and training) are applicable to recovery and serve as elements in the proposed policy implementation framework and theory of recovery discussed later in this chapter.

DEFINING DISASTER RECOVERY

Key terms and definitions are described next, in order to establish a baseline understanding of disaster recovery, followed by a review of the sustainable recovery literature. Emphasis is placed on several important premises and our evolving understanding of this complex topic, including the construction of a new definition that describes the potential to attain sustainable recovery. Early definitions of recovery emphasized that recovery was predictable, made up of identifiable parts occurring in a sequential manner; choices and decisions were value driven; and outcomes (i.e., paths to recovery) emphasized a return to normalcy or the incorporation of those actions that have become more recently associated with sustainability—a reduction of future vulnerability (post-disaster mitigation), equity, and amenity (Haas, Kates, & Bowden, 1977, p. xxvi). However, this definition is an oversimplification of reality and fails to recognize that recovery is not uniformly achieved by all members of society, nor does it always follow a clearly defined path (Quarantelli, 1989a; Sullivan, 2003; Wilson, 1991). In reality, recovery is messy and uncertain. Factors such as power, race, class, gender, past disaster experience, and access to resources, including information, can all play a role in shaping the process for social units ranging from households to societies (Barry, 1997; Bolin, 1985; Francaviglia, 1978; Peacock, Morrow, & Gladwin, 1997; Platt, 1999).

Several definitions of recovery have focused on the repair and restoration of the built environment as well as the temporal differentiation between short- and long-term recovery or reconstruction, including an appreciation of pre-disaster actions such as land use and recovery planning (Rubin & Barbee, 1985; Schwab et al., 1998). Other scholars, such as Nigg (1995a), have argued that recovery involves more than the reconstruction of the built environment. Rather, it is more appropriately defined as a social process shaped by both pre- and post-disaster conditions. Thus, an alternative definition of disaster recovery is one that describes the numerous challenges faced by people and the impacts of disaster on human constructs (i.e., families, groups, organizations, communities, governments, and economies) as well as a description of how natural systems are impacted and "recover" from disaster. It is therefore suggested that disaster recovery can be defined as *the differential process of restoring, rebuilding, and reshaping the physical, social, economic, and natural environment through pre-event planning and post-event actions*. While this definition describes the outcomes associated with a sustainable disaster recovery, it also recognizes that people, groups, and institutions are affected differently by disasters, and as a result, the overall recovery process is not necessarily linear, nor is it driven predominantly by technical challenges, but rather by social parameters (Nakagawa & Shaw, 2004; Nigg, 1995a.) As a result, people, groups, organizations, communities, governments, economies, and the environment often recover at differing rates, and in some cases fail to reach their pre-disaster condition. Conversely, opportunities exist to recover in a manner that results in recognizable (social, economic, and environmental) improvements over those conditions that were prevalent prior to the event.

SUSTAINABILITY AND DISASTER RECOVERY

Recovery is described next within the context of the new definition provided in the previous section, emphasizing how the concepts of restoration, rebuilding, and reshaping affect sustainable development outcomes. The concept of restoration has historically implied getting back to normal, as Haas, Kates, and Bowden (1977) suggest. Traditional examples include the repair of damaged housing, infrastructure or commercial buildings. As defined here, restoration also applies to the psychosocial conditions found post-disaster, including the ability of an individual or family to regain a sense of well being or to reconnect disrupted social networks. Disasters often precipitate the creation of issue-specific emergent groups, including social networks intended to address perceived shortfalls in the distribution of assistance (Bolin & Stanford, 1999), or those who seek to educate disenfranchised populations about risk and appropriate preparedness activities (Lindell & Perry, 1992).

Understanding the relationship between sustainability, hazards, and disasters requires recognizing both the destructive and regenerative forces of nature. Attempts to restore or protect natural systems must be done in a manner that respects the importance of allowing them to function properly (Beatley, 1998; Burby, 2001; National Science and Technology Council, 1996; Phillippi, 1994; Thieler & Bush, 1991). A review of history and an extensive body of research clearly demonstrates how poor decision making has lead to more damaging disasters (May & Deyle, 1998; Mileti, 1999; Pilkey & Dixon, 1996; Platt, 1998, 1999). The use of levees to modify the Mississippi River floodplain and the intensive armoring of our shorelines represent stark examples of how our actions can result in long-term costs including greater hazard vulnerability and less sustainable communities. Restoring natural systems may involve the removal of existing structures or placing limits on future growth in known hazard areas, thereby maintaining a small "ecological footprint" as Rees (1992) suggests.

An important part of disaster recovery involves the physical reconstruction of the built environment. Specific examples include rebuilding or repairing damaged infrastructure (including water, sewer, and electrical service delivery systems) homes, businesses, and community assets such as parks, public buildings, and community icons. During the reconstruction process, key questions emerge and decisions must be made regarding how this will occur. Numerous options exist, including the repair of damaged structures and supporting infrastructure to their pre-disaster condition, or the incorporation of sustainable redevelopment principles, including hazard mitigation, energy efficiency, or improved local aesthetics (Geis, 2000; Skinner & Becker, 1995). Those that choose to rebuild in a manner that embraces these principles may require changes to past construction practices and land-use patterns, including the type, location, and density of development (Burby et al., 1999; Mader, Spangle, & Blair, 1980). While local, state, and federal laws governing the location and type of development that may occur in hazard areas exists, the standards and enforcement mechanisms vary widely across the country (Berke & Beatley, 1992; Burby, 1998; Burby & French, 1981; Godschalk, Brower, & Beatley, 1989; Olshansky & Kartez, 1998).

Reshaping a community implies changing the way things were before the disaster. Specific actions taken during the recovery process can enhance or hinder sustainability. The failure to establish clear recovery goals and an effective implementation strategy can lead to shoddy reconstruction, a loss of jobs, a reduction in affordable housing stock, missed opportunities to incorporate mitigation into the rebuilding process, and an inability to assist the neediest recover (Bolin & Bolton, 1986; Comerio, 1998; Peacock, Morrow, & Gladwin, 1997). According to Vale and Campanella (2003), historical evidence suggests that cities recovering from disasters are unlikely to make significant changes to the built environment during reconstruction. Shaw, Gupta, and Sarma (2003) have shown that meaningful change can occur under the appropriate circumstances.

Communities can choose different paths to recovery. In reality, choices are often constrained because of a lack of awareness of the options before them and the failure to involve a wide range of stakeholders in the decision-making process. Recovery practice traditionally emphasizes the management of federal assistance programs rather than a systematic identification of community needs and the development of a comprehensive strategy for long-term recovery and reconstruction (Kartez, 1991; Schwab et al.). As a result, communities often fail to return to their pre-disaster condition, or worse, actions may increase their exposure to hazards, worsen economic conditions, damage natural systems, or exacerbate racial and ethnic tensions. Conversely, the post-disaster environment provides savvy communities with an unprecedented opportunity to improve (sometimes dramatically) the overall quality of life for its residents, enhance local economies, and improve environmental conditions.

One of the best examples of reshaping a community involves the incorporation of hazard mitigation into the reconstruction process. Hazard scholars have emphasized the need to add mitigation into pre- and post-disaster recovery decision making, thereby facilitating disaster resilience, which implies an ability to "bounce back" more quickly following a disaster than those who fail to adopt this approach (Beatley, 1995; Burby, 2001; Olshansky & Kartez, 1998).

Scholars and practitioners from other disciplines are often unaware of hazard resilience or the role it plays in the broader sphere of sustainability. For these concepts to be put into practice on a larger scale, hazards researchers and those who have successfully implemented sustainable recovery principles or incorporated mitigation into other community initiatives need to promote this connectivity. The ability to enlarge coalitions of sustainable development proponents to include those supporting the concepts of hazard resilience and sustainable disaster recovery enhances the likelihood of communities adopting and institutionalizing these principles.

In the United States, a number of tools have been developed to assess and reduce the impacts of hazards. Examples include sophisticated meteorological models, loss estimation software, warning systems, grants management programs, education and outreach efforts, land-use planning, and various construction techniques. While the opportunity exists to take advantage of these tools, communities have largely failed to recognize how current development patterns affect the long-term sustainability of our communities. As Timothy Beatley notes: "Natural disasters dramatically illustrate the ways in which contemporary development is not sustainable in the long run" (1998, p. 237). Mileti notes that disasters frequently occur in areas where unsustainable development is prevalent and disasters limit the ability of communities to move toward sustainability (1999, p. 13). While this perspective is an unfortunate reality in many cases, it does not fully recognize the ability of communities to plan for sustainable recovery.

PLANNING FOR SUSTAINABLE RECOVERY

Following disasters, the pressure to quickly resume services, repair damages, and rebuild is intense. In many communities, powerful pro-growth coalitions comprised of landowners, development interests and governmental units strive to maintain land use practices that serve to profit a small interrelated "growth machine," regardless of their impacts on less powerful interests (Logan & Molotch, 1987). Conversely, research and practice suggests that planning and the use of public sector dispute resolution techniques can play a role in addressing imbalances of power and long-standing community needs and concerns (Forester, 1987, 1989; Godschalk, 1992; Susskind & Cruikshank, 1987). In the context of sustainable disaster recovery, returning to the way things were before the disaster is not always the best approach. Disaster recovery presents a significant, albeit limited, window of opportunity to rebuild damaged structures stronger than before the event, alter land-use patterns, and reshape the existing social, political, and economic landscapes.

A large body of research has shown that disasters tend to differentially impact individuals and groups because of pre-disaster levels of social vulnerability (Blaikie et al., 1994; Bolin & Bolton, 1986; Bolin & Stanford, 1999; Peacock, Morrow, & Gladwin, 1997). To bridge the gap between maintaining the status quo and taking advantage of post-disaster opportunities to enact beneficial change, including actions taken on behalf of less powerful groups, it is incumbent on planners and others to involve all relevant stakeholders and seek consensual approaches that elicit mutual gains across potentially conflicting groups. Past research has shown that disaster policy is less salient to local officials, who tend to experience disasters less frequently than state and federal personnel (Wright & Rossi, 1981), whereas Geipel found that resistance to change can be overcome through the rapid development of inclusive recovery strategies (1982). Oliver-Smith (1990), in his study of earthquake recovery in Peru, found that sustainable recovery objectives such as addressing issues of social inequality and the adoption of hazard mitigation practices during recovery were evident when planning strategies met local needs, local capabilities were considered by those responsible for the distribution of external aid, and the community understood programmatic assistance requirements. More recently, research suggests that individuals and organizations may be more willing to consider changes in the status quo following disasters (Birkland, 1997), including planning for disaster recovery and the adoption of sustainable recovery and reconstruction practices as a result of local, state, and federal leaders who advocate this approach (Smith, 2004; Smith, forthcoming).

The importance of recovery planning has been documented in several communities in the United States (Berke & Beatley, 1992; Geipel, 1982; Schwab et al., 1998; Spangle, 1987; Spangle and Associates, 1991), and abroad (Berke & Beatley, 1997; Bolin & Bolton, 1983; Oliver-Smith, 1990). Yet it is not widely used as a post-disaster decision-making tool. Further, the extent to which planning is utilized, including the methods used to shape recovery decision-making processes, remains largely unknown. In reality, recovery planning-related research has focused on a limited number of communities rather than a nationwide or global analysis. Nor has a comparative study been conducted to assess the merits of comprehensive pre-disaster planning versus the post-disaster adaptive planning approach that is practiced today by the majority of local governments in the United States. Lessons learned through a comparative cross-cultural analysis of recovery planning practice in the United States and other countries should be undertaken to assess key factors affecting a sustainable recovery.

The effectiveness of pre-disaster emergency response planning on post-disaster response has been conducted by Quarantelli (1993b), who notes that sound planning does not always equate with the effective managing of disaster response activities. Similarly, Clarke (1999) found that some communities seemed to respond effectively to a disaster when they failed to plan or disregarded existing planning documents altogether. More recent work suggests that sustainable recovery can be achieved using an adaptive planning approach (Smith 2004; Smith, forthcoming).

CHARACTERISTICS OF SUCCESSFUL LOCAL RECOVERY PLANS

Mileti (1999) has identified several underlying characteristics of successful local recovery plans. They include:

Community involvement. Stakeholders who will be affected by post-disaster decision making should provide input and policymakers should obtain buy-in from them before a disaster occurs. This will reduce conflict and aid in the development of a plan that reflects local needs.

Information. The effectiveness of a plan is driven by the information used to establish policy and spur action. Specific information needed to develop a recovery plan includes hazard characteristics (e.g., ground motion, high wind, and storm surge) and areas likely to be impacted; population size, composition, and distribution; local economic factors; resources available post-disaster; powers, programs, and responsibilities of local, state, and federal governments as well as nonprofits, businesses, and other relevant stakeholder organizations; current and projected land-use patterns; the type and location of existing and projected building stock and infrastructure, including its interconnectivity to existing and projected development. A Geographic Information System (GIS) provides a meaningful analytical tool to graphically display, overlay, and analyze data and is being increasingly used by local governments and emergency managers to plan for hazards and disasters.

Organization. A recovery plan should identify relevant groups and organizations that can provide specific or assigned types of assistance. A recovery and reconstruction committee can spearhead post-disaster efforts and regularly convene to engage in pre-event planning and policy making. This type of organizational structure should include not only governmental agencies but also seek out nonprofits and emergent organizations that are often the most effective when trying to aid the disenfranchised or those who seem to "fall through the cracks" following disasters.

Procedures. Recovery plans should be action oriented. In the post-disaster environment, existing policymaking procedures must be modified to account for the need to make rapid decisions. For example, recovery plans should incorporate hazard mitigation into the repair of damaged facilities and the chosen location of future development relative to identified hazard areas. In the short run, post-disaster reconstruction permitting and code review procedures may be streamlined or a temporary building moratorium placed on reconstruction until the community can assess its recovery objectives.

Damage evaluation. The recovery plan should clearly articulate operational tasks associated with the mobilization, deployment, and coordination of those assigned to conduct damage assessments. The information should be gathered in such a way that it can be rapidly assimilated and used to assess local needs and assist in the implementation of pre- and post-disaster reconstruction strategies.

Finances. Post-disaster recovery and reconstruction costs money. In many cases, major disasters can result in costs greatly exceeding local municipal budgets. Federally declared disasters can trigger the provision of substantial funding. The ability to link identified needs (gathered as part of the damage assessment) to existing funding sources, technical assistance and appropriate policies is crucial to successfully implementing identified objectives. Local needs may not always match program eligibility criteria, and alternative implementation strategies should be identified. In the case of localized disasters that do not meet federal disaster declaration criteria, state and local governments may need to develop contingency budgets.

STATE AND FEDERAL RECOVERY PLANNING

The evaluation of state and federal recovery planning remains virtually nonexistent and represents a fertile area of needed research (Waugh & Sylves, 1996). Nor has the role of federal and state agencies in local recovery practice been adequately described. Anecdotal evidence suggests that states are more likely to develop recovery plans than local governments. Yet their quality, including the degree to which they provide the tools necessary to coordinate state recovery efforts, assist local governments to develop sound plans, or embrace the concepts of sustainable recovery remain uncertain. A nationwide analysis of local and state recovery plans is needed to more accurately assess their effectiveness. The practice of content analysis has been performed on both local (Berke & Beatley, 1992; Godschalk, Brower, & Beatley, 1989) and state hazard mitigation plans (Godschalk et al., 1999). The findings of Godschalk et al. make a compelling argument for strengthening many of the weaknesses identified in this chapter regarding recovery planning. Specific issues and concerns include ineffective implementation strategies, poor plan quality, unclear federal policy directives, organizational fragmentation, the need to foster intragovernmental actions (e.g., training and plan evaluation) that lead to a higher level of capacity and commitment among state and local governments, the value of developing a mitigation ethic, and the use of sustainability as a framework for guiding mitigation planning decisions.

States are typically ill prepared to provide meaningful advice and training in recovery planning. Emergency management planners at the state level have tended to emphasize local response and preparedness workshops and exercises, while recovery efforts have focused on the administration of federal aid programs following disasters rather than helping local governments devise a pre-disaster strategy emphasizing proactive planning and self-reliance. More recently, state emergency management agencies across the country are providing guidance on the creation and implementation of hazard mitigation plans, in large part because of the passage of the Disaster Mitigation Act.

The failure to develop sound pre-disaster recovery plans is particularly troublesome, considering that the majority of hazard events do not trigger federal disaster declarations, leaving state and local governments to address recovery concerns without a clear plan of action. There is, however, some evidence of state participation in the recovery planning process. Florida, for example, has linked hurricane recovery planning to coastal management guidelines, yet their effectiveness as a recovery tool has been questioned by Deyle and Smith (1996) because of a low level of commitment among local governments.

The majority of federal recovery "planning" remains focused on the management of disjointed federal programs and an ad hoc provision of technical planning assistance driven by political pressure or provided in isolated areas that have received significant damages (Smith, forthcoming). Improving the existing federal delivery system will require a major emphasis on state and local capacity-building that is not currently in practice today. There is some evidence that this is changing (Schwab, 2005). FEMA has begun to provide more post-disaster recovery planning assistance, as evidenced by the actions taken following the Florida hurricanes. It remains unclear whether this was a response to political pressure or indicative of a major policy shift within FEMA. One indicator suggesting that the agency is adopting a more active stance includes the development of a new emergency support function titled "long-term recovery," which is now part of the National Response Plan (NRP). The NRP provides broad functional guidance for federal agencies assigned emergency management roles and responsibilities in the post-disaster environment (FEMA, 2004a). It remains unclear whether this will result in a more formal institutionalization of federal recovery planning assistance. It does not, for example, address the need to proactively develop pre-disaster plans for recovery, nor does the NRP outline the means to adequately train federal, state and local officials. Following hurricane Katrina, for example, large numbers of contractors were hired by FEMA to assist Louisiana and Mississippi communities develop local recovery plans, yet the majority of those involved were largely inexperienced in disaster recovery.

The current disaster recovery policy framework can be substantially improved through planning. The primary emphasis of state and federal efforts should aim to assist local communities more effectively plan for recovery. In 1998, a collection of federal and state government officials and nonprofit representatives met to discuss the creation of action items intended to foster the incorporation of sustainability into the disaster recovery process. The conference resulted in the "wingspread principles," which focused on the education and training of stakeholders, the importance of sustainable redevelopment planning, the creation of incentives (including financing), the elimination of disincentives to sustainable recovery, and building local capacity. Proposed ideas included a proposed 1% allocation of disaster funding to support sustainable recovery assistance, the development of pre- and post-disaster training workshops and materials, outreach efforts in hazard-prone areas, the creation and deployment of sustainable redevelopment "strike teams," the assignment of sustainable redevelopment experts to Disaster Recovery Centers (DRCs), encouraging the development of pre-disaster sustainable redevelopment plans, the provision of financial incentives based on meeting established performance standards tied to prevention, the creation of more flexible funding mechanisms, the adoption of model redevelopment codes, and the facilitation of locally empowered decision making (U.S. Department of Energy, 1998). Three factors limited the success of this effort: the principles were not widely shared with government officials and other relevant stakeholders; an implementation strategy was not established; and the long-standing separation of mitigation and other recovery programs within FEMA was not addressed.

Based on the findings of the conference and past recovery planning research, state and federal plans should include the following principles:

- A concepted effort to obtain buy-in from state and federal emerging management officials, including those who may not recognize the merits of recovery planning
- An emphasis on the importance of pre- and post-disaster recovery planning, including long-term recovery and reconstruction;
- The clear identification of stakeholders and their roles in a sustainable recovery;
- A strategy to identify and address local needs in both the pre- and post-disaster environment;
- An emphasis on the concept of disasters as opportunity (to incorporate sustainable development strategies into post-disaster recovery and reconstruction); and
- The establishment of an education and training agenda focused on building and sustaining local capability, self reliance and commitment, leading to the creation of a sustainable recovery ethic.

A sustainable recovery ethic implies a moral code of conduct that is incorporated into the day-to-day actions of those who embrace the set of guiding principles outlined in this chapter. A sustainable recovery ethic is comprised of three primary components—self reliance, hazard resilience, and, multi-objective planning. Access to disaster recovery assistance has increasingly become recognized as an entitlement (Platt, 1999). Sustainable communities strive toward self-reliance. That is, communities take action to reduce dependence on state and federal assistance following a disaster. This is accomplished, in large part, by embracing hazard mitigation and disaster resilience. Taking action to reduce identified vulnerabilities before a disaster speeds recovery and limits social and economic disruption. Taking advantage of pre- and post-disaster opportunities to achieve multiple objectives is also vitally important. Achieving this aim requires reaching out to a wide range of individuals, most of whom are not emergency management officials. To facilitate the creation of a sustainable recovery ethic, communities must be held accountable for their actions, particularly those that continue to develop in known hazard areas and seek federal assistance following disasters. Accountability implies that individuals and local governments must bear a greater proportion of disaster recovery costs and invest in locally driven sustainable recovery options.

Local governments have the greatest stake in recovery and must bear the responsibility of long-term reconstruction efforts, yet they are typically the least knowledgeable about recovery programs when compared to FEMA and state emergency management agencies. On the surface, local governments may seem unaware of the potential to achieve sustainable recovery. During a disaster, local officials are often overwhelmed by the tasks associated with response activities, the provision of temporary and long-term housing, grant administration, and the tracking of financial reimbursements. The idea of creating a post-disaster recovery plan can be viewed as a time-consuming exercise by people who are already taxed to their physical and emotional limits. In reality, many local government officials are more aware of the tools that *could* be used to facilitate a sustainable recovery than federal and state emergency managers.

Sustainable development practices are becoming increasingly utilized by local governments. Land-use planners are frequently the primary proponents of these techniques. When viewed in the context of disaster recovery, the concepts of sustainability are often foreign to state and federal emergency management officials. Local land-use planners can play a key role in achieving a sustainable recovery if they are invited to participate in pre- and post-disaster recovery planning activities. Kartez and Faupel (1994) have shown that a great deal of work remains to be done to improve the level of coordination between these groups. Comprehensive land-use planning, economic development, subdivision regulations, zoning, capital improvements planning, greenways design, and other commonly used approaches represent techniques employed at the local government level that are directly relevant to recovery (Schwab et al., 1998; Topping, 1991). This suggests that training and educational methods should emphasize the reciprocal exchange of information including meaningful policy dialogue and the use of participatory planning techniques among federal, state, and local stakeholders that is not fully utilized in the current recovery framework.

NEXT STEPS AND NEW DIRECTIONS: TOWARD A THEORY OF RECOVERY AND THE CREATION OF A NEW RECOVERY IMPLEMENTATION FRAMEWORK

Improving the likelihood of achieving sustainable recovery at the community level requires a reevaluation and modification of the implementation framework in place today. To achieve this result, two interrelated issues must be addressed. First, a theory of sustainable recovery for communities must be developed. Second, embedded within the understandings derived from theory and past research, a new policy implementation framework should be introduced. This chapter concludes with a discussion of these two issues.

Toward a Theory of Sustainable Disaster Recovery

A significant portion of this chapter has described the nature of sustainable recovery and examined the existing research literature in light of that concept. What we have not discussed, *because it does not exist*, is a comprehensive theory of sustainable community disaster recovery. The development of such a theory is beyond the scope of this chapter. What will be discussed is the importance of theory development for both hazard researchers and practitioners; the scale of theory construction; the nature of the dependent variable; and a presentation of critical contextual, facilitating, and inhibiting variables that can influence the achievement of sustainable community recovery.

The Importance of Theoretical Development

The development of a theory of sustainable community recovery is of great importance both to researchers and practitioners. As a proposed explanation, theory has the potential to guide substantive, integrated research. Currently, we have accumulated a body of research findings and conceptual variables that is beginning to verge on being rather impressive. However, we lack a guiding theory or searchlight to lead our investigations.

The research community is increasingly aware of this lacuna. At the 1st International Conference on Urban Disaster Reduction in Kobe, Japan, a session was devoted to the issues of developing a theory of disaster recovery. Indicative of the current state of the research literature, a variety of topics were discussed, including comparative financial approaches (Johnson, 2005); the use of existing, consensus-based findings (Olshansky, 2005); metrics for measuring disaster recovery (Comerio, 2005); the application of the theory of complex self-organizing systems to recovery (Alesch, 2005); and the quantitative modeling of the recovery process (Chang, 2005). Although they brought discrete and disparate pieces to the theoretical puzzle, the participants unanimously agreed that it is time to integrate what is known into a comprehensive, theoretical explanation of disaster recovery that can be examined through future research.

However, the importance of developing theory is not limited to researchers. Practitioners also benefit from having a verified, theoretical model of disaster recovery. The actions of local, state, and national officials and representatives from financial, insurance, and other private sector institutions can be enlightened and guided by theoretically grounded findings. In addition, a comprehensive theory of disaster recovery can provide a solid foundation for the development of a sustainable recovery implementation framework that is discussed later in the chapter.

The Scale of Theoretical Development

One of the difficulties in producing a comprehensive theory of sustainable recovery is that it must integrate current findings and theoretical concepts that bridge the micro (household, business, and neighborhood) to mid-range (community, region) to macro (society) levels. It has yet to be determined if this formidable task is achievable. The current work of Chang (2005) and

Alesch (2005) represents initial attempts at bridging the micro and mid-range levels. However, their efforts are not based on notions of sustainability.

Our task is more modest. The theoretical formulation suggested here focuses on the community level. The focus on the community is based on the traditional notion of communities as social institutions that solve problems inherent in geographically confined localities. It is that arrangement of social units and systems whose activities, be they consensual or conflictive, form the social, economic, political, built, and natural environmental contexts for daily existence. It is also that social arrangement, because of legal mandate and issues of shared governance, that most directly impacts the achievement of sustainable, community disaster recovery.

The Nature of the Theoretical Dependent Variable

In this proposed theory, we are not interested in traditional notions of disaster recovery that focus on reconstruction or restoration. Instead, we are interested in the concept of sustainable disaster recovery at the community level. Previously we defined sustainable disaster recovery as *the differential process of restoring, rebuilding, and reshaping the physical, social, economic, and natural environment through pre-event planning and post-event actions.* This orientation focuses on processes. It sees sustainable disaster recovery as a holistic, nonlinear series of actions taken by community-level social units and systems that result in alterations to the built, social, economic, and natural environments. Both pre-event and post-event actions are part of the process, including the role state and federal organizations, non-profits, emergent groups, corporations, and others play in local recovery.

Operationalizing such a concept presents some severe problems. The focus on process means that measures of activities and involvement of various social units and systems must be developed. In addition, since the definition assumes through "reshaping" that alterations in systems will occur, some measures for assessing these changes, for example, implementation of new structural and nonstructural mitigation measures, economic growth, heightened local capacity, and so forth must be developed. Further, since there is no clear end to the recovery process and the distinction between short-term and long-term recovery is arbitrary, the question of "when" to measure the progress toward sustainable recovery varies. Any movement toward the development of such a theory must address these gnarly measurement issues.

Some Suggested Contextual, Facilitating, and Inhibiting Variables

Based on the existing research literature, the following are suggested as key variables that may be included in the theoretical model (Table 14.2).[1] These variables are not exhaustive, but are offered as examples of the types of endogenous and exogenous conditions that should be included in any proposed theoretical model of sustainable community disaster recovery. Further, for practitioners to take action, the model should identify a clear set of conditions that facilitate or impede the implementation of this approach. The conditions identified here are intended to stimulate dialogue, including the formulation of additional research questions.

---

[1] The facilitators and impediments of sustainable recovery identified in Table 14.2 are representative of research conducted as part of the FEMA Higher Education Project college course, Holistic Disaster Recovery: Creating a Sustainable Future (Smith, 2004), and the text Inter-organizational Relationships and Policymaking: Key Factors Shaping Sustainable Disaster Recovery in the United States (Smith, forthcoming).

TABLE 14.2. Suggested Elements for a Theory of Sustainable Community Recovery

Pre-Disaster, Community-Level Contextual Variables

- Local capacity, including population size, social economic status, economic viability
- Previous disaster experience
- Leadership and advocacy
- Nature and extent of horizontal ties among locality based social units and systems
- Nature and extent of vertical ties of locally based social units and systems to external resources, institutions and centers of power
- Level of local governmental viability and effectiveness
- Level of local public participation in collective action
- Condition of critical infrastructure and housing
- Level of local disaster vulnerability (including social vulnerability)

Characteristics of the Disaster Agent

- Intensity of the impact
- Scope of the impact
- Speed of onset of the disaster
- Level and adequacy of warnings
- Duration of impact

Facilitators of Sustainable Disaster Recovery

- Leveraging resources
- Self-reliance and self-determination
- Commitment to disaster resilience
- State and federal capability and commitment to sustainable disaster recovery
- Capacity-building approaches
- Multi-party recovery committees
- Pre- and post-disaster recovery planning
- Use of dispute resolution techniques
- Identification of local needs
- Program flexibility

Impediments to Sustainable Disaster Recovery

- Viewing disaster recovery programs as an entitlement
- Over reliance on disaster programs that result in more vulnerable communities (moral hazard)
- Narrowly defined recovery programs
- Low capability and commitment
- Lack of federal, state and local recovery planning

Dependent Variable

- Sustainable community disaster recovery

The contextual variables refer to conditions inherent in the community prior to the disaster. They reference the general economic, social, political, organizational, and environmental character of the community. In general, with the exception of the level of local community vulnerability, we would expect these dimensions to be positively related to attaining sustainable disaster recovery. Local capacity, which references the general economic, political, and technical strength and viability of the community to resolve issues and handle problems, is an important component. Similarly, communities that have strong local or horizontal relationships between their constituent social units and systems should be able to achieve sustainable recovery more easily than those communities that lack such cohesion. Likewise, communities with strong vertical ties to state, regional, and national organizations and institutions have access to external resources that can assist in the recovery process (Berke, Kartez, & Wenger, 1993).

The second set of variables refers to the actual characteristics and magnitude of the disaster. Disasters that are more intense, impact a broader geographic area, have limited forewarning, have a rapid speed of onset that allows for little pre-impact protective activity, and impact the community over an extended period of time will likely produce greater damage and disruption of the local community and may work against the achievement of sustainable disaster recovery. In other cases, widespread damage, for example, may result in a greater willingness to take action to address past practices that are not sustainable.

The facilitators and impediments listed in Table 14.2 represent a preliminary set of variables to consider. Others may be uncovered through further case study analysis. The conditions cited are interrelated and may require the use of multivariate analysis and case study research to explain the strength of hypothesized relationships.[2] For example, the ability to leverage resources beyond those associated with FEMA programs to include other federal, state, or local sources, requires a certain degree of self-reliance. This is particularly true when recovering from localized events that may not result in the release of federal assistance. Lessons learned from developing countries, whose communities routinely implement localized recovery strategies with limited or nonexistent governmental assistance, should be studied further and applied in the United States, when possible.

Similarly, pre- and post-disaster recovery planning relies on the meaningful involvement of multiple stakeholder groups and the use of participatory tools, including dispute resolution techniques (e.g., policy dialogue, negotiation, and group facilitation). Relationships among impediments include the expectation that federal funding will be available post-disaster and a low level of capability and commitment to plan for recovery. Is achieving a sustainable recovery a realistic outcome for many communities given disparities in local capabilities, access to external resources and lack of commitment and leadership? Further, to what extent has "sustainability" become a pejorative term, associated with liberal policies and programs, thereby limiting its widespread adoption among governmental units? Can the emphasis on community-level capacity building be achieved as the United States continues to move toward more formalized policy regimes, including those that address hazard mitigation (Aguirre, 2002)?

Stated in the context of the proposed theory, to what extent can one facilitator affect an impediment to sustainable recovery and vice versa? For example, to what extent can pre- and post-disaster recovery planning be used to increase local capability and commitment, effectively bridging the gap between national objectives, self-reliance and the implementation of strategies addressing local needs? Can the formation of a multiparty recovery committee address the complex issues associated with balancing the use of federal assistance with a long-term vision to reduce the over-reliance on those programs that can increase hazard vulnerability in the long run? Can self-reliance overcome narrowly defined federal assistance programs that are not designed to facilitate a sustainable recovery? As additional facilitators and impediments are identified and the relationships between them are described, a growing body of knowledge will emerge in an area that remains one of the least understood in emergency management. As our understanding of recovery improves, it is incumbent on researchers to disseminate these findings to those who stand to benefit the most from the results.

---

[2] The quantitative modeling of disaster recovery processes and outcomes remains limited (see Chang & Miles, 2004; Miles & Chang, 2003, 2004).

SUSTAINABLE RECOVERY IMPLEMENTATION FRAMEWORK: CREATING A DISASTER RECOVERY ACT?

Based on an analysis of the existing literature and an anecdotal review of recovery planning practice, it is clear that the policy implementation framework must be changed to facilitate the widespread adoption of sustainable recovery principles. It is suggested that this may be achieved by the development of a training, research, and education agenda, focused on strengthening the nascent core of sustainable recovery advocates. The findings of applied research, including policy lessons learned from the implementation of the Disaster Mitigation Act of 2000 and the current state of recovery planning practice at the federal, state, and local levels, analyzed through the proposed theory of recovery, should provide meaningful insight into the means necessary to create a new policy framework (Table 14.3).

The intent of this chapter was to describe the concept of sustainable disaster recovery, propose a policy framework to achieve this end (based, in part, on the work of past hazards research), identify specific issues and concerns associated with this approach, and outline a theory of recovery that describes key factors that facilitate or hinder the ability of communities to achieve this aim. Key factors are intended to serve as the basis of a future research agenda. One of the most pressing issues among practitioners and policymakers involves the development of an improved intergovernmental framework focused on the means to assist communities achieve a sustainable recovery. Important subelements of this approach include developing a recovery ethic based on building state and local capacity and self-reliance through an educational, training, and research regimen focused on the role of recovery planning.

Training, Research, and Education

Training and applied research represents a critically important part of developing and sustaining an improved recovery framework. For a training, research, and education program to be effective, six factors should be present:

1. Training in recovery planning should occur before and after a disaster.
2. Training approaches must involve those who are likely to be involved in recovery and reconstruction, while reaching out to those who are often excluded from the process.

TABLE 14.3. Sustainable Recovery Implementation Framework

I. Training, Research, and Education	II. Policy Change	III. Creation of a Sustainable Recovery Ethic
Recovery planning: training and education Pre- and post-disaster; federal, state, and local	Advocacy coalition framework	Reducing moral hazard: hazard resilience

Conduct research
    Analysis of the Disaster Mitigation Act
    Nationwide assessment of recovery planning
	Disaster Recovery Act
	
	Other policy and program options
		Beyond liberal bias
		    Movement toward self-reliance

Disseminate findings		

3. Training methods should emphasize local empowerment, including the means to identify and address local needs.

4. Research focused on addressing unanswered recovery questions should be conducted before and immediately after disasters.

5. A greater emphasis should be placed on answering questions posed by practitioners.

6. The methods used to disseminate research findings should be improved to reflect the needs of the practitioner, incorporated into appropriate training materials, and used to educate those tasked with recovery.

Pre- and Post-Disaster Training for Recovery Planning

The current system of recovery training emphasizes how to implement FEMA grant programs. Courses tied to recovery planning are extremely limited.[3] To advance recovery planning, FEMA and appropriate state agencies and organizations should develop and conduct training courses across the country. A greater effort should be made to educate those who are drawn into the recovery process, including land-use planners, public works officials, city managers, building inspectors, business owners, and economic development interests as well as nonprofit officials and representatives of community organizations. State and federal emergency management agency personnel should be required to take recovery planning courses, emphasizing their role as a facilitator of local recovery. A stated intent of the program should be to develop a cadre of trainers that can be used on a regular basis to teach courses before and after a disaster.

Dissemination of Research Findings

Improving our ability to more effectively link research findings and the needs of the emergency management professional represents a major challenge (Cochrane, 1991; Fothergill, 2000; Gori, 1991; Quarantell, 1993; Yin & Moore, 1985;).[4] The current method used to conduct and disseminate information is inadequate. Effectively sharing research findings with practitioners requires developing the institutions capable of receiving unanswered questions posed by practitioners, disseminating research results in a readily accessible and user-friendly format, and

---

[3] The Emergency Management Institute offers three hazard-specific disaster recovery planning courses. The courses, which are tailored for individual communities are infrequently conducted. Two FEMA guidebooks, *Planning for a Sustainable Future: The Link Between Hazard Mitigation and Livability* (2000a) and *Rebuilding for a More Sustainable Future: An Operational Framework* (2000b), were created to provide a broad overview of sustainable recovery principles and more specific guidance to "sustainability planners" who were to be deployed in federal Disaster Recovery Centers following disasters. The positions, proposed as part of the Wingspread Principles, were never created. In 1998, *Planning for Post-Disaster Recovery and Reconstruction* (Schwab et al., 1998), a collaborative effort between the American Planning Association and FEMA, was written. The text represents perhaps the best existing document linking disaster recovery research and practice. The materials are not used by FEMA as part of a training curriculum, nor have they been systematically disseminated to practitioners.

[4] The definition of the emergency management professional is evolving. The creation of emergency management associations (i.e., the International Association of Emergency Managers and the National Emergency Management Association) and the development of accreditation standards have led to a nascent, but growing recognition among local and state officials of the emergency management profession. Smith (2002) argues that following disasters, the definition of an "emergency manager" becomes blurred. This is particularly evident in the case of disaster recovery, when public works officials, planners, financial analysts, and others are drawn into the complexities of recovery planning and policymaking, grants management, and reconstruction.

establishing an effective university reward/incentive system for conducting applied research. Numerous research questions linked to achieving sustainable recovery remain unanswered.[5] It is imperative that the gaps in the literature are studied and the findings shared with those who can put the lessons learned into practice. The measurement of fundamental assumptions in disaster recovery (e.g., mitigation works, pre-disaster planning improves recovery outcomes, and adaptive planning can result in a sustainable recovery) has been done on a surprisingly limited basis. A new research agenda requires the systematic analysis of these and other questions, focused on the development of applied research findings that are useful to the practitioner and policymaker, while advancing our knowledge of recovery.

Developing interagency agreements between practitioner-based organizations like the National Emergency Management Association, the International Association of Emergency Managers, and the National Association of Floodplain Managers and research centers such as the Natural Hazards Research and Applications Information Center, Disaster Research Center, or the Hazard Reduction and Recovery Center could provide a vehicle to collect unanswered research questions. Once distributed to individuals or teams, the researcher(s) would agree to develop reports highlighting results, emphasizing a succinct writeup of specific actions or policy recommendations. Research centers could publish quarterly newsletters comprised of research findings and distribute them to practitioner-based organizations. Another option involves the creation of a "hazards extension service" operated through existing land grant universities. Agricultural extension agents have a long history of transferring the latest knowledge and techniques to farmers and ranchers, for example. Information sharing has resulted in a major shift in behavior over time (i.e., the regular use of crop rotation to sustain soil fertility, the implementation of techniques limiting soil erosion, and the use of seed types suitable to local conditions). Perhaps this organizational framework can be used to share the latest research findings with state and local government officials, nonprofit agencies, or other stakeholders (including individual citizens) involved in disaster recovery and emergency management.

Policy Change: The Advocacy Coalition Framework

A number of policymaking models exist that provide insight into the current disaster recovery implementation framework including choice theory (Jones, 1994; Simon, 1977) agenda setting (Baumgartner & Jones, 1993; Braybrooke & Lindblom, 1970; Kingdon, 1984; Lindblom, 1959), economic game theory (Chong, 1991; Stoker, 1991), and policy and social learning (Friedman, 1981; Rose, 1993; Sabatier & Jenkins-Smith, 1993). Baumgartner and Jones (1993) as well as Chong (1991) provide substantial evidence that incremental change can be followed by brief periods in which major policy transformations can occur. These findings have been supported when analyzing emergency management policy change as Claire Rubin's (2001) Disaster Timeline suggests.

The Advocacy Coalition Framework describes the means by which policy change can be purposefully achieved through the identification of champions or "policy entrepreneurs" who sustain advances via policy learning (Birkland, 1997; Olson, Olson, & Gawronski, 1999). Sabatier and Jenkins-Smith (1993) argue that policy change is explained by "advocacy coalitions" that drive policy adoption and learning. Evaluated in the context of disaster recovery

---

[5] The book *Disasters by Design* notes several pressing disaster recovery research questions, most of which have not been addressed and remain worthy of study (pp. 310–311).

policy implementation, this requires building a diverse and powerful coalition of stakeholders, many of whom do not understand the benefits of a pursuing a sustainable recovery. Most local government officials do not recognize the opportunities lost during recovery and reconstruction, while state officials routinely face ongoing constraints associated with maintaining a cadre of recovery experts and federal agency officials manage narrowly defined programs whose rules serve to limit coordination across administrative units and hinder sustainability.

Those who currently support the concepts of a sustainable recovery include hazard scholars; multinational organizations; and a narrow band of federal, state, and local government officials who have employed these techniques on a limited basis. The views of hazards researchers are evident throughout this chapter. Multinational organizations such as the World Bank, Organization of American States, and United Nations have begun to address the connectivity between hazard mitigation and sustainable development in earnest, yet hazards are still not widely recognized in the larger sustainable development policymaking arena (Berke & Beatley, 1997). This being said, steps have been taken to draw attention to the problem, including the United Nations declaration of the 1990s as the International Decade for Natural Disaster Reduction.

During this time period, FEMA attempted to push forward the creation of grass-roots support for hazard mitigation and an improved level of preparedness at the local level through the creation of Project Impact, the limited development of sustainable recovery education materials, and the selective provision of post-disaster recovery planning assistance. These federal activities resulted in the establishment of strong advocates (particularly among local governments) as well as some who viewed the programs as overtly political, thereby limiting the breadth of support. The creation of Project Impact and the wingspread principles did not include a wide political spectrum in their formulation, nor were all members of the emergency management community, including stakeholder groups traditionally tasked with mitigation and recovery at the state and local levels, involved in the early phases of the process. In the case of Project Impact, this resulted in a degree of hostility among FEMA staff from other program areas who viewed the initiative as a drain on limited resources. Several state emergency management agencies expressed concerns that they were not involved in the program's formulation. Following a change of federal leadership, the Project Impact program was discontinued. A coalition of support remains, primarily among local governments who received seed money from FEMA. At the community level, research suggests that the program helped to foster an enhanced level of pre-disaster preparedness through the assessment of hazard vulnerabilities and the adoption of mitigation practices (Wachtendorf & Tierney, 2001). The wingspread principles never moved beyond the conceptualization stage.

In a limited number of cases, sustainable recovery and reconstruction principles have been put into practice at the community level. This has occurred predominantly in high hazard states such as California, North Carolina, and Florida, where regulations encourage or require it. This is, however, the exception rather than the rule. In the post-disaster environment, FEMA has selectively provided recovery planning assistance to communities based on political factors (i.e., media attention) and the extent of damages rather than institutionalizing the means necessary to provide widespread training and technical assistance in both the pre- and post-disaster environment. As mentioned previously, there is some evidence to suggest that this may be changing. States, such as North Carolina, have attempted sustainable recovery initiatives with moderate success, driven in large part by the infusion of federal and state assistance following major disasters. The degree to which this has had the unintended effect of limiting the long-term commitment needed to build local capability and self-reliance remains worthy of future study (Smith, forthcoming).

Initiating a coordinated change in current practice requires the reformulation of the existing recovery policy framework. To be effective, the lessons learned from past federal, state, and local initiatives should be considered. Following a groundswell of support for improving the nation's mitigation efforts, Congress passed the Disaster Mitigation Act of 2000, which codified mitigation planning through a collection of incentives and penalties for compliance and noncompliance, respectively. The Disaster Mitigation Act was created in large part because of identified shortcomings in the implementation of state and local hazard mitigation strategies. More specifically, members of Congress and the Office of Management and Budget questioned why millions of post-disaster Hazard Mitigation Grant Program funds remained unspent, often years after an event (Godschalk et al., 1999). The Disaster Mitigation Act of 2000 mandated the development of state and local hazard mitigation plans as a precondition for receiving federal pre- and post-disaster mitigation funding. This has resulted in the creation of thousands of hazard mitigation plans across the country. While the Act is still in its infancy, and the overall quality of the plans have yet to be evaluated (beyond the requirements established by FEMA), the Act represents an important step forward in the attempt to tie specific rewards (i.e. federal funding) to pre-disaster planning. The assessment of Disaster Mitigation Act-compliant state and local plans represents an important area of continued research, building on the work of Burby (1998), Burby and Dalton (1994), and Godschalk et al. (1999). The plans provide a rich, nationwide dataset that is directly comparable across communities and regions because of standardized planning elements and uniform requirements.

Should we consider the creation of a Disaster Recovery Act to aid states and local governments plan for a sustainable recovery? Emergency management planning mandates have been widely criticized, particularly those that emphasize a top-down approach (Berke & Beatley, 1997; Tierney, Lindell, & Perry, 2001). It has also been shown that federal emergency management policy initiatives must more fully recognize the interrelationships across our system of shared federal, state, and local governance in order to be effective (May, 1994; May & Williams, 1986). These findings do not mean that mandates cannot provide an important means to achieve local, state, and national policy objectives. For example, research demonstrates a nexus between local comprehensive planning mandates, reduced disaster losses, and the establishment of vehicles for local input in decision-making processes that affect a community's level of disaster resilience (Burby, 2005; Burby & Dalton, 1994). Similarly, Berke, Beatley, and Wilhite (1989) have identified specific factors that influence the local adoption of hazard mitigation planning techniques.

There is widespread evidence demonstrating that federal, state, and local governments are unprepared to address long-term disaster recovery. The challenge then becomes developing a *process* that balances the legitimate concerns of local empowerment and self-determination with the need to provide local communities with the tools they need to more effectively and comprehensively recover from disasters. A primary purpose of a recovery act, or other policy options for that matter, should include the reworking of the existing federal–state–local partnership and the redesign of the current set of uncoordinated programs and policies. This approach would require significant changes in the way pre- and post-disaster recovery planning occurs; state and local needs are identified; recovery assistance is provided; and federal, state, and local capability is maintained over time.

Any attempt to change the existing policy framework should involve an analysis of the Disaster Mitigation Act in order to apply relevant policy lessons. Since the Disaster Mitigation Act has been in existence since 2000, numerous questions posed throughout this chapter can be studied and used to craft a more robust recovery framework reflecting current conditions and realistic policy objectives and outcomes. Specific areas of research should include an analysis of the type and quality of federal and state assistance (i.e., education and training programs), the breadth of stakeholder involvement (i.e., land-use planners, environmental and social justice groups) in local mitigation planning, the degree to which the Act's policy objectives have been met (i.e., speeding the implementation of mitigation projects and an aggregate reduction in hazard losses), the degree to which the Act has resulted in the formulation of a state and local mitigation ethic, and the degree to which a diverse and powerful advocacy coalition capable of sustaining mitigation as a key practice within state and municipal government was achieved.

Few states and local governments have developed disaster recovery plans, owing in part to the fact that states and local governments have not been shown the tangible benefits of doing so, nor have specific incentives or penalties been established. To be effective in the long run, the reward system must be balanced with the need to build local capacity, thereby avoiding the rich get richer syndrome—namely the tendency of those communities (and individuals living within those jurisdictional boundaries) with a high degree of technical, administrative, and fiscal capability to gain access to federal assistance, while those with lesser capabilities fail to do so. This would have the unwanted effect of reducing assistance to low-income communities, which are often the most vulnerable to the effects of disasters (Cutter, 1996, 2001; Peacock, Morrow, & Gladwin, 1997).

Creating a Sustainable Recovery Ethic

The creation of a sustainable recovery ethic should represent a long-term aim of the Advocacy Coalition Framework, based on an extensive training, research, and education agenda leading to a shift in the current policy implementation framework. In a review of the book *Disasters by Design*, Aguirre (2002) argues that hazard scholars and planners are not capable, nor willing to advance this agenda as it relates to hazard mitigation. Further, forcibly changing social norms associated with how societies address natural hazards could result in a form of social engineering, potentially discrediting the profession. In reality, it is too early to tell the breadth and depth of influence that hazard scholarship, including *Disasters by Design*, has had in shaping the behavior of local governments, businesses, and individuals. A clear connection can be made already, however, on its impact on the thinking of FEMA and the ultimate creation of the Disaster Mitigation Act. While political pressure to expedite the expenditure of federal mitigation funding was a key factor associated with the formulation of the Act, the role of hazards scholars and practitioners should not be discounted. The scientific analysis of social problems often represents the genesis of policy change. It should also be noted that the influence of any advocacy coalition can increase or decrease over time, and an argument can certainly be made that the role of mitigation, and sustainable recovery for that matter, is becoming lost in the highly politicized homeland security milieu. This does, not, however, discount the importance of changing the manner in which we address disaster recovery.

Like in the case of mitigation, convincing policymakers and government leaders to adopt a sustainable recovery ethic will necessitate clearly demonstrating the benefits in a way that appeals to a broad range of interests. Historically, the concept of sustainability has been associated with a more liberal political philosophy, owing in large part to its roots in the environmental community. In reality, increasing self-reliance and reducing the outlay of federal assistance appeals to a broader network, including those espousing a more fiscally conservative viewpoint. The implementation of hazard mitigation measures represents a widely recognized component of a sustainable recovery and one that can produce quantifiable outcomes (i.e., future monetary losses avoided). Other, sometimes more intangible benefits, including an improved quality of life, social equity issues, a sound economy, the protection of environmental resources, and improved public health, have not been quantitatively assessed in the context of sustainable recovery. Qualitative "success stories," which are often written post-disaster and represent an important tool to share information with other practitioners, are not nearly as influential among federal policymakers as those reports that clearly document specific monetary benefits. The initial inability of FEMA to effectively demonstrate the quantitative benefits of hazard mitigation to skeptical members of Congress nearly led to the elimination of the Hazard Mitigation Grant Program. Were it not for the strong support of members of Congress whose districts benefited from the funds following past disasters, the program may have been discontinued.

SUMMARY, CONCLUSIONS, AND RECOMMENDATIONS

The intent of this chapter was to suggest that the principles of sustainability represent a valid means to improve the way we currently approach disaster recovery. A growing number of researchers and a select group of practitioners are increasingly demonstrating the merits of this model (Beatley, 1998; Burby, 1998; Mileti, 1999). Yet fundamental recovery questions remain unanswered. Given our limited understanding of key recovery concepts, it should not be surprising that the current approach used by the majority of practitioners does not facilitate sustainability—rather it systematically hinders it. Advancing the cause of sustainable recovery will require expanding the network of support to include local government planners, for example, who frequently implement sustainable development initiatives.

A review of past research found that while a number of dimensions of sustainable recovery had been investigated, they had not been integrated into a meaningful theoretical framework. Operationalizing a sustainable recovery agenda will require the development of a broad coalition of advocates who can articulate the benefits of altering the status quo. Hazard scholars can play a key role in this effort, similar to that achieved in advancing a hazard mitigation agenda that ultimately led to the passage of the Disaster Mitigation Act of 2000. A modified research agenda is needed—one that more closely links research and practice. A central aim should be to address the gaps in the existing research literature (as identified in this chapter), assess the policy lessons associated with the implementation of the Disaster Mitigation Act of 2000, and share these findings with practitioners. As studies are conducted and the findings disseminated to practitioners, a growing awareness of how the current recovery framework can be improved should emerge. A suggested agenda is tied to five actions:

1. *Conduct a nation-wide assessment of recovery planning.* The study should evaluate the factors listed in Table 14.2 as well as broader questions such as the extent and quality of recovery planning as practiced by local and state governments; an assessment of direct (quantifiable) benefits and missed opportunities across local, state, and federal planning efforts; and the degree to which pre- and post-disaster planning leads to sustainable outcomes. To a large extent, disaster recovery research has focused on natural hazards. More work needs to be done to assess how communities plan to recover from other hazards including technological accidents, terrorism, and medical disasters. To assist practitioners, specific recommendations for action should be provided, based on the results of the assessment.

2. *Assess the policy lessons learned from the implementation of the Disaster Mitigation Act of 2000.* The proposed recommendations for action must reflect the political realities of

the current emergency management policy implementation framework. An analysis of the Disaster Mitigation Act merits attention for several reasons. One, the Disaster Mitigation Act includes requirements (i.e., linking state and local planning to rewards and penalties) that may be applicable to disaster recovery planning. Two, the timing of the assessment should allow researchers to determine the degree to which planning requirements led to identifiable outcomes (i.e., an expedited expenditure of post-disaster mitigation funding and a reduction in hazard vulnerability). Three, understanding the historical and political underpinnings of the Act can provide lessons for those seeking to improve the current disaster recovery implementation framework.

3. *Use the information obtained through research to build an advocacy coalition supporting the passage of the Disaster Recovery Act.* The Advocacy Coalition Framework literature suggests that meaningful policy change can occur over time (generally a decade or more) given the development of advocates (including researchers and policy analysts) who maintain a set of core beliefs and seek to modify the political system to meet their aims (Sabatier & Jenkins-Smith, 1993). Viewed in the context of developing a new sustainable recovery implementation framework, policy advocates must be prepared to act following the results of the proposed research agenda (Quarantelli, 1993b). Attempts to push for meaningful policy change may also be considered following major disasters given their heightened political salience. A review of the emergency management literature clearly demonstrates that significant policy change has occurred in the United States following a number of major disasters (Barry, 1997; Rubin & Renda–Tanali, 2001). Hurricane Katrina, perhaps the worst disaster to strike the United States, is representative of the type of event that can trigger significant policy change. The extent to which the hurricane affects changes in federal, state, and local response and recovery policy and practice merits extensive study.

Any attempt to foster change must take into account prevailing political and organizational conditions. For example, the creation of the Department of Homeland Security, the organizational changes within FEMA, and the national emphasis on combating terrorism all play a part in how a coalition should be created and the means used to push a given policy agenda. Can FEMA function effectively within a department whose primary aim is to combat terrorism? What impact will organizational changes within FEMA have on the delivery of key functions such as hazard mitigation? Has the emphasis on terrorism resulted in a shift away from an all-hazards approach to emergency management? For researchers to play a greater role in the current policy dialogue, a greater understanding of how these changes impact the delivery of pre- and post-disaster recovery assistance (across both natural and human-caused hazards) is required.

4. *Evaluate the merit of other policy options.* The passage of a Disaster Recovery Act represents one of several potential methods to improve the current system that is best characterized as a disjointed array of recovery programs without a clear set of guiding principles. Regardless of the policy option(s) chosen, a central theme should include attempts to foster a greater measure of local self-reliance, moving away from the existing model which has created an over-dependence on federal aid. Other approaches emphasizing bottom-up techniques should be considered as the international disaster recovery and sustainable development literature suggests (Berke & Beatley, 1997; Harrel-Bond, 1986; Oliver-Smith, 1990; Uphoff, 1986). Options may include the creation of local sustainable recovery incubators in selected communities; the establishment and implementation of sustainable recovery training programs; the modification of current funding streams to complement sustainable recovery efforts and the placement of experts in Disaster Field

Offices as suggested in the wingspread principles; the integration of recovery practices into existing federal, state, and local programs that currently embrace sustainable development initiatives (e.g., coastal management, community development, environmental planning, etc.); or the creation of collaborative planning networks (Mileti, 1999; Nakagawa & Shaw, 2004) comprised of professionals (e.g., planners, engineers, etc.), nonprofits, community and environmental groups, and businesses that have successfully implemented sustainable recovery programs and are willing to share their experiences with others. The approaches mentioned here should be further studied and the results applied in the field in order to assess their effectiveness.

5. *Create a nationwide sustainable recovery ethic.* Sabatier and Jenkins-Smith note that the ability to successfully implement major policy change through the use of the Advocacy Coalition Framework can take upwards of a decade. It is suggested here that the eventual widespread adoption of a sustainable recovery ethic will require a robust training, research and education agenda and the development of a cadre of advocates capable of maintaining this effort over time. One possible objective of this coalition may include the passage of the Disaster Recovery Act. An important aim of any approach should include facilitating the incorporation of sustainable recovery principles into state and local policy; planning; and the day-to day activities of local governments, organizations, businesses, and citizens. It will be incumbent on the Advocacy Coalition to continually improve the recovery process through training and education programs based on policy lessons learned through practice and applied research.

CHAPTER 15

Sheltering and Housing Recovery Following Disaster*

WALTER GILLIS PEACOCK, NICOLE DASH,
AND YANG ZHANG

Reestablishing housing is a critical factor for understanding recovery processes, whether one is addressing the phenomenon at the household or community level. Researchers examining household or family recovery, for example, have utilized a variety of measures or indicators to capture different dimensions of recovery including psychological or perceptual measures related to stress, and sense of loss and recovery to more objective indicators such as regaining income, employment, household amenities, and household assets (Bates, 1982; Bolin, 1976, 1982, 1993, 1994; Bolin & Bolton, 1983; Bolin & Trainer, 1978; Peacock, Killian, & Bates, 1987). However, this research also suggests that fundamental to an overall assessment of household recovery is reestablishing permanent housing, or in the vernacular, home, because without establishing home, the ability of a household to carry out normal activities and reestablish a routine is limited and hampered (Bates & Peacock, 1987, 1993; Bolin & Trainer, 1978; Quarantelli, 1982). In short, delays in reestablishing housing all too often delay all other dimensions of recovery (Bolin, 1986).

Communities, as complex networks of social systems, often require more of a multidimensional perspective when considering recovery (Bates & Pelanda, 1994; Dynes, 1970; Lindell & Prater, 2003; Lindell, Prater, & Perry, forthcoming; Wenger, 1978). An important complex element of community recovery is associated with infrastructure and lifelines that are fundamental for the operations of other systems dependent upon transportation, electricity, water, and waste disposal to carry out their normal activities. Getting business up and moving again is also critically important for resuscitating economic activities within communities that provide economic resources in the form of wages and salaries as well as goods and services. Communities without businesses providing economic opportunities, jobs, goods, and services will in short order lose their populations. Yet, if the population lacks housing would they stay or

*This work was supported by grants funded by the National Science Foundation (CMS-0100155) and Mid-America Earthquake Center through funding received from the National Science Foundation under Grant No. EEC-9701785. Any opinions, findings, and conclusions or recommendations expressed in this material are those of the authors and do not necessarily reflect the views of the National Science Foundation or the Mid-American Earthquake Center.

return in the first place? Without housing, the individuals necessary to populate the economy, fill the jobs, and restart and reopen businesses as well as consume the services and purchase the goods will be absent. Indeed, the ability to house, not just professionals, business owners, CEOs, and managers, but also line workers, service workers, and staff personel is critical. In other words, housing recovery is critical and all types and forms of housing recovery including affordable housing are important. There is of course a chicken and egg element to this—which should come first, business recovery or housing recovery?

In 1975, Mileti, Drabek, and Haas noted that there was little in the way of research focusing on what was termed the post-event reconstruction phase of disaster. Two years later Haas, Kates, and Bowden (1977) published *Reconstruction Following Disaster*, beginning the process of redressing this shortfall by focusing directly on reconstruction issues, drawing on four case studies, two historical (the San Francisco and Anchorage Alaska earthquakes) and two more recent for that period (Managua earthquake and Rapid City flood). In tackling the problem of reconstruction, Kates (1977, p. 262) declared that "the reconstruction process is ordered, knowable and predictable," suggesting that cities basically recover in four phases termed *emergency response, restoration* of the restorable, *reconstruction (I)* of the destroyed for functional replacement, and *reconstruction (II)* for commemoration, betterment and development with each period lasting approximately 10 times the previous period (Kates & Pijawka, 1977). Housing recovery issues relating to emergency sheltering, repairing, and restoring of homes only partially damaged, and ultimately rebuilding of severely damaged and destroyed structures were hypothesized to occur primarily during the first three periods, with the entire reconstruction lasting 100 times the emergency period (Kates & Pijawka, 1977, p. 20). While a number of graduate students in this work became key players and contributors to the growing literature throughout the next 30 years, the formulation of an ordered process of successive stages has not.

Quarantelli (1982), noting that housing victims in the aftermath of major disasters involves complex social processes made even more difficult to study in light of the conceptual confusion in the literature, offered a typology of distinctive forms of sheltering and housing. Drawing from three case studies in the Disaster Research Center archive, he suggested that there were four more or less distinct forms of sheltering and housing that are of particular relevance: emergency sheltering, temporary sheltering, temporary housing, and permanent housing. Emergency sheltering "refers to actual or potential disaster victims seeking quarters outside their own permanent homes for short periods: hours in many cases, overnight at most" (Quarantelli, 1982, p. 2). Temporary shelter "refers to peoples' displacement into other quarters, with an expected short or temporary stay" (Quarantelli, 1982, p. 2). The critical element for establishing temporary housing is not simply occupying some form of housing with an at least initial expectation that it will be temporary, but also reestablishing normal household routines, responsibilities, and activities to the extent possible. Finally, permanent housing "involves disaster victims returning either to their rebuilt homes or moving into new quarters . . . occupying permanent, residential facilities" (Quarantelli, 1982, p. 3). This typology is not without its problems, particularly if viewed as phases in which households are expected to progress. The latter does of course happen, but even Quarantelli (1982, 1995) noted that there can be many repetitive steps and jumps in the process. Further, the distinctions are not always clear as when, again noted by Quarantelli (1982, 1995), temporary housing becomes permanent or when emergency shelters transition into temporary shelters out of necessity. In addition, in any disaster, members of a community's population of households may be found in every form of shelter or housing simultaneously. Despite these problems, the typology has often been employed in subsequent research.

While Quarantelli's typology might have proven to be useful, the paucity of research noted in 1975 by Mileti et al., has remained. In 1986, for example, Drabek noted that long-term household recovery issues, of which housing recovery is so central, is one of the least studied and understood by disaster researchers. Further, as late as 2001, Tierney, Lindell, and Perry noted that much of what is known about post-disaster sheltering and housing was undertaken in the last 15 years and that the entire "process remains significantly understudied, and little research has looked at post disaster housing patterns across social classes, racial/ethnic groups, and family types" (Tierney, Lindell, & Perry, 2001, p. 100). This chapter pulls together the strands of research that has been undertaken focusing on shelter and housing following disaster, with particular attention to permanent housing recovery and to research focusing on these issues in the United States. Indeed, not only has there been little overall research focusing on housing and sheltering, but with the exception of a few studies there also has been little integration of international and U.S.-based research. We will structure our discussions of the literature utilizing Quarantelli's shelter and housing typology. While our focus is on the process of reestablishing permanent housing, the discussion must, at times, focus on how households negotiate the different steps along the way. This is followed by a discussion of issues related to linking this typology together to better understand the processes of housing recovery following disaster and with comments regarding linking international and U.S.-based research. The final section addresses the future of research on these topics, where it might lead, and some potential issues that should be addressed.

SHELTERING AND TEMPORARY HOUSING

Understanding the phenomena of emergency sheltering as Quarantelli (1982, 1995) defines it focuses on the immediate response disaster victims take to shelter themselves for short periods of time either before a hazard (in the case of a tornado or hurricane) or immediately after impact (such as after an earthquake). The period of time ranges from a few hours to overnight depending on specific hazard conditions. Emergency sheltering is often spontaneous and focused on locational convenience and immediacy of need (Alexander, 2002b; Bolin, 1993; Bolin & Stanford, 1998b; Tierney et al., 2001). Pre-impact emergency sheltering is particularly common during wind events, especially hurricanes, where a period of warning accompanies the hazard threat. Research has found that those who perceive their risk are more likely to take emergency shelter even if taking protective measures is accompanied by inconvenience (Dash & Morrow, 2001). However, it is important to realize that it is not limited to pre-impact needs. Emergency sheltering also includes locations of refuge after all types of disasters particularly as a result of damage, fear of further damage, and utility outage (Bolin, 1993; Morrow, 1997; Phillips, 1993). After earthquakes, for example, emergency shelter may include individuals sleeping in their yards, parks, or cars for fear of additional aftershocks or undetected damage (Bolin, 1993; Bolin & Stanford, 1991, 1998b; Phillips, 1993).

In fact, where pre-impact sheltering fits into Quarantelli's topology is not very clear. While Quarantelli (1982, 1995) argues that emergency sheltering usually happens spontaneously by victims themselves for their immediate safety, some confusion exists as to what types of sheltering belong in this category. If we assume, as Quarantelli does, that emergency sheltering is spontaneous individual or household protective measures, then it is consistent that planning would be challenging and rarely involve organizational activities. On the other hand, emergency sheltering also includes planned activities particularly related to wind events. The State of Florida and Texas, for example, focuses a significant part of their evacuation planning to the provision of emergency sheltering for those who flee their homes before a tropical system makes landfall. While such evacuation sites may also be used for longer term sheltering (Bolin, 1994), until a hurricane makes landfall with known damage, such sheltering is clearly planned emergency sheltering. Planned tornado shelters, such as designated areas in airports, government building, or schools, are also examples of emergency sheltering.

Using the airport as an example, those who take protective action by following signs designating shelter location are taking emergency shelter, even though it is at least partially organized and planned. When the threat passes, the need for the shelter is gone, and people resume their normal activities. The process is dynamic. As conditions pre- and post-disaster change, emergency sheltering also changes rapidly (Tierney, Lindell, & Perry, 2001). Indeed, individuals may return to their undamaged permanent homes shortly after the threat has passed. On the other hand, emergency sheltering may transition to temporary sheltering when the hazard event creates temporarily uninhabitable housing (Bolin, 1994).

Temporary shelters are places victims can stay for a longer period of time before it is safe to return to permanent residences. Unlike emergency sheltering, daily necessities such as food, water, sleeping arrangement, and other needed services (i.e., security) must be provided in temporary shelters, and thus requires more significant preparedness by nonprofit and governmental agencies. However, temporary sheltering is never intended to replace primary housing. Quarantelli (1982, 1995) argues that households in temporary shelters make little attempt to reestablish their normal household routines.

While considerable attention by emergency responders is given to public sheltering such as the use of the Superdome in Hurricane Katrina or public schools during other types of events, the majority of those seeking temporary shelter use public sheltering as a refuge of last resort (Drabek, 1986; Perry, Lindell, & Greene, 1981; Quarantelli, 1982). Research has found that less than a quarter of those seeking sheltering use large-scale public facilities (Bolin & Stanford, 1990; Lindell et al., 1985), and those who do, are more likely to have lower socioeconomic status, live in rental housing, own homes in disrepair (prior to the hazard), and have few familial resources (Drabek & Boggs, 1968; Morrow, 1997; Tierney, Lindell, & Perry, 2001). One complication with temporary sheltering is that often disaster victims compete with disaster responders and even the homeless for housing (FEMA, 1994; Phillips, 1993; Yelvington, 1997), or as Hurricane Andrew emphasizes, extended family members in the area may also experience damage (Morrow, 1997). Those with more resources, both socially and financially, are more likely to shelter with friends and family or in hotels/motels (Whitehead et al., 2000). For those whose homes are damaged or whose utilities are out for an extended period of time, the same location of emergency sheltering may become temporary sheltering. The physical location does not change; rather, its purpose shifts to focus on longer term, but not permanent, needs.

The pre- and immediate post-impact of Hurricane Katrina in the New Orleans area in 2005 illustrates the tenuous differences between emergency sheltering and temporary sheltering. For many, particularly the poor, emergency sheltering can extend in time to temporary sheltering (Bolin, 1994). As Hurricane Katrina approached New Orleans, many residents took refuge in locations outside of the city, but a significant number, including those with special needs, took emergency shelter at the Superdome. These early evacuees sought emergency shelter—safe space to ride out the storm. If the levees protecting New Orleans and surrounding areas remained intact, the majority of individuals would have simply returned home when the winds were over.

However, no one can forget the images from the city where hundreds of people remained in their homes during the storm for a variety of reasons, including lack of transportation to safer locations, responsibility for ill or disabled family members, or because they themselves were infirmed or disabled. While their homes survived with little damage from the wind, the subsequent flooding from breaches in protective levees surrounding the city required households to find safer sheltering. Using a variety of mechanisms such as walking through flood waters, traveling by boat, or rescue by helicopters, thousands of individuals found themselves sheltered at the Superdome with little to no supplies and deteriorating conditions. Whereas the first wave of evacuees used the Superdome as emergency shelter, those fleeing their flooded homes used it as temporary shelter, finding themselves waiting for further rescues to safer locations. Consistent with the literature, it appears that the majority of those in the Superdome were those who were more socially marginal in that they had little to no resources to leave the city on their own. What began as a protective measure from the approaching storm (emergency shelter) became the refuge for those fleeing the effects of the storm to stay for a longer time before they were taken and dispersed, often without knowledge of their destination, to safer locations (temporary shelter).

As with emergency sheltering, temporary sheltering is a social process that is not static; the needs of those seeking shelter vary across individuals and through time. Temporary sheltering is expected to be short term; however, no one has defined exactly what short term entails. While emergency preparedness focuses the most attention on this phase of post-disaster recovery (Tierney, Lindell, & Perry, 2001), little research has focused on issues such as population dislocation, temporary shelter demand, location, and duration following a large-scale natural disaster. Research after Hurricane Andrew focused on understanding how social position affected temporary sheltering location. As expected, those with higher incomes were more likely to stay at hotels and motels, while those with lower incomes stayed with family (Morrow, 1997). More significant is that logistic regression results indicated that "among low-income households who had relatives move in with them, the chance of them still being there four months later was nearly three times higher" than for higher income groups (Morrow, 1997, p. 152).

One of the few in-depth studies of temporary sheltering focused on the implementation of tent cities by the U.S. military after Hurricane Andrew. While many of the 180,000 individuals who found themselves homeless after the storm had resources to relocate to homes of family or friends, many found themselves with few options. Lack of financial resources, transportation, and friends and relatives outside of the damaged area limited their options. More than 3500 individuals were sheltered at four tent cities in south Florida during the two months they were open. However, it is important to note that the tent cities did not immediately fill (Yelvington, 1997). Instead, as homes were condemned, renters evicted, and rains made uninhabitable the barely habitable damaged homes, the number of individuals increased during the first few weeks after the storm. In addition, population at the tent cities increased as deportation fears of undocumented immigrants diminished and relief information was released in both Spanish and Creole (Yelvington, 1997). For the most part, individuals did not choose tent cities as their first choice of sheltering, but rather ended up there when other options were not available.

Although the conditions were not normal for any of those who lived in these makeshift cities, the U.S. military who oversaw the day-to-day functioning of these new communities tried to integrate fun activities such as a 5-day tour by a Disney troupe to reduce the everyday stress people were experiencing (FEMA, 1994). The goal, however, always remained to close the tent cities as soon as possible by shifting temporary shelters to temporary housing. This shift began about 6 weeks after Hurricane Andrew as the first tent city closed and gave way to the Federal Emergency Management Agency (FEMA) sponsored travel trailer parks (FEMA, 1994).

These tent cities, however, were not planned for in advance. The use of the military to house disaster victims was an adaptive response to the overwhelming need in south Florida after Hurricane Andrew. Similar adaptive responses occurred after Hurricane Katrina since little or no planning seems to have focused on having significant populations in need of temporary sheltering. While the response after Hurricane Andrew was relatively successful, the response to Hurricane Katrina failed to meet the needs of those who were displaced. Families were separated as individuals were transported to locations throughout the United States with little or no tracking in place to reunite households. With sections of the City of New Orleans significantly damaged, particularly socially vulnerable areas, significant number of individuals and households require longer term solutions in order to reestablish routine. What is clear is that while time plays a role in the transition from sheltering to housing, the amount of time varies, with those with more resources often able to transition from sheltering to housing more quickly.

The key distinction between sheltering and housing is the resumption of household activities and responsibility (Quarantelli, 1982, 1995b). With temporary housing, routine day-to-day household activities are reestablished, and those in temporary housing wait for permanent housing, either return to their pre-disaster homes or some type of alternative housing solution (Tierney, Lindell, & Perry, 2001). For those with the most extensive damage, temporary may be anywhere from weeks to months to years. According to a review of research done by Tierney, Lindell, and Perry (2001, p. 102) for the second assessment of natural hazards research, little is known about how households negotiate this stage of their journey to permanent housing. A significant feature, however, is that in the United States, temporary housing arrangements after disaster are usually funded by the FEMA or the Department of Housing and Urban Development (HUD) through cash grants for temporary rental housing or the provision of mobile homes (Bolin, 1993, 1994; Bolin & Stanford, 1991, 1998a, 1998b; Comerio, 1998; Quarantelli, 1982).

Temporary housing can transition to permanent housing when displaced households cannot return to or refuse to return to their pre-disaster home (Bolin, 1994; Bolin & Stanford, 1991; Haas, Kates, & Bowden 1977). Often difficulties arise when trying to transition some households to more permanent housing options. FEMA mobile homes after Hurricane Andrew, for example, were expected to house displaced households for 6 months; however, the last family moved from their mobile homes 2.5 years after Hurricane Andrew (Morrow, 1997). While the provision of travel trailers and mobile homes, both after Hurricane Andrew and other storms such as Hurricane Charley in 2004, offered temporary housing for those in need, the conditions can be difficult, with parks often riddled with crime and violence (Enarson & Morrow, 1997; Wilkinson, 2005). The problems after Hurricane Andrew were not unique, as research in other disaster settings found mobile homes to be a problematic form of temporary housing (Bolin, 1982, 1994). Important to note is that some families who were hard to place in permanent housing because of family size or socioeconomic status were given their FEMA trailers and relocated to a different mobile home park that became their permanent housing (Morrow, 1997). For some households, these structures may represent a significant improvement in housing, but in other conditions such structures can inhibit housing recovery (Bolin, 1993; Peacock et al., 1987). In addition, these mobile homes become vulnerable housing in wind hazard situations. Less than one year after Hurricane Andrew, a major northeaster killed a Hurricane Andrew survivor who was living in a FEMA mobile home.

The problems and issues regarding temporary housing are not isolated to the United States. Research conducted in Italy, for example, after the Friuli earthquake found that the nature of temporary housing can significantly disrupt the nature of communities, social networks, and livelihoods, and had negative consequences for the psychological health of inhabitants (Giepel, 1982; Hogg, 1980). Bates (1982) and colleagues found that in Guatemala temporary housing can have potentially debilitating impacts for long-term housing recovery (see also Bates & Peacock, 1987; Peacock et al., 1987). Specifically, they found that many households simply transitioned temporary housing into permanent housing, because they lacked sufficient resources to procure or reconstruct permanent housing. The failure to recognize that the severe limitations many households face when addressing housing issues in normal situations can result in a failure to transition out of temporary housing into permanent housing is a message relevant in nearly all post-disaster situations globally.

PERMANENT HOUSING

In the United States, permanent housing recovery is primarily a market driven process (Bolin, 1985, 1993; Comerio, 1998; Peacock & Ragsdale, 1997). With the exception of the 1964 Alaskan Earthquake where the federal government was actively involved in the management and reconstruction of residential housing (Kates, 1970; NAS, 1987; Quarantelli & Dynes, 1989), the federal government does not take an active role in housing recovery processes. The basic tenets of federal and state policy is to fill the gaps or, as Comerio (1998, p. 197) notes, provide a "safety net" by supplementing individual resources such as private insurance and nonprofit charity. This laissez faire approach at the federal and state level was noted by Quarantelli (1982, p. 77), who also suggested that the "matter is almost totally ignored at local community level disaster planning," a theme also echoed by others (Bolin, 1985, 1993, 1994; Peacock & Girard, 1997). Allowing the market to "manage" housing recovery in the United States has led a number of researchers to characterize the results as essentially conservative in nature with restoration of the status quo ante as the goal (Bates & Peacock, 1989b; Bolin, 1982, 1985). Haas et al. (1977) takes this a step further by suggesting that the "market is a suitable mechanism in disaster recovery if one wishes to maintain or increase pre-disaster social inequities" (quoted in Bolin, 1985, p. 712). While it is a generally held assumption that pre-disaster social patterns will shape permanent housing recovery (Bates, 1982; Bates & Peacock, 1987; Blaikie et al., 1994; Oliver-Smith, 1990; Quarantelli, 1982), some have also suggested that this is particularly likely where market based recovery scenarios as suggested by Haas, may in fact accentuate pre-disaster inequities (Bolin, 1982, 1985; Bolin & Stanford, 1991, 1998b; Peacock & Ragsdale, 1997). In light of this, it will be worthwhile briefly discussing the nature of housing markets and housing related issues in the United States.

As Foley (1980, p. 460) suggests, housing in the United States operates as a trickle-down process: "New housing is provided for those who can afford it, and successively older housing is passed along to other households that seek to make incremental improvements in their situation." On the whole, housing markets systematically fail when it comes to providing quality housing to low-income households and this failure disproportionately impacts racial and ethnic minorities (Alba & Logan, 1992; Bratt, Hartman, & Meyerson, 1986; Horton, 1992; Lake, 1980). Low-income households and racial and ethnic minorities tend to reside in poorer quality housing and that housing is often segregated into low-valued neighborhoods (Logan & Molotch, 1987; South & Crowder, 1997; Stinchcomb, 1965). Minorities, particularly blacks, still find major problems with racial discrimination when buying, selling, and renting housing in the forms of racial steering, redlining, hostile white attitudes, and lender discrimination (Feagin & Sikes, 1994; Guy, Pol, & Ryker, 1982; Horton, 1992; Oliver & Shapiro, 1995; Sagalyn, 1983). Minority households that are able to achieve sufficiently high incomes often find purchasing a home will still demand overcoming additional obstacles. For example, black households are more likely to be denied a mortgage, must make larger down payments, and when accepted, they often pay higher interest rates; after purchase, their homes are likely to appreciate at lower rates (Flippen, 2004; Oliver & Shapiro, 1995). One of the hidden factors in successfully obtaining a mortgage is finding insurance. Minorities often have problems obtaining homeowners insurance in general and quality insurance in particular, which can make procuring a home mortgage impossible (Squires, 1998; Squires, O'Connor, & Silver, 2001; Squires & Velez, 1987). Finally, we still find high levels of racial segregation, and black households in particular are substantially less likely than whites to escape poor neighborhoods and, when they do, they are more likely to relocate to poor areas again (Charles, 2003; Iceland, Weinberg, & Steinmetz, 2002; Massey & Denton, 1993; South & Crowder, 1997).

Low-income and minority households face many challenges dealing with housing recovery as we discuss later, but the simple trickle down nature of housing in the United States often predisposes these vulnerable populations to higher levels of damage in the first place. Research has found that such households often live in the structures that were built according to older, less stringent building codes; used lower quality designs and construction materials; and were less well maintained (Bolin, 1994; Bolin & Bolton, 1983; Bolin & Stanford, 1998b; Peacock & Girard, 1997). As a result, one of the most consistent findings in the disaster literature, whether discussing findings in the United States or abroad, is that low-income and minority households tend to suffer disproportionately higher levels of damage in disasters (Bates, 1982; Bates & Peacock, 1987; Bates, Fogleman, Parenton, Pittman & Tracy, 1962; Blaikie et al., 1994; Bolin, 1982, 1986, 1993; Bolin & Bolton, 1986; Dash, Peacock, & Morrow, 1997; Drabek & Key, 1984; Haas et al., 1977; Peacock & Girard, 1997; Quarantelli, 1982). In light of the differential damage impacts, it can be anticipated that permanent housing recovery, unless supplemented with higher levels of recovery resources for housing occupied by low-income and minority households, is likely to also be an uneven process.

With the preceding discussion in mind, attention is turned directly to permanent housing recovery. On the whole, there is almost no literature that focuses on permanent housing recovery itself; instead the focus is generally on homeowners and hence partially on owner-occupied housing. In addition, most research on homeowners generally addresses single-family housing, ignoring potential unique issues associated with other forms of housing such as condominiums. Permanent rental housing recovery is even less well researched and is generally limited to households occupying rental-housing units of unknown form. Researchers have also noted that pre-impact homeless populations are also ignored (Phillips, 1996; Wisner, 1998) and yet can represent sizable numbers in large urban centers, often becoming policy and moral issues when officially determining who "deserves" post-disaster shelter, housing, and other forms of aid. Our discussion begins with the primary resources drawn upon to finance housing recovery.

Permanent housing recovery is dependent on financial resources for repairing or rebuilding housing. One might also consider labor and expertise as critical for rebuilding, particularly in areas where household and family members are actively involved in the actual repair and rebuilding process. Clearly, this can be important in the developing world, but can also play an important role among some in the United States, as was found among low- to moderate-income households in Miami where many family members worked in construction and were able to donate their skill, expertise, and labor in the reconstruction process. However, more often than not, labor and expertise are purchased, hence the importance of financial resources. These resources primarily come from two broad sources: private and public funding (Bolin & Stanford, 1991; Comerio, 1998; Comerio, Landis, & Rofe, 1994; Quarantelli, 1982; Wu & Lindell, 2004). Private funding includes insurance, household savings, commercial loans, and, in some cases, funds from family and friends. Public funding also includes a variety of sources such as low-interest loans from the Small Business Administration (SBA), grants from FEMA such as minimal home repair (MHR) or individual or family grants (IFG, often administered by the state), and additional funding from the Department of Housing and Urban Development (HUD) in the form of Community Development Block Grants (CDBGs) and HOME program funding. While individual homeowners cannot use the latter, they can be employed by community agencies to facilitate rebuilding, particularly for low- and moderate-income housing. In addition, some states might also have programs to facilitate rebuilding (Bolin & Stanford, 1998a, 1998b; Comerio, 1998). There are also a host of public programs such as FEMA's temporary rental housing program, SBA's rental housing loans, and HUD's Section 8 Voucher program which provide temporary housing through rent subsidies/payments or mobile homes or travel trailers that can be employed by renters and homeowners. While not directly focused on rebuilding, these programs can facilitate the rebuilding process. For example, some households obtain travel trailers that they move onto their property while their homes are being rebuilt.

In keeping with the market-based logic of housing recovery in the United States, private insurance is the primary source of most private funding for repairing and rebuilding homes (Comerio, 1998; Kunreuther & Roth, 1998; Wu & Lindell, 2004). There can, however, be considerable variations in the relative importance of private insurance for housing recovery across natural hazards and states. For example, according to Kunreuther (1998, p. 39), earthquake coverage can be included in a general homeowner's policy for an additional premium in most states, except in California where residential earthquake policies are purchased through the California Earthquake Authority, a state agency. Flood insurance, on the other hand, is never covered as part of a normal residential policy and must be purchased separately. The National Flood Insurance Program (NFIP) established by Congress in 1968 underwrites flood insurance, which is administered jointly by private insurance industry and the federal government. Wind hazards associated with hurricanes, tornadoes, and other storms are generally covered by basic wind coverage as part of a normal residential policy (Kunreuther, 1998, p. 40). However, this is not always the case. For example, in some coastal areas in Florida insurers have been allowed to split wind coverage from basic residential policies, requiring it to be purchased separately. The literature has consistently found that earthquake and flooding insurance policies are much less likely to be purchased than normal residential policies (Palm, 1995; Palm, Hodgson, Blanchard, & Lyons, 1990; Pastrick, 1998; Roth, 1998). As a consequence, the federal role in funding housing recovery from earthquakes and flooding tends to be much larger.

This mosaic of coverage patterns means that the actual contribution of private insurance to the housing recovery efforts can vary considerably dependent upon the nature of the hazard. Comparing the relative contributions of private versus public funding following the Northridge earthquake and Hurricane Andrew easily conveys this variation. Wu and Lindell (2004, p. 69), employing data from a variety of sources, determined that 65.3% of housing reconstruction funds came from private insurers, followed by the SBA at 20.7%, with FEMA and HUD grants contributing 7% each following Northridge. Utilizing data presented by Comerio (1998, p. 90) on residential housing claims paid by private insurers and public funding of housing assistance, repair, and reconstruction following Hurricane Andrew, we calculated that private insurance funded 89.9% of residential reconstruction, followed by SBA loans at 3.3%, FEMA minimum assistance grants at 2.8%, HUD at 3.1%, and other sources such as the National Flood Insurance Program at 1%. If focus is narrowed to aid directly related to repair and reconstruction, removing, for example, FEMA IFG, SBA temporary rental loans and HUD Section 8 vouchers, the percentage of residential recovery funded by private insurance increases to nearly 95%. Clearly, there can be major variations across hazard and potentially disaster events; nevertheless, private insurance funds a majority of residential housing recovery efforts.

To better establish the roles various private and public funding play in permanent housing recovery, we must draw from the literature on household/family recovery. It is difficult to compare research findings related to household "recovery" because recovery is measured in many different ways including psychological perceptions of recovery, satisfaction with recovery levels, income recovery, house size recovery, domestic assets restoration and recovery, and household amenities recovery to name a few. At times, recovery is met when pre-disaster levels are reached, while at other times this is defined as restoration with recovery defined as reaching levels a household might have achieved had no disaster occurred. In addition, analysis techniques employed are as varied as are measures of recovery including qualitative/ethnographic methods, simple cross-tabulations, Chi-squared testing, difference in means and proportions testing, discriminate analysis, path analysis, ordinary least squares regression, lagged residualized regression, logistic regression, and interrupted time series. Thus, generalizing can be problematic. Nevertheless, throughout this discussion we draw upon household recovery research findings that are related to overall housing recovery.

Research focusing on household recovery, particularly of homeowners, suggests that insurance and public funding are indeed important for housing recovery and in many cases, perhaps even in a majority of cases, homeowners do generally receive the assistance they need to repair and rebuild. For example, Peacock and Girard (1997, p. 188) reported that in the Hurricane Andrew case, the vast majority of homeowners had homeowners insurance, with only 5% reporting no insurance. This figure represents a substantial improvement in coverage, particularly when compared to some historical studies dealing with hazards likely covered by general residential policies (cf. Bolin, 1982; Cochrane, 1975; Drabek & Key, 1984; Moore et al., 1964; Quarantelli, 1985). On the other hand, as can be expected, when dealing with earthquake and flood insurance, a different picture of much lower rates of coverage generally is found (Kunreuther & Roth, 1998; Lindell & Perry, 2000; Palm, 1995). The research literature also suggests that households having insurance generally report receiving sufficient settlements or at least what they consider fair/adequate settlements. Peacock and Girard (1997), again for example, reported that nearly 76% of homeowners following Hurricane Andrew received sufficient settlements and were on the whole satisfied. While this percentage is high compared to some prior research settings, the general pattern appears to hold (Bolin, 1982; Bolin & Bolton, 1986; Drabek & Key, 1984; Quarantelli, 1985). And, in the event that insurance is not sufficient, or there is no policy in effect, public assistance, particularly in the form of low-interest SBA loans and Minimum Housing Assistance from FEMA, become critical.

Research focusing on household recovery following earthquakes, for example, tends to find that these forms of assistance become highly important for recovery in earthquake disasters (Bolin, 1993; Bolin & Bolton, 1986) and can also be important in other situations such as flooding (Quarantelli, 1985). Unfortunately, the direct analysis of the impacts insurance and public funding play for housing recovery itself is difficult to assess, given (1) the limited research that actually focused on housing recovery, (2) the great variability in measures, (3) variability in techniques employed, (4) hazard variability in the relative roles of public and private financing, (5) data limitations, and (6) a host of complexities related to analysis decision, subsample selection, and data constraint interactions. On the whole, the results do suggest general positive impacts; however, assessments of the relative contributions, particularly for subpopulations, are difficult to ascertain.

Despite these overall patterns suggesting favorable outcomes, it is sometimes what Drabek and Key (1984, p. 93) termed the "patterned neglect" that is equally important for understanding the full complexities of household and housing recovery. Just as we saw with normal housing market operation, low-income and racial/ethnic minority homeowners often have limited access to both private and public resources important for permanent housing recovery. Poor language skills and educational backgrounds can leave many minorities, low-income households, and even female-headed households at a distinct disadvantage in the protracted qualification and negotiation processes often necessary to obtain public financial resources such as SBA loans or minimum housing assistance (Bolin, 1985; Bolin & Stanford, 1990; Morrow, 1997; Morrow & Enarson, 1997; Phillips, 1993). With less economic power and political representation, marginalized racial/ethnic groups are often excluded from community post-disaster planning and recovery activities (Bolin & Bolton, 1983; Morrow, 1997; Morrow & Peacock, 1997; Phillips, 1993; Prater & Lindell, 2000; Quarantelli, 1985; Tierney, 1989) and may be taken advantage of by private businesses. For example, a group of low-income Hispanic homeowners in southern sections of Miami-Dade County had little success at negotiations with their insurer whom they felt had not properly compensated them for damage to their homes. It was only after a community-based organization pleaded their case to the insurance commissioner that the company increased their payout. Other low-income minorities did not fair as well (Dash et al., 1997; Morrow, 1997; Peacock & Girard, 1997).

Households and neighborhoods that are poorer prior to disaster often fall far short of receiving necessary aid to jump start the recovery process, particularly for housing (Berke, Kartez, & Wenger, 1993; Bolin & Stanford, 1991; Dash et al., 1997; Phillips, 1993; Rubin, 1985). Low-income households are often limited in transportation options and this limitation may increase following a disaster when public transportation is extensively disrupted and personal transportation is destroyed. Lack of mobility may slow down the effort of recovery for these households and even jeopardize their employment (Morrow, 1997; Peacock & Girard, 1997). In addition, low-income households are less likely to qualify for governmental reconstruction programs because of their weak capability to repay (Bolin, 1982, 1986; Bolin & Bolton, 1983; Tierney, 1989). It must be remembered that the primary governmental program for those without insurance or with insufficient insurance coverage is the SBA's low-interest loan program. However, this is a loan program, not a grant program, and as a consequence, low-income and marginalized households, such as those on fixed or limited incomes, find it difficult to qualify. Indeed, the research has clearly shown that low-income and minorities are much more likely to fail to qualify for an SBA loan than are higher income and Anglo or white households (Bolin, 1982, 1986, 1993; Bolin & Bolton, 1986; Bolin & Stanford, 1998a, 1998b; Drabek & Key, 1984; Quarantelli, 1982). FEMA's minimum home repair program is exactly that, minimum. This program is designed to fund limited emergency repairs, in the interest of preventing further damage, and no more.

Similar patterns emerge when examining private insurance claims. Earlier research tended to consistently show that low-income and minority households were more likely to report not having insurance in the first place (Cochrane, 1975; Drabek & Key, 1984; Moore, Bates, Layman, & Parenton, 1963, Moore et al., 1964). Later research found that it was not just the lack of insurance, but that poor and minority households were also more likely to report insurance payments that were not adequate to meet repair and reconstruction needs (Bolin, 1982; Bolin & Bolton, 1986). Peacock and Girard (1997) found a similar pattern in Miami-Dade County following Hurricane Andrew, where minority homeowners, both black and Hispanic, were more likely to report insufficient insurance settlements for repairs and reconstruction. These differentials, however, were in part a function of the companies underwriting the policies. Households not covered by one of the top insurance companies were many more times likely to report insufficient insurance payments, and one of the most important determinants of having coverage by a top three company was the proportion of blacks residing on the block where the home was located. In other words, there was evidence suggesting that insurance redlining prior to Hurricane Andrew resulted in lower insurance settlements. The overall results found that black and lower income households were significantly more likely to report insurance settlements that were not sufficient to meet housing recovery needs (Peacock & Girard, 1997).

The picture that emerges from the household recovery literature clearly suggests that while both insurance and public funding are important for household recovery, access to these resources is far from equal. While the majority do indeed have access to both private and public recovery resources, lower income and minority homeowners appear to have much greater difficulty procuring access to adequate insurance and qualifying for SBA loans. While this research tends to focus only indirectly on housing recovery itself, the findings suggest that housing recovery is uneven at best and leads to significantly lower rates of housing recovery and increasing housing inequality at worse. The parallels to normal housing attainment processes do appear to play out in the post-disaster period; unfortunately, there is little systematic research that directly addresses and assesses uneven recovery rates in housing recovery. The picture for renters follows the same general pattern.

Rental properties have unique recovery problems. In the aftermath of a natural disaster, renters are much more likely to be displaced, for they have few if any rights to the property, only to the contents within them, whereas single-family homeowners can often choose to stay despite the damage. Renters are much less likely to have insurance to cover their assets (Kunreuther & Roth, 1998), and the range of government programs open to them is much more limited as discussed in the preceding text (i.e., IFG, Section 8 rent vouchers; SBA rental loans, food stamps) (Bolin, 1982; Bolin & Stanford, 1998a, 1998b; Comerio, 1998; Quarantelli, 1985). Low-income and minority households often have particular difficulty finding alternative housing, in no small measure because affordable housing is likely to be in short supply prior to the disaster (Bolin, 1982, 1985, 1993; Quarantelli, 1982). As a consequence, they are much more likely to find themselves in various forms of temporary sheltering and housing options (Bolin, 1985, 1993). Of course, renters are, in some sense, more mobile and less constrained than perhaps homeowners who often feel compelled to secure and guard their property. Hence, renters, at least theoretically, are free to move on to other rental opportunities. However, their ability to locate permanent housing will depend upon a number of factors such as transportation; economic resources such as savings, job, and family locations, and, most importantly, rental vacancies.

In addition, while they may be freer to relocate, they are often as tied to a location because of employment, schools, and social networks, as homeowners. For lower income households these factors are all in question and, as noted earlier, racial discrimination in housing can also limit possibilities of minorities (Girard & Peacock, 1997; Morrow, 1997). In addition, as has been noted by a number of studies, rents often increase in the post-impact period, and higher income and more affluent households often occupy the vacant rental properties that are available (Bolin, 1993; Bolin & Stanford, 1998a, 1998b; Comerio, 1998; Quarantelli, 1982). The net effect is that in major natural disasters, the opportunities can be very limited, which places those most vulnerable in a very untenable situation. This is clearly being played out in the aftermath of Hurricane Katrina for the many low-income renters who find themselves scattered to the winds.

What can exacerbate this situation tremendously is that rental housing can be difficult to bring back on line. The owners of rental properties, whether individuals or commercial entities, are responsible for recovery duties such as inspecting buildings and repairing damage to ensure safe occupancy. Rental properties often take significantly longer to rebuild and in the rebuilding process these projects rarely target low-income affordable housing, a continuation of normal

TABLE 15.1. Housing Characteristics in Six Disaster-Prone Cities

	Los Angeles	San Francisco	Houston	New Orleans	Miami	Charleston
Housing units	1,337,668	346,527	782,378	215,091	148,554	44,143
1 unit/detached (%)	39.2	18.1	46.6	41.9	30.6	50.5
1 unit attached	6.6	14.1	5.4	15	11.5	4.6
2 units	3.2	10.9	2.1	13.7	6	7.2
3–4 units	6.4	12.5	4.2	9.6	6.5	9.3
5–9 units	9.4	11.3	6	5.6	9.3	11.5
10–19 units	10.4	10.1	8.3	4.2	8.4	7.1
20 or more	24.1	22.9	26.4	9.3	26.7	8.6
Mobile home	0.6	0.1	1	0.3	1	1.1
Boat, RV, Van	0.1	0.1	0	0	0.1	0
Owner occupied (%)	38.6	35.0	45.8	46.5	34.9	51.1
Renter occupied	61.4	65.0	54.2	53.5	65.1	48.9
Vacant	4.7	4.9	8.2	12.5	9.6	8.5

housing processes. In their research after the Whittier Narrows, Loma Prieta, and Northridge earthquakes, Bolin (1986), Bolin (1993), Bolin & Stanford (1998a, 1998b), and Comerio et al. (1994) found evidence that some landlords delay repairs to damaged housing because of limited financial assets and developers seeking to establish new multifamily units are often blocked by local officials or residents. The typically slower reconstruction of rental properties places neighborhoods with a high proportion of rental properties at risk of failing to recover and potentially becoming blighted areas typically referred to in the literature as post-disaster ghost towns (Bolin & Stanford, 1998b; Comerio, 1998; Morrow & Peacock, 1997).

The difficulties for renters, particularly low-income renters needing affordable housing, is made much more difficult because of the nature of post-disaster policy. As Comerio (1998) and Comerio et al. (1994) note, there is seemingly a distorted image of whom the federal and state government needs to help. Policy is focused on the American dream household, as if the populations of households are all the owners of single-family detached housing. The effect has been that post-disaster policy has been biased in favor of homeowners, particularly single-family middle-income homeowners, at the expense of renters, the owners of rental properties, and low-income households (Comerio et al., 1994, p. 37). This bias is particularly evident in major urban centers likely to experience a major natural disaster. According to the 2003 U.S. Census estimates, 68.3% of households are in owner-occupied housing and 56.4% of all housing is owner-occupied single-family detached housing, these figures are at least somewhat consistent with the bias found in policy. However, a very different picture emerges from Table 15.1.

Table 15.1 presents housing characteristics data drawn from the 2000 Census for six cities that are likely candidates for future disasters given their histories; the first two are of course probable earthquake candidates and the last four are hurricane candidates. In fact, New Orleans is currently living its disaster nightmare. Only in Charleston are single-family detached housing units a majority and only in the same city is owner-occupied housing a majority. Indeed, in Los Angeles, San Francisco, and Miami, sizable percentages of housing units are renter occupied and in four communities between onefifth and one quarter of all housing units are located in buildings with 20 or more units. Clearly, at least in these metropolitan areas, the logic of a post-disaster housing policy that is biased against renters and rental unit owners (particularly large apartment buildings) must be brought into question. In addition, in all but one of these cities the vacancy rates are all below 10%. It is likely then that there would be a housing shortage following a major event.

While research focused on individual household recovery shows variations in the abilities of households to marshal reconstruction financing and other resources, the direct consequences for trends in owner- and renter-occupied permanent housing recovery have not been explored. Indeed, it is only at the aggregate levels that overall housing impacts and recovery are addressed. Housing recovery is usually characterized as generally being completed within 2 to 3 years after the event (Bolin, 1993; Comerio, 1998). Comerio (1998, p. 92) suggests that 75% of the single-family stock that was lost was restored to within 90% of its pre-Hurricane Andrew value within 2 years. Following the unprecedented efforts at modifying normal housing recovery funding patterns, following the 1994 Northridge earthquake which saw the federal government working with Los Angeles, to target special supplemental programs focusing on multifamily and lower-income housing, Comerio (1998, pp. 109–113) suggests remarkable success within 2 years as well. However, all of these findings are "estimates" based on very limited if any data, often times as questionable as local housing authorities claims. The simple fact is that there are no systematic studies. One now famous attempt, using aggregate level Census data for two decades (1960 and 1970), found that disasters have no significant long-term impact on housing stocks in the disaster-stricken community, particularly when examining broader countywide or regional impacts (Wright, Rossi, Wright, & Weber-Burdin,1979). However, in light of the literature on household recovery and early stages in the restoration process, one might well expect the distributive effects at the individual level to be quite different than aggregate level statistics suggest.

In an attempt to model and track permanent housing recovery following Hurricane Andrew, Peacock, Zhang, and Dash (2005) used property tax data from Miami-Dade County to assess differential recovery patterns in single-family housing that might be invisible at aggregate level analysis. While they too reported that in general single-family housing had reached, on average, pre-Andrew levels in 2 years, 32% of properties were still below their pre-impact levels nearly 2 years later and even 4 years later 16% were still below their pre-impact levels. They undertook a panel analysis of more than 60,000 single-family detached housing units from 1992 through 1996 and found considerable variation in recovery trajectories. Specifically, they found that rental housing was significantly slower recovering when compared to owner-occupied housing. Furthermore, their findings also suggest that single-family detached housing located in lower income neighborhoods and in neighborhoods with higher concentrations of non-Hispanic blacks and Hispanics had significantly slower recovery trajectories.

SHELTERING AND HOUSING SUMMARY

As evidenced in the preceding text, a review of the literature emphasizes that historically little research focuses on systematically understanding the four stages of Quarantelli's (1982) typology of sheltering and housing after disaster. While useful, more recent literature, particularly on hurricane disasters, suggests that the typology may be dated and need revision. For example, pre-impact sheltering, such as sheltering for hurricanes, does not fit cleanly into Quarantelli's categories. Even more complicated is trying to disentangle household recovery and housing recovery. As this chapter has shown, while our emphasis is on housing recovery, a complete understanding of this process must also be couched in terms of household recovery since it is the household, in part, that is negotiating the stages leading to permanent housing and receiving or as the case may be, not receiving, adequate assistance or resources to return to permanent housing. The other substantial part relates to rental housing itself, little research, and policy for that matter, has focused on this important component of housing recovery.

What is clear is that regardless of the type of shelter or housing being addressed, preexisting social processes related to housing attainment or, more broadly, the social construction of vulnerability, play important roles in shaping outcomes. Specifically, the above discussion highlights the consequences class and racial/ethnic differences play in the complex social process of returning to permanent housing after disaster. Whether considering differential levels of damage caused by natural hazard events, the ability to insure property and household assets, the availability of adequate emergency and temporary sheltering and temporary housing, or the challenges faced when garnering adequate resources to recover, the process from disaster impact to permanent housing recovery is complicated, particularly for low-income and minority households. The housing recovery process is rife with challenges for those with few personal, social, and financial assets.

The market "managed" recovery scheme upon which the United States depends is structured to favor those most likely to have resources to recover in the first place. Disaster recovery policy focuses on offering single-family homeowners assistance in rebuilding their homes, and thus, their lives, while leaving renters and the most financially marginal homeowners who cannot secure subsidized loans with few options. The safety net is flawed. Yet, because little systematic research has highlighted these inequities and problems, policy continues to focus on owner-occupied single-family housing recovery even though, as Census data show, in many areas the majority of households would be left to recover on their own. Only through a clear research agenda focused on the reality of disaster impact and recovery for all types of housing and households can we inform public policy and suggest change that will better meet the needs of all households.

While our focus has been primarily on housing issues in the United States, it is clear that the literature has gained from research conducted in international settings. Much of the work cited in the preceding drew extensively from research conducted in Latin America (Bates, 1982; Bates & Peacock, 1987, 1992, 1993; Bolin & Trainer, 1978; Bolin & Bolton, 1983; Haas et al., 1977; Oliver-Smith, 1990, 1991; Peacock et al., 1987), the Caribbean (Berke et al., 1993; Morrow, 1992), Europe (Bates & Peacock, 1992, 1993; Geipel, 1982; Hogg, 1980), and Japan (Wisner, 1998). Indeed, the insights related to social vulnerability and linking disasters with normal developmental processes, which have so fundamentally shaped recent, albeit limited, research that has been undertaken on housing recovery, were greatly influenced by international research (i.e., Blaike, Cannon, Davis, & Wisner, 1994). In addition, the international literature is relatively more well developed in the areas of emergency and temporary sheltering and to a certain extent on issues related to temporary housing (e.g., Davis, 1978, 1981), and U.S. researchers might well gain from it. In addition, to the extent that market phenomena are readily spreading with marked increases in globalization, the lessons learned in the United States regarding housing market failings, insurance, and their consequences for housing recovery are likely to find increasing relevance internationally. What is clear is that the broader sheltering and housing literature is emerging in both the United States and international context and much can be learned, gained, and fruitfully shared.

DISCUSSION AND FUTURE RESEARCH

We began this chapter with a focus on housing recovery following disasters and in so doing adopted the shelter and housing typology introduced by Quarantelli (1982) in an attempt to clarify the various forms of shelter and housing individuals and households often find themselves in need of or involved in as they cope with the displacement that is associated with natural disasters. For some households, this displacement is very limited, perhaps better termed temporary dislocation, as they flee their homes because of an acute hazard threat, or, in the immediate aftermath, as a result of limited damage to their homes or lifeline disruption. However, for households that are displaced because they are victims of a major natural disaster that has destroyed or otherwise left their homes uninhabitable, as we saw unfolding before us in the wake of Hurricane Katrina, seeking emergency shelter becomes only the first step in what may well be a long and protracted process of reestablishing permanent housing.

This chapter has highlighted research findings associated with each form of sheltering and housing, paying particular attention to what is generally considered the goal, reestablishing permanent housing, or again, in the vernacular, reestablishing home. This undertaking has made clear that some solid research has been undertaken in the 20 years since Quarantelli introduced his typology. It is indeed ironic that in addition to the typology, Quarantelli also offered twenty-two topics, seven of which he defined as high-priority topics, for future research. Of the seven he singled out as high priority, two have received no attention, four have received limited attention, and only one has received, relatively speaking, a good deal of attention albeit by only a few researchers. That one topic was "how pre-disaster conditions affect the post-disaster recovery operation in housing" (Quarantelli, 1982, p. 80). Rather than restate his list, we urge researchers to pay it heed, for most if not all deserve attention even today. Instead we offer the following general suggestions.

- While the emergency shelter–permanent housing continuum is not meant to suggest a progressive linear process, it does provide an interesting framework for examining the process of housing recovery. A recent dissertation by Cole (2003) perhaps represents a first step in mapping out and examining the complexities of households transitioning this process, sometimes moving forward, falling back, and even skipping over forms.
- Solid ethnographic/qualitative research needs to be undertaken following panels of household through the process of housing recovery, paying particular attention to transition points in the process. Ethnographic decision tree analyses would be particularly fruitful in helping the research and policymaking communities better understand factors shaping household decision making in the complex housing recovery process.
- Solid ethnographic/qualitative research also needs to be undertaken on developers, rental property owners, and managers, to better understand the decision-making process related to post-disaster repair, rebuilding, and redevelopment decisions. This should examine not only owners and developers of properties that existed prior to a disaster, but also those that consider such activities following a disaster.
- Longitudinal panel studies of households—both renter and homeowner households—transitioning through the housing recovery process following a major natural disaster. In light of future demographic trends, focusing on populations in large multiethnic metropolitan areas would be particularly important as well as considering all dimensions of social vulnerability (i.e., gender, age, etc.), not simply class and race/ethnicity.
- Longitudinal panel studies of different forms of housing (single-family, multifamily, condominiums, etc.) and the difficulties experienced by households occupying these structures having varying tenure status should be undertaken.
- Consistent and appropriate quantitative multivariate analysis of future, existing, and historical datasets should be undertaken. Advances in generalized linear models, hierarchical linear models, and panel analytic techniques provide a greater range and

flexibility for researchers to undertake appropriate analyses with all forms of recovery measures. Revisiting and reanalyzing historical datasets might be particularly fruitful.

- Displacement of individuals and households from their permanent homes, as noted by Quarantelli, is the first step setting into motion shelter and housing process. Displacement itself will be a function of not only disaster damage to the structure or lifelines, but also a host of social factors such as tenure status and access to resources. Displacement/dislocation itself should also be a subject of research.

- Clearly, insights have been gained from the international research arena that have been fruitfully applied in the United States context. However, we have not seen concerted efforts to integrate research between these settings. As research focusing on housing recovery emerges, more efforts must be undertaken to share and exchange insights and thereby promote transferability.

- Finally, and perhaps most importantly, we return to Quarantelli's (1982, p. 80) final admonition: conceptual rigor and clarity. As researchers, we must strive for conceptual and theoretical clarity in our work. This may involve the creation of distinctive concepts as tools for the development of our theories and research or the refinement of existing concepts; but unless we are clear in our theorizing about the phenomena under study, we cannot hope to cumulatively develop as a mature area of research.

CHAPTER 16

Businesses and Disasters: Vulnerability, Impacts, and Recovery

KATHLEEN J. TIERNEY

As units of analysis in disaster research, businesses have only recently begun to be studied. Far more research has been conducted on public sector organizations such as local emergency management agencies, public safety agencies, and other governmental organizations. Researchers studying the economic impacts of disasters have tended to focus on units of analysis that are larger than individual firms and enterprises, such as community and regional economies. Until fairly recently, very little was known regarding such topics as business vulnerability, loss-reduction measures adopted by businesses, disaster impacts on businesses, and business recovery. Systematic research was lacking despite the singular importance of businesses for society. Private businesses provide a vast array of goods and services that literally make life possible in our complex global economy. A recent governmental report on the U.S. critical infrastructure points out that "[t]he lion's share of our critical infrastructures and key assets are owned and operated by the private sector" (White House, 2003, p. 32)[1]. Businesses are the foundation of local, regional, and national economies; when businesses are affected by disasters, that disruption produces not only direct business losses, but also indirect losses and economic ripple effects. Destruction of and damage to businesses, along with disaster-related closures, result in the loss of jobs, negatively affecting incomes and creating even greater challenges for households, neighborhoods, and communities as they attempt to recover from disasters. After disasters, business owners face a host of challenges, including how to finance business recovery, and often how to cope simultaneously with damage to both business and residential property. Disasters can produce both psychological distress and additional debt burdens for business owners. At the community level, business destruction and damage can result in lost tax revenues for communities and can undermine the viability of business and commercial districts.

---

[1] In the United States, the "critical infrastructure" is defined as composed of the following elements: agriculture and food; public health; emergency services; the defense industrial base; telecommunications; energy; transport; banking and finance; chemical production and hazardous materials; and postal and shipping enterprises. It is commonly said that about 85% of the U.S. critical infrastructure is in private hands.

This chapter reviews social science research on businesses and disasters, focusing on business vulnerability, the ways disasters affect business operations, and post-disaster business recovery. In this discussion, the term business is used to refer to organizations that are operated for profit, as opposed to public sector and nonprofit organizations. The term applies to a range of business types, including sole proprietorships, partnerships, and corporations, irrespective of the goods and services they supply, and whether they do business in one location (establishments) or multiple locations (enterprises). The concept covers both large and small businesses, including owner-operated businesses with no employees. The chapter is heavily weighted toward U.S. research and to English-language publications, in part because of the attention U.S. researchers have paid to disaster-related business issues. The chapter closes with recommendations for future research, including a recommendation centering on the need for more systematic, comparative research on these issues.

BUSINESS VULNERABILITY TO EXTREME EVENTS

How and Why Businesses Are Vulnerable to Disasters

Business vulnerability to disasters stems from a variety of interrelated factors that include physical location, the conditions under which businesses operate, and business and community characteristics. Consistent with the *social vulnerability* paradigm, business vulnerability can be thought of as stemming not only from exposure to the potential physical impacts of hazards, but also from societal conditions and trends that render certain businesses and types of businesses less able to cope with "environmental shocks," including disasters (Cutter, 1996; Cutter, Mitchell, & Scottal., 2000; Dahlhamer, 1998). Vulnerability thus has both physical and social dimensions; like communities and households, businesses are differentially vulnerable to disaster impacts.

Vulnerability of Place

In the most general sense, business vulnerability to disasters is related to the hazardousness of the locations in which business and economic activity take place. Around the globe, many primate cities and "megacities"—the urban places that serve as economic engines for entire societies—are located in areas with high hazard exposure. Tokyo, Istanbul, Caracas, Manila, and Tehran are examples (Parker & Mitchell, 1995; Solway, 1994; Wisner, n.d.). In the United States, many cities that account for a substantial amount of the nation's economic activity, including Greater Los Angeles, Miami, Houston, San Francisco, and New York City, are vulnerable to both natural disasters and terrorist attacks. When hurricane Katrina struck Mississippi, Alabama, and Louisiana, it resulted in the closure of tens of thousands of businesses, the shutdown of one of the nation's busiest ports, and massive disruption of the petrochemical industry in the impact region. Just weeks later, Hurricane Rita threatened comparable impacts for Houston and the oil facilities in the western Gulf of Mexico.

While virtually all communities are vulnerable to hazards to some degree, within individual communities some locations are more vulnerable than others. However, business owners are typically more concerned about finding the best locations for generating business revenues than about the disaster vulnerability of those locations or of the buildings they occupy. For many retail and service businesses, the most desirable business properties may be located in older downtown commercial areas where structures do not meet current codes. Historic downtown shopping districts are good places for some businesses to locate from a purely financial standpoint, but such locations may also be more vulnerable to hazards when disasters strike. The California cities of Coalinga, Whittier, and Santa Cruz all had historic commercial districts that were heavily damaged by earthquakes that occurred in 1983, 1987, and 1989, respectively. In the 1992 Nisqually earthquake, commercial damage was heaviest in Seattle's historic Pioneer Square area (Chang & Falit-Baiamonte, 2003). Memphis and Shelby County Tennessee face the risk of a major earthquake owing to their proximity to the New Madrid Fault. A survey conducted in the early 1990s with a randomly selected, representative sample of Memphis/Shelby County businesses found that 24% of the businesses in the sample were located in non-earthquake-resistant brick buildings,—that is, the types of buildings most likely to collapse or sustain serious structural damage in an earthquake—and that small businesses in the service and the finance, insurance, and real estate sectors were more likely than others to be housed in these types of structures. Overall, small businesses in Memphis and Shelby County, as opposed to large ones, were more likely to be located in hazardous structures (Tierney & Dahlhamer, 1997).[2]

Business Choices and Disaster Vulnerability

Business decisions also affect vulnerability to disasters. In their efforts to locate near needed resources, such as raw materials, transportation routes, and skilled and able workers, as well as to take advantage of synergies that come about through co-location, businesses and business sectors may inadvertently put too many of their assets at risk from hazards. In the late 1970s, concern with mitigating and managing earthquake hazards in the United States began to intensify, partly out of recognition that so many defense-related research and development and production facilities were located in vulnerable areas in Southern California. For this reason, the earthquake hazard also began to be seen as a national security threat (Federal Emergency Management Agency [FEMA], 1980). California's Silicon Valley is another example of industry concentration in a high hazard area. A major center for the computer and semiconductor industries, Silicon Valley also sits in a very vulnerable location with respect to earthquakes. Recognizing this problem, some Silicon Valley firms have been making their facilities and business operations more dispersed geographically in order to reduce vulnerability. In many cases, businesses choose to stay in hazardous locations but upgrade their facilities to make them more disaster resistant. In other cases, owners choose to hope for the best, rather than undertaking costly loss-reduction projects.

Renting a business property, as opposed to owning the property outright, can also be a factor in business vulnerability. Renting is often a necessity, rather than a choice for businesses. However, businesses that rent space typically have fewer options with respect to the loss-reduction measures they can undertake. They cannot, for example, decide to make their buildings more flood, wind, or seismically resistant through structural upgrades (although they can take steps to protect inventory and equipment). Instead of being able to act independently,

---

[2] Another study conducted around the same time found that, based on square footage, 45% of the commercial and industrial space in Memphis and Shelby County was located in buildings that were vulnerable to earthquake damage (Jones & Malik, 1996). The business survey, however, focused on individual businesses, rather than buildings.

renters are often subject to the mitigation choices made by building owners. Similarly, when disasters strike, renters are dependent on building owners for needed repairs, particularly when there is structural damage. If the landlord has difficulty financing repairs, those renting or leasing space may be forced to relocate or to operate their businesses under adverse conditions. Research suggests that when lease agreements are made between businesses and landlords, leases do not adequately address the circumstances in which both tenants and landlords may find themselves in the event of a disaster (Alesch, Holly, Mittler, & Nagy, 2001).

Market Characteristics and Vulnerability

Market diversification and the degree of competitiveness within different market niches are also factors that affect business vulnerability. There is evidence suggesting that, other things being equal, businesses that are primarily dependent on local markets can experience greater financial difficulty than those that serve a more diversified market base, in part because disasters affect consumer behavior (Chang & Falit-Baiamonte, 2003; Webb, Tierney, & Dahlhamer, 2002). Businesses that depend heavily on discretionary spending by local residents, who are themselves disaster victims, may be especially vulnerable.[3]

When businesses experience disruption, such as forced closure, their competitors are in a position to benefit. Consumers who need to replace lost items quickly will turn to whatever business—either within or outside their communities—that can provide those items. Extensive disruption of operations can result in permanent losses for businesses. For example, the Port of Kobe, Japan was one of the largest container ports in the world at the time that the Great Hanshin-Awaji earthquake struck in 1995. The port was severely damaged, and during the period in which it was being repaired and restored, shippers turned to other container ports in the region. When the Kobe port returned to capacity, which also entailed making a number of important post-earthquake improvements, there was still no particular reason for shippers to bring their business back to Kobe. The port, which had already been experiencing revenue declines before the earthquake, never regained its position (Chang, 2001).

Community-Level and Infrastructure Influences on Vulnerability

The vulnerability of individual businesses is also determined in part by what communities choose to do—or not do—with respect to disaster loss-reduction. The fates of businesses following disasters are influenced by such community-level factors as whether their communities had been effectively managing hazards through prudent land-use strategies; whether they had adopted up-to date codes for new construction; whether they required retrofitting for structures that do not meet codes; and whether steps had been taken to reduce disaster-induced lifeline service disruption. With respect to codes and retrofitting, for example, the earthquake-stricken communities of Coalinga, Whittier, and Santa Cruz California, which were discussed

---

[3] One possible exception is the case of businesses that supply items that disaster victims need to replace, such as carpeting and window glass. However, local businesses can lose their inventories of items like these when disasters occur, and they can also be undercut by outside providers of needed goods and services that see an opportunity to increase their profits in the aftermath of disasters. It appears that following Hurricane Katrina, numerous goods and services are being offered by businesses from outside the impact region, since such a large proportion of affected businesses simply could not reopen. In any case, whatever benefits businesses reap from disasters are short lived; once lost and damaged articles are replaced, subsequent demand for those articles drops.

above, either had no seismic retrofitting programs for older unreinforced masonry buildings such as those that sustained heavy damage, or had not gotten started on implementing such programs.

Many businesses fail to recognize how much their operations depend on uninterrupted lifeline services. The critical infrastructure that enables individual businesses to operate is a "system of systems" characterized by various interdependencies and vulnerabilities. Despite efforts to understand and map these interdependencies, the consequences of local infrastructure failures for larger infrastructure systems, as well as for businesses and business sectors, may become apparent only when disaster strikes. For example, Mendonca, Lee, and Wallace (2004) have shown how failures in electrical power and telecommunications systems following the World Trade Center (2001) attacks had a major impact on the banking and finance sector, another component of the critical infrastructure.

Among various lifeline services, electrical power is often considered most critical, since so many of the other infrastructural systems and resources that make it possible for businesses to function depend in one way or another upon electricity (Tierney & Dahlhamer, 1997). Business losses in disasters are influenced significantly by steps lifeline service providers have taken to mitigate damage and rapidly restore services. In the 1993 Midwest floods, for example, business interruption losses were extensive. During the floods, almost half of the businesses in Des Moines, Iowa were forced to close for at least some period. However, only about 15% of all Des Moines businesses experienced direct flood damage. Instead, businesses were required by the city to close because lifeline services were disrupted after vulnerable water and sewage facilities were flooded out (Tierney, Nigg, & Dahlhamer, 1996).[4] In this case, businesses suffered losses not so much because of direct damage, but rather because of decisions (and non-decisions) that had been made at the community level with respect to lifeline protection. Des Moines subsequently undertook a mitigation project to avoid such problems in the future. When underground flooding occurred in downtown Chicago in 1992, the "Loop," the city's main business district, was forced to shut down because the flooding caused a loss of electrical power. The lack of power in turn affected water service (including water for fire suppression) and public transportation in downtown Chicago.

Businesses are dependent on governmental capacity to undertake pre-disaster mitigation measures and to respond effectively following disasters—and they are vulnerable when communities are unable to do so. Hurricane Katrina is a dramatic case in point: business and residential losses stemmed directly from government's failure to provide sufficient protection for the city against large hurricanes. After disasters strike, businesses again rely on government-initiated loss-containment measures—for example, responding to secondary threats such as fires and hazmat spills, providing security, and rapidly clearing debris and restoring transportation so that businesses can reopen. Government actions with respect to allowing business owners to reenter damaged areas to retrieve inventories and business records, as well as policies for condemning and demolishing damaged business properties, can also create additional burdens on business owners.

As discussed later in this chapter, the fates of individual businesses also depend on local capacity to manage the recovery process, which includes the ability of the community, to undertake pre-disaster recovery planning; gain access to, package, and leverage different

---

[4] This disaster also showed what a small factor insurance can be in assisting businesses in recovering from disasters. Of the businesses that were flooded, only one fourth had any flood insurance coverage. Few businesses had business interruption insurance capable of paying for the costs of closure, and many owners who did have insurance did not use it because their losses were not covered.

sources of aid for businesses; and take advantage of knowledgeable experts both from within and outside the community during the recovery process.

Broader Business and Economic Trends and Disaster Vulnerability

Businesses are sensitive both to general economic trends and to the economic climate in particular business sectors. Disasters can exacerbate "everyday" vulnerabilities, while pre-disaster economic health can cushion the impacts of extreme events. Eighteen months after the Northridge earthquake, for example, firms in industries that had been experiencing growth in the 2-year period just before the earthquake were significantly less likely than firms in declining industries to report being worse off than before the disaster (Dahlhamer, 1998). In studies on the longer-term impacts of Hurricane Andrew and the Loma Prieta earthquake, business owners who considered the general economic climate to be positive for their firms were significantly more likely to report positive recovery outcomes (Webb et al., 2002).

Regulations, Standards, and Vulnerability

The existence of and compliance with mandates, regulations, and standards are also factors that affect business vulnerability to disasters. Generally speaking, there are few outright mandates governing business disaster mitigation, preparedness, response, and recovery. Exceptions to this pattern include businesses in the highly-hazardous nuclear and chemical industries. The Nuclear Regulatory Commission places strict requirements on nuclear facilities, including requirements related to in-plant safety, public education, and emergency planning in areas surrounding those facilities (see, e.g., Nuclear Regulatory Commission, 2005). Laws such as the Emergency Planning and Community Right to Know Act and the Clean Air Act regulate safety and emergency preparedness for chemical facilities in the United States Since the terrorist attacks of September 11, 2001, security procedures at such facilities have received even greater scrutiny (Government Accountability Office, 2005; White House, 2003).

Loss-reduction requirements are also relatively strong for businesses in the finance, insurance, and real estate sectors, and there is some evidence suggesting that businesses in that sector tend to do more to prepare for disasters (Dahlhamer & D'Souza, 1997). However, most safety measures that businesses undertake are done voluntarily. For example, NFPA 1600 (National Fire Protection Association, 2004) is a comprehensive set of standards recommending steps that businesses and other types of organizations should take to reduce their vulnerability and prepare for, respond to, and recover from disasters. First promulgated in 1995, the standard has been updated twice, most recently in 2004.[5] While NFPA 1600 provides guidance on best practices that should help all businesses better cope with hazards and disasters, it is nevertheless a voluntary standard, not a requirement that all businesses must meet.

No systematic data currently exist regarding factors associated with business adoption of NFPA 1600, nor is it clear how effective the standard will be in reducing business losses following disasters. Such research is badly needed. In the meantime, however, given the

---

[5] Both businesses and public sector organizations are being urged to adopt the standards by FEMA and by the Department of Homeland Security. The 9/11 Commission Report also recommends its adoption, stating that "[t]he experience of the private sector in the World Trade Center Emergency demonstrated the need for these standards" (9/11 Commission Report, 2004, p. 398).

comprehensiveness of the standard and the difficulty involved in implementing many of the recommended measures, it is safe to assume that it will be more readily adopted by very large and prosperous corporations that have the expertise to implement such large-scale programs.

Unfortunately, it is quite common for business interests to actively fight proposed loss-reduction measures out of a concern for how such measures will affect their profits. For example, landlord associations were perhaps the strongest opponents to the seismic retrofit program for unreinforced masonry buildings that was put forward by local officials (and eventually adopted) in Los Angeles, because landlords were unwilling to bear the expense of retrofitting their rental properties (Alesch & Petak, 1986).

Business and Owner Characteristics

Business size is a factor that has been consistently shown to be associated with business vulnerability. Small businesses are often described as the engines that drive the economy, both through job creation and through innovation. The small business sector in the United States is extremely large, and most small businesses are extremely small. Of the approximately 7.1 million business establishments covered in the most recent "Statistics of U.S. Business" survey, about 5.1 million had fewer than 20 employees (U.S. Department of Commerce, 2001a).[6] While they represent the majority of U.S. businesses, small businesses are inherently more vulnerable to disasters than their larger counterparts. Even under non-disaster conditions, small businesses generally experience more financial stress than larger ones; many are undercapitalized and may be operating with only marginal profits. The economic sectors in which the majority of small businesses are located—specifically the service and retail sectors—are also highly competitive sectors that generally see more business failures and turnover among firms during non-disaster times.

Size is to some extent a proxy for resources: larger enterprises generally have a greater ability to cope with misfortunes of all types because they have larger cash reserves. Larger firms can afford to hire specialists, such as risk managers and emergency management professionals, to reduce their vulnerability to extreme events. The vast body of research that has been conducted on businesses indicates that overall larger businesses do more to prepare for disasters than smaller ones (see, e.g., Dahlhamer & D'Souza, 1997; Mileti et al., 1992; Webb, Tierney, & Dahlhamer, 2000). Even though the adoption of standard recommended preparedness measures may actually have little to do with post-disaster business outcomes, as discussed later in this chapter, researchers concur that size conveys many advantages for businesses, both during normal times and in disasters. However, the vast majority of businesses are small ones.

Size is also frequently associated with business owner characteristics that are in turn associated with business vulnerability. Minority- and woman-owned businesses, which are particularly vulnerable to shifting economic trends, tend to be concentrated in the small business sector; 82% of minority-owned businesses are single proprietorships, as opposed to partnerships or corporations (U.S. Department of Commerce, 2001b). Minority- and woman-owned businesses are currently increasing at a faster rate than the national average for businesses in general. The number of woman-owned businesses grew 20% between 1997 and 2002; during that same period, Hispanic-owned businesses grew by 31%. It is worth noting that

---

[6] About 10% of this number had no employees at all—that is, the businesses were operated by self-employed individuals.

minority-owned businesses constitute a high proportion of the businesses in high-risk states such as California and Florida and in high-risk metropolitan areas in those states, such as Los Angeles and Miami (U.S. Department of Commerce, 2002).

Even within the fragile minority-owned business sector, businesses are differentially vulnerable. Recent data indicate that businesses owned by African Americans are more likely to fail than other ethnic businesses (Hocker, 2005). Nearly two thirds of black-owned businesses are in the service and retail trade sectors, both of which see relatively high rates of business failure during non-disaster times. About 40% of African-American businesses are woman-owned, a far larger proportion than among other minority-owned businesses (U.S. Department of Commerce, 2001c). Research on ethnic economies suggests that African-American entrepreneurs reap substantially fewer economic benefits from their businesses, compared to both whites and other minority business owners (Light & Gold, 2000).

WHEN DISASTER STRIKES: IMPACTS ON BUSINESSES

Negative Impacts of Disasters

The degree of physical damage businesses sustain in disasters is but one in a series of factors that affect the ability of businesses to survive when disasters strike. In dealing with disasters, businesses face a variety of challenges, many of which are unrelated to the magnitude of damages they experience. As the following sections show, many of these challenges stem from the interdependencies that exist among businesses, their customers, and their communities.

Direct, Indirect, and Ripple Effects

Direct impacts of disasters on businesses include structural damage to business properties, damage to nonstructural elements in those properties (e.g., windows, lighting systems, utility pipelines inside business structures, telecommunications and computer services, and equipment), and damage to or loss of contents, inventories, and business records. Direct business impacts resulting from disasters also include impacts that result from disaster-induced failures in critical systems both within and outside the business property itself, including in particular utility service losses.

Direct impacts also include losses that occur due to business interruption. As discussed elsewhere in this chapter, business interruption may result from direct physical damage to the business or from a range of other factors, including utility loss, transportation system damage, or governmental action, such as cordoning off highly damaged areas. Thus, even if a business remains undamaged in a disaster, it may still be forced to close. As noted earlier with respect to the city of Des Moines during the 1993 floods, the majority of businesses in Des Moines had to close because they lost lifeline services, not because of flooding.

Indirect impacts and economic ripple effects consist of "downstream" effects that result from disasters, such as the disruptions in the flow of goods and services and supply-chain problems. These types of second-order effects can also create additional business interruptions and job losses, over and above those resulting directly from initial disaster impacts. Analyses of economic ripple effects highlight the fact that disasters affect not only individual businesses and business districts, but also larger units of aggregation, such as regional economies (Okuyama & Chang, 2004; Rose & Guha, 2004; West & Lenze, 1994).

Researchers who focus on assessing the aggregate economic losses resulting from disasters have developed methodologies for estimating and measuring those losses. Much of this research depends critically on understanding what happens to individual businesses during disasters and how firm-level damage and losses contribute to business interruption, other indirect losses, and economic ripple effects (see Rose, 2004 for a recent example).

Post-Disaster Operational Problems and Owner Burdens

Other problems that accompany disasters can negatively affect both business operations and aggregate-level economic activity. Such problems include difficulties businesses experience because customers cannot reach the business location owing to disaster damage, or because customers have left the area, either temporarily or permanently. Other problems include downtime associated with business clean-up, difficulties with shipping products to clients, the need to find a property to which to relocate, and loss of employee productivity because of difficulties employees experience following disasters. Business owners may also be torn between family-related post-disaster needs (such as having to make home repairs or find a new place to live) and getting the business back on its feet. Owners must also cope with complicated disaster assistance requirements, insurance reimbursement applications (if they are fortunate enough to have insurance), and additional financial pressures, such as increased debt, brought on by the disaster (for more detailed discussions on the impact of these sorts of difficulties, see Webb et al., 2000; Alesch et al., 2001).

Indirect Effects on Nondamaged Businesses: Examples from the World Trade Center Disaster

As indicated throughout this chapter, businesses may be adversely affected even if they have not experienced direct disaster impacts. This is particularly true for businesses whose fortunes are closely linked to those of damaged businesses, business districts, and residential areas. The World Trade Center (WTC) attacks dealt a devastating blow to businesses located in the Trade Towers and in nearby structures. In addition to these direct impacts on businesses in the WTC complex, many businesses located near Ground Zero experienced a variety of different types of losses. Business revenues were affected initially, for example, by security measures designed to keep residents and tourists from entering lower Manhattan; retail businesses trying to operate in blocked-off sections adjacent to the Trade Center complex abruptly lost customers unless they were able to relocate their operations. According to a 2002 report by the Asian American Federation of New York, businesses in nearby Chinatown experienced a variety of persistent negative impacts. The report estimated that in the first 2 weeks after the September 11 attack, 75% of the Chinatown workforce was without work, and 3 months later, 25% were still unemployed. Chinatown tourist revenues for the summer of 2002 were 40% lower than for the summer of 2001, and the Chinatown garment industry lost an estimated $500,000,000 in revenues in the year following the attacks (Asian American Federation of New York, 2002). Negative effects were especially pronounced for businesses in the restaurant, retail trade, hotel, air transport, and building services (Fiscal Policy Institute, 2001). Many businesses located near the Ground Zero reconstruction area are still being affected by the fact that tens of thousands of people who once needed the goods and services they offered are working elsewhere. When the Trade Towers and other structures were lost, many of these businesses, especially those dependent on local foot traffic, effectively lost their markets.

Other Negative Effects

Businesses—even those that do not suffer direct losses—can be negatively affected in still other ways. For example, following disaster, insurance may become more costly and more difficult or even impossible to obtain. Again focusing on September 11 and its impacts on businesses, a survey of insurance agents and brokers serving businesses in all five New York City boroughs found that insurance providers had increased their premiums for all lines of insurance after the terrorist attacks, with increases ranging from 39% to 73%. Increases were particularly steep for businesses operating in high-rise structures in Manhattan, especially businesses located in or near landmark and "iconic" properties. Insurance also became significantly harder for businesses to obtain at any price following 9/11 (Thompson, 2002). Other disasters, most notably Hurricane Andrew in 1992 and the 1994 Northridge earthquake, caused insurance providers to either raise premiums significantly or withdraw completely from offering both residential and commercial insurance.[7] Impacts on insurance markets can affect businesses nationwide. Current projections suggest that homeowners and businesses throughout the nation will see a hike in their premiums, both as a direct consequence of Hurricanes Katrina and Rita, and also because the insurance industry now recognizes that it must prepare for future hurricane losses that will result in escalating damage in the coming years.

BUSINESS DISASTER RECOVERY AND LONGER-TERM IMPACTS

As noted in the introduction to this chapter, it is only recently that social scientists have begun to study businesses as units of analysis affected by disasters. Most research on disaster recovery processes and outcomes has focused on other units of analysis, such as households and communities. Research in economics and regional science did shed some light on the macroeconomic and regional impacts of disasters (see, e.g., Albala-Bertrand, 1993: Jones & Chang, 1995; Kunreuther & Rose, 2004; Rose, Chang, Szczesniak, & Lim, 1997), but again individual firms were not the focus of that research. However, because of the substantial amount of research that has now accumulated on business disaster recovery, it is possible to provide at least provisional answers to questions related to recovery processes and outcomes. Unfortunately, because so little research has been conducted outside the United States, it is not clear how generalizeable findings from U.S. research may be to other societies. Cross-nationally, there will likely be significant differences in business recovery processes and outcomes owing to societal differences in forms of economic organization, the availability of risk management instruments such as insurance, and the types of recovery assistance provided to businesses. A second important caveat is that most of what is currently known about business recovery

---

[7] Following the Northridge earthquake, the crisis in insurance availability was so acute that in 1996 the State of California formed a new agency, the California Earthquake Authority, as a means of making insurance available. New policies now differ from those offered before the earthquake in terms of rates, deductibles, and exclusions.

is based on studies of "typical" disasters, rather than catastrophic events such as Hurricane Katrina. The need for further research in these two areas is discussed later in the chapter.

Do Businesses Recover?

The answer to this question depends in part on how the question is asked: how recovery is conceptualized, how the concept is operationalized, what types of businesses are selected for study, and how studies are conducted. A series of studies on short- and longer-term business recovery following four different disasters—the Loma Prieta earthquake (1989), Hurricane Andrew (1992), the Midwest floods (1993), and the Northridge earthquake (1994)—were conducted by the University of Delaware's Disaster Research Center (DRC) during the 1990s. These studies, which were carried out through mail surveys with owners of randomly selected, stratified samples of all businesses in the disaster-affected regions, asked owners to assess business well-being, compared with how well the business had been doing prior to the disaster. Specifically, owners were asked to indicate whether the business was "worse off," "better off," or "about the same" as before the disaster. The surveys covered both short-term (the 1993 floods and the Northridge earthquake) and longer-term business outcomes (Loma Prieta and Andrew; for a summary of this research, see Webb et al., 2000; Tierney & Webb, forthcoming, 2006).

These studies showed that even in the short-term (i.e., a year to 18 months after a disaster event) most businesses do at least return to pre-disaster levels of economic performance. For example, a little over a year after the Midwest floods and the Northridge earthquake, 12.2% and 23.3% of businesses, respectively, reported being worse off, and comparable numbers actually reported being better off. With respect to the longer term, 21% of businesses in hard-hit Santa Cruz County reported being worse off, but 37% said they were better off than before the earthquake. Findings were roughly the same for businesses in South Dade County 6 years after Hurricane Andrew; while 34% of businesses surveyed reported being worse off, 31% were better off than before the hurricane.[8]

Even in an event as devastating as the World Trade Center attack, businesses show great adaptability. In a 1-year follow-up, *New York Times* reporters located 500 businesses (out of an estimated total of 600 to 700) that had been operating in the Trade Center complex on September 11, 2001. Only 39 were no longer in business, and 30 more were operating out of private homes. More than 350 were continuing to do business in Manhattan, some very close to Ground Zero. The majority of businesses were still struggling with many challenges, but they had at least managed to relocate and stay afloat during the first year after the attack (*New York Times*, September 11, 2002).

Other research on the prospects businesses face following disasters paints a slightly different picture. Daniel Alesch and his collaborators (Alesch & Holly, 1997; Alesch et al., 2001, n.d.) have engaged in studies on short- and long-term business recovery following several disaster events, including Hurricane Andrew; the Northridge earthquake; the severe 1997 flooding on

---

[8] These surveys were conducted on business "survivors"—that is, businesses that were operating before the disasters occurred and that were still in operation when contacted at a later date. Businesses that failed or disappeared completely where thus not included in the Disaster Research Center (DRC) studies. However, despite urban legends indicating that a large proportion of businesses fail following disasters, that does not appear to be the case. Moreover, quitting business after a disaster may be a prudent choice for some business owners, rather than an indication of disaster induced failure (Alesch et al., 2001).

the Red River of the North that caused extensive damage in communities such as Grand Forks, North Dakota; and floods caused by Hurricane Floyd in 1999. Unlike the Disaster Research Center studies, which focused on randomly selected representative samples of businesses, their work concentrated specifically on small businesses and nonprofit organizations in communities and neighborhoods that experienced high levels of damage and disruption following disaster events. Such businesses were thus prime candidates for experiencing poor outcomes following disasters.

Also in contrast with the DRC questionnaire surveys, the studies conducted by Alesch and his colleagues involved in-depth, open-ended interviews with business owners, many of whom were interviewed more than once over time. These more qualitative studies focused on the lived experiences of business owners as they attempted to recover following severe disaster losses. Among the findings from this research was that the idea of "recovery" as the reconstitution of business activity as it had been before the disaster, had little meaning for these business owners. Even years after suffering disaster losses, owners were still struggling and still trying to come to terms with the "new normal" ushered in by disaster. Indeed, Alesch and his colleagues argue that those struggles—and ultimate outcomes for businesses—may be far more painful for owners who cling to the past instead of attempting to innovate, change their business operations, and seek new opportunities. Noting that for many the disaster experience never really ends, they conclude that (Alesch et al., 2001, p. 15):

> ...long after the physical evidence of the destruction is gone, long after water is being distributed and sewage collected, long after new buildings are built, and long after the grass grows over scars on the land, the effects of the disaster linger. They linger economically, socially, and psychologically. We have come to believe that, for organizations that suffer significant losses from a natural hazard event, return to the *status quo ante* is a chimera—a mythical illusion that can never be achieved.

Alesch et al. (2001) nevertheless argue that business owners do recover following even very severe disaster impacts, although to varying degrees. Their criteria for assessing the extent of business recovery include the following: (1) the organization is still in business and is doing at least as well as it was before the disaster; (2) even though it may not be as profitable as before, the business has successfully adapted to the new post-disaster economic environment; (3) the business is at least surviving, even if it is not totally viable; and (4) the owner is able to maintain his or her financial resources, even if he or she has been forced to branch out into another type of economic activity. These recovery indicators allow for the fact that an *owner* can continue in business and even eventually make a profit, despite the fact that the original *business* may no longer be in existence. The Alesch et al. research also emphasizes that permanent closure following disasters is not, in and of itself, an indicator of disaster-induced failure; rather, in light of new post-disaster circumstances, it can be a wise strategic business decision. Unfortunately, however, according to their studies, many business owners simply refuse to acknowledge that their circumstances have been radically altered by disaster, Instead of adapting, they continue to pump money into enterprises that have essentially no possibility of success—a pattern that Alesch et al. refer to as the "dead business walking" syndrome.

Factors Affecting Business Recovery

Business recovery outcomes following disasters can be thought of as the result of a combination of vulnerability and resilience factors. This conceptualization recognizes that even among businesses that are vulnerable and that suffer loss and disruption, recovery trajectories can differ because some businesses are more able than others to cope with losses and to adapt during the recovery process.

Vulnerability Factors for Poor Post-Disaster Business Outcomes

The existing literature on businesses and disasters has identified several factors that appear to make businesses more vulnerable to negative outcomes (for more general discussions on these factors, see Alesch, Taylor, Ghanty, & Nagy, 1993; Alesch et al., 2001; Dahlhamer, 1998; Drabek, 1994; Tierney & Webb, 2006; Webb et al., 2000). As discussed earlier in the section on business vulnerability, some types of firms are more vulnerable than others even during non-disaster times, as indicated, for example, by their higher propensity to fail. Disasters only serve to exacerbate these inherent vulnerabilities. Thus, studies show that smaller businesses are at larger risk for poor recovery outcomes than larger ones. Dahlhamer (1998) suggests that the difficulties that small businesses experience following disasters are related to a pattern that has been identified in the broader literature on organizations, termed the "liability of smallness" (see Baum & Oliver, 1991), which makes small businesses more likely to fail and less likely to be profitable than their larger counterparts.

Also showing continuity with general research on more general business risk factors, it appears that post-disaster recovery outcomes also differ according to economic sector. Businesses in the wholesale and retail sectors seem particularly vulnerable to disasters, no doubt owing in part to the high competitiveness and normally high rates of business failure and turnover within that sector. Construction-related businesses tend to enjoy higher revenues in the aftermath of disasters even though those effects may be short-lived (Dahlhamer & Tierney, 1998).

With respect to post-disaster recovery, it is again important to point out that recovery processes and outcomes are affected not only by the direct physical impacts businesses experience at the time of the disaster, but also by the ways in which disasters create longer-term problems for business owners. Those problems can include extended periods of business interruption, difficulties with shipping and receiving products, revenue declines due to loss of customers, and other operational problems. Research on long-term recovery following the Loma Prieta earthquake and Hurricane Andrew indicated that such problems were very common after both disasters and that they were significant predictors of poor recovery outcomes years after those events (Tierney & Webb, 2006, in press).

In a related vein, even undamaged businesses can experience recovery-related difficulties if they happen to be located in especially hard-hit areas where damage is extensive (Dahlhamer, 1998). This is particularly true in situations in which businesses are interdependent with one another—as many businesses are—and when businesses depend on local foot traffic for their livelihoods. For example, if a large grocery store is the "anchor" business in a shopping center that contains other smaller businesses people typically visit when they shop for groceries, and if that store is destroyed, those smaller businesses will also suffer. One of the most serious recovery-related problems in New Orleans following Hurricane Katrina is that for many individual businesses, future survival will depend on the extent to which not only residents and workers, but also other businesses, return to the city. Individual businesses depend critically on robust local business ecologies. The initial returnees to the city will face an uphill battle to recover, and without critical mass of consumers, workers, and other enterprises that are back in operation, business recovery outcomes will likely be very poor.

Business Resilience Factors

Few studies on businesses directly address the question of what makes some businesses more resilient than others in the face of disasters. Nonetheless, based on the literature, it is possible to identify in at least a preliminary way a number of resilience factors that seem to make a difference for recovery processes and outcomes. Following Rose (2004), resilience can be seen as having two components, which he terms inherent and adaptive. Inherent resilience factors consist of business characteristics that help to cushion or mitigate the effects of disasters on business operations. The concept of adaptive resilience refers to other factors, including decisions made by business owners, that increase business options and business adaptability in the aftermath of disasters.

Some proportion of inherent business resilience stems simply from being less vulnerable in the first place—that is, businesses can be said to be more inherently resilient if they possess fewer of the vulnerability factors discussed above. Inherent resilience can thus be associated with larger business size; being in better financial condition when the disaster strikes; doing business during periods of economic expansion and in more robust economic niches, rather than fragile ones; having a diversified market base, as opposed to an exclusively local one; and taking steps to mitigate damage and disruption and ensure business continuity, rather than simply engaging in workplace preparedness.

Inherent resilience is also related to the relationship between business disruption and income streams. Certain types of businesses, such as those that provide unique, nonsubstitutable services, are more resilient than those that provide substitutable ones. In this respect, establishments such as restaurants and hotels lack inherent resilience; losses from rooms not rented and meals not served can never be recovered. In contrast, many businesses can recoup their losses through stepped-up production once their operations resume.

Adaptive resilience, which Rose defines as "ability in crisis due to ingenuity or extra effort" (2004, p. 42), consists of factors that increase owners' ability to contain negative disaster impacts and increase recovery options. In his research on resilience, Rose (2004) points to such factors as a business's ability to overcome lifeline service disruption by instituting conservation measures or by locating alterative sources for needed services (generators when electricity is lost, bottled water when water systems fail, etc.), noting that "[i]n the aftermath of a disaster, people behave in a more urgent manner and are more likely to call forth ingenuity" (2004, p. 46). In other words, they cope, improvise, and innovate.

In their research, Alesch et al. (2001) also address issues of inherent and adaptive resilience—but more explicitly from the point of view of the business owner and actions he or she may take before, during, and after disasters. With respect to the inherent dimension of resilience, they underscore, for example, the importance of what they term "management mitigation," or "management techniques used to reduce both exposure and vulnerability through smart business practices" (p. 25). Such techniques include seeking to increase customer diversity, storing inventories in multiple locations, doing business out of more than one location, and backing up and otherwise protecting critical business records.

Alesch et al. (2001) place equal emphasis on adaptive resilience, or business owner capacity to innovate and respond realistically to new economic conditions following disasters. They emphasize that while virtually all businesses struggle to remain viable after they experience disaster-related losses and disruption, many struggle while at the same time failing to recognize how the disaster event itself has altered the operating climate for the business. For example, if there has been so much residential damage that the business's clientele has moved elsewhere (perhaps never to return), it makes little sense to reopen in the same location. If a business enterprise depends on selling luxury items, when customers have no or only limited funds for discretionary purposes, the business will be in jeopardy. Alesch et al. stress that owners must objectively assess their post-disaster chances of survival and profitability. The more resilient businesses are those that are alert to adverse changes and able to adapt—even if that means ceasing operations or moving into an entirely new line of business. Owners who succumb to the "dead business walking" syndrome will likely find themselves much worse off, both with respect to business viability and with respect to their own personal finances.

Governmental Action and Business Recovery

As noted earlier, businesses are dependent in many ways on actions that their communities undertake (or fail to) before, during, and after disasters. To appreciate the significance of governmental and community capacity, one only needs to think of the immense additional losses suffered by businesses in New Orleans following Hurricane Katrina that were due not to the disaster event but rather to the city's lack of fire-fighting capability and its inability to provide even minimal security protection in the first days after the hurricane. In contrast, following the 1989 Loma Prieta earthquake, the San Francisco fire department was able to contain fires that were burning in the city's Marina district, despite broken water lines, low water pressure, and the failure of the city's auxiliary fire-fighting water supply system through the innovative use of a portable water system, thus saving both residential units and business properties (Scawthorn, Porter, & Blackburn, 1992).

As noted earlier, many business losses stem directly from damage and loss of capacity in lifeline systems, including transportation lifelines. Following the Northridge earthquake, for example, Gordon, Richardson, and Davis (1997) found that approximately 23% of overall business interruption losses were attributable to transportation system disruption.[9] Businesses are critically dependent upon community-wide mitigation, preparedness, response, and recovery strategies for their own survival. Indeed, business owners should be very concerned about the status of their communities' comprehensive emergency management efforts, since their livelihoods depend on such efforts.

Just as businesses benefit from community adoption of pre-disaster mitigation and preparedness measures and from community-level response effectiveness, they also benefit when their communities employ knowledge and foresight during the post-event recovery process. Unfortunately, while most communities have developed disaster *response* plans, the vast majority have done little in the way of *pre-disaster recovery planning*. Such planning is badly needed, because once a major disaster occurs, there is little time to develop such plans de novo, as well as a greater potential for poor decision making. Currently, except for a very small number of exceptional cases—Los Angeles, for example, has been engaged in pre-event planning for post-event recovery for nearly 20 years—communities will have no choice but to improvise and engage in ad hoc decision making for recovery. In such situations, businesses will be faced with having to press to have their post-disaster recovery needs met, even as they struggle to stay afloat.

---

[9] These same researchers estimated that total business interruption losses following Northridge totaled approximately $6.5 billion—a substantial sum even when compared with the estimated $30 billion in structural damage that was caused by the earthquake.

More than 20 years ago, based on their analyses of recovery following fourteen different disaster events, Rubin, Sapirstein, and Burbee (1985) developed a series of empirical generalizations regarding factors that affect community recovery outcomes. Their work emphasized the importance of three general attributes—personal leadership, knowledge of appropriate recovery actions, and the ability to act—that local governments must possess in order to facilitate community recovery. Recovery chances for individual businesses and business districts depend in important ways on appropriate government action. With respect to post-disaster recovery strategies, Berke, Kartez, and Wenger (1993) emphasize that recovery processes and outcomes are influenced by a range of factors, key among which are (1) public participation in recovery decision making; (2) horizontal community integration, or the extent to which strong networks exist among various community organizations and institutions; and (3) vertical integration, or the extent to which strong ties exist among local communities, higher levels of government, and other extra-community resource providers. Obviously, communities possessing strong networks along both horizontal and vertical dimensions are in a much better position to successfully manage post-disaster recovery—including business recovery. Other studies suggest that the implementation of community-wide pre-disaster recovery plans following disasters both speeds up the process of housing recovery and also helps to ensure that mitigation of future hazards is integrated into the recovery process (Wu & Lindell, 2004; see also Spangle and Associates, 1991). Although no comparable research has been done on business recovery, it can be hypothesized that pre-event planning also has a positive effect on business recovery.

Other recent research points to the ways in which businesses depend upon early recovery decisions made at the local community level regarding repair and restoration priorities. Stephanie Chang and her collaborators (see Miles & Chang, 2003) have recently begun research to explore ways of optimizing the recovery process through organizational and community decision making that takes into account interdependencies among infrastructural elements, households, neighborhoods, businesses, and local economies. Based on extensive reviews of the literature and analyses of their own data on disaster recovery, they have developed agent-based simulation models that show how both pre-disaster community policies (e.g., policies regarding code adoption, pre-disaster recovery planning) and response and early recovery decisions affect recovery trajectories (and their interrelationships) at various levels of analysis. Their simulations indicate, for example, that pre-disaster mitigation measures directed at lifeline systems significantly shorten the recovery period for both businesses and households. Another finding points to the importance of transportation system restoration following disasters, because so many other early recovery activities depend upon having transportation access to affected communities.

These models and scenarios represent the first-ever attempt to analyze recovery processes and outcomes across various domains, including critical infrastructure elements, housing, neighborhood viability, jobs, and business and economic recovery, and to understand interrelationships among these different domains throughout the recovery process. The aim of this research is to develop decision-support systems that will enable those who attempt to manage post-disaster recovery to visualize the outcomes of different pre- and post-event decisions. Unless and until such models are improved, refined, and adopted by local communities and other levels of government, communities—and their businesses—must rely either on (practically nonexistent) pre-disaster recovery plans or on post-disaster improvisation.

Hurricane Katrina was the first catastrophic disaster event to strike the United States in a century. It will be important to chart business recovery processes and outcomes following this unprecedented disaster event. As of this writing, there is little evidence of systematic, integrated, comprehensive planning for short- and long-term recovery needs in New Orleans and other heavily-damaged communities—either with respect to households and neighborhoods or with respect to businesses and business districts. Some early news is quite discouraging. For example, outside contractors are routinely being employed to engage in recovery activities that businesses in the affected region are quite able to undertake. These contract arrangements, many of which have been made on a no-bid basis, run counter to Stafford Act provisions stipulating that strategies should be put in place to ensure job and livelihood recovery in disaster-affected areas.[10] Practices such as the use of outside contractors do nothing to help local businesses get back on their feet following disasters, and they also create resentment among victim populations. And again, had the intergovernmental response to the hurricane been more rapid and effective, damage, disruption, and losses could have been contained, and businesses would have a better chance of recovering.

What Should Make a Difference for Business Recovery, But Does Not

Some factors that might be expected to have an influence on business recovery outcomes make essentially no difference. Although it seems intuitive that the greater the damage to a business property, the more difficulty the business will have in its struggle to recover, this is not the case. As discussed elsewhere in this chapter, business recovery is determined by a broad set of factors that go well beyond the degree of physical property damage. On the one hand, a business whose property has been completely destroyed but that has access to an alternative business location may suffer little disruption as a consequence of a disaster. On the other, businesses can experience little or no direct damage but still suffer prolonged disruption and high losses. Moreover, at least some research suggests that, as odd as it may seem, physical damage per se is not even a significant factor in business *losses*, let alone recovery. In a study of businesses affected by the 2001 Nisqually earthquake, for example, important determinants of total business losses included size, with small businesses being more vulnerable to loss; occupancy tenure, in which renters are more vulnerable; and neighborhood effects, such as loss of foot traffic or the stigma of being located in a high-damage area. This study found that physical damage was not a significant predictor of business loss (Chang & Falit-Baiamonte, 2003).

Another factor that fails to predict recovery outcomes is the degree to which businesses engage in preparedness activities prior to the occurrence of the disaster. This is not to say that no anecdotal examples can be found of businesses that survived and thrived as a result of good pre-event planning, nor is it an argument against enhancing business preparedness for extreme events. Rather, research finds that *in the aggregate and controlling for other factors*, standard recommended preparedness measures have little impact on short- and long-term business recovery outcomes (Webb et al., 2000). There are likely several reasons for this counterintuitive effect. One possible reason is that, as indicated in various studies (see, e.g., Dahlhamer & D'Souza, 1997) the majority of businesses actually do very little to prepare for disasters—so much so that in surveys even the "more prepared" businesses typically score quite low on preparedness measures (Cavanaugh, 2000). However, the lack of association between workplace preparedness and recovery outcomes is more likely due to a combination of other factors. As noted above, at the most fundamental level, preparedness appears to have no impact on the size of actual disaster losses (Chang & Falit-Baiamonte, 2003). In addition, as

---

[10] See Robert T. Stafford Disaster Assistance and Emergency Relief Act 42 U.S.C. (307) 5150, "use of local firms and individuals."

discussed earlier, many sources of business loss, disruption, and negative recovery outcomes, such as infrastructure failures, residential dislocation, and the quality of community-level response and recovery efforts, are essentially beyond the control of the individual business owner. Moreover, recommendations for what businesses should do to prepare for disasters may themselves be flawed. As Alesch et al. (2001) note, most business preparedness guidance stresses protecting the business property and its contents, developing disaster response plans, stockpiling supplies, and taking other steps designed to protect life-safety and reduce direct property losses. The DRC surveys on businesses suggest that these are the types of measures businesses are most likely to undertake, if they do anything at all in the way of preparedness. Guidance on planning and worker safety generally does not address other issues, such as what to do in the event that a disaster radically alters the overall business climate or results in a decline in demand for the goods and services a business offers. Nor does most preparedness literature provide suggestions on how to cope through months and perhaps even years of disaster-induced community disruption. In short, most guidelines for business disaster preparedness do little to help prepare business owners for the large array of real-world problems they will face in the aftermath of disasters.[11]

Although the stated purpose of post-disaster assistance is to help businesses recover, the various forms of assistance that are available to help recover also appear to have little impact on how businesses fare in the aftermath of disasters. Neither formal sources of aid such as Small Business Administration disaster loans and insurance nor informal sources of assistance, such as financial help from relatives, make much difference in recovery outcomes for disaster-affected businesses. Indeed, surveys following the Northridge earthquake even suggested that the more aid sources businesses used following the earthquake, the less likely they were to report positive recovery outcomes (Dahlhamer & Tierney, 1998).[12] The lack of a relationship between post-disaster aid and business recovery, which has been found consistently across a range of studies, is likely due to several factors. First, the types of aid that are available to businesses generally come in the form of loans, either from agencies like the Small Business Administration or from banks. This automatically leads to increased debt for the business owner. Second, even if aid is obtained, it typically covers only a portion of the losses businesses experience in disasters. Third, no amount of assistance can offset problems such as a loss of customers, disaster-induced declines in demand for goods and services, or losses associated with the disruption of local business ecologies. Nor can assistance reverse pre-disaster trends that affect business fortunes over the long term.[13]

Many businesses, particularly small ones, do not carry insurance that provides protection in the event of a disaster. In other cases, owners believe that they have adequate insurance coverage, only to find that the damage and disruption they experience in disasters is not included in their insurance policies—or worse yet, that they have been misled by insurers. For example, based on their interviews, Alesch et al. (2001) recounted numerous problems business

---

[11] There are, of course exceptions. Alesch and his colleagues have developed more-comprehensive guidance for business owners, and the "Open for Business" program developed by the Institute for Business and Home Safety highlights numerous factors businesses should consider in seeking to survive the impacts of disasters.

[12] One likely reason for this relationship is that businesses that are having the most difficulty following disasters continue to struggle and seek multiple forms of assistance—even when such assistance ultimately does nothing to help the business recover.

[13] For example, if a business is located in a damaged central business district, and if even before the disaster occurred, customers had already begun to shop in outlying areas, perhaps for lower prices and better parking, that pattern will continue, and may well intensify, after the disaster. Aid to individual businesses will have no effect on business recovery under such circumstances.

owners experienced with respect to insurance, such as finding out belatedly that they had been sold the wrong type of policy—one that did not cover their losses; being covered but never compensated because the insurance company went out of businesses; and having insurance that covered only a fraction of business losses. Even businesses that are adequately covered with respect to damage may lack business interruption insurance. Insurance problems will be numerous and complex following Hurricane Katrina, since so many property owners who had insurance were only protected from wind damage, but not from hurricane-related flooding, and since business interruption is likely to be very protracted for many business enterprises.

FUTURE RESEARCH NEEDS

Impacts, Recovery, and Issues of Scale

As the U.S. Gulf region and Florida struggle to recover from Hurricanes Katrina, Rita, and Wilma, it is important to recall that most knowledge on disasters, their impacts, and household, business, and community recovery is not based on studies of truly catastrophic disaster events. It is widely recognized in the field of disaster research that just as disasters are not just "big emergencies," catastrophic events are not just "big disasters." As Quarantelli indicates with respect to disasters and catastrophes (2005a, p. 333–334):

> ... there are both qualitative and quantitative differences in the references of the two terms .... In a catastrophe, most/all of the total residential community is impacted, making it impossible for the homeless to go to friends and relatives who are in a similar situation ... most of the facilities and operational bases of emergency operations are themselves impacted ... local officials are unable to undertake their usual work roles not only in the crisis period, but also into the recovery period ... most of the everyday community functions are sharply and simultaneously interrupted across-the-board.

These are the exact conditions that Hurricane Katrina produced. With so much infrastructure and property damage, disruption, and displacement of victims, and with such immense mitigation-related challenges, recovery will be extremely difficult.

Well-informed decision making is needed that can take into account interdependencies among critical infrastructure elements, as well as among units within the social structure. Investments in recovery much be prioritized and coordinated—a massive challenge with which this nation has had little experience.

More research is needed on Katrina and other catastrophic events and their broader effects on communities and regions. Such research could reveal that what is currently known about businesses and disasters may not be scalable to catastrophic events. If we do not develop a knowledge base on the distinctive challenges presented by catastrophic and near-catastrophic disasters, we have little chance of managing the consequences of such events.

Cross-Societal and Comparative Research on Businesses and Disasters

With the exception of discussions on the economic impacts of the Kobe earthquake, this chapter has focused almost exclusively on research that has been conducted on U.S. disasters by U.S. researchers. This could give readers the mistaken impression that businesses have not been studied in any societies except the United States and Japan. There has been a good deal of research on private-sector enterprises in other societies. However, a considerable amount of that work has focused on how business enterprises have contributed to disasters, especially environmental ones, rather than on business preparedness, response, recovery, and other topics discussed here (see, e.g., Shrivastava, 1987, on Bhopal). On the basis of studies that have been translated into English, it appears that research in other societies has tended to consist of onetime studies on specific disasters, making it difficult to amass cumulative findings and discern patterns over time. International periodicals, such as the *Journal of Contingencies and Crisis Management*, published by Blackwell, occasionally publish studies on businesses and disasters, but they also include studies on many other topics not related to business issues.

As this chapter has shown, research on U.S. businesses has uncovered a number of factors that appear to work fairly consistently to make businesses either more or less vulnerable to disasters. However, this research cannot be generalized to other societies because societies differ along so many dimensions, including economic systems, business–state relationships, financing mechanisms, availability and types of hazard insurance, societal capacity to manage hazards and disasters, and the availability of post-disaster aid for businesses. Without a great deal more comparative, cross-societal research, it will be very difficult to reach conclusions regarding business vulnerability and resilience and other topics discussed in this chapter.

Integrating Disaster Studies and Organizational Research

As preceding discussions show, there is a great deal to be gained by analyzing issues facing businesses in disasters in the context of broader research on organizations. For example, the concept of the "liability of smallness," which predicts that small businesses are more fragile and less resilient during normal times, is also applicable to the study of disaster-stricken businesses. However, other streams of research on business vulnerability and on how organizations manage risks and cope with turbulent environments have not been integrated into business disaster research. In the field of organizational safety and risk, the contrasting theoretical perspectives of "normal accidents" (Perrow, 1999) and "high-reliability organizations" (Roberts, 1989; Roberts, Rousseau, & La Porte, 1993) appear to be directly related to questions of business vulnerability and resilience in disasters, but disaster researchers tend not to employ such frameworks or cite the sizable literature on these opposing perspectives (for a direct empirical comparison of these paradigms, see Sagan, 1993). Do the factors that make business enterprises vulnerable to normal accidents also make them more vulnerable to disasters? Can normal-accidents concepts such as linearity and tight coupling help us better understand how and why some systems fail during disasters and how such effects might be mitigated? Can the study of the normal accidents literature provide insights on how to prevent cascading failures that could result from disasters of all types, including those produced by willful acts? Is the high-reliability concept applicable to both organizational safety and disaster resilience?

Similarly, general social science theories on organizations and organizational processes are seldom employed in studies on organizational behavior during and after disasters. One important exception is Lee Clarke's book *Acceptable Risk: Making Decisions in a Toxic Environment* (1989), which employed "garbage can" theory, framed at the interorganizational level, to explain how organizations responded following a hazardous materials release in a state office building. Another exception is Diane Vaughan's acclaimed study on the factors that contributed to the space shuttle Challenger accident, *The Challenger Launch Decision* (Vaughan, 1996), which attempts to explain how and why organizations claiming to be committed to safety drift gradually begin permitting unsafe practices. Despite the fact that Vaughan's perspective is highly applicable to both public- and private-sector organizations, it seems to have had only a small impact on the disaster research field.

Focusing on other research in the organizational literature, research on businesses and disasters indicates that the decisions that business owners undertake before, during, and after disasters can be critical for business viability. Yet disaster studies tend not to draw upon research in fields such as business administration and organizational behavior that focus on leadership and decision-making styles within business organizations, particularly with respect to risk management and crisis-related decisions (see, e.g., Mitroff, Pauchant, Finney, & Pearson, 1989; Mitroff & Pauchant, 1990; Pauchant & Mitroff, 1992). What can disaster researchers learn from the crisis management literature that might provide insights on how businesses approach and manage disaster-related problems? If organizational leaders have a high tolerance for risk during normal times, do they also make riskier decisions regarding disaster loss reduction? Do businesses that are recognized for their good management practices fare better in disasters? Is a business entrepreneur who has a track record of innovation and adaptability to changing business environments also better equipped to cope when disasters strike? How can the literature on management and business leadership inform the study of businesses in disasters?

Knowledge Transfer and Applications: The Practical Literature on Business Disaster Management

For decades, consultants and consulting companies have offered guidance on business disaster preparedness and business continuity and recovery planning. Government agencies such as FEMA have also sought to raise awareness and suggest best practices for business disaster management. The field of disaster business consulting grew by many orders of magnitude in the years and months prior to December 31, 1999, as businesses worldwide struggled to reduce and cope with potential problems associated with Y2K, or the "millennium bug." Y2K forced many businesses to think for the first time about how to identify and protect their most critical business functions and how to address supply chain vulnerabilities. Under the scrutiny of the U.S. Congress and regulators, both public-sector organizations and private businesses associated with elements in the critical infrastructure, such as transportation, utility lifelines, and banking and finance, undertook massive programs to ensure continuity of operations during the Y2K turnover.

The September 11 attacks provided a further stimulus for business preparedness and continuity planning. While the Pentagon was also targeted, the 9/11 attacks focused primarily on businesses and on the iconic Twin Towers; this caused great alarm among many businesses that also considered themselves potential targets, particularly those located in tall structures. Like Y2K, 9/11 further stimulated business loss-reduction efforts.

As a result of these previous crises, books, manuals, toolkits, checklists, and training programs have burgeoned in recent years (for representative publications, see FEMA, 1998; Gustin, 2004; Hiles, 2000; Institute of Business and Home Safety, 2005; Laye, 2002; Shaw, 1999; Wallace & Webber, 2004). Those who provide business loss-reduction solutions have their own professional association, the Association of Contingency Planners, and a number of professional journals, such as the *Disaster Recovery Journal*. Despite the fact that guidance now exists in great quantity, there have been essentially no empirical studies regarding the quality and potential effectiveness of such efforts in actual disaster situations. There are, of course, anecdotal accounts and single case studies on "success stories," but testimonials are not the same as systematic research.

The activities and visibility of the business loss reduction industry raise many questions for further research. What types of businesses are most likely to use special consulting services, and what types of services are typically offered? For example, do consultants tend to provide more assistance with IT-related issues, such as data backups and "hot sites," or is the guidance they offer more comprehensive? How do businesses choose among alternative services and service providers? On what criteria do they base their decisions? To what extent does current business preparedness practice draw upon empirical research on businesses and disasters or on studies of organizational crisis management?

It would be useful to carry out research on randomly selected businesses that followed particular types of guidance or used particular consulting services, and then later experienced disasters, in order to determine the extent to which selected loss-reduction measures actually made a difference for business continuity and viability. Perhaps some measures are more effective than others. Along other lines, guidance to businesses may have unintended consequences. Perhaps steps taken to reduce disaster losses bring additional benefits even if no disasters occur. If that is the case, it would be important to document those additional contributions to business organizations. Since businesses and particularly large ones frequently spend substantial amounts of money on business consulting and continuity services, it would be interesting to conduct research on the extent to which various measures businesses adopt turn out to be cost-effective when assessed over the long term.

CHAPTER 17

Organizational Adaptation
to Disaster

GARY A. KREPS AND SUSAN LOVEGREN BOSWORTH

> Organized responses which may range from small emergent work groups to large, complex, and
> bureaucratic organizations are not only the primary agencies through which communities respond
> to disasters, they also provide the shaping contexts for most individual responses. (Kreps, 1978,
> p. 67)

The major focus of this chapter is twofold. We first consider what has been learned about organizational adaptation to disasters from original field studies by the Disaster Research Center (DRC) during the initial 20 years of its existence (1963–1983). We then examine a series of secondary data analyses (1982–2001) that we, along with our graduate and undergraduate students, completed using data archives produced primarily from these studies and maintained by the DRC. The groundwork established by what amounts to several decades of original field studies and follow-up archival analyses has continued to inform DRC field research on preparedness for and response to natural, technological, and willful disasters by organizations in both the public (e.g., Tierney, 1985, 1993) and private sectors (e.g., Webb, Tierney, & Dahlhammer, 2000). Arguably the most compelling example of continuity from the earliest to the most recent work within the DRC tradition is the Center's major study of organizational adaptation following the September 11, 2001 terrorist attack on the World Trade Center (Kendra & Wachtendorf, 2003; Kendra et al., 2003; Wachtendorf, 2004).

What has been learned about organizational adaptation within the DRC tradition provides an excellent foundation for implementing what we propose later in this chapter as an integrated research strategy to increase readiness for anticipated and improvised responses to disasters. That strategy captures organizational adaptations at role, organizational, and multiorganizational levels of analysis. The audience for the proposed integrated strategy includes both hazards and disaster researchers and emergency management practitioners. The first and longest section of the chapter argues that knowledge about organizational adaptation has evolved continuously from original DRC field research to follow-up archival studies of our own, and to more recent DRC primary research through reliance on core sociological concepts (Bosworth & Kreps, 1986; Dynes, 1970; Kreps, 1985; Kreps & Bosworth, 1993; Wachtendorf, 2004; Webb, 1998; Weller & Quarantelli, 1973). These concepts include formal organizing, collective behavior, and role enactment and their underpinning in even more basic conceptualizations of social action and social order (see in particular Kreps, 1989c and Wachtendorf, 2004). The initial

DRC TYPOLOY OF ORGANIZED RESPONSES

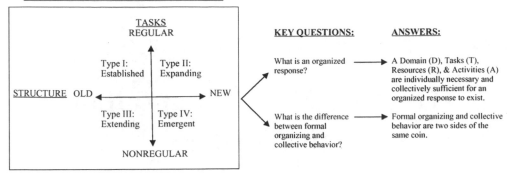

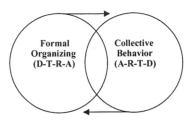

FIGURE 17.1. From a simple typology to a formal structural code.

DRC tool to capture organizational adaptation was a deceptively simple typology of organized responses. What has come to be known as the DRC typology (see Fig. 17.1) has not only stood the test of time (Brouillette & Quarantelli, 1971; Dynes, 1970; Kreps, 1978, 1985; Quarantelli, 1996; Stallings, 1978; Wachtendorf, 2004; Webb, 1998; Weller & Quarantelli, 1973), but it has also led to more elaborate understandings about how organized responses emerge, link with each other, and flexibly adapt during disasters in both planned and improvised ways. The second section of the chapter connects briefly what continues to be learned about organizational adaptation from DRC-based studies to broader research issues about disaster preparedness and response (for recent summaries of the broader research literature see Mileti, 1999, Chapter 7; Tierney, Lindell, & Perry, 2001).

By building on the foundation of what is known about organizational adaptation to disasters, both within the DRC tradition and more generally in hazards and disaster research, the final section of the chapter offers an integrated strategy for research and application that connects most directly Gary Webb's contemporary work on role improvisation within our own research program (Webb, 1998, 2002a) with related recent research on planned and unplanned organizational improvisations by, respectively, David Mendonca (2001, in press; Mendonca & Wallace, 2002, 2004) and Tricia Wachtendorf (Kendra & Wachtendorf, 2003; Kendra et al., 2003; Wachtendorf, 2004). Noteworthy is that Webb's research includes archival studies of primarily natural disasters as well as some technological events and major civil disturbances; Mendonca's work combines both more selective archival studies of natural and technological events with primary data collection on the September 11, 2001 terrorist attack on the World Trade Center; and Wachtendorf's work is based on a major DRC study of the same 9/11 World Trade Center attack. Given the broad range of complementary data captured by Webb,

Mendonca, and Wachtendorf, we believe a firm foundation has been established to expand and codify knowledge about organizational adaptation through more highly structured studies and computational models of disaster preparedness and response. Such knowledge, we also believe, can be used productively by emergency management practitioners in preparing for both anticipated and improvised responses to natural, technological, and willful events (Kreps, 2001).

ORGANIZED RESPONSE TO DISASTER: FROM THE DRC TYPOLOGY TO A FORMAL STRUCTURAL CODE

There was a tendency in most disaster research within the social sciences from World War II until the founding of the Disaster Research Center (DRC) at the Ohio State University in 1963 to describe disaster responses at either the individual or overall community levels of analysis (Kreps, 1981, 1984; Quarantelli & Dynes, 1977). But both the founders of the DRC and those funding its studies believed that learning more about distinct types of organizational adaptations and their interconnections was essential. Structurally speaking, major disasters exhibit stunning complexity as existing groups and organizations restructure to meet disaster demands, new groups and organizations emerge, and both existing and new entities become parts of broader social networks of collective action. Unraveling that complexity was and remains a central issue at the DRC and within the broader hazards and disaster research community.

The Emergence of Organization: Formal Organizing and Collective Behavior Are Two Sides of the Same Coin

An important start was made on what, as noted earlier, has historically been called the DRC typology of organized disaster responses. As noted in Figure 17.1, the typology clusters into a simple fourfold table the range of discrete organized responses that can be observed within a community during a disaster. Type I organized responses are termed established because they exist prior to an event and much of what they do is expected (e.g., hospitals; law enforcement and fire fighting units; public utilities; departments of public works; mass media; military units; and specialized units dealing with chemical, biological, or radioactive hazards). Type II organized responses are called expanding because while much of what they do is expected as well, their core structures change from a small cadre of professional staff to a much larger unit of volunteers (e.g., local community emergency management agencies, Red Cross chapters, Salvation Army units). Type III organized responses are called extending because while they exist prior to an event, much of what they do is not predetermined (e.g., other governmental agencies, small businesses, larger firms, social clubs, public service organizations, religious organizations). Finally, type IV organized responses are termed emergent because both their existence and activities are ad hoc and therefore unique to the event.

Studies of all four types of organized responses have been undertaken under DRC auspices as well as by many other researchers over several decades (for summaries see Drabek, 1986; Dynes, 1970; Mileti, Drabek, & Haas, 1975; Quarantelli & Dynes, 1970; Tierney, 1985, 1993;

Tierney, Lindell, & Perry, 2001; Wenger, Quarantelli, & Dynes, 1989). Much has been learned about what they do and how they relate structurally to each other as parts of broader community response systems. As noted in Figure 17.1, of particular interest to us in reconstructing hundreds of cases of organized responses during the immediate emergency periods of natural, technological, and willful disasters have been two key questions. While these questions are most directly relevant to emergent organized responses (type IV), we think they apply whenever the existence of an organized response cannot be taken for granted. The first question is: What is an organized response? Building on the DRC typology, the answer we have developed during our archival research program is simply this: A fully organized response must have a Domain (D), Tasks (T), Resources (R), and Activities (A). A domain is an external representation of a self-contained unit and its reason for being. Tasks are an internal representation of a division of labor for the enactment of human activities. Resources are individual capacities and collective technologies of human populations. Activities are conjoined actions of individuals and social units in chronological time and physical space.

It is because "organization" is such a fundamental concept in Sociology that definitions of its core properties must be subjects of sustained academic discussion and debate (see, e.g. Kreps, 1989c, Chapters 7, 8, and 10; Kreps, 1994). While a series of theoretical and methodological issues remain critical, their consideration does not belie the necessity for disaster researchers and emergency management practitioners alike to know what, in fact, an organized response is, how an organized response is different from other types of collective action, and how organized and other types of collective action interrelate. It is not a matter of being organized or disorganized at community, regional, or societal levels. It is not a matter of being organized formally or informally at any level of societal response. It is a matter of systemic adaptation to disaster that includes both organized and many other forms of collective action that, depending on the circumstances at hand, are more or less efficient and effective.

We believe that disaster researchers and emergency management practitioners would agree that an organized response requires at some point external recognition as a purposive and self-contained entity (D), that an organized response requires clarity within that entity about a division of labor (T), and that an organized response cannot be contemplated without reference to human and material resources (R) and the conjoined actions of both individuals and small to larger social units. Simply put, a structural code of (D), (T), (R), and (A) builds on what is both basic to social scientists and highly familiar to emergency management practitioners about the concept of organization.

The second question is: What is the difference between formal organizing and collective behavior? Building on the DRC typology, the answer we have developed from our archival research program is that capturing how an organized response evolves during a disaster requires drawing simultaneously on classic sociological ideas about formal organizing and collective behavior. These ideas predate modern disaster research of the post-World War II era and they remain central to this research specialty and the social sciences generally (Kreps, 1985, 1989c; Quarantelli & Dynes, 1977; Weller & Quarantelli, 1973). Using the structural code described above, formal organizing begins with clear understandings about domains and tasks (i.e., what is being done, by whom, and how) before resources are mobilized and activities take place. The sequencing of organizational elements is D-T-R-A. With collective behavior, activities take place and resources are mobilized before such understandings exist. The sequencing of organizational elements is A-R-T-D. The structural differences between formal organizing and collective behavior are depicted graphically in Figure 17.1. These structural arrangements illustrate a continuum between formal organizing (D-T-R-A) and collective behavior (A-R-T-D) that captures the essential relationship between these two ideas. As each element comes into

TABLE 17.1. A Formal Organizing/Collective Behavior Continuum

Organizational Forms	Logical Continuum (0 midpoint)	Number of Forms	Organized Responses Identified Through Archival Analysis	
D-T-R-A	6 (+3)	(1)	167	(167)
D-T-A-R			5	
D-R-T-A	5 (+2)	(3)	53	(59)
T-D-R-A			1	
D-R-A-T			27	
D-A-T-R			2	
T-R-D-A	4 (+1)	(5)	4	(100)
T-D-A-R			—	
R-D-T-A			67	
D-A-R-T			1	
T-R-A-D			21	
T-A-D-R			—	
R-D-A-T	3 (0)	(6)	12	(39)
R-T-D-A			4	
A-D-T-R			1	
T-A-R-D			—	
R-A-D-T			15	
R-T-A-D	2 (−1)	(5)	13	(31)
A-D-R-T			1	
A-T-D-R			2	
R-A-T-D			13	
A-T-R-D	1 (−2)	(3)	4	(22)
A-R-D-T			5	
A-R-T-D	0 (−3)	(1)	5	(5)
	Totals	(24)	423	(423)

DOMAIN   An external representation of a self-contained unit and its reason for being
TASKS   An internal representation of a division of labor for the enactment of human activities
RESOURCES   Individual capacities and collective technologies of human populations
ACTIVITIES   Conjoined actions of individuals and social units in chronological time and physical space

place, an organized response reflects varying degrees of formal organizing and collective behavior. The continuum is more fully elaborated on Table 17.1 as a structural code and metric scale. The code and the metric scale depict all possible forms of organizing with D-T-R-A at one end and A-R-T-D at the other.

The key requirement in constructing the code and metric scale is to capture all of the transitivities (i.e., gradations) between formal organizing (D-T-R-A) and collective behavior (A-R-T-D). This can be done in the following way: At the formal organizing end of the continuum D precedes T, R, and A (3 points), T precedes R and A (2 points), and R precedes A (1 point). By giving one point for each conforming transitivity (3 + 2 + 1), formal organizing (D-T-R-A) receives a score of 6 and its direct obverse, collective behavior (A-R-T-D), receives a score of 0. Thus, for example, an organization that begins with a clearly understood domain (D), followed by the implementation of activities (A) then the mobilization of resources (R), and finally the establishment of a task structure (T) is a D-A-R-T form of organizing. Using formal organizing (D-T-R-A) as a reference point in calculating the metric score for a D-A-R-T form, D precedes T, R, and A (3 points), T does not precede R or A (0 points), and R does not precede A (0 points). On the Logical Continuum of Table 17.1, the D-A-R-T form receives three points. This sequencing of elements represents an organizational form that is a blend of formal organizing and collective behavior. Beginning at the collective behavior end of the continuum would simply reverse the scores but not change the distribution in any way. For the six forms that fall in the middle of the continuum, the score remains 3. These forms highlight the balance of formal organizing and collective behavior. By subtracting a constant three points from each derived level of formal organizing or collective behavior, the resulting metric is $+3$ to -3 with a 0 midpoint. A 0 midpoint is useful for highlighting where logically a balance between formal organizing and collective behavior is greatest. Note that each end of the continuum includes one form, but there are increasingly more forms as formal organizing and collective behavior become more balanced.

The metric scale depicted in Table 17.1 has been used over the years during our research program to provide a quantitative measure for describing the process of organizing as we have been able to reconstruct alternative patterns from the DRC archives (see, e.g., Bosworth & Kreps, 1986; Kreps, 1985, 1989c, 1991a; Kreps & Boswoth, 1993; Noon, 2001; Saunders & Kreps, 1987; Webb, 1998, 2002a). The number of each organizational form we have identified through archival analysis is reported in the right column of Table 17.1. Disasters serve as catalysts for observing how individuals and units organize in response to a disaster. The types of organizational forms have been mapped to the DRC typology and have been used to describe and explain social response to disasters (see Kreps & Bosworth, 1993, 1994). A useful illustration of the relationship between an original DRC study and our archival research is Noon's recent (2001) application of the above structural code to the same set of interviews used in an earlier study by Forrest (1973) of an emergent organized response (type IV in the original DRC typology).

> Empirical Case: Following a major urban riot in the United States what came to be called the Interfaith Emergency Center (IEC) evolved from an information hotline to serving as a broker distributing food, clothing, and other services to riot victims. As Noon (2001, pp. 493–497) describes the IEC from Forrest's original case study and his own reconstruction of the same transcribed field interviews used by Forrest, an informal group of local clergy wanted to create an information hotline service that people could access 24 hours a day, 7 days a week. The service was to be staffed by them and housed in a diocesan building offered by an Episcopalian representative of the group because of its adequate telephone set-up, parking, kitchen, and office space (Resources). A news release was prepared announcing the availability of the information service (called the Interfaith Information Center) and then broadcast on the evening news by local television stations (Resources-Domain). Shortly after the local television broadcast calls started coming into the hotline for processing (Resources-Domain-Activities). While it was originally assumed that the majority of calls would simply be requests for information, it quickly became apparent that what was required was a brokerage that could connect individual requests for assistance with community resources and services. With the assistance of a local AFL-CIO (a federation of national and international labor unions) council, an assistance distribution system was set up within the center to dispatch volunteer drivers to 25 collection centers and 21 distribution centers (Resources-Domain-Activities-Tasks). Further departments were also set up and the hotline changed its name (now the Interfaith Emergency Center) to more accurately describe what it was actually doing.

The IEC (an R-D-A-T form in the above structural code) was ad hoc rather than planned: Human and material resources were mobilized before there was clarity about what was going to be done, and activities drove the development of tasks rather than the other way around. The case therefore reveals classic features of collective behavior (Drabek, 1987a; Smelser, 1962; Turner, 1964; Weller & Quarantelli, 1973; Wenger, 1987). On the other hand, the emergence of the IEC was clearly influenced by existing social arrangements, revealing classic bureaucratic features of formal organizing (Drabek & Haas, 1974; Hall, 1962; Scott, 1991; Thompson, 1967; Weber, 1947). In other words, explicit and shared understandings of what was being done and how it was being done evolved quite rapidly during the emergency period (see Thompson, 1967, pp. 51–53 on synthetic groups). The resulting balance between collective behavior and formal organizing represented by this emergent organized response (type IV) is reflected in its metric score. The existence of a domain precedes activities and tasks, but not resources (2 points), tasks follow rather than precede resources and activities (0 points), and resources precede activities (1 point). A total score of 3 minus the constant 3 (see Table 17.1) places the case appropriately at the precise midpoint of the formal organizing-collective behavior metric (R-D-A-T) represented on Table 17.1.

During our archival studies we documented 52 cases of emergent organized responses; the spread of these cases covers the entire range of the formal organizing-collective behavior continuum (14 of the 24 types identified one or more times); and the average score of the 52 cases, falls at the midpoint of the metric (see Saunders & Kreps, 1987). Thus for emergent organized responses (type IV), disaster researchers can rightly conclude that neither formal organizing nor collective behavior dominates the process. Emergency management practitioners can rightly conclude that flexibility is essential because there are many different ways organized collective actions can be improvised.

Both researchers and practitioners are well aware that emergent organized responses represent only a small albeit important part of what goes on during a disaster. In our own archival studies, for example, only about 13% of the well over 400 cases of organized responses we were able to reconstruct from field interviews and documents were emergent (type IV) in the original DRC typology. Another 22% were extending (type III) or expanding (type II), and the remaining 65% were established (type I). While the predominance of data on established organized responses in the DRC archives reflects the primary focus of the original field studies, it also reflects the importance and predetermined involvement of type I responses during disasters. Two conclusions are certain, however: first, describing the range of organized responses during a disaster requires attention to all four types in the DRC typology; second, capturing the interconnections among the four types of organized responses within broader networks of organized responses is essential. The above structural code provides a means of capturing the processual qualities of these multiorganizational response networks.

Multiorganizational Response Networks and the Process of Organizing

Empirical Case: With little forewarning a tornado cut a 7-mile swath through a Northwestern city. The State Air National Guard facilities and planes were badly damaged, as were several blocks of homes and a trailer park. Emergency personnel began responding even before the tornado left the city. Two voluntary agencies were both distributing food, and independently of each other. By the second day after impact their lack of coordination resulted in emergency personnel and victims missing meals. At this point a local emergency management official met with representatives of both agencies, suggesting that they develop a more cooperative effort. The two agencies then worked out an arrangement in which each would be responsible for food distribution on alternative days (Tasks). This resolution was successful and the two units continued to operate separately during the emergency.

Empirical Case: A major volcanic eruption in the northwestern United States created enormous damage from ash fall and flooding. Within minutes of the initial blast the sheriff's office of a less devastated region sent vehicles and deputies to assist the sheriff's office of a severely impacted county with roadblocks (Resources). There is no evidence that the two offices worked in the same locations of a quite large impact area. Several days later the two county sheriffs met with a third county sheriff and officials from numerous local, state, and national organizations for the purpose of coordinating search and rescue regionally. A resulting division of labor linked the two sheriff's offices and other responding organizations engaged in ground search and rescue, flight search and rescue, ground security, debriefing, and developing missing persons lists (Resources-Tasks). Within a short period of time this broader social network became recognized as having responsibility for search and rescue operations in the region (Resources-Tasks-Domain). Despite some external criticism, this entity served as an authoritative decision-making body for 12 days.

The preceding empirical cases are part of a sample of 592 cases of multiorganizational response networks we have reconstructed from archival data, with 462 cases coming from the DRC archives and an additional 130 cases from archival data provided by Thomas Drabek (see Drabek et al., 1981). In the first example, and facilitated by a local emergency management official, two expanding organized responses (type II) reach agreement on a simple division of labor, but otherwise operate separately. With respect to the structural code, then, agreement about tasks (T) links the two units in social space but their activities are not conjoined in chronological time or physical space (absence of A), no joint resources are mobilized (absence of R), and the two units never merge (absence of D). In the second example, two established organized responses (type I) are linked initially by the need for and availability of resources, then become parts of a complex search and rescue domain (D), but operate separately in physical space (absence of A) before and after that operation is set up (T). Indeed, all of the units involved in search and rescue are linked in social space through the presence of a common domain and tasks, but in this case their respective activities are not conjoined in physical space. With respect to the structural code, social space is defined by what organized responses of whatever type do in relation to each other. This is quite different from ideas about conjoined actions in chronological time and physical space (Bates & Peacock, 1989a; Kreps, 1991a; Warriner, 1981).

Four structural questions can be asked about simple to larger and more complex multiorganizational response networks. Does the network involve conjoined action in chronological time and physical space (A)? Does the network evidence a mobilization of human and material resources (R)? Does the network evidence a division of labor that is agreed to by network members (T)? Are the units identified and legitimated externally as parts of an inclusive entity (D)? Our research suggests that affirmative answers to one or more of these four questions reflect different types of organizational adaptation during a disaster (i.e., one to three element types in the structural code), but not necessarily organization itself (i.e., four element types in the structural code).

Developing answers to these questions is not simply an academic exercise. Answers are essential if emergency management practitioners are to understand and plan for the involvement of discrete organized responses (of whatever DRC type), on the one hand, and broader response networks that connect them on the other. And just like the discrete organized responses themselves, while some response networks are predetermined, others are improvised during the emergency period. The more severe the disaster is, such as the September 11, 2001 terrorist attacks on New York and Washington, the more important do these improvisations become. Improvisation is specific to the definition of emergent and extending organized responses within the DRC typology and most certainly relevant to response networks linking all four types.

As graphically represented in Figure 17.2, the greater the number of elements present in a multiorganizational response network, the greater the evidence of organizing as a process. The vast majority of the almost 600 response networks we have reconstructed from the archives have only one or two elements present (about 90%), and the clear majority of these cases

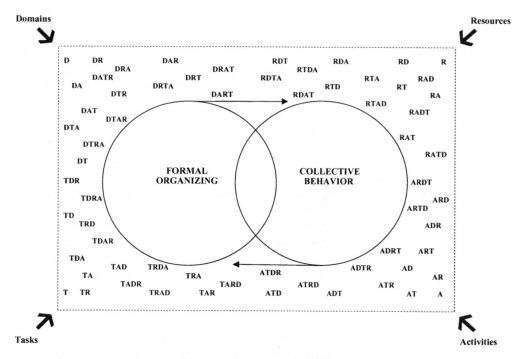

FIGURE 17.2. The process of organizing and reorganizing.

involve only resources and/or activities (about 85%). Thus the modal circumstances involve transfers of exchanges of resources (R), conjoined actions (A), or mobilization of resources in association with conjoined actions (R-A or A-R). Only a minority of the cases (about 25%) evidence (in most cases) an explicit division of labor (T) or (in a very few cases) an explicit merging or inclusion of network members within a self-contained entity (D). These findings suggest that there are potential parallels between response networks and collective behavior as both relate to the process of organizing (Kreps, 1991a). The various combinations of conjoined action and transfers or exchanges of resource (A, R, A-R, R-A) are elemental forms of collective action that create the potential for organization, however, in the vast majority of cases a fully developed organized response does not emerge from a multiorganizational response network. The structural code allows distinguishing when response networks become more fully organized and when they do not.

It is reasonable to infer from these findings that the demand for self-containment and internal control by existing organizations constrains their merging with each other or being absorbed by more inclusive entities (Aldrich, 1979; Gillespie, 1991; Gillespie, Colignon, Banerjee, Murty, & Rogge, 1993; Kreps, 1991a; Starbuck, 1983; Stinchcombe, 1965). But such a result is not inevitable because emergent organized responses (type IV) of various forms and sizes do arise and are consequential. And even when the lives of these emergent organized responses are relatively short, once formed they exhibit all of the basic characteristics taken for granted about organizations that exist prior to disasters. Findings about organized responses and multiorganizational response networks are familiar to both experienced disaster researchers and emergency management practitioners. Such findings support a core principle: that planned and improvised disaster responses are core foundations of emergency management (Kreps, 1991b).

Internal demands for self-containment and control are arguably greater for established and expanding organizations, first, because their involvement during a disaster is anticipated, and second, because they have a preparedness mandate. The result for them is greater predictability about domains and tasks, the resources and activities that will be needed to implement them, and the relevance of other responding organizations to their missions. But that predictability is far from complete, and it decreases as the magnitude and scope of impact become greater.

The September 2001 terrorist attacks on the United States, the December 2004 international tsunami, and the August 2005 hurricane (Katrina) on the United States Gulf Coast are dramatic cases in point. Improvisation is an essential component of emergency management during these and other major events, not only in terms of what is being done and how by established and expanding organized responses, but also in terms of developing essential response networks with each other as well as extending and emergent organized responses. Fortunately, being prepared does not decrease the ability to improvise as conditions warrant. Indeed, disaster researchers and emergency management practitioners increasingly concur that disaster preparedness and prior experience increase the ability to improvise. What is needed, however, is the development of practical decision-making tools that support both preparedness and improvisation within the emergency management system (Kendra & Wachtendorf, 2003; Kendra et al., 2003; Mendonca, 2001, in press; Mendonca & Wallace, 2002, 2004; Wachtendorf, 2004; Webb, 1998, 2002a).

One need never worry about threatened communities being overprepared for disasters (Tierney, Lindell, & Perry, 2001, Chapter 2). The obstacles (e.g., lack of resources and technical expertise, concerns about organizational autonomy and control, limited and selective experience with major disasters as opposed to more routine emergencies) are formidable and they impact preparedness at both organizational and multiorganizational response network levels (Auf der Heide, 1989; Gillespie & Streeter, 1987; Gillespie, et al., 1992; Tierney, 2005; Waugh, 1988). Moreover, it is simply impossible to prepare for every possible contingency, and disaster plans that are too detailed become unworkable. But there is a more pressing constraint on preparedness: while most communities face multiple hazards, the resources needed for sustained disaster planning, training, and public education are more often than not diverted to what seem to be more pressing everyday concerns. In the face of limited resources and political commitment, particularly at the local level, only a modest level of preparedness is a reasonable expectation.

A growing consensus between disaster researchers and emergency management practitioners is that a modest yet sustained level of preparedness should not be based on an inflexible command and control model, but on a flexible resource coordination model. Prototypical examples of the resource coordination model are emergency operations centers which, whether planned or not, will emerge in some form (Dynes, Quarantelli, & Kreps, 1972; Kreps, 1991b; Wenger, Quarantelli, & Dynes, 1987). The various combinations and permutations of domains, tasks, resources, and activities documented in our archival studies of response networks clearly support the conclusion that they are as likely as not loosely coupled (Weick, 1981). Quite simply, loose coupling demands flexibility.

The Process of Reorganizing

Empirical Case: Located in the heart of the impact area, the reorganization of a counseling intervention agency began one hour after a major tornado struck the heart of a small Midwestern city.

The agency's predisaster major mission included drug education and treatment, suicide prevention, family counseling, and venereal disease and birth control counseling. The agency also maintained a small emergency hotline service related to these counseling intervention tasks. The agency's available staff began responding to disaster related information needs because, by chance, it was one of the few units in the immediate impact area that maintained telecommunications. That, combined with public knowledge of its hotline service, resulted in phone calls related to the disaster. The volume of calls was quite high and there was initial uncertainty about what to do about them. The result was a decision to suspend all routine counseling intervention activities (Activities), and to develop new procedures for monitoring calls, referring requests or offers of assistance to the proper authorities, and transmitting messages by phone or by messenger (Activities-Tasks). The agency then recruited volunteers to help staff the new hotline service (Activities-Tasks-Resources). The resulting message center and referral service continued for about 2 weeks, by which time most telecommunications in the impact area had been restored.

Here an Extending organized response (type III) reorganizes temporarily its operations in response to an immediate need for emergency related communications. When an existing organization restructures itself, the basic question becomes: What can change? Once again, answering this question requires a basic conception of what an organization is. Our conception is a structural code that can be used to define organization as both a thing and a process. Using that code earlier, it was shown how emergent organizations, on the one hand, and multiorganizational response networks among emergent and existing organizations, on the other, represent a more fundamental process of demonstrably more or less organizing. But as this example shows, various combinations of changes in activities, resources, tasks, and domains can also allow for descriptions of what happens when an existing entity restructures its routines. In this instance of reorganizing, the routine activities (A) of a counseling intervention agency are suspended temporarily, new tasks are developed (T), and additional resources are mobilized (R). Interestingly enough, this reorganization was only the first of several undertaken by the agency over a six month period, ultimately leading to its merger with another local mental health unit (see Linn & Kreps, 1989, pp. 115–119).

We have examined more than 500 cases of reorganizing by established, expanding, and extending types in the DRC typology, including more detailed analyses of 167 cases of reorganizing related to the above Midwestern tornado and an equally severe Northeastern flood. Within the smaller sample, about 60% of the reorganizations involved only one or two elements of the code, and of these the clear majority (more than 66%) were (A), (R), (A-R), or (R-A) types. Another 28% of the reorganizations involved three elements, and only changes in tasks were added to the mix in over 88% of these cases. The remaining 12% of the cases involved complete reorganizations, and it is only here where changes in domains became central. Thus the modal types of reorganizations were changes in activities, resources, tasks, and various combinations of these elements.

Similar to response networks that connect them, reorganizations of existing units are bounded largely by activities, resources, and to a much lesser extent tasks. While these findings point again to internal demands for self-containment and control (i.e., the constraining effects of existing domains and tasks), they suggest also the continuing importance of collective behavior (i.e., the momentum of changes in activities and resources on, in particular, the reorganization of tasks). Thus as depicted graphically in Figure 17.2, regardless of whether the research issue is the reorganization of existing organizations, multiorganizational response networks, or the emergence of new organizations from multiorganizational response networks, formal organizing and collective behavior are two sides of the same coin. Organizational adaptation during a disaster is most certainly complex, but that complexity is neither incomprehensible nor unmanageable.

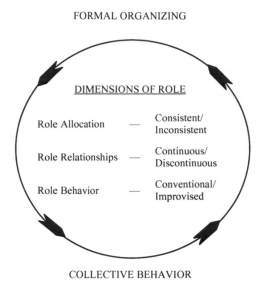

FORMAL ORGANIZING

DIMENSIONS OF ROLE

Role Allocation — Consistent/Inconsistent

Role Relationships — Continuous/Discontinuous

Role Behavior — Conventional/Improvised

COLLECTIVE BEHAVIOR

FIGURE 17.3. Role enactment within the context of organizational adaptation.

Role Enactment Within the Contexts of Organized Responses and Multiorganizational Response Networks

Organized responses and multiorganizational response networks are important on their own terms and, as noted in the lead statement of this paper, they provide structural contexts for the responses of individuals. We suggested in the preceding text that capturing these contexts requires dual reference to formal organizing and collective behavior. Capturing individual responses within and among organizations, however, requires focused research on how individual roles are enacted (Barton, 1969; Dynes, 1987). Figure 17.3 highlights three sociological dimensions of role enactment we have examined during our archival studies: role allocation, role relationships, and role behavior (Barton, 1969; Bates & Harvey, 1975; Bates & Peacock, 1989a; Merton, 1957; Turner, 1980a, 1989).

With role allocation, the question is whether disaster roles, (i.e., what people are actually doing during a disaster such as search and rescues workers as opposed to a search and rescue leader), are consistent or inconsistent with predisaster occupations of the individuals enacting them. Members of a fire department searching for survivors in damaged or destroyed buildings would have consistent role allocations, but an architect who happens to be at a disaster site leading a search and rescue operation would have an inconsistent role allocation. The relevant preparedness issue is the extent to which disaster roles can be formally assigned beforehand, or at least predictably assumed.

With role relationships, the question is whether direct links between individuals enacting disaster roles are, on a case-by-case basis, continuous or discontinuous in terms of their predisaster occupations. A police chief and a mayor having direct contact at an emergency operations center (EOC) would have a continuous role relationship, but a college professor and a director of public works having similar contact at an EOC would have a discontinuous relationship. The relevant preparedness issue is the extent to which it reasonably can be assumed that disaster role links will be extensions of everyday relationships among occupations, or whether new role relationships are forged on an ad hoc basis.

With role behavior, the issue is whether disaster roles are performed in a conventional as opposed to an improvised manner. The performance of a disaster role (e.g., search and rescue leader or head of an EOC) is quite different from the role allocation issue outlined earlier. When a disaster role is performed conventionally there is familiarity with how it is to be accomplished and little or no departure from expected performance. When a disaster role is improvised, there is some to greater deviation from routine performance. As documented systematically by Webb on a broad range of disaster types (1998, 2002a), the deviation can range from procedural and equipment changes conventionally related to the role enactment, to changes in the conventional location of the role enactment, to expansion of a disaster role by taking on activities that are not authorized, to the issuing of orders to others over whom one has no formal authority, and to the commandeering of supplies and equipment without legal mandate. The relevant empirical issue here is the extent to which anticipated performances of disaster roles are complemented by improvised performances as they relate to unanticipated contingencies, response problems, or special opportunities to innovate.

In completing archival studies of well over 550 role enactments that occurred during natural, technological, or willful (e.g., urban riots like the example discussed earlier in the chapter) disasters, our core findings about role enactments across two large subsamples are as follows: first, at least two thirds of the role allocations were consistent rather than inconsistent; second, on average over two thirds of the role links of individuals enacting disaster roles were continuous rather than discontinuous; and third, the roles were performed conventionally in slightly more than half of the cases in one large subsample (Kreps & Bosworth, 1993) and about three quarters of the cases in a second large subsample (Webb, 1998). Where improvisations occurred in at least one or more behavioral components of disaster roles, most of them (about 80%) involved changes in procedures, equipment, or the location of the role performance. The remaining improvisations (about 20%) most often involved an expansion of the role or the issuing of orders that was not previously authorized. The primary reasons for these improvisations were human and material resource needs, intra- and interorganizational operational issues, time pressures to get things done, and frequently mixes among these kinds of problems and opportunities.

Because of oversampling of established and expanding organized responses in the original DRC field studies, disproportionately more cases of inconsistent role allocation, discontinuous role links, and improvised role behaviors occurred in these types. However, all three dimensions of role are strongly related to the DRC typology. Established and expanding organized responses, whose involvement during disasters is anticipated, are more likely to have consistent role allocations and continuous role relationships. Extending and emergent organized responses, whose involvement is not anticipated, are more likely to have inconsistent role allocations and discontinuous role relationships. We have also found that role improvisation is more likely to occur in extending and emergent organized responses, with the association being much stronger in one large subsample (Kreps & Bosworth, 1993) than in the other (Webb, 1998).

Distributions on the three dimensions of role enactment as well as findings relating them to the DRC typology point to an important theme about the emergency periods of disasters. While the allocation of roles, relationships among roles, and actual role behaviors tend to be patterned in terms of pre-disaster routines and anticipated involvement, there is compelling evidence that exceptions to these routines occur quite often (Stallings, 1998). These exceptions—in this case inconsistent role allocations, discontinuous role links, and improvised role behaviors—happen in all four types of organized responses and they arise in response to very specific problems and opportunities (see also Mendonca, 2001; Wachtendorf, 2004). These problems and opportunities reflect the inherent complexity and fluidity of disaster situations.

Preparedness of established and expanding organized responses necessarily serves to increase predictability about what roles are to be performed, by whom, with whom, and how. In so doing, preparedness serves to enhance the resiliency of disaster-threatened communities, regions, and societies. That is why disaster planning, training, and public education are such important components of emergency management. But the ability to adjust and react flexibly as conditions warrant is also a core foundation of emergency management, one that is evidenced by all four types in the DRC typology as well as both preexisting and emergent multiorganizational response networks. The question is whether individuals who necessarily will or even may be involved in emergency situations can become better prepared to change their respective roles as conditions warrant. We think they can through the development of research based decision-making models that support role enactment preparedness and training (Mendonca, forthcoming; Mendonca & Wallace, 2004). We will suggest an integrated research strategy that highlights the importance of such models in the last section of the chapter.

DRC-BASED STUDIES AND BROADER
RESEARCH ISSUES ON DISASTER
PREPAREDNESS AND RESPONSE

Disasters are non-routine events in societies or their larger subsystems (e.g., regions, communities) that involve conjunctions of physical conditions with social definitions of human harm and social disruption. (Kreps, 2001, p. 3719)

The above entry from the latest edition of the *International Encyclopedia of the Social and Behavioral Sciences* draws on the rich traditions of hazards and disaster research within the social sciences since World War II. As defined previously, disasters are social catalysts that relate to community and societal adaptations before, during, and after they occur (Birkland, 1997; Dubin, 1978; Kreps, 1998; Kreps & Drabek, 1996). Those researchers focusing on potential disasters (hazards) study conditions of physical and social vulnerability, the risks associated with these conditions, and efforts to mitigate these conditions before they become disastrous. Those researchers focusing on actual events (disasters) study the dynamics of disaster preparedness, emergency response, and long-term recovery. Hazards and disaster researchers alike increasingly are taking an inclusive view of their subject matter. Over time they have become keenly interested in comparing adaptations to a broad range of natural, technological, or willful events (Cutter, 2001, 2003a; Tierney, Lindell, & Perry, 2001).

Our archival studies summarized above were stimulated by the DRC typology and bounded by the focus of the original DRC field work. Accordingly, they have been focused almost exclusively on emergency response and disaster preparedness topics and not on those related to hazard vulnerability, mitigation, and disaster recovery. Summarized most recently by Tierney, Lindell, and Perry (2001), early to more recent disaster response and preparedness studies have highlighted, on the one hand, major obstacles to achieving anything more than sporadic to modest levels of preparedness at all levels of analysis (household, organizational, community, regional, national), and on the other hand, the remarkable absorptive capacities of communities and societies during and after natural, technological, and willful events. In so doing, research over decades has contradicted myths that during a disaster people will panic, that those expected to respond will abandon occupational and disaster roles, that community systems will break down, and that antisocial behavior will be rampant. Having systematically debunked such myths, the more interesting research questions have become where, when, how, and why communities, regions, and societies are able to leverage anticipated (and perhaps planned) and improvised post-impact responses in coping with the circumstances of disaster.

Building on the DRC typology and archives, our secondary research has tried to address systematically these questions. Anticipated and improvised organized responses, multiorganizational response networks, and disaster roles of various types and levels of complexity are the primary means through which communities respond to disasters on their own terms, and also are linked with response systems at regional, state, and national levels. Disasters are local events in the United States, and treated as such, but it is also clear that societal-wide adaptations become increasingly important as the magnitude and scope of impacts become greater (Birkland, 1997; Drabek, 1991a; Drabek, Mushkatel, & Kilijanek, 1983; Dynes, Quarantelli, & Wenger, 1990; Kreps, 1991a; May & Williams, 1986; Sylves, 1991; Wachtendorf, 2004). And while political and cultural differences must always be taken into account, the strength of community and societal adaptations of all nations directly contributes to their resiliency in the face of human harm and social disruption (Berke, Kartez, & Wenger, 1993; Mileti, 1999; Tierney, Lindell, & Perry, 2001 Wenger, 1978).

As documented in the preceding text and in a host of other studies, the adaptations of disaster relevant organizations and the performance of disaster roles have been important foci of disaster research for decades, such that the knowledge base on these topics is increasingly amenable to codification (e.g., Barton, 1969; Drabek, 1986; Dynes, 1970; Kreps & Bosworth, 1993; Webb, 1998, 2002a). Far less research has been completed on multiorganizational response networks. However, findings at the response network level of analysis have expanded rapidly during the past two decades, and they are based on state-of-the-art methods and models. Needed now are systematic comparisons of organized responses, multiorganizational response networks, and disaster roles across multiple types of disasters. Such comparisons will require the use of standardized data protocols, for which complete research designs are not yet available. Needed also are more sustained efforts to formally disseminate and use findings about anticipated and improvised post-impact responses of disaster relevant organizations.

Knowledge about crisis relevant organizations, multiorganizational response networks, and disaster roles must be placed side by side with findings on adaptations by households, firms, other community-based organizations, and government agencies at all levels. A fairly solid knowledge base has been developed at the household level of analysis with respect to such topics as risk communication, warning dissemination and response, evacuation, and other forms of protective action. But serious knowledge gaps remain on these topics and, just as with adaptations at the organizational level, there are essential requirements for standardized measurements of household responses across different types of events. Far less is known about the behavior of firms, other community-based organizations, and intergovernmental relationships during disasters. Most notably, very little work has been completed on how national government structures, policies, and political cultures influence preparedness and disaster responses at regional and local levels, and most of what little research that has been done is confined to the United States and other highly industrialized democracies (see Tierney, Lindell, & Perry, 2001, Chapter 6).

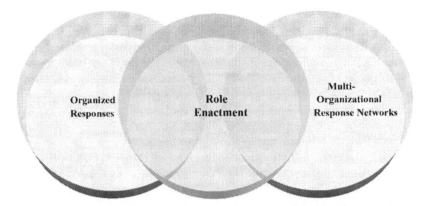

FIGURE 17.4. An integrated research strategy to increase readiness for anticipated and improvised post-disaster responses.

AN INTEGRATED RESEARCH STRATEGY TO INCREASE READINESS FOR ANTICIPATED AND IMPROVISED DISASTER RESPONSES

Organizational adaptations to disaster have enormous range and complexity. As depicted graphically in Figure 17.4, hazards and disaster researchers are attempting to unravel that complexity at essentially three distinct levels of analysis: within organized responses (emergence and reorganizing), among multiorganizational response networks, and in terms of disaster roles that are nested within organized responses and multiorganizational response networks. Anticipated and improvised disaster responses can be distinguished at all three levels of analysis. The above structural code and formal organizing–collective behavior continuum provides one way to make that distinction for organized responses and their associated response networks, and the above three dimensions of role serve the same purpose at the individual level of analysis. The result is that each of the three levels of organizational adaptation is important on its own terms and worthy of further research on an inclusive range of natural, technological, and willful disasters. Indeed, DRC-based and a host of other previous studies on organizational adaptation, broadly defined, have contributed greatly to the development and dissemination of knowledge about how communities and societies respond to disaster.

But much more research is needed. The conceptual tools summarized in this chapter (the DRC typology, a structural code, formal organizing-collective behavior continuum, and role enactment framework) can reduce the inherent complexity of organizational adaptation during disasters to a more intelligible research problem and a more solvable emergency management problem. For that to happen, however, disaster role enactments, organized responses, and multiorganizational response networks must be combined within a more highly structured approach to research and application.

With that goal in mind, we propose an integrated research and application strategy that is based most directly on Gary Webb's (1998, 2002a) systematic research on role improvisations, a very powerful methodology being developed by David Mendonca to describe the broader structural contexts within which role improvisations occur, that is, what he terms organizationally situated improvisations (Mendonca, 2001; forthcoming; Mendonca & Wallace, 2002, 2004), and a superbly illustrated typology developed recently by Tricia Wachtendorf to describe what she terms organizational improvisations (Wachtendorf, 2004; Kendra & Wachtendorf, 2003; Kendra et al., 2003). By blending the conceptual tools and empirical approaches of Webb, Mendonca, Wachtendorf, and their collaborators, we believe improvised disaster responses at the role, organizational, and multiorganizational levels can be isolated more precisely in future research from those responses that are anticipated. Once described and distinguished from each other, anticipated and improvised disaster responses can then become key dependent variables in, first, structural models of organizational adaptation to disasters, and second, complementary cognitive models of individual decision making in these same contexts. The application yield of the integrated research strategy we propose, we believe, will be preparedness support tools for emergency management practitioners.

As highlighted by its centrality in Figure 17.4, the core foundation of our proposed strategy should be studies of role enactments by key participants (at executive and operational levels) in established and expanding organizations. Selection of these two types does not mean that extending and emergent responses from the DRC typology are less important. It ensures, however, that expected involvement of individuals (and therefore direct disaster relevance) can be taken for granted. That being the case, any unexpected role allocations, or development of new role relationships, or improvised role behaviors by key participants in established and expanding organizations document changes in anticipated role enactments. While such role changes have been chronicled in greatest detail by Webb, of common theoretical interest to himself, Mendonca, and Wachtendorf are improvised role behaviors. Simply put, it is essential to the research strategies of all three scholars and their collaborators to document the following about such role behaviors: when improvised role behaviors occur relative to the time of impact; where they occur relative to the location(s) of impact; how they occur, namely, as nonconventional uses of resources, procedures, status, or authority; and why they occur, namely, as improvised responses to unanticipated contingencies, problems, or special opportunities.

Having located and documented short-term role changes within established and expanding organizations, with particular attention given to improvised role behaviors, there are two additional core data requirements. First, any evidence of reorganizing by established and expanding organizations studied can be documented with reference to either the above structural code or the typology of organizational improvisations (reproductive, adaptive, creative) developed by Wachtendorf to document organizational improvisations (discussed in another paper in this handbook). For Kreps and Bosworth, the more elements of the structural code (1-4) implicated by the substance of a respective reorganization (i.e., what was actually happening), the greater the degree of potential improvisation at the organizational level of analysis. But potential and actual improvisations must be distinguished analytically and empirically. For Wachtendorf, it is essential to isolate reorganizations that are planned from those that are improvised. The relative presence of reproductive, adaptive, and creative improvisation during any reorganization (however documented) clearly allows such determinations. Second, and using Mendonca's methodology, any documented improvisations at either role or organizational levels must then be colocated within the multiorganizational response networks of which established and expanding organizations are members. Documenting the niches and overall centrality of respective established and expanding organizations within these response networks requires use of state-of-the-art social network methods and detailed data on the flow of communications among network members. Assuming such data are collected and stored, the above structural code may be useful also for documenting the organizational qualities of the network itself. The more elements of the code (1-4) represented substantively within a multiorganizational response network, the greater the evidence of organizing in process at that level of analysis. And once documented, Wachtendorf's typology can be used productively to distinguish between planned and improvised adaptations by the multiorganizational networks themselves.

The primary research objective, in effect, is to document and nest individual role behaviors within established and expanding organizations and their associated response networks. In so doing, both improvised role behaviors and other organizational adaptations can be distinguished from those that are anticipated. Associated structural models can then be developed to predict discrete and contingent probabilities of improvised and anticipated role behaviors and organizational adaptations as a function of disaster events characteristics as well as any number of standard variables that have been used to measure structural characteristics of organizations and social networks. There is no question that building these structural models has major associated data requirements. The DRC archives that have been analyzed in detail only scratch the surface in meeting these data requirements (see, e.g., Kreps & Bosworth, 1994, Chapter 7 and Appendix C). But the respective studies of Webb, Mendonca, and Wachtendorf illustrate beautifully the rich descriptions of organizational adaptation that ultimately will be required. We therefore conclude that the conceptual and empirical foundation has been established for developing standardized data protocols to distinguish planned and improvised post-impact role enactments, organized responses, and multiorganizational response networks.

While research at the individual level of analysis is arguably easier, conventional and improvised role behaviors never occur in a social vacuum. That is why it is essential to document also disaster role allocations and role relationships and then, in effect, situate data on all three dimensions of role enactment within both broader organizational and response network contexts (Gillespie, 1991; Gillespie & Streeter, 1987). Only then can powerful structural models of improvised and conventional role behaviors be produced. Such models can and we think should be complemented by cognitive models of decision making by individuals who are enacting disaster roles. Cognitive models of decision-making are also of common interest to Webb, Mendonca, Wachtendorf, and their collaborators. Building them, however, is a major research problem in its own right, one with associated conceptual issues and essential data requirements.

Cognitive models require measurement of what those enacting disaster roles are thinking about in relationship to their behaviors. We concur with our above colleagues that conventional or improvised role behaviors relate directly to how people make sense about what is happening around them during a disaster and what they themselves are doing. Weick (1993) argues that making sense of things during crisis situations is a muddy process that involves vague questions, vague answers, and negotiated agreements to reduce confusion. One way individuals make sense of things is by drawing on prior knowledge of or experience with the roles they are enacting either from routine circumstances or (perhaps) from comparable crisis situations. The biographies of role incumbents are, therefore, essential to document in the development of cognitive models of decision making. Another way people make sense of things is through communications with other participants enacting similar or related disaster roles. That is why role relationships are one of the three core dimension of roles we have identified. Still another way people make sense of things is by observing what their respective organizations are doing independently and in relationship with what other organizations are doing. That is why role enactments must be nested within the contexts of organized responses and multiorganizational response networks.

In effect, decisions to enact disaster roles conventionally, by improvising, or by some combination of convention and improvisation serve as individual adaptations that reduce ambiguity about what is happening, what needs to be done, where, when, how, and why. Sometimes these adaptations are compelled by contingencies and problems over which people performing disaster roles have very little control. Other times they result from proactive decision-making wherein role incumbents exercise considerable control. While the former circumstances are no less important to document than the latter, the labeling of proactive decision-making as novel, opportunistic, creative, or entrepreneurial seems particularly apt (e.g., Mendonca, forthcoming; Wachtendorf, 2004; Weick, 1998). Rest assured, however, that both compelled and proactive decisions and actions do not arise out of thin air; they are contextually based within organizations and social networks.

Like structural models of improvised and conventional role behaviors, cognitive models are feasible to develop, particularly if there is a standardized cataloguing of data on the decision-making processes of individuals enacting disaster roles. Once constructed, structural and cognitive models are highly complementary and have two important applications to emergency management. First, the models can provide logical preparedness frameworks to increase readiness for conventional and improvised role behaviors during a disaster. Second, findings from the models allow for the development of empirically based training simulations on conventional and improvised role behaviors. Existing emergency operations centers are very appropriate for either of these modeling applications, first, because they are routine venues for preparedness and training activities, and second, because they have strong representation from established and expanding organizations. Some limited modeling application is possible now using current frameworks and findings on organizational adaptation. But maximizing the use of structural and cognitive models requires more highly structured data protocols, more adequate data, and more readily retrievable data. The increasing use of state-of-the-art computer technologies is essential for these data management activities.

A CLOSING COMMENT

When the Disaster Research Center was established during the mid-1960s, its research program included both field studies and laboratory simulations of organizational adaptation to crisis events. The field studies have continued for decades and over time there has been increasing use of survey research techniques. But after a very creative early application (see Drabek & Haas, 1969), the simulation work was largely suspended because of its related cost and complexity. At its founding, DRC's leadership (Russell Dynes, Henry Quarantelli, and J. Eugene Haas) made the wise decision to create a data archives and a rudimentary system of cataloguing and retrieving data collected on specific events. The early combination at the DRC of field work, disaster simulation, and data archiving serves as a template for what is needed for future research and knowledge application on organizational adaptation. Developing standardized data protocols, building structural and cognitive models, using these models as preparedness and training tools, and maintaining an effective data management system are all non-trivial problems. Solving these problems will require interdisciplinary teams that include (at the very least) social scientists, cognitive and decision scientists, and computer scientists. Given the growing global importance of natural, technological, and willful hazards and disasters, work on and support for the collaborative effort that is needed should begin now.

CHAPTER 18

Community Innovation and Disasters

James M. Kendra and Tricia Wachtendorf

Much is made of the American spirit of innovation, yet innovation is certainly not a process isolated to the United States nor is it always embraced in American communities. How do we come to understand community innovation, particularly as it concerns practices related to disaster mitigation, preparedness, response, and recovery? Indeed, innovation is a much-studied subject with a vast corpus of research literature that is, unfortunately, conflicted and contradictory. Community, too, is a troubled and often imprecise term, its colloquial meaning often at odds with the complex and sometimes antagonistic social relationships existing in a place. Yet much of disaster research and practice is grounded in at least an implicit recognition of the importance of both community and of innovation.

One of the principal definitions of disaster (Fritz, 1961, p. 655) implicitly recognizes community in the very concept of disaster: "an event, concentrated in time and space, in which a society, or a relatively self-sufficient subdivision of a society, undergoes severe danger and incurs . . . losses to its members and physical appurtenances . . . " Contained in this definition, in the idea of self-sufficient systems, are communities that are understood as politically bounded entities, and most disaster research has looked at disasters via their impact on sociopolitical collectives—cities, towns, states. Innovation, too, is a recurring theme of disaster studies, though often more implicitly understood than explicitly mentioned. If people are under threat from a known hazardous condition, what do they do to change that condition? And if people do, indeed, experience a disaster, what do they do to manage its effects? Hence the study of innovation in communities is central to the study of disaster, and innovation in communities is itself central to mitigating hazard, responding to emergencies and disasters, and recovering afterward.

In this chapter we examine community innovation. We begin by conceptualizing community and innovation as they relate to hazard—understood as a mismatch between human, natural, and technological systems (Mitchell, 1990)—and disaster. We identify the difficulties inherent in the terms *community, innovation,* and *community innovation*, presenting some working concepts that seem to align best with overall disaster research experience. We examine the characteristics of communities that make innovation both necessary and difficult, using examples of innovations drawn from the United States and internationally, including the mitigation-oriented Project Impact, elements of response to the 2001 World

Trade Center disaster, as well as recovery following the 1976 Tangshan earthquake, the 1989 Loma Prieta Earthquake in California, and the 2004 Indian Ocean tsunami. This discussion will point toward some directions for future research, including an understanding of community that might be suitable for newer, complex, and diffuse hazards, such as bioterrorism or cyberterrorism. The discussion will also point to some needed reorientations in policy that might proceed from either subsequent research or from what is already known.

CONCEPTS AND DEFINITIONS

Before considering community innovation as a feature of pre-disaster mitigation and preparedness and of post-disaster response and recovery, we must first consider carefully what we mean by each of these terms. The terms not only have conventional uses but they also take on different technical meanings in the research literature. Moreover, *community innovation* itself requires some explanation. It barely exists as a term in disaster research. Lindell and Perry's (2001) work on Local Emergency Planning Committees (LEPCs) is a noteworthy exception, but they make little use of the innovation literature in their analysis of the effectiveness of LEPCs. Community innovation is, however, a subtext of most work in the hazard and disaster area, and when used elsewhere has a broad diversity of meanings, emphases, and implications.

Community

The word community evokes an image of people in a certain geographical setting, socially organized via the mechanism of a local government for the good of the people who live in that place. The fundamental assumption is that the people who live there share common interests, needs, or aspirations. But there are really many more kinds of community: professional communities, linguistic communities, ethnic communities, and religious communities that may or may not be tied to certain locations but that are instead linked by interests apart from geography. Moreover, socially organized groups sharing a certain geographic setting are often comprised of many such communities within its boundaries. However, as Peacock with Ragsdale (1997) point out, the warm and positive connotations of community are often more wishful thinking than reality. They see community as a collection of competing interests. Their concept of a *sociopolitical ecology* holds that various groups—themselves shifting continually in composition—negotiate with each other for power and resources. Given this conception, community is characterized as much by conflict as by consensus, and the outcome of this process may lower the community's overall resistance to disaster. Moreover, it may result in distributions of risk that are unequal across the various residents. Coordination, defined as "agreed-upon relationships between independent organizations" (Gillespie, 1991, p. 55), is generally regarded as an important feature of emergency management. Comfort, too, strongly emphasizes coordination in the development of systems adaptive to threat, characterized by such features as sense of shared risk, and "common understanding" about remedial measures (Comfort, 1999, p. 31). Yet the coordination, mutual understanding, and information exchange that are necessary to respond to threat are undermined by the fractious nature of communities, and innovators may struggle for expression in such places.

Innovation

Survival requires innovation. This statement is regarded as axiomatic in the corporate world, where organizations must respond to constant shifts in the competitive landscape with new products or services; more efficient communications and information technology; and streamlined, flexible, "organic" structures. Innovation itself, of course, has a reflexive quality, since it is innovations or changes occurring elsewhere in the operational environment that compel other organizations in that environment themselves to seek new strategies or methods. Innovation, then, is a key survival attribute, but it is one with a central paradox—though it denotes a break or departure from customary methods or structures, the break itself is necessary for the continuity of the organization in question. This could include either the continuity of their reputation or perceived legitimacy; the continuity of socially constituted parameters of performance; or in extreme cases, the continuity of the organization's existence: its survival.

We are looking principally at innovation as a capacity or a process, rather than at the product, and the unit of analysis is a community (again, not necessarily linked by geography or political boundaries) that does something new in the face of crisis, either a crisis that is potential or one that is realized. The emphasis is on a departure from an established way of conceiving danger. This departure could include new ways of thinking about potential perils, developing strategies for mitigating them in advance, becoming better prepared for threats that eventually result in disaster, and responding to disastrous events when they occur.

Much work on innovation has been done at the organizational level, and some of these findings have applicability to our consideration of community innovation. Researchers generally distinguish between innovation and change, looking at change as "the adoption of a new idea or behavior by an organization [whereas in contrast, organizational innovation is seen as] the adoption of an idea or behavior that is new to the organization's industry, market, or general environment" (Daft, 2004, p. 404). However, Daft (2004, p. 404) goes on to note that when managing change in organizations, "the terms ... can be used interchangeably because the *change process* within organizations tends to be identical whether a change is early or late with respect to other organizations in the environment." We also will not make a distinction between whether the innovation is completely new, never before seen anywhere, or instead is new to that locality. In looking at creativity, for example, a concept closely allied to innovation, Amabile (1997) considers organizations that do new things to be creative, even if the idea was also thought of elsewhere. The key issue is doing something new, not being first. Similarly, Damanpour and Gopalakrishnan (1998, p. 3) argued that innovation can be brought into the organization; that is it can originate in the organization or can be imported after being developed elsewhere.

Not only is the research literature on innovation large, it is also fraught with conflict and contradiction. For example, Bigoness and Perreault (1981, p. 69) commented that studies tend to be "inconclusive or contradictory," and they note that other researchers have arrived at a similar assessment, stating that "factors found to be important for one innovation in one study are found to be considerably less important, not important at all, or even inversely important in another study." Levi and Lawn (1993, p. 226) found a "lack of integrating theories," and suggested that fully developed widely applicable theory may actually be impossible, while Damanpour and Gopalakrishnan (1998, p. 2) argued, "Despite their efforts ... researchers still cannot identify with certainty the causes and effects of organizational innovations." The principal challenge is the great differences in such variables as organization type, size, configuration, and environment. Even organizations which appear to be similar may differ enough to defeat attempts at generalizing factors relating to innovation. These challenges are arguably more complex at the community level where members may be less formally bonded to each other than members of a highly structured organization or alternatively be comprised of multiple organizations. There is a further difficulty in applying existing research to the problem of community innovation, and that is that most research looks at private-sector companies (see Kreamer & Dedrick, 1997). There is less literature on innovation in public sector organizations, and what there is suggests that innovations follow a somewhat different trajectory with different factors of facilitation or obstruction, especially because different demands are placed on organizations in these contexts. The same may be true for communities based around non-private sector definitions.

COMMUNITY INNOVATION

The literature on innovation, as noted earlier, is quite sizable. However, much of this literature is concerned with technical or industrial innovations, in particular how new products circulate through different markets. Community innovation, as such, is not much covered in the general sociological literature; it is very conspicuous in urban studies and planning, and management and organization science, but again there is a marked technological or industrial focus, looking at the distribution of new products or services, or the uptake of new technology in firms. The literature explicitly on community innovation follows a similar approach, looking at how communities or regions attract or retain certain industries or become known for producing new goods and services. However, there are many community innovation *programs*. These consist of community innovation grants and sponsorship activities associated with community social or economic development. These are themselves vast topics and include accessible technology, social entrepreneurship, sustainability, low-income support and antipoverty initiatives, and numerous of other such enterprises. For example, the Institute for Community Innovation at Florida International University emphasizes the viability of community-based organizations such as art groups in the South Florida area, but it also has an international reach. One project focuses on rural economic development in the agricultural sector of Central America (Institute for Community Innovation, ND). Elsewhere, the Sustainable Community Grants program, a partnership of the Southern Region Sustainable Agriculture Research and Education (SARE) Program and the Southern Rural Development Center (SRDC), provides grants for projects that connect agriculture, industries, local or regional economic development, and sustainable agricultural practices (Southern SARE and SRDC, 2005). Some suggested projects include those that foster local leadership capability, public–private partnerships, and entrepreneurship. Similarly, the United Way of The Lower Mainland, Vancouver (2003) in its grant funding programs, sponsors such initiatives as youth development, suicide prevention, and computer training for seniors. The significance for this chapter is that community innovation is a concept filled with whatever meaning potential innovators want to put in it; there is no consensus as to its content, though invariably there is a positive connotation. Initiatives are meant to work some improvement in their locales. Since all the literature at issue here is profoundly vexed, it seems reasonable to place attention on innovations that hold both illustrative and instructional value.

INNOVATING IN COMMUNITIES

Given Peacock with Ragsdale's (1997) formulation, the characteristics of community can be opposed to the characteristics of social relationships that are required for innovative action. For example, Comfort (1999) has highlighted the importance of a sense of shared risk in order for communities to be able to organize to minimize the risk. Yet, if the risks are differentially distributed across the terrain of the community, then mobilizing attention and resources is likely to be more difficult. Moreover, differential distribution may result in disparities in risk perception which in turn may weaken community will or present barriers to decisive action.

Of course, many of the conflicts that Peacock and his colleagues identified are very deeply rooted in systems of production, of economic exchange, or in the debilitating persistence of racism or sexism. The difficulty of communities to deal with problems that crystallize locally but whose ingredients swirl in the social mix nationally or even globally is well documented (e.g., Patterson, 2002). In particular, the most profound social vulnerabilities—those rooted in macrostructural systems of organization—often equate to the most serious risks (Wisner et al., 2004). Thus public officials are, in their effort to reduce risk, compelled to try to take account of vulnerability as well. Reducing such vulnerability is sometimes possible at the local level, though the root causes are in conditions usually far beyond the power of local officials to affect.

The significance of Peacock with Ragsdale's conception of community, though, is that "communities" do not innovate; individuals, groups, and organizations innovate. These might be government agencies, nongovernmental organizations (NGOs), citizen groups, pressure groups, or other collectives. And this means that it is appropriate to look at community innovation from an organizational perspective, because communities, fractured and schism-filled as they are in the sociopolitical ecology model, are conglomerates of organizations, whether acting individually or working together. *Community innovation*, therefore, takes place as *innovation in communities*.

Much of the job of public officials, as a consequence, is to try to bring about the processes of coordination that Comfort outlines while functioning in the environment that Peacock with Ragsdale's (1997) have described. Peacock et al's conception is of the conditions that *exist* in a certain time, and Comfort's analysis shows what *ought to exist* in order to identify goals that the community as a whole can work toward. Given the differences in what *is* versus what *ought to be*, some aspects of the social organization of the community may have to be changed, on at least some functional level, in order to be aligned with the capacities that Comfort has outlined. Innovation and change, however understood, are necessary in this effort; in other words, innovative thinking and organizational arrangements are needed for innovative action.

INNOVATION ACROSS THE DISASTER PHASES

Disaster scholars and emergency managers customarily divide the concept of disaster into four phases: mitigation, preparedness, response, and recovery. Some argue that this is not the most conceptually sound breakdown (Neal, 1997) and, more recently, concern about national security embodied in the U.S. National Response Plan has yielded an additional stage of the disaster cycle: prevention. Borrowing from a division of the disaster timeframe used by Quarantelli (1980b) in a different sort of study, we find it useful in discussing innovation to divide the disaster time frame into three phases: pre-impact, trans-impact, and post-impact.

The time that is available for innovating is perhaps the single greatest difference in the nature of innovation across the disaster phases. In the pre-impact phase, there is time for weighing options, considering different strategies for reducing disaster, and evaluating and adjusting new methods or techniques as their effects are observed. Sometimes these can include more modest programmatic efforts, but often these are large-scale, policy-level shifts intended to change people's perception of risk or risk-reducing action that they can take, or to actually change the way people understand and interact with the natural environment. Innovations in the trans-impact phase (immediately before, during, and after impact) include not just those that are policy oriented but also those that are operationally oriented, made under great time pressure and sometimes more appropriately referred to as certain forms of improvisations (see Kendra & Wachtendorf, 2004; Wachtendorf, 2004; Wachtendorf & Kendra, 2005). The post-impact phase, early and long-term recovery, also includes operationally oriented innovations but may in addition include innovative approaches for handling some of the difficult decisions to be made during this phase, such as whether or how to rebuild damaged areas. In the next section, we consider innovations in these three phases, but recognize that the boundaries between them are not distinct and that they may blend into each other at different times.

Pre-Impact

Most conceptions of hazard are now gathered around the premise that hazards do not exist as "things" by themselves or only as forces of nature. Rather, the idea of hazard includes to a large extent the choices that people make, especially in terms of where they live. Understanding those choices, particularly from the cognitive dimension, was the motivation behind much of the early hazards research (White, 1973). Later work (e.g., Hewitt, 1983) argued that the "choices" people make were often not real choices, but were the narrowed options resulting from social, economic, and political marginalization. From these research directions, however, emerged an understanding of hazard as a mismatch of social, natural, and technological systems (Mitchell, 1990). Human needs, particularly with respect to land for settlement, clash with the climatic or geophysical forces of certain places. Mitigation then can take either or both of two directions: to modify the natural environment to redirect or contain the earth's processes, or to modify the human uses of space that are incompatible with the natural events that occur there. Examples of the former, termed structural mitigation, include such engineered systems as dams and levees but might also include more personalized devices such as home lightning rods. Nonstructural mitigation involves redirecting human uses, such as keeping development out of hazardous areas through land-use regulations, bracing furniture to walls in earthquake prone areas, or education and information campaigns to alert people to local dangers.

As Cannon (1994) stated, mitigation is too often hazard-centered rather than people centered. Because disasters are tied to social processes, strategies that aim to reduce disaster vulnerability must pay attention to vulnerabilities in both the built and the social environment. Among scholars and emergency managers, structural mitigation has fallen out of favor as a principal strategy. White's (1973) early work showed that flood losses continued to increase even after the establishment of an elaborate flood management system on the western rivers. Development simply increased, placing more life and property at risk and, as the 1993 Midwest floods and the 1997 Red River Flood revealed, very extreme events can surpass the design parameters of such vast systems and lead to even greater flood losses. Thus, while the spectrum of mitigation strategies includes a mix of both structural and nonstructural programs, the preferred emphasis is now more toward nonstructural methods. Given the understanding of hazard as a mismatch of human–environment relations, nonstructural mitigation requires adjusting human action. This involves, from the perspective of the hazards paradigm founded by Gilbert White, shifting people's choices away from hazard and, from the vulnerability perspective emphasized by Hewitt, ensuring the capacity of individuals, groups, and communities to understand and minimize the risks of decisions, especially with respect to location and land use.

The fundamental requirement of hazards mitigation—moving people away from areas that threaten particular land uses or, when those uses are urgent enough to merit tolerating some risk, to promote awareness and foster protective measures—are straightforward in concept but surpassingly difficult to achieve in practice. Indeed, disaster scholars often regard localities' failure to move people away from hazard as a principal shortcoming of local mitigation strategies. Yet the challenge should not be understated. For the prelude to Hurricane Katrina, several hundred thousand residents did, indeed, depart from a hazardous location. Their departure—for the short or long term—has provoked multiple economic crises in the host areas, amounting to a serious national problem. Land use is inextricably connected to social and economic patterns. Adjusting land use decision making or adjusting other behaviors that bear on risk in communities requires modifying how people perceive the character of their environments and the potential danger to which they might be exposed. This often necessitates helping people to see their environment in new ways, and to do new things. In short, it requires innovation, at all levels of community life, to enact the social changes that are reflected in different land uses or different organizational relationships that can increase the overall capability of various members to mitigate the impacts of hazards.

An example of such a program directed at sustained change in human–environment relations was Project Impact (PI). This initiative, introduced by the Federal Emergency Management Agency (FEMA) in 1997 under the Clinton administration, provided seed money to local communities in the broad area of funding disaster mitigation and building disaster resistance. In addition to fundamental efforts to facilitate local adoption of hard mitigation projects, the initiative—where most successfully implemented—was a large-scale programmatic effort to affect the alignment of community social organization with the capacities needed for change. The program began with just seven pilot communities, each eligible for up to $1 million in seed money, though ultimately some 250 communities participated. The Disaster Research Center (DRC) at the University of Delaware completed a multiyear evaluation of Project Impact, concluding that many communities were successful in elevating local awareness of hazards and their willingness to implement mitigation measures (see Wachtendorf, Connell, Tierney, & Kompanik, 2002).

Project Impact stressed education, outreach, partnership building, and a sustained emphasis on measures that individuals as well as government could take to reduce their risk. Part of the emphasis was first to identify and publicize risks in the community. Certainly, leveraging financial resources within the community toward mitigation efforts was a central component of the initiative, but it also involved (though not explicitly expressed as such) leveraging of awareness to create shared identities of mutual exposure that could cut across the various group boundaries established by the ongoing competitions that normally exist among community groups. After the hazard was identified it was publicized through brochures, public service announcements and advertisements, educational programs in the schools, and even through direct communication, such as door-to-door public awareness campaigns by local scout troops or other organizations, inserts in pay stubs and electric bills, sporting events through partnerships with NASCAR, and disaster expos.

Although implemented to varying degrees of success across the country, effective communities attempted to transcend conflict between their constituents by emphasizing shared risk. PI coordinators made explicit efforts to build alliances, especially between the public and private sectors. These could take the form of bidirectional relationships between the PI office and business, public agencies, or community based-groups, or could involve multidirectional relationships among and between several organizations or businesses at the same time—for example, through the involvement of the local Chamber of Commerce or other consortiums of organizations. Some PI communities were able to build upon mutual interests between departments, developing innovative approaches to achieve common goals. For example, one community identified ways to leverage funds from environmental groups, leisure groups, a parks department, a planning department, and emergency management to buy out flood-prone property and develop green space for recreational use.

The programs that were initiated under Project Impact were not necessarily, in themselves, new ideas. They were often the kinds of ground-level efforts that most disaster researchers have come to believe are important in community-level mitigation, and they often did not differ from other kinds of community development initiatives. Education, building partnerships across government agencies and the public and private sectors, and developing programs to fund various projects or to encourage people to take self-help measures are not new. And, taken as a class, these activities were not necessarily new in these communities, either. Public–private partnerships have previously tackled other kinds of public problems. The use of other trappings of Project Impact—such as mascots, advertisements, and school education programs–had been done before. But all these aforementioned initiatives were deployed in new ways, and for new purposes, and their ambition was to foster new thinking within the community. At the same time, many projects were quite innovative when realized at the local level and, in most of the communities involved, the various initiatives marked real departures from customary ways of regarding and using the natural environment, and from established norms of individual, group, and organizational relationships. Some local PI communities made commendable strides in fostering what they called a synergy on mitigation issues

Trans-Impact

In this chapter, we have adopted a fairly broad definition of innovation, essentially referring to any new and creative program, procedure, or technique that a community implements to meet the demands of their environment. In the period before a disaster, this demand is registered as a sense of risk—the belief that some aspect of the community's condition is dangerous and needs to be addressed. The change, following Amabile's (1997) definition of creativity or Daft's (2004) specifically relating to both innovation or change, does not have to be totally new, never seen anywhere before. It only has to be something that is new to the community.

Response involves "Actions taken immediately before, during, or directly after an emergency occurs, to save lives, minimize damage to property, and enhance the effectiveness of recovery" (Godschalk, 1991, p. 136). This phase of the emergency management cycle puts a premium on timely action. The temporal scale for mitigation and preparedness spans months or even years. In the trans-impact phase, minutes, hours, or a few days is the more likely span for innovating, as emergency managers assess the situation and adapt plans for the general disaster envisioned in advance to the specific disaster unfolding before them. Or, as might also happen, they must develop plans for contingencies not imagined at all. Responding to disaster is likely to yield innovative techniques or procedures that are new to those people, but given the urgency of time they are likely to also be, more accurately, *improvisations*, or combinations of new and existing knowledge made in real time (Weick, 1998). One may be tempted to say that large complex disasters generate more improvisations than smaller events, but lesser events require improvisation, too. In fact, Tierney (2002a) argues that if an event does not require improvisation, it is not a disaster, so that improvisation is actually a distinguishing feature of disaster. Wachtendorf (2004) and Wachtendorf and Kendra (2005) have identified several types of improvisational actions, based on the extent to which structures, activities, resources, or tasks serve as substitutes for a missing capability, adapt an existing capability, or create a capability that had not existed before. We note here that discussion of innovation and improvisation brings us into potentially confusing questions of scale and the boundary between what is established or old and therefore not innovative, and what is new and thus innovative. New York City's effort to reconstitute its Emergency Operations Center (EOC) following the September 11, 2005 terrorist attacks serves as an example of *reproductive improvisation*. After the original EOC was destroyed as a result of the attacks, it was reproduced within days at a cruise ship facility on the Hudson River. In this sense the EOC as an organizational structure, as an emergency management function, and as a place (Perry, 1991) was not an innovation, though the original might have included innovative equipment and, indeed, the new facility required considerable innovation in its equipment and operations (see Kendra & Wachtendorf, 2003a, 2003b). The September 11 attack on the World Trade Center did, however, yield many innovations in technologies, organizations, and strategies for accomplishing multiple response-related needs. One such *creative improvisation* strategy was the emergent waterborne evacuation of several hundred thousand commuters and others from Lower Manhattan using a wide range of vessels not previously involved in any evacuation planning efforts or schema. After the attack, residents and workers from Lower Manhattan fled, mostly by foot, in all directions—uptown, or over the Brooklyn Bridge, or south. Those fleeing south were halted at the waterfront. Even before the towers collapsed, some ferries turned around with their passengers, while others returned to pick up their regular clientele. Simultaneously, tugs and other craft moved toward Manhattan. Some vessels asked and waited for permission from the Coast Guard, but others acted on their own.

This was an unplanned use of resources. Although segments of existing crisis management plans were available for some participants (the U.S. Coast Guard [USCG] had contingency plans for a water parade in 2000), most participants were unaware of this or any other contingency planning. In fact, significant dimensions of the operation were developed in the earliest stages of the response, as when the USCG and local harbor pilots developed a traffic management plan for vessels around the tip of Manhattan. At the same time, many participants reported no external direction for their actions (Kendra, Wachtendorf, & Quarantelli, 2003). Hence this effort was not merely innovative, it was collectively innovative on the part of the harbor community, with a set of goals, norms, and procedures that emerged across a large number of participants. Such an effort requires what Weick, Sutcliffe, and Obstfeld (2005) term "distributed sensemaking," or "the collective induction of new meaning" in a situation that had not previously been defined. How this happens is the subject of current research (Kendra & Wachtendorf, 2004), but shared collective identity (based on Weick, 1995), shared knowledge (as in Comfort, 1999), recognizing the limits of knowledge, and reworking norms according to an emerging ethos appear to be significant features.

Post-Impact

Innovation during the recovery stage tends to encounter conditions of support and resistance that are similar to those seen in the mitigation phase. During the mitigation phase, public officials, emergency planners, and the community in general must *imagine* the threat they are facing. Even if it is one that has transpired before, memories of such events are often short. The issue in this phase is one of perceived risk, and in trying to foster the sense of shared risk that Comfort argues is urgent for community action, public officials are often engaged in what Gioia and Chittepedi (1991) have termed "sensegiving," imparting a comprehension of events that should inform the actions of others. As community consensus, fleeting though it may be, emerges after impact, it is possible to see processes of collective or distributed, sense*making* (Kendra & Wachtendorf, in preparation; Weick, Sutcliffe, & Obstfeld, 2005) as multiple individuals and organizations read changing events through their congruent identities that foster similar interpretations and sets of possible actions. Innovations, many of them tactically oriented, appear at a rapid pace. But as has been seen after all disasters—especially after technological disasters (Marshall, Picou, & Gill,2003)—previous divisions and lines of conflict reemerge. The therapeutic community (Barton, 1969) gives way to the previous order as groups compete not just for resources, but for legitimacy and hence for a voice in the recovery. In terms of innovation, this phase looks something like the mitigation phase, politically charged and contentious. Indeed, since ideally the recovery phase should include mitigation, this is not totally surprising. But, while preparedness and response are devoted to crisis, mitigation and recovery are devoted to a vision of what the community should look like. Such visions are never achieved collectively without struggle. The ongoing debates in New York City regarding the appropriate use of the former World Trade Center site—or Ground Zero—epitomize the way competing interests can clash regarding appropriate recovery strategies. Whether or not office space should be part of the rebuilding plans, whether or not the footprints of the towers should remain relatively untouched, the aesthetics of site buildings, and the proper way to memorialize the site and those who died there have all been heatedly debated.

There are examples, however, of successful recovery innovations. One such short-term recovery approach was undertaken by the City of Santa Cruz, California after the 1989 Loma Prieta earthquake. The city suffered widespread damage to both structures and infrastructure, but also damage to its downtown business district. Faced with the need to reestablish commerce for local businesses in the short term, at first in response to business closures and later in reaction to customer leakage, the city countered the leakage trend by establishing pavilion tents to temporarily house dislocated businesses. Added support from labor unions and Vision Santa Cruz—a downtown recovery group with representatives from the private and public sector, as well as the community at large—was instrumental in the pavilion's quick construction and overwhelming success. Indeed, the pavilions allowed businesses to take advantage of important holiday season sales. Respondents reported a synergy and market-like or "festive" atmosphere in tent pavilions. Santa Cruz engaged in numerous promotional activities to attract customers to the city and to rebuild community spirit, including a promotional Christmas rally and a "Shake, Rattle, and Roll" celebration. Customer leakage was a phenomenon that proved difficult but not impossible to reverse because of the innovative recovery approaches of the community. As we have discussed in other sections, the innovations implemented in Santa Cruz are not necessarily new in their concept. The creation of temporary locations for businesses was not unique to this community. What was innovative, however, was the festive atmosphere created through the way those temporary locations were constructed and promoted in this particular community.

The emergence of Tangshan, China as an economic center displays a number of large-scale innovative aspects. The city was nearly completely destroyed by an earthquake in 1976, but Mitchell (2004) notes a number of new initiatives incorporated into the rebuilt city. For example, considerable care was devoted to the long-term treatment of people with very severe injuries, including psychological treatment, vocational readjustment, and social reintegration. This latter point includes marriage and new family life, but also having the survivors help to preserve memories of the event through writing about it and working with youth groups. The city has established a museum for the event with displays highlighting the recovery and growth since then, and implemented a number of mitigation and preparedness initiatives—a seismic monitoring system; projects considering the significance of water level and animal behavior; trained civilian observers; and anti-seismic construction techniques (Mitchell, 2004, pp. 4–6).

Innovation is important in communities' efforts to be less vulnerable or more resilient. Consider an example of community innovation following the Indian Ocean tsunami. A community education and development group, Disaster Mitigation Institute (DMI), worked closely with a number of communities in the weeks following the disaster. From their perspective, vulnerability to hazard was a development issue. Homes were destroyed that were not insured; boats, motors, and fishing equipment were destroyed that were not insured; and moreover, some fishers had outstanding loans on boats that were now gone. Given that the government assistance package included loans (albeit low-interest) for replacement equipment, deepening debt was the likely prospect. Even setting aside the serious vulnerability inherent in coastal living, economic vulnerability was deeply implicated in this disaster, largely through reliance on a single industry.

DMI's approach was to broaden the economic base, by building the earning capacity of women. Many women had worked in small manufacturing or other jobs; capitalizing on these existing skills would strengthen the community's capacity. Diversifying resources is a key element of resilience because it promotes redundancy, a vital component of resilience (see Bruneau et al., 2003; Kendra & Wachtendorf, 2003). At the same time, it decreases vulnerability. And in communities with a strong patriarchal social structure, involving women is a compelling social innovation as well, bringing their skills into the resource mix. Though perhaps the monetary sums are small, the magnitude of change in social relationships may be quite large if the communities follow through.

FACILITATING AND OBSTRUCTING INNOVATION

Damanpour and Gopalakrishan (1998, p. 4) argue that, "Innovation adoption is a means of changing the organization to facilitate the adaptation to changing environments in order to sustain or increase organizational effectiveness." External requirements often spur innovation; these relate to the survival or viability of the organization and are generally tied to some aspect of competitiveness, including such metrics as profit or market share or more hard-to-measure but still important features as reputation. Some sort of a perceived need is generally, as depicted in most research, a principal requirement for innovation in an organization. Of course, in the corporate realm, the need generally relates to productivity or profit requirements, either in an absolute sense—the company is falling behind in profit or market-share—or relative, in terms of how the organization's performance is measured against expectations of major constituents, such as shareholders. In this sense, the need for innovation is really a response to preserving or enhancing competitive stature. While competitiveness itself is a troubled term, as Schoenberger (1998) noted, and few companies can define what is competitive enough, most commercial organizations have a sense of competitiveness tied to their prosperity and even survival.

Public organizations do not face exactly the same competitiveness demands. Their role is generally to provide a service and thus they do not have to show a profit and, except in spheres of activity that are being privatized (prisons, package delivery) they rarely face an open market of potential competitors. This does not mean, though, that they do not face demanding stakeholders or that efficiency and effectiveness are of no consequence. Maintaining legitimacy and the public trust are the public sector analogs of competitiveness and are often the reasons for the adoption of new equipment or procedures. Having the latest technology in an emergency management office, for example, conveys the image of preparedness and competence that emergency managers' desire.

In a broad way, researchers group the factors that bear on innovation into those that are either internal to the organization or external to it (Levi & Lawn, 1993). Internal characteristics relate to the structure of the organization or to the size and composition of the workforce. External factors are those relating to the organization's environment, especially competitive pressures. This general categorization is reflected in Daft's (2004, pp. 404–406) assessment of five required elements of change: *"novel ideas"; recognition of need; adoption; implementation;* and *resources* (of people, skill, and money). Of these, *need* is probably most associated with externally oriented demands and may dominate other considerations; ideas, according to Daft, may be either internal or external to an organization. Forces spurring the adoption of innovations are generally, though not exclusively, external to the organization; forces impeding innovation tend to be, though are not always, internal to an organization. Levi and Lawn (1993) found that firms are generally more alert to external factors but are less attentive to internal forces that can hinder innovation. Daft (2004, p. 426) outlined a number of potential impediments, including *"excessive focus on cost"; "failure to perceive benefits"; "lack of coordination and cooperation"; "uncertainty avoidance";* and *"fear of loss"*. These factors are based on research on organizations; however, similar factors are evident at the larger community scale. These various elements of change and of potential obstruction are not precisely opposites of each other, but they share some opposing characteristics. For example, when resources are plentiful, or needs are more easily recognized, there may be less concern about cost. At the same time, some elements are clearly related to and affect each other. If perceived benefits are low, costs may seem too great. In this next section, we discuss principal elements of innovation facilitation and obstruction in the context of communities.

Recognition of Need

Successful mitigation initiatives, for example, require a reconstitution of a population's environmental perception, but if the hazard has not presented as a disaster, then those who advocate mitigation strategies are arguing about, essentially, a phantom menace, which a few recognize but which must be made evident to others. When a disaster has occurred in a community, the lingering risk and hazard has been laid bare for the citizens. Often, the need is not as obvious to all stakeholders or, even if they are aware of the threat, they may not know what can be done about it. Innovation always requires a recognition of need, but that recognition may not always exist, especially across the various stakeholder groups in a community. And here we include public officials and government as stakeholders. For example, the need to develop innovative approaches to warning and evacuating a migrant segment of a city's population may be recognized by those in that particular community, while at the same time the need may not be recognized by public officials, those with a greater access to decision-making power, or other communities of individuals not exposed to the same risk, even if the heightened vulnerability contributes to the city's overall vulnerability. What makes community innovation particularly challenging compared to organizational innovation is that individuals can be a part of multiple communities, each with different interests, priorities, abilities to mobilize others, and degrees of access to power.

A need must be both identified and clearly communicated. Even those who understand the need are generally not able to implement innovations single-handedly. Rather, what is often required are persons who can build a constituency; a (growing) group of people who share that perception of a situation that change is needed. Daft (2004) refers to these people as *champions*—those who take on the job of fostering change in technology, procedures, or organizational structures.

In the mitigation or preparedness phases, the emergency manager virtually by definition is required to champion community change in the direction of reducing risk. The emergency manager's job is to identify the existing "need"—the sources of potential emergencies that remain in the community (or communities) and to develop programs to reduce them. This is, often, a highly evangelical activity, in which the emergency manager must continually work to make the community aware of lingering risks and what can be done about them. Other ideal champions include citizens who are members of community-based organizations who have a keen relationship with their constituents, private sector leaders who have a visible role in the community, or members of environmental advocacy groups, which often focus their attention on hazards (particularly industrial hazards). In some cases, a champion may be appointed, but often a champion emerges, someone who perceives a need and is inspired and inspiring to others. Lois Gibbs, who founded the Love Canal Homeowners' Association, was one such champion who emerged following discovery of toxic waste leaks at Love Canal and who campaigned for financial assistance for nearby homeowners.

Groups who are not traditionally emergency response organizations can make a substantial contribution to the development of innovative emergency management approaches within the community. For example, some NGOs are better able to act as watchdogs and enact political pressure on governments and the private sector; some groups adopt a neutral stance and run education campaigns; still others are successful in attracting funding from sponsoring agencies. Just as NGOs vary in their functions, perspectives, and what they can achieve, so too do public and private sector organizations differ from each other and from groups within the same sector. By bringing together organizations that can offer a variety of resources, ideas, perspectives, and sources of knowledge, the collaboration can result in innovative broad-based mitigation strategies that could not be achieved if one sector or group were to work in isolation.

Again, the activities in some Project Impact communities provide excellent examples. The most successful Project Impact initiatives at the local level not only included traditional disaster planning partners, but also brought to the table leaders of such groups as senior citizen organizations; organizations that work with people with disabilities or with immigrant communities; and organizations such as Habitat for Humanity, the Boy Scouts, the Sierra Club, the Humane Society, and Neighborhood Watch. These are just a few examples of the types of groups that provided a clearer understanding of the needs of different segments of the populations but that also had their own resources, skills, and expertise to add to the tool chest of the community's capacity.

Excessive Focus on Costs

Costs are usually mentioned among the challenges impeding innovation and available financing is so often a limit to action that it hardly seems necessary to mention. Communicating risk; and persuading or forcing people to take steps to avoid risk. Expenses are generally cited as impediments to the adoption of new strategies for reducing hazards in a place. For example, acquiring land in a floodplain is one way that communities have been able to lessen hazards, by simply not allowing dwellings to remain in flood-prone areas. There are, however, a number of financial implications to consider in such a strategy. Platt (1996, pp. 333–335) noted several, such as initial purchase prices or loss of tax revenue when property becomes publicly owned.

The post-disaster period is often described as a "window of opportunity" in which a community, alerted to the particular dangers of its setting, might try to mitigate some of the hazards that are prevalent there. Mitigation grants that are included in association with a federal disaster declaration can help communities lessen their risk, and communities are now required to have mitigation plans. In this sense, innovation is mandatory after a disaster, and moreover, *thinking about innovation* has to occur before disaster strikes. Of course, Project Impact also showed that some innovative steps do not have to cost money, or may require only relatively small sums of public funds or can be supplemented through donations or other sources. Classes on hurricane-proofing one's home, taught at a hardware or building-supplies store, require just a bit of goodwill from the company (which will benefit when people purchase their materials there). While financial considerations undeniably present limits on what a community can accomplish, an excessive focus on cost can stifle the imaginative consideration of novel approaches for which funding from novel sources can later be acquired. Indeed, sometimes imagination and merely a willingness to start somewhere are key attributes in launching new risk-reducing initiatives.

Avoiding Uncertainty and Fear of Loss

In the community context, avoiding uncertainty and fear of loss are related to longstanding social and cultural norms and expectations. Ownership of property is a cherished principle of liberty in the United States, and ownership of land and homes is a principal means of securing wealth, especially for intergenerational transfer, at several income strata. Buy-out programs provide an example of cultural challenges, confronting residents both with uncertainties and the loss of cherished community patterns. Some are undertaken via the eminent domain power, but those that are sponsored under the FEMA post-disaster Hazard Mitigation Grant Program must be voluntary; FEMA will not extend the program to facilitate the exercise of eminent domain. As a consequence, public officials must engage in a substantial process of persuasion and negotiation. Even so, some homeowners occasionally hold out. The town of Valmeyer, Illinois, for example, voted to move away from the floodplain (see Rozdilsky, 1995, for an extended discussion of the case of Valmeyer). Mitigation funds through FEMA enabled the buy-out of properties. However, a few landowners resisted the program, criticizing the sums offered them for their properties. It is generally understood that people form extremely strong locational attachments but even so, the strength of that attachment is often underestimated. Indeed, the symbolic value of property is a strong determinant in decisions to remain in hazardous areas for homeowners as well as those with a more fragile hold on physical place. Veness (1993) found that "homeless" people become very attached to their dwellings, however rudimentary, and find moving to be quite personally disruptive regardless of the paucity of their possessions. The ability to implement innovative strategies requires confronting existing social norms and may demand further innovations that allow for more appropriate, or accepted, solutions.

There is an extreme and very politically charged cultural element of resistance to change and the uncertainly that change brings. Other elements might lie in certain expectations of who is responsible for disaster management—a belief that "the government" is both responsible for and able to provide a complete restoration of community life. This is always impossible. Indeed, counteracting a persistent sense that a higher level of government will continually provide assistance has become a project in policy-oriented hazards research. Scholars such as Platt (1999), Mileti (1999), and Cutter (2001) have argued that local communities have become far too dependent on federal disaster assistance and should take on more responsibility for lessening the hazards. From this perspective, local communities are the principal sites for identifying the climatological, geophysical, or industrial hazard agents and ensuring that human activities take these into account. What these researchers are calling for is essentially a large-scale social change, a shift in *national* disaster policy to be realized at the *local* level and involving a sizable shift of expectations and substantial new norms of accountability. To the extent that communities have not attended to their local circumstances, innovation will be necessary.

The discussion of innovation adoption and implementation extends internationally. Several initiatives proposed following the Indian Ocean tsunami are likely to be extremely difficult to implement. Both India and Sri Lanka governments announced an intention to enforce existing regulations that prohibit construction in the coastal zone or to establish new ones. These regulations were originally intended both for hazard mitigation and as conservation measures, but they will now conflict with the post-tsunami recovery ambitions of dozens of coastal communities. These residents desire reconstruction of their communities in their existing locations, even though such reconstruction will reproduce the locational component of their overall vulnerability. At the heart of their vision is the maintenance of long-established patterns of community life, closely associated with fishing and proximity to the water. There is thus the potential for two competing goods: reducing vulnerability to hazard and preserving traditional practices. Clearly, innovative thinking will be required, though it is not clear what direction that might take.

The fundamental conflict transcends international boundaries: What changes should communities make in order to lessen their risk, and what degree of change should communities be expected to make so that they do not require assistance from other communities or from larger scales of social organization? What is the acceptable risk? In Valmeyer, much of the community moved, and there was significant transformation of community life. In India and Sri Lanka, there would also be significant upheaval. There, however, the recurrence interval will probably be much longer than that of floods in Valmeyer though without warning systems the danger to life is greater. Balancing the economic advantages of a place, the desirability of preserving established rhythms of social life, and reducing hazard are difficult in any setting. Concerted community action will require a consensus on the acceptable collective risk of living there. At a minimum, in areas impacted by the tsunami, mitigation should begin with a new awareness of the environment, and it is likely that large-scale social changes will be required to lessen the risk of future such events. Innovations do not always lead to positive changes for a community, or certain segments of a community. The uncertainty of whether or not those new approaches or large-scale social changes will better or worsen community life can work to impede any innovation at all.

Coordination and Cooperation

Even when communities share overall goals, there may be disagreements about how progress is to be made toward those goals, either in terms of timeframes, expectations, or means of achieving goals. As a result, conflict with or between communities may ensue. Much of the writing on coordination involves some use of the concept of a shared vision, so much so that some writers, such as Weick (1995) show some impatience with the term, stressing that it does not really go far enough in explaining just what is needed in harmonizing people's actions. Nevertheless, while the concept of shared vision has not been fully reconsidered in the literature given Weick's concern, its general contours remain generally accepted and important.

One of the important aspects of how individuals, organizations, and communities make sense of new situations and determine courses of action is their ability to "extract cues" from the environment (Weick, 1995). But they do not all extract cues at the same rate, nor do they extract the same ones since, as Weick also noted, a large part of how people make sense of their environment is based on their identities. That is, as participants are exposed to different environmental and social situations, they may come to determine that different courses of action are necessary. After the September 11, 2001 attack on the World Trade Center, emergency management officials had to cope with the clearance of vast amounts of debris, much of it asbestos and other harmful materials. How to wash the debris from the transport vehicles became a point of contention between two New York City agencies, the Department of Health and Mental Hygiene (DOH) and the Department of Design and Construction (DDC). A DOH official wanted to develop a functional washdown system that would be in place immediately; a DDC official wanted to carefully design a structure that would be suitable throughout the duration of the operation, including in the freezing winter weather. One's identity as a health official, concerned about toxic exposure, conflicted with another's identity as an engineer, concerned about quality work and long-term solutions. Faced with the need to innovate, they both "made sense," but it was different sense, leading to a very different innovation trajectory.

FUTURE RESEARCH

The act or process of collective innovation would seem to be a useful line of inquiry. Virtually from the founding of the hazards field, in geography's human ecological tradition, the emphasis was on understanding how communities got themselves into trouble and suggesting what had to be done about it. These suggestions were for innovations—changes in how communities understood and acted in their natural surroundings. Yet the dynamics of human–environment interactions, in the United States and worldwide, have hardly been static. The world's population has increased dramatically; economies have grown and faltered; new dependencies have been created; new needs have evolved; and resources of energy and space have been strained. Innovation is needed to meet change but it also sparks the need for innovation elsewhere. Innovation in the entire disaster milieu is rarely and perhaps never carried out by a single person. Even when one person has a flash of creative insight, other people modify it during implementation. In our research on the interorganizational response to the World Trade Center, we encountered several officials who each claimed to have initiated a particular action. Were all but one of them wrong? Maybe. But maybe they were *all right*, so that collective innovation can emerge from multiple individual thoughts directed toward a shared goal. Research taking this approach would then come into view of the growing body of work on sensemaking, and would thus likely contribute to several fields.

In this chapter, we have taken a fairly positive stance toward innovation, emphasizing the virtues of change when confronting environmental hazard. Such a stance follows from the meaning of hazard—"a threat to people and what they value"—and the normative requirement that the situation be rectified. Innovations can, however, go awry. The project of controlling flooding along the Western rivers, study of which was the subject of much of Gilbert White's (1973) work, was relatively maladaptive. The National Flood Insurance Program has earned criticism for encouraging settlement in dangerous areas (Platt, 1999) and for payouts for repetitively damaged properties. Note that these were not innovations *in* communities, but innovations *for* communities, but still there were unintended negative spin-off effects. The principal challenge to innovations, even those that are salutary to begin with, is that they are set in a particular social and economic context. The context may change, faster than that which was innovative can be adjusted, so that in later years the innovation can actually become detrimental. Clearly more research is required for better anticipation, and also for understanding innovations as part of larger systems of social and economic activity.

In examining Tangshan, Mitchell (2004, p. 15) indicates that it is necessary for recovery planners "to hone their capacities for managing surprising contingencies." He further suggests (2004, p. 2) that the emphasis of recovery has changed over the last decades, "from the compassable goal of retrieving a known world that *was*, towards the much more uncertain task of achieving a projected, predicted or imagined world that is *yet to be*." Such a statement suggests that innovation is "squared"—that it is necessary to be able to innovate over innovations to take account of changing circumstances. Even with the apparent success of the recovery in Tangshan, Mitchell notes certain complicating factors. First, he argues that the city's recovery plan emphasized structural and economic concerns but subordinated more social needs of the community, the consideration of survivors with disabilities being, perhaps, an exception. Moreover, he suggests that an important element of successful recovery was not anticipated— the simultaneous opening and expansion of the Chinese economy. Meeting unanticipated developments will thus become a necessary capacity of officials who are managing recovery as well as those working in other disaster phases. In the case of Tangshan, shifts in circumstances were beneficial; with the National Flood Insurance Program they were not. While emergency managers have to be alert for unexpected transformations that affect their plans, is it possible to plan for innovation? In some senses, yes. It is clearly possible to plan attempts to innovate, by setting up in advance the necessary preconditions (Daft, 2004) that facilitate the exchange of information and also risk-taking, and by enacting policies that limit the conditions that stifle creativity (Amabile, 1997; Woodman, Sawyer, & Griffin, 1993).

Project Impact demonstrates something else about the effect of unexpected changes on innovation: it can be quite transient. Project Impact was dismantled at the national level by the Bush administration when they assumed office, to be replaced by a competitive grant program. Just as communities are split by conflict, so too do they fit within a larger political universe where there are many different views about the proper relationship of local and national scales of economic and political activity. In certain places, Project Impact lives on among some dedicated devotees who advance its principles in their communities and have worked to institutionalize these innovations in their local practices. Of course, the flow of federal funding would not have lasted indefinitely; the program's durability in spite of the early termination of funding points even more strongly to its larger success. Nevertheless, the transience of Project Impact shows that we need ways of decoupling innovative programs from their political provenance, and we need ways of sustaining interest in initiatives over many years. In the United States there is very little track record for sustained large-scale ambitions. The space program might be one example, though its fortunes, too, have been quite variable.

Finally, we may need to fully reconsider what is meant by community. Aguirre, Dynes, Kendra, & Connell, (2005) argued that such diffuse hazards as bioterrorism or cyberterrorism disrupt the accustomed scale of viewing community and that it may, for some hazards, be more useful to look at institutions that might be under threat, such as hospitals. Such hazards may spread quickly and surreptitiously and appear very far from their point of origin. Increasing travel and globalized economies also disrupt sociospatial connections. Owing to the growth of the South Asia tourist industry, European countries became stakeholders in the recovery and identification of victims following the 2004 Indian Ocean tsunami. And many of the victims of the 2001 World Trade Center attack lived in other cities; their relatives' desires for memorialization clashed with the more proximate residents' desires for a return to normal neighborhood rhythms. What is considered "community" can truly transcend physical linkages and create a demand for community innovation that mirrors the social rather than physical connectivity of its members.

CONCLUSION

It is impossible in a single chapter to account for all aspects of innovation in communities. Innovation is, as noted earlier, a vast area filled with conflicting theories on initiating and being successful at, change in various types of organizations. The purpose in this chapter, rather, was to highlight a number of points that seem relevant to community innovation for reducing risk and for responding to disaster. Money is certainly at issue, as is recognizing a need, though what "need" really means depends on the community's environment and the particular imperatives that it must respond to. A challenge facing communities is when the need for action is a response to a threat that is distant, speculative, unlikely, or of unknown magnitude. Prior to such an event, coordination and cooperation may be impeded because all of the required participants in the change do not see the same necessity. Even with an organizational entity such as city government (itself composed of many organizational units) disagreements can erupt over interpretations of needs, possibilities, action, and consequences. Information technology has provided an example of such discord, as city agencies have clashed over software type and specifications. The possibilities for discord become even more numerous as one looks beyond local government to the diverse organizations and interests that comprise a community. Yet at the same time, organizing against disaster requires alignment of these interests, either via their direct involvement and participations or via the action of legitimate intermediaries (e.g., elected officials).

One of the greatest needs for innovative thinking is in establishing consensus, even if merely a grudging, functional agreement, across multiple community interest groups. Often such a consensus emerges upon a disaster event, as observed, for example, by Barton (1969). Many innovative strategies and uses of resources occur in the response phase whose implementation in non-disaster times would be slowed or precluded. Urgent need, which is plainly evident, overcomes most objections. This period, however, is short lived and, moreover, though many important innovations may occur, others will prove to be maladaptive. In the urgent environment of disaster, some suboptimum innovations are an acceptable risk, and generally everyone agrees on the need for action. Such need is much less obvious in other disaster phases, and the need is not merely for innovation, but just in establishing a sense that there is a need at all. Even then, certain irreconcilable interests may be at issue.

Innovation in communities occur at multiple scales of social activity; individual organizations in the community can be innovative, so if their innovation is realized to the benefit of the community as a bounded socioeconomic and political entity, then in a sense the whole community receives the "credit" for that innovation. The reverse is also possible. Silicon Valley innovations don't make the local communities innovative, though obviously innovative and very successful people live there. A community innovation has to emerge from the same social–political ecology that creates the collective that is known as the community, from entities that are participating in that ecology. One of the principal requirements for successful innovation in communities, either before or after disaster, is coordination among various member groups. The waterborne evacuation of Manhattan, for example, involved public agencies such as the United States Coast Guard, commercial organizations such as the various tour boat and ferry companies, and private individuals acting together in a shared interpretation of the best interests of the city at that time. As Comfort (1999) emphasized, a sense of shared risk is essential. But as Peacock et al. (2000) argued, our communities are anything but coherent groups of like-minded people. It is an axiom in the hazards research field that hazards are "mismatches" of natural and social systems (Mitchell, 1990), but devastating events such as the Kobe earthquake, the Indian Ocean tsunami, and more recently Hurricane Katrina demonstrated all too ably that communities do not "share" the risk that natural forces and social systems combine to create. Innovations to benefit the community must transcend the fractures in community relationships at all scales; the most successful ones will be those that can reengineer those relationships as well as their precarious interactions with the natural environment.

CHAPTER 19

Disaster and Development Research and Practice: A Necessary Eclecticism?

MAUREEN FORDHAM

Those concerned with disaster and development represent a diversity of interests including the academic/theoretical, the policy-related, the practitioner-oriented, and the political. This results in the generation of different theories and literatures, varied budgets, disparate organizational structures, and diverse constituencies and worldviews. Perhaps, not surprisingly, there can be conflicting expectations, and even degrees of hostility and incomprehension, among those who deal in some way with disaster and/or development.

Exhortations to appropriate action can suggest that the melding of disaster and development is a matter of simple common sense but this deceptive simplicity masks both conceptual and practical complexity. Who could deny the appropriateness of ensuring that disaster risk reduction and response should take due note of long-term development initiatives and concerns? Furthermore, who could deny that development policy makers and practitioners should avoid increasing people's disaster vulnerability through inappropriate programs? While the bringing together of disaster and development is called for by a growing number of researchers, donors, and activists, the categories persist in many cases as stubbornly separate areas of practice and enquiry.

This chapter can only touch upon some of the many possible elements of this complex field. It explores some of the meanings of disaster and development in both research and practice; explores why they have followed divergent paths and why there are increasing calls for union; proposes some possible research areas; and finally suggests some common ground may lie in the application of theories of social capital.

WHAT DO WE MEAN BY "DISASTER" AND "DEVELOPMENT"?

Viewed simplistically, development is a positive term (but see the discussion below): it is forward-focused on improving economic and social conditions and tends towards long-term processes. It can be separated from the term disaster, which has negative connotations and typically tends toward a short-term, backward, focus on the response to, or the management of, extant, somewhat localized, catastrophic events. These simplistic conceptualizations are expanded below to show how theories and practices of development and disaster have their own histories and cultures and present a challenge to those who would wish them more closely allied. Further, the two terms are slippery and defy any but the most generally agreed definition by those who call themselves disaster researchers (Quarantelli, 1998).

DEVELOPMENT

Development, in its commonly understood sense of an increasing standard of living through, initially, economic processes, programs, and projects (Hodder, 2000, p. 3), was envisioned after World War II when U.S. President Truman advocated (in 1949) a "fair deal"—not just for the United States but for the whole world—to be achieved through the application of capital, science, and technology. However, this vision appears increasingly tarnished in the face of widespread *under* development and impoverishment (Escobar, 1995), which partly reflects the nonsustainability of primarily economic development trajectories of the neoliberal form. In the 1950s and 1960s, dominant forms of development based on modernization theory held traditional forms of social organization (e.g., the community-based structures and relations currently regarded so highly) to be regressive and a barrier to capitalist progress trajectories (Moore, 1997 in Woolcock & Narayan, 2000, p. 4).

A more people-centered, social vision developed subsequently and is inherent in the longer-term, future-oriented, and now classic, definition of sustainability from the United Nations' Brundtland Commission Report, "Our Common Future: Development that Meets the Needs of the Present Without Compromising the Ability of Future Generations to Meet Their Own Needs" (WCED, 1987, p. 43).

While this was primarily stimulated by concerns for intergenerational equity arising from the exploitation of natural resources, its viewpoint has been internalized by a much wider range of interests concerned with taking a longer term approach to the interrelated spheres of environment, economy, and society.

Development studies (or international development studies as it is also known) is, like disaster studies, a multi- or interdisciplinary field of studies rather than a single discipline but can generally be assumed to have a normative focus, at the heart of which is poverty reduction in developing countries. As commonly understood in the present context, development is deemed to be the provision of aid from the developed to the developing countries of the world to enable them to reach levels of economic, social, and political development similar to that of the donors. In this light, development is assumed to be a "good thing" but post-development theorists have undermined this romantic and uniform view with a representation of development as vulgar modernization, controlled by elites, and leading to the creation of underdevelopment (see, e.g., Corbridge, 1990, 1986; Escobar, 1995).

Development studies and development practice share with disaster studies and disaster management a similarly complex and varied history and diversity of identities. Wijkman and Timberlake (1984) assert that there is even less agreement on the definitions of development than there is on the meanings of disaster (p. 123) about which there is considerable discord. However, the focus of this chapter is on the interface between disaster research and development rather than on development per se.

DISASTER

The 1980s was a significant decade for advancing our thinking on disaster and development (see Cuny, 1983) but Quarantelli (1998, p. 260) notes the dissimilarity in subject matter and literature between disaster researchers and development researchers arising most probably from an early North–South divide. This split is apparent in the exclusion from the purview of disaster sociology, of famines, droughts, and epidemics (Quarantelli, 1998)—not exclusive to, but more common in, the global south—which effectively excludes much that concerns researchers and workers in and on the developing world. For example, Sanderson (2000, p. 96) notes that disaster management strategy in an African context is almost synonymous with food security and thus immediately puts it outside the commonly allowable sociological definition. Attempts to define disasters have a theoretical basis grounded in substantial theoretical and empirical research on organizational and collective behavior which has tended to rule out inclusion of conflict and slow-onset events (see the Disaster Research Center Web site). Therefore, the appropriate subject range for disaster researchers has also been affected. While these subject areas are not strictly proscribed, the vast majority of work within the disaster sociology area eschews them (Dynes, 2004; Quarantelli, 1998), because chronic and acute forms of collective stress result in sociologically distinct processes (see Merton in Barton, 1969, p. xxv). Arguably it is also because they are not so amenable to management by professional disaster management organizations (a more frequent focus of disaster sociological inquiry) but reflect more saliently the underlying political power structures, the study of which has been the focus for a different set of researchers/actors (see the vulnerability approach below).

Disaster sociology is of course but one subset of the disasters field. Others include those who work under the banner of hazards research and sit on one side of a traditional environment–society divide, although it has become more generally accepted that focusing on the (physical) hazard alone will not reduce disaster risk or subsequent impacts. The once dominant hazards paradigm (with its primary focus on the "natural" and the geophysical, and its characterization of disaster events as exceptional (extreme) and separate from the everyday), met a significant critique in Hewitt's 1983b edited collection, which adopted an avowedly political economy approach and took its examples and case studies, not only from the Third World but also from the perspective of the victims. This position was more closely allied to development theory than disaster research and inevitably paved the way for different recommendations, solutions, and methods of enquiry. These tended away from the technical fixes of the hazards paradigm, or the advancement of expert systems and command and control structures of organizational sociology (Hewitt, 1998), and toward participatory, community-based approaches (Maskrey, 1989), and the alternative perspective of, what has been called, the vulnerability approach (Blaikie, Cannon, Davis, & Davis, 1994; Cannon, 2000; Comfort et al., 1999; Hewitt, 1997; Varley, 1994b; Wisner, Blaikie, Cannon, & Davis, 2004). The vulnerability perspective is anchored in political economy and analyses that identify the root causes of disaster vulnerability (Wisner et al., 2004) and the social geography of harm (Hewitt, 1997). It identifies the social, economic and political structures underpinning societies which create inequalities and vulnerabilities, and—through "development gone wrong"—disasters. The disaster definition used is expansive and blurs the exceptional and the everyday.

An example of this would be Lavell's (2002, 2003) analysis of the flood problem in the Lower Lempa River Valley in El Salvador which highlighted the everyday risks and hazards faced by the local population—the vast majority of whom live below the poverty line. Lavell's paper presents a project that included land-use planning and health and risk management among other wide ranging responses to the flood risk and thus integrated development with disaster risk reduction. He also refers to the transformative potential, even necessity, of the disaster-development nexus when he argues that isolating disaster mitigation initiatives from the transformation of social and economic conditions simply perpetuates inadequate conditions of everyday life (Lavell, 2003, p. 3). Another important conclusion of the work was that *social organization* was the key to empowerment and sustainability (Lavell, 2002, p. 13) and this is discussed further below under *social capital*.

The preceding discussion has referred briefly to just three competing/complementary approaches to disaster studies: natural hazards, disaster sociology, and vulnerability; but there are numerous others, each with their own subject matter and literature. They cross over many disciplinary fields such as sociology, geography, anthropology, and politics; in fact Alexander (1997) has claimed some 30 disciplines have an interest in the disasters field. While the variety of disasters research is presented elsewhere in this volume, two others are mentioned here because of their more frequent overlaps with disaster sociology and vulnerability approaches. These are, respectively, the risk and humanitarian fields. They are mentioned here for further examination by those interested in disaster and development research and practice because each has developed considerable bodies of case material, theories, and practices (for some recent examples of risk literature see Beck, 1992; Boin, Lagadec, Michel-Kerjan, & Overdijk, 2003; Comfort, 1999; Horlick-Jones, 2001; Pidgeon, Kasperson, & Slovic, 2003; and for the humanitarian approach see Clay, 2005; Macrae, 2000; Macrae & Zwi, 1994; Turner and Pidgeon, 1997; Yamin & Huq, 2005; the Humanitarian Practice Network Web site). For a more detailed exposition than can be presented here, the interested reader is referred to Dynes (2002) for a discussion of the two separate streams of disaster and development literature.

DISASTER AND DEVELOPMENT

Wijkman and Timberlake point to the cause of most Third World disasters in unsolved development problems (1984, p. 122). Anthony Oliver-Smith (1994, 1999c) provides a long historical view of an unsolved development problem in Peru that led inevitably to disaster. This is development as colonization where the coming of the Spanish in the 1530s was itself a disaster. Peru was always a hazardous place but traditional adaptations had tended to minimize these effects. The Spanish conquerors located towns in hazardous areas previously avoided and ordered the migration and concentration of people into fewer, larger settlements that would be easier to control but also vulnerable to disaster. Spanish building techniques and settlement plans concentrated people into a grid pattern of narrow streets where previously settlements had been spaced out; they built houses taller with second stories and heavy tiled roofs, making them more dangerous in a collapse. The Spaniards extracted surpluses, leaving nothing for storage and to provide for the survival of people following disaster. All this could be seen as advancement and development for Peru but the result, hundreds of years later, was that more than 65,000 people died in the earthquake that struck in 1970. Disasters do not suddenly occur: they are constructed over time—sometimes many centuries—and are closely related to societal development.

There is now a growing body of both First and Third World examples showing positive and negative outcomes of disaster and development, and the relationship between the two. This can be seen schematically in Table 19.1.

The following are some generic examples for each cell of this disaster–development matrix:

TABLE 19.1. Disaster and Development Linkages

	development		
negative	(a) Development increases vulnerability to disaster.	(b) Development reduces vulnerability to disaster.	positive
	(c) Disasters impede development.	(d) Disasters provide development opportunities.	
	disasters		

Adapted from UNDP/DHA, 1994, p. 10.

1. *Development increases vulnerability to disaster.* Tourism development in scenic yet hazardous areas (e.g., coasts, floodplains, mountains, etc.) can place many more people at risk (e.g., from hurricanes and tsunami, from flash floods, from avalanches, and mud and landslides). Specific development projects can increase risk (e.g., digging tube wells in Bangladesh tapped into arsenic contaminated water; ineffective building codes were the cause of many earthquake deaths in Turkey in 1999). Campbell (1990) discusses how a Pacific Island community became more vulnerable to disasters through development processes that modified social, economic, and resource management systems and undermined their traditional mechanisms for coping with disasters. This approach would be of interest in analyzing the 2004 Indian Ocean earthquake and tsunami which demonstrated the manufacture of vulnerability through global tourism development.

2. *Development reduces vulnerability to disaster.* Housing projects that incorporate safe design and follow building codes can reduce damage in the next storm or earthquake (see ITDG, 2005, for earthquake-resistant housing design in Alto Mayo region of Peru). Tree planting and terracing can reduce landslide risk while simultaneously strengthening livelihoods and improving agricultural output.

3. *Disasters impede development.* The AIDS/HIV pandemic is having major, long term impacts on development in many African countries. Major disasters frequently destroy school buildings and children's education. It may be many months before children can return to education. Sometimes they never do because they are needed to rebuild household livelihoods and cannot be spared from the effort.

4. *Disasters provide development opportunities.* Post-disaster livelihood development programs (in place of simple relief) increase the ability of households and communities to rebuild not only what was lost in disaster but also their everyday coping capacities and household incomes. Women's empowerment can be stimulated by post-disaster programs that incorporate gender equality requirements (see also SEWA's microfinance initiatives for women [Patel & Nanavaty, 2005]).

Another conceptualization is presented in DFID (2005) where the possibilities for either negative or positive outcomes is characterized as either a vicious spiral of disaster risk and development failure or a virtuous spiral of risk reduction (pp. 24–25). Mary Beth Anderson (1991) identifies three reasons why disasters should be integrated in development planning:

1. Disasters and poverty are closely linked.
2. Development itself can create or exacerbate disasters.
3. Failure to factor in disasters can mean development resources are wasted.

Anderson provides a sound economic argument for the linking of disaster—and more importantly, disaster risk reduction—with development: in its minimization of damage it "promotes a stable environment, incentives for investment and enterprise, and the sense that people can control their own economic destiny" (Anderson, 1991, p. 27). These she regards as fundamental to sustainable long-term development.

This reasoning is apparent in more recent work by Benson and Twigg (2004a, 2004b), who also point out that the achievement of the Millennium Development Goals and poverty reduction initiatives are threatened by a recent escalation in the occurrence of major disasters. Hurricane Mitch in 1998 provided an unwanted example of the impact on development gains that major disasters can bring. The President of Honduras, Carlos Flores, remarked that Mitch destroyed in 72 hours what it had taken more than 50 years to create (Tearfund, 2004). However, Benson and Twigg point out that despite the rhetoric linking disasters and development, many of these same organizations are hesitant about making risk reduction—rather than disaster response—their focus.

When disasters occur they force their own dynamic in which the *speed* of delivery is dominant over the *form* of delivery. This, as it relates to gender needs, has been described as the "tyranny of the urgent" (BRIDGE, 1996). The response is framed in the short-term context of the disaster with all its attendant pressures to be seen to be doing something quickly in an attempt to return to normality/normalcy. It can mean that long-term development principles (particularly related to working with local people in a truly participatory and egalitarian manner) may be overturned (Anderson & Woodrow, 1998).

It is common for considerable resources and attention to be focused on the response stage, less frequently on the recovery stage (Berke, Kartez, & Wenger, 1993), and least represented of all are the activities that come before the disaster: prevention, mitigation, preparedness, and risk reduction. These are also the areas for which donor funding is scarcer. It is hard to demonstrate the benefit of work that results in the *absence* of something (Annan, 1999), but preparedness that makes communities resilient to disasters or that prevents disasters occurring is—or should be—at the heart of sustainable development. In its recent (2002) global review of disaster risk—Living with Risk—the UNISDR has argued that disaster reduction, social and economic development, and sympathetic environmental management are inseparable conceptually and must be in practice if future development is to be truly sustainable. However, while it is hard to argue with the rhetoric, the reality comprises disparate agencies, budgets, cultures, and practices that represent seemingly insurmountable barriers to integration.

An example that identifies some of the disaster-development linkages and schisms is Walker's (1990) discussion of contingency planning for future famine crises in Ethiopia. He refers, for example, to the importance of monitoring changes in people's total asset bundle rather than the more limited monitoring of local food availability and sale of peasant assets. This necessitates agencies with long-term commitments to an area and these are usually long-term, program focused development agencies/nongovernmental organizations (NGOs) rather than short-term, single project focused disaster/relief agencies (p. 114). He concludes that the way ahead lies in vulnerability reduction through appropriate development (p. 116). This conclusion is echoed by Kelly and Chowdhury (2005, p. 3), who examined disaster, poverty, and environment linkages in Bangladesh and found that poverty contributes to disaster impact with the poor being more affected and taking longer to recover than the wealthier. However, they also found that non-disaster shocks can outweigh disaster impacts on poorer people over the long term (related to this see the Web sites of La Red and DesInventar). Thus, a focus on disaster (relief or response) here would not necessarily protect poor Bangladeshis from livelihood impacts (see below) unless it incorporated development-oriented capacity building.

THE PRACTICES OF DISASTER PLANNING/MANAGEMENT, AND DEVELOPMENT PROGRAMMING

Those who would work in disaster and/or development must contend not just with varying disciplinary and political perspectives but also with the tension between academic/scholarly endeavor and practitioner-led interests. Robert Chambers has described the two differing cultures of practitioner and academic development professionals as focused respectively on action and understanding (Chambers, 1997, pp. 33–35).

This is something that faces all disciplinary areas that attempt the crossover and the dichotomy can also be identified within the natural hazards community. White and Haas (1975) recognized the need to bring together research and practice and disseminate it to researchers and practitioners alike and it is made concrete in the Annual Workshop run by the Natural Hazards Research and Information Applications Center in Boulder, Colorado (Myers, 1993). A Special Issue of the *International Journal of Mass Emergencies and Disasters* is a good starting point for exploring these issues with a set of papers concerning bridging the gap between disaster research and practice (IJMED, 1993, Vol. 11, No. 1). Despite these, and other, initiatives, there are still tensions between these two cultures. Guarnizo argued in 1993 that researchers' understanding of disaster-development linkages was ahead of institutional practice, although here she was referring specifically to NGO responses in the Third World. However, appreciation of the linkages has not just been seen in theoretical work but also in the focus of donors and major agencies. For example, significant recent documents include UNDP's (2004) "Reducing Disaster Risk: A Challenge for Development" and DFID's (2005) "Disaster Risk Reduction: A Development Concern." The World Summit on Sustainable Development (WSSD) highlighted disaster risk reduction; the UNISDR (despite its genesis in the International Decade for Natural Disaster Reduction [IDNDR] which was criticized for its overly physical and technical approach), has a development, most particularly a *sustainable* development, focus very much to the fore of its recent work (see "Living With Risk," 2002); the United Nations Environment Programme (UNEP) has highlighted a "vulnerability gap" within and between countries and regions (2002); the International Federation of Red Cross and Red Crescent Societies (IFRC), perhaps the quintessential humanitarian relief agency, has progressed to include a more recent focus on the development context. Its 2002 World Disasters Report (IFRC, 2002) has as its theme "reducing risk" in which it asks: "Does development expose more people to disasters?"

However, changes in policy direction at the international level do not seamlessly manifest themselves in national level activities. A Philippine National Red Cross (PNRC), integrated, community disaster planning program on the island of Leyte attempted to reduce the passive receipt of aid and facilitate a more active role for local communities as disaster and development actors but a truly sustainable livelihoods approach was blocked by the PNRC's own project design and implementation systems and also donor conditionality (Allen, 2003). As Sanderson (2000) notes, disasters are rarely included in urban development strategies and vice versa. Completely different ministries are involved with little knowledge of each other's activities. Indicative of this yawning gap is his example of India's Ministry of Urban Affairs' 1999 Draft National Slum Policy which has no reference to the vulnerability to natural disaster of slum dwellers. Yet the Ministry's own documents record that 1% of India's total housing stock is destroyed by natural disasters every year (Sanderson, 2000, pp. 95–96). These constitute evidence of the complexity of the disaster-development environment.

Alongside this growing recognition of disaster development linkages, considerable separation still remains. Many humanitarian organizations have identified themselves as either development- or disaster-focused. Indeed, professionals in one are sometimes hostile to those in the other, regarding the others' operations as disruptive to their own and sometimes finding the other's professional culture alien and even offensive. While some personnel remain dominantly in one or the other, most are now realizing that there is more that connects disaster and development than divides them. Disasters "turn back the development clock" (Sanderson, 2000, p. 95). Furthermore, it is increasingly common for academic courses related to disaster or development (which many newer members of staff in humanitarian organizations may have studied) to draw out the connections as a result of the growing recognition of the way disasters are a manifestation of failed development (Lewis, 1999).

THE CONTRIBUTIONS OF SUSTAINABLE DEVELOPMENT

While "development" traditionally was seen as something to be carried out largely in developing countries, "sustainable development," coming out of the World Conference on Environment and Development 1987, has more recently become firmly embedded in the developed world's consciousness. In the present context, a significant research milestone, albeit with a U.S. focus, was the publication of Dennis Mileti's edited work, *Disasters by Design*. This reassessment of natural hazards placed the increasing losses from U.S. disasters at the door of short-sighted or ill-conceived development. Sustainable development is popularly seen as even more of a "good thing" than ordinary development. However, McEntire (1998a, 1999) and Aguirre (2002b) raise some concerns with the concept as it is applied to disasters, in particular the primacy given to the environment and its relative silence on disaster risk reduction.

Can *development* be sustainable? Cuny remarked in 1983 on the link between vulnerability and people's desire for modernity in which the least able to cope with disaster are those who have begun to change their socioeconomic status and left behind their less sophisticated but self-reliant societies (p. 4); how much more so in the context of processes of globalization which have advanced in the intervening years (Fordham, 2003; Wisner, 1999)? Cuny's observation concerning self-reliant societies, while still having analytical strength, appears strangely archaic in the context of globalization and regionalization which, through international/transnational institutions and market forces, are charged with overtaking the role of the nation state or society—"the standard unit of development" (Pieterse, 2001, p. 1). Yet, the undermining of the autonomy of the nation state has simultaneously reawakened interest at the level of smaller communal units. Community-based approaches have become the new norm in both disaster and development and the community is recognized as the locus of disaster response and disaster resilience (Dynes, 2005). Community-based approaches attract support from across the political spectrum, appealing (paradoxically) to both a radical activist sensibility as well as a neoliberal rejection of modernist grand development projects (Rapley, 2004, p. 353).

THE CONTRIBUTION OF THE LIVELIHOODS APPROACH AND SOCIAL CAPITAL

A useful progression in sustainable development thinking has been the livelihoods approach (see Ashley & Carney, 1999; Chambers & Conway, 1992; Sanderson, 2000). According to DFID (http://www.livelihoods.org), sustainable livelihoods are about putting people at the center of development which could be read as a rebalancing of development, less in favor of macroeconomics and more in favor of the social. Sanderson argues that "sustainable livelihoods methodologies provide a valuable opportunity for combining disaster reduction and development interventions in one unifying approach." (2000, p. 96). This approach views people in a vulnerability context as prone to various shocks and stresses, but also recognizes a range of poverty-reducing (and, by implication, disaster resilience creating) assets—in the form of different "capitals" of which social capital is one (see DFID's Livelihoods Connect Web site). Although this approach has grown out of work on rural natural resources and food security (African drought-induced famine in particular) its utility is much wider and it is a valuable tool for linking poverty with disasters (Sanderson, 2000, p. 97); indeed, Woolcock and Narayan argue that social capital is the capital of the poor (2000, p. 240).

In the disasters context, while not referring to social capital as such, Berke et al. (1993) highlight the importance of horizontal integration between community/citizen groups and vertical integration between them and external governmental and other agencies in recovery after disaster. The language of social capital would call these horizontal and vertical networks "bonding" and "bridging" social capital respectively (see Woolcock & Narayan [2000, pp. 7–8] for more on this and, for its origins, Georg Simmel's work on insiders and outsiders).

Nakagawa and Shaw (2004) have used social capital to examine post-disaster communities in Kobe, Japan and Gujarat, India. They conclude that the communities' social capital and leadership were the most effective elements in enhancing collective action and disaster recovery. This analysis exemplifies that conceptual shift noted by Portes and Landolt whereby social capital is regarded as an attribute of the community (following Putnam), not as an attribute of the individual, as originally formulated by Bourdieu, Coleman and others (cited in Portes and Landolt, 1998, pp. 534–535). It is, however, the conceptualization that is most common in the more recent disaster and development literature discussed here.

While community-based approaches have perhaps now become the dominant paradigm in both disaster and development, communities can represent both inclusion and exclusion and thus cannot be regarded as an undiluted social good. Social capital must be recognized as also having a "downside" (e.g., group membership that enables privileged access to resources also bars others from the same assets; see Portes & Landolt, 1998, pp. 532–533). Further, social capital concepts are prone to overly simplistic readings that are reminiscent of the early inclusion of gender in development, characterized by the WID (Women In Development) approach which simply added "women" into the development mix and ignored the gendered social relations that were later conceptualized in the GAD (Gender And Development) approach. Social capital theory is thus open to abuse through its purely technical application to disaster and/or development field-study. Similarly, in policy making or programming it is just one of many tools or community attributes and "contrary to the expectations of some policymakers, social capital is not a substitute for the provision of credit, material infrastructure, and education" (Portes & Landolt, 1998, p. 547) nor is it a replacement for poor governance (see Woolcock & Narayan, 2000, referring to Tendler & Uphoff on pp. 234 and 238, respectively).

WHAT SHOULD RESEARCHERS IN DISASTER AND DEVELOPMENT STUDY AND HOW?

There is much to be learned from the interchange of ideas between the various disaster and development research and practitioner communities. For example, both disaster and development are highly *gendered domains* (see Mueller, 1991, p. 1 cited in Escobar, 1995, p. 180 regarding the development apparatus as male-dominated and world-dominating) but development work, workers, and policymakers employed a gender lens far sooner and to greater effect than their equivalents in disaster (see Enarson & Morrow, 1998a; Morrow & Philips, 1999). Disaster practice and disaster scholarship has had to learn from development and this has meant the import of ideas from the global south into northern theory and practice. This has been responsible for some of the most fruitful advances in disaster and sustainable development thinking. There is much that still needs to be done in examining disasters and development through a gender lens and the gap in application of this approach to the developed, particularly European, milieu is significant.

As already outlined above, the *livelihoods approach* and *social capital* in particular are fruitful conceptual frameworks for the analysis of disaster and development in both developed and developing countries. The role of "livelihood relief"—which aims to support people's economic development and not just provide static, potentially dependency-engendering, relief aid—is a newly emerging disaster response which could be explored in a developed world context also. So far it appears largely confined to India (see the All India Disaster Mitigation Institute Web site) but has wider currency and can be seen to have its beginnings in Cuny's work in 1983. As yet, while practical application may be growing, there is little research and literature on the subject (Twigg, 2004).

Much more remains to be explored through social capital and its relationship to other capitals. Methodologically, a shared resource of research tools is available at the World Bank Social Capital Web site (http://www.worldbank.org/socialcapital). It is important to explore its "downside" in terms of exclusionary practices and negative, as well as the more widely trumpeted, positive benefits of "the community." A review of the "community studies" literature would be beneficial, particularly as it met a significant critique because of its overly sympathetic portraits of localities (Bell & Newby, 1971, p. 55).

Much attention has been focused on large-scale disasters or catastrophes but less on *lower level impacts*, the conventional preserve of development. The cumulative damage of these chronic events that are never included in disaster statistics can be significant, and ultimately have a similarly negative development impact, especially in poor or marginalized communities (Hewitt, 1983b; Lavell, 1999). Although this challenges some of the core definitions of the disaster field, the extent to which unsolved problems of development were significant factors in disasters and lesser events is worthy of further exploration in a range of settings.

It is not just the subject of research (the "what") but also the method (the "how") that must be considered. Methodological approaches will be determined by the way the reality of disaster and development is understood. There has been a fundamental conflict between positivist and critical approaches: for the former, reality is observable and social facts can be explained and predicted. For the latter, reality is ideological and explanation must lead to social and political change. However, the breadth of the disaster and development terrain and the range of people with an interest in it are such that no single position can claim overall dominance, yet all have much to learn from the interchange of ideas.

CONCLUSION

More and more agencies are realizing the linkages and are crossing the disaster-development divide. They are being encouraged to do so by organizations such as the United Nations in many of its constitutive divisions, offices, programs, and funds (and the UNISDR in particular). Thus, many organizations formerly seen to be disaster agencies are now incorporating development work into their programs and activities. Similarly, development agencies are becoming

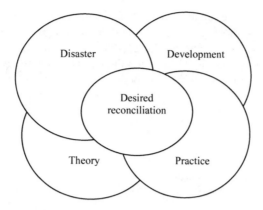

FIGURE 19.1. Desired reconciliation of disaster and development.

increasingly involved in disasters. The Millennium Development Goals (not notable for their attention to disasters) are not likely to be met by many countries and the country reports often refer to disasters as the major contributing cause (see MDGs Web site). There is thus a desired reconciliation of these different elements (see Fig. 19.1).

However, while it may be legitimate to argue that policy and so-called real world practice should bring together disaster and development, in research and scholarship the issue is not so clear-cut. There are fundamental differences between different research paradigms to which there is no simple technical solution such as more empirical evidence or a more elegant theoretical model to convince those of another disposition. The information deficit model (Irwin, 1995) is not sufficient to bridge this divide. It represents different—sometimes conflicting, sometimes complementary—worldviews and ideological positions. There is a politics inside disaster studies as well as outside in the subjects of the research. Within the academic sphere it represents, at its extreme, a clash between descriptive/explanatory and normative approaches; between the intentionally separated, and the inescapably linked, realms of fact and value. It is characterized respectively by the objective scientist as disinterested observer and the radical activist operating from a critical, action-oriented, perspective for whom, in Marxist terms, the purpose is not just to understand the world but to change it. At its less extreme it represents differing disciplinary traditions and professional expectations that place limits on the extent to which researchers can step outside conventional boundaries.

Pieterse has said: "Development is too complex to allow partial approaches to have their way" (2001, p. xii). The law of requisite variety would suggest that the complexity of the disaster-development nexus demands at least a degree of multidisciplinarity and preferably interdisciplinarity, and points to a necessary eclecticism in the field. However, each paradigm potentially brings its own particular contribution to knowledge and is therefore legitimate in its own right. While research and scholarship demand broad familiarity with the field(s), individual research outputs may not make all aspects explicit. These exclusions of what others regard as critical may stimulate further epistemological confrontation but arguably that is symptomatic of a dynamic research field. It is hard to see how a widespread move to the middle ground (with an inevitable withering of the more radical extremes) would necessarily improve either research output or social change.

Social capital theory is one possible unifying framework for the disparate interests of disaster and development, theory and practice. Woolcock and Narayan (2000) note how the literature has embraced all the social science disciplines and offers researchers, policymakers, and practitioners opportunities for cooperation and dialogue regarded as crucial for both conceptual and operational advancement (pp. 228 and 242). Co-evolution with fruitful interchange using such a framework is one way to maintain the richness and diversity of the disaster and development fields while offering scope for cooperation.

CHAPTER 20

National Planning and Response: National Systems

NEIL R. BRITTON

The notion of a "national system" evokes an image of unity, perhaps even coherence and integration, which many in the disaster management field would query. The assumption that through orderly arrangements, disaster risk goals are being achieved in the best possible manner is not a reality yet. To be fair, disaster management is not the only field of endeavor that falls short, although it is true that disaster management coordination has long been a problem. The term "national system" also directs attention to different governance levels and mechanisms to secure systematic action. In this context the role of central government comes to the fore, and this is the focus of attention in this discussion. Studying national-level planning and response systems requires analyzing the role of central governments: "national" disaster management calls for specific actions at a central government level. Some general observations about governmental classifications and the role of government will set the scene for a review of this system level.

In the context of this discussion, national system refers to enduring unitary central governmental arrangements. In such a system all authority to make laws is vested in one principal governing body whose legality embraces the entire country. While subnational legislatures may exist, their roles are subordinate to and are determined by the central government. The generic term "government" encompasses a wide range of agencies, departments, and institutions in executive, legislative, and judicial branches comprising elected and appointed officials who can be either full- or part-time and permanent or temporary employees. Other types of central governmental systems that are distinct from unitary systems, such as transitional governments (states with governance systems passing from one condition to another, sometimes referred to as hybrid regimes) and federal governments (wherein central and local governments have a measure of guaranteed autonomous decision-making authority), are discussed by other contributors.

While the statement conceals more than it reveals, it has been said that government provides services that are not exchanged on economic markets but are justified on the basis of general social values, the public interest, and politically imposed demands of groups. Governments and their public organizations thus perform crucial functions, a major purpose of which is to ensure the maintenance and well-being of a sovereign society. It does this through offices staffed with functionaries who have legitimate authority to make decisions on behalf of their respective communities; to establish frameworks within which decisions can be made and/or implemented; and to carry out (or cause to carry out) specific tasks. In general, responsibilities for these actions are divided between national (the term "central government" is used interchangeably in this chapter) and subnational (or local) government. Within this distinction central governments typically maintain systems of law, justice, and social organization. They maintain individual rights and freedoms; provide national security and stability; and give direction to the nation and its constitutive communities. By contrast, subnational government normally provide the basic services, amenities, and controls necessary for the health and overall well-being of the community, as well as the mechanisms for enhancing the quality of life of its citizens through leadership, advocacy, and representation.

Within this overall arrangement, and following Curtice (1985), national governments can be classified on the basis of the relationship between government and the governed. Here, the focus revolves around the extent to which government attempts to achieve its aim by coercion rather than persuasion, and the extent to which limits are placed on the legitimate authority of government. A distinction is often drawn between liberal democratic governments, on the one hand, which are responsive to the wishes of society and have clear limits placed on their ability to coerce or mold society in a particular way, and totalitarian governments that have fewer limits on either their authority or methods of coercion. Based on their underlying democratic relationships, Kamrava (1996) further suggests four distinct governmental types: first world democracies with historical longevity; more recent governments born out of the 1970s–1980s democratization process; proto- or quasi-democracies in which democratic mechanisms such as elections and political parties exist but the spirit of democracy does not extend beyond elite circles; and nondemocratic governments that often take the form of either bureaucratic-authoritarian regimes or inclusionary populist ones.

Within this broad tapestry, central government has a special role in relation to disaster management and has specific responsibilities to ensure that appropriate risk reduction, disaster preparedness, and response activities are adopted and implemented. How governments deal with risk says a lot about a nation's institutions and political culture (Waugh, 2006). Appendix 1 outlines some key tasks that central governments should, in an ideal world, pursue although it must be noted that while laws, institutions, and systems for managing disaster around the world follow certain patterns there is no universal model and hence the 10 attributes highlighted in Appendix 1 will be pursued in different ways and under different structural and procedural arrangements. Studies in various countries have identified approaches that range from exclusive "top-down" central government-only directed efforts, to styles that encourage "bottom-up" all-of-nation cooperative- measures, as well as versions in between. However, detailed analyses of specific national approaches to the management of disaster risk that go beyond mere structural description (e.g., explaining organizational "wiring diagrams") and legal narratives (e.g., providing an account of key sections from relevant statutes) are few and far between, especially with respect to effectiveness against specific criteria, strategic development, or links to other areas of significant national-level actions. Cross-cultural studies of disaster management systems are also relatively rare. These conditions have led researchers Tierney, Lindell, and Perry (2001) to state that not only does little systematic research exist to compare organizational features, policies, and practices of central governments, but there is also an absence of research on how governmental structures and policies influence preparedness and recovery activities. A recent endeavor by the Inter-Agency Secretariat of the International Strategy for Disaster Reduction (ISDR) has gone part way to resolve this by compiling descriptive material of national disaster management planning systems written by government officials that include examples of what individual nations consider to be "best practice" (available in the national platform section of the ISDR Web site).

Moreover, it is still commonplace that national governments do not automatically recognize disaster management as a core function, although it is true that its significance is moving up government agendas. Nevertheless, cumbersome administrative procedures, shortages of funds, and low levels of political commitment are still cited as outcomes from disaster's lack of political salience, along with poor and unsustainable development practices, a lack of community participation and many other factors that either divert or prevent actions that have been widely agreed and accepted in principle (Burton, 2005).

Governments, however, are not theoretical but empirical in orientation. Moreover, governments tend first to address their legislated mandates and act from political self-interest rather than looking beyond their traditional processes for solutions (Newtown, 1999, p. 264). They form positions and policies on the basis of reflection and reaction to occasions that impact on the lives of the citizens they are obliged to protect. Disasters, as social disruptions, are one such category of occasion that demands governmental attention. How government defines disaster is therefore important because this starts the process of policy development that leads to the domain, tasks, resources, and activities mix described by Kreps (1998), the combination of which helps to frame social action in a disaster. Moreover, disaster management practitioners tend to operate within action frameworks that are handed down and enshrined by governments through legislation.

HISTORICAL ROOTS

For most of the 20th century, and in particular between the late-1930s until the late-1970s (prompted initially by the civil defense movement in the United Kingdom in preparation for World War II and boosted in the post-Korean War era by the United States), if central governments had any systematic disaster management program at all, it was typically based on a military "command and control" model (Dynes, 1994), staffed by former or serving armed forces personnel, located as an outpost within the nation's department of defense, focused on preparing for the next impact, and preparations were backward-looking based on the assumption that solutions to the next problem would be found in the last. This representation went relatively unimpeded until the 1980s, when the National Governor's Association (1979) made inroads with a call for focused policy initiatives and wider skills among relevant staff.

Although the attention of social science research and government policies has been on planning for preparedness, response, and short-term relief, the total amount of effort overall was modest. One reason why early investigations tended not to focus on the national level was because research at the time indicated that major benefits were to be found by bolstering community level efforts and the national thrust should be to enhance local level activities and skills. Existing material tended to deal with ways in which governmental structures and policies influenced planning and response. Moreover, most was conducted in the United States, although some work was pursued elsewhere, for example in Australia (e.g., Britton, 1984, 1986b, 1991; Britton & Wettenhall, 1990; Wettenhall, 1975), both federal systems. Drawing on what was available, while noting that the pickings were slim, Drabek (1986) concluded that national level preparedness initiatives were formed mainly following major impacts: it was somewhat exceptional for a country to progress disaster management contingencies unless an actual hazard impact had revealed deficiencies in existing planning and/or response arrangements. Hence, "planning reflects the unevenness of growth spurts stemming form a short-lived consciousness of risk" (Drabek, 1986, p. 60).

Based on understandings such as these, Drabek (1986) postulated that, "in all societies disaster planning will be uneven and non-uniform across hazard types, reflecting cultural values, assumptions and power differentials" (1986, p. 60). Drawing on the U.S. experience, Tierney et al. (2001) referred to this approach as the "fix upon failure" arrangement, which was characterized by a massive mobilization of material aid following impact to be replaced soon after by a period of restoration that, more often than not, was undertaken without incorporating risk reduction measures designed to reduce the prospects of similar impacts occurring in the future. This scenario, recognizable throughout most of the world, supported Dynes and Drabek's "universal view" (1994, p. 12) of how disaster was conceptualized, including the typical central government position wherein, "disaster planning was to enhance the national government's ability to reestablish social order and to facilitate recovery" (1994, p. 12). These researchers noted in addition that disasters were considered as collective misfortunes rather than objects of specific study or for public policy (1994, p. 5).

One early study, repeatedly cited, that focused on national systems in a comparative context (which is another neglected field of inquiry) is McLuckie's (1970) treatment of the public administration systems in Italy, Japan, and the United States. Using an ecological perspective, his central theme was that the economic, political, and sociocultural systems will affect the structure and performance of disaster response functions. In particular, he noted how centralization has an affect on disaster response. A centralized system (portrayed in varying degrees by Japan and Italy) was defined as one in which the highest level of government retains power to itself with the result that there are relatively fewer decision makers (McLuckie, 1970, p. 50). Centralization makes lower-level officials reluctant to take initiatives since to do so would be tantamount to overstepping authority. This resulted in decisions being passed upward, causing a slowing down of the decision-making process, although McLuckie noted this depended on the disaster phase and the tasks performed. McLuckie further qualified this observation by stating that a focus on formal structures of decision making tends to give the impression of greater centralization than actually occurs.

The adoption of a holistic approach in disaster research and practice started to make headway from the 1990s, which coincided with the United Nation's International Decade for Natural Disaster Reduction (IDNDR). Until then, risk assessment and hazard mitigation activities were typically on the fringes of national level response planning. Studies of the type conducted by May and his colleagues (May et al., 1996), a quarter century after McLuckie, looked at intergovernmental approaches to environmental and hazard management, and helped broaden the disaster planning approach. These researchers undertook a trination assessment (Australia, New Zealand, and United States) and distinguished between coercive and cooperative policy mandates that entailed the imposition of procedural and/or substantive requirements by higher-level governments on subnational levels, either as conditions for assistance or as direct orders. While both approaches attempted to achieve vertical consistency and congruency within national systems, "the different mechanisms may possibly result in long-term solution variance" (1996, p. 3). They concluded that no matter what the approach taken to induce local governments to deal with environmental and hazard management issues, a "commitment conundrum" prevailed: when forced under coercive mandates (such as in parts of the United States), participation is either half-hearted or political back lash can result; however, when encouraged to take on these problems but not forced to do so under a cooperative mandate (as the case with New Zealand and some Australian states) local governments tend to drag their feet. In either case, it leaves a challenge for policy makers to figure out how to build commitment to hazard management and sustainable environmental goals.

A good summary of the status of national systems is Hays' assessment of governmental actions prior to the advent of the International Decade of Natural Disaster Reduction (IDNDR). Hays (1999) stated that, "in hindsight, few nations had policy makers and stakeholders ten years ago who knew how to change their natural disaster reduction culture and make natural disaster reduction a national and worldwide public value" (p. 276). He identified six conditions that captured the prevailing situation:

- No legal or social mandate from the citizens and stakeholders to evaluate existing research and research applications programs, plans, and public policies and to make major changes in the natural disaster reduction culture.
- A lack of overall understanding of the complex interrelations between the hazard, built, and policy environments of their nation.
- A lack of technical capacity to conduct a national risk assessment.
- A lack of technical capacity to develop improved monitoring, forecasting, and warning systems.
- A lack of political will to initiate a national mitigation strategy.
- Existing science, technology, and traditional knowledge was not enough to effect these kinds of major changes in their natural disaster reduction culture (Hays, 1999, p. 277).

While this brief review of historical roots might appear, on balance, to be more negative than upbeat, the significance of these early studies was nevertheless considerable. In particular, as Dynes and Drabek (1994) point out, at the commencement of the 1990s the consequences of the disaster research tradition transformed policy approaches to disaster at national level and internationally, although the effect was more nascent than actual outside the United States. The research reinforced the need to bolster local community resources and to reduce the moral hazard issue created when national level agencies took responsibility of local hazard problems. It helped create national-level bureaucratic disaster focal points and assisted in bringing together administrative, planning, and operational functions that were previously scattered. Disasters started to be regarded as nonroutine social problems (Kreps & Drabek, 1996) and were pursued from socioeconomic and political environmental perspectives rather than just a technical one.

This period also identified a series of policy, legal, and institutional arrangements that were indispensable for effective disaster management, namely, a strong legal basis, a capable nodal agency, mechanisms for interinstitutional coordination, ongoing planning and capacity-building processes, public policies that protect people's lives and economic and natural resources, community and stakeholder participation, and the development of an overarching strategic framework outlining how disaster management links with other governance requirements. Moreover, some national-level policymakers and practitioners started to comprehend the aptness of turning away from previous disasters as the sole means for developing future policies, while also coming to an understanding that disasters are embedded in routine decisions and behavior, and the consequences of everyday actions resulting from many small decisions that can cumulatively lead to disaster (Burton, 2005; Hewitt, 1997).

REVIEW OF CONTEMPORARY RESEARCH

For decades governments and their agencies accepted notions implicit in the definitions at the time that the real task of organizing for disaster was to concentrate on preparedness and response. This approach seriously hampered addressing underlying causal issues, and it weakened hazard mitigation efforts. Even now, practitioners tend to focus on the consequences of disasters, but many do so in a way that has shifted their thinking from a response-focused to a consequence-based analysis. In this respect, their judgment reflects a definitional shift that incorporates political, economic, and cultural ecological perspectives. Disaster management planners are now more likely to ask themselves, "What will the overall societal effects of impact be?" The interest in sustainable hazard mitigation that characterizes contemporary approaches (see Burby, 1998; Mileti, 1999; United Nations, 2005), will consolidate this, although some (e.g., Aguirre, 2002a) point out there is still some serious theoretical thinking to do on this. National-level disaster managers in some countries have spent a great deal of effort thinking about disaster resilience and what it means for social stability.

The approaches used by different nations to manage hazards and their consequences reflect the distinctive characteristics of those societies. Planning and response activities take place within particular governmental systems and are shaped by larger cultural, economic, and political forces, which are starting to be better understood as researchers and practitioners recognize their significance. Situating hazards and disaster management policies in their social contexts can lead to a better understanding of the extent to which both research findings and practices may be generated from one society to another (Tierney et al., 2001, p. 199). However, the point needs repeating that there is a "void in the empirical data base" (Drabek, 1986, p. 79) concerning disaster planning and response on the national level.

To illustrate the distinctiveness of approaches within their contextual settings, three national-level systems—Japan, New Zealand, and the Philippines—will be looked at in detail. All three countries fall into Curtice's (1985) category of liberal democratic governmental systems and Kamrava's (1996) first world democracies. All three countries are multiple island nations roughly similar in size. The countries differ in terms of size of economy and economic indicators, living standard, population size, and density (Table 20.1). While each country straddles the Circum-Pacific Rim of Fire, an ironically poetic label for the sequence of highly active seismic and volcanic sites along plate boundaries surrounding the Pacific Basin, recent studies indicate national differences with respect to natural hazard exposure (World Bank, 2005). Furthermore, there are visible differences in national-level disaster management attributes (Table 20.2). While not portraying the full range of approaches to be found, the three modes illustrated below nevertheless depict the disaster management approaches of, respectively, an affluent, a small, and an emerging economy, and hence should be instructive. The first study, Japan, is currently the world's second largest economy and approaches national disaster management from a strong technology application position that relies heavily on legislation. Each major disaster impact typically results in a new enactment, often with an accompanying requirement to set up a new science-based group to solve the problem (see also Table 20.3). Existing legislation is not rescinded, and a cumbersome legal code has developed. This reinforces Japan's reactive management style and emphasizes development of products (mainly engineering) rather than processes or social structural realignment, which seldom occurs. The use of legislation as a primary vehicle also perpetuates a hazard-specific orientation. By contrast, New Zealand approaches disaster management from an all-hazards risk management perspective that builds on prior institutional reform and instigated in anticipation that a major disaster is inevitable. Based on a national strategy for disaster management, policies are strongly linked to hazard management as a means of avoiding unintended disruptions to national development priorities. This small OECD economy is an example of a country using a process outlook that engages its people and its social structures as the prime resource base. The third case study of the Philippines provides a style that is evident, in part or in whole, in many emerging economies. Here, disaster management decision-making is centralized; international agencies

TABLE 20.1. Context Factors for Three National Systems[a]

Attributes	Country		
	Japan	New Zealand	The Philippines
Area	• 377,727 km^2	• 270,534 km^2	• 300,000 km^2
Population	• 127.5 m	• 3.8 m	• 78.6 m
Population/km^2	• 337.5 ppsk	• 14.0 ppsk	• 262.0 ppsk
Urban population per 1000 population	• 78.9%	• 85.9%	• 59.4%
Population <15 years/ >60 years	• 14.6% • 23.3%	• 22.9% • 15.7%	• 37.5% • 5.5%
HDI[b]	• 93.2	• 91.7	• 75.1
GDP ($US)	• $3,993 bn	• $58.6 bn	• $78.0 bn
GDP per head	• $31,320	• $15,420	• $990
Hazard exposure[c]	• 10.5% total area exposed to multiple hazards • 15.% total population exposed to hazards • 84% of population in multiple hazard areas at relatively high mortality risk	• 4.3% total area exposed to multiple hazards • 1.7% total population exposed to hazards • 22.4% of population in multiple hazard areas at relatively high mortality risk	• 22.3% total area exposed to multiple hazards • 36.4.% total population exposed to hazards • 88.6% of population in multiple hazard areas at relatively high mortality risk

[a] Source: The Economist (2005). For Japan, see pp. 168–169; New Zealand, see pp. 184–185; for The Philippines, see pp. 194–195.
[b] HDI = Human Development Index, developed by UNDP and combines statistics on average years of schooling, adult literacy, and life expectancy with income levels. Countries scoring higher than 80 are considered to have high human development, those scoring 50–79 medium, and >50 are low (see *The Economist*, 2005, p. 30)
[c] Hazard exposure figures derived from Tables 1.1a and b and Table 1.2b in The World Bank (2005).

are central actors; practices are reactive being primarily focused on responding to impact and a lack of coordination is apparent. In many ways it could be said that Filipino politicians have learnt from several decades of international disaster assistance that a good strategy is to do nothing. However, changes taking place externally will require internal modification, and Philippines decision makers are slowly coming round to appreciate the benefits that effective disaster risk management can have on national development planning.

JAPAN

Since the 1950s the Government of Japan has invested significant financial resources in natural hazard mitigation and prevention. Japanese observers have reported that the government routinely spent between 5% and 8% of the annual national budget (about 0.8% of gross domestic product [GDP]) in disaster reduction, with most of this directed to structural mitigation developments (Sudo, Kameda, & Ogawa, 2000). The most recent figures, for fiscal year 2003, identify a budget of ¥2.7 trillion, about 5% of the total general account budget dispersed by various government departments for research development, disaster preparedness, national land conservation (all for structural mitigation schemes), and disaster recovery and reconstruction.

Japan's first disaster related legislation was enshrined in 1880, although its first attempt to prepare a comprehensive national disaster management system can be traced to the 1961 Disaster Countermeasures Basic Act, prompted in 1959 by a destructive typhoon that left more

TABLE 20.2. Disaster Management in Three National Systems

	Country		
Attributes	Japan	New Zealand	The Philippines
Overall approach	• Centralized/directive	• Decentralized/ cooperative	• Centralized/ hierarchical
	• Fragmented	• Inclusive/all-of-nation approach	• Fragmented
	• Reactive	• Proactive	• Reactive
Supporting platform	• Incremental	• "Greenfields approach" to develop best fit	• Ad hoc
Legislation characteristics	• 1961 *Disaster Countermeasures Basic Act*	• 2002 *Civil Defence Emergency Management Act*	• 1978 *Presidential Decree 1566*
	• 15 generic Acts	• Risk-based	• Reactive
	• 28 hazard-specific Acts	• Proactive	
	• Reactive	• Empowering	
Disaster management approach	• Product-focus	• Process-focus	• Task-focus
	• Impact-based	• Consequence-based	• Impact-based
	• Technical research/response	• Mitigation/response	• Response-focus
Decision-making style	• Reactive	• Proactive	• Static-reactive
Level of specificity	• Hazard specific	• All-hazard	• Nonspecific
	• Structural mitigation dominates	• Integrated mitigation	
		• Promote risk reduction	
Focal agency attributes	• Cabinet Office	• Ministry within Department of Internal Affairs	• Department of Defence
	• Nonmilitary head	• Nonmilitary head	• Military head
	• Policy-advice	• Policy advice	• Operational control (OCD)
	• Operational advice	• Operational control	• Policy coordination (NDCC)
		• Warning advice/ responsibility	

than 5000 dead. This keystone legislation defines essential administrative policies at each level of government and for 60 designated public corporations under the Disaster Countermeasures Basic Plan. Both instruments are periodically revised in incremental fashion following major impact, the most recent of which took place following the 1995 Hanshin-Awaji earthquake, the 2004 Niigata-ken Chuetsu earthquake, and the 2004 typhoon season; at the time of writing a further revision was under consideration following the 2005 Fukuoka-ken Seiho-oki earthquake. Before 1961, Japan "had an improvised policy focused on rendering aid and providing financial assistance to victims" (Palm & Carroll, 1998, p. 87). Under the 1961 law, national level councils, ministries and agencies are responsible for updating the Basic Plan and developing operational guidelines. At the next tier, Prefectural governments are charged with the execution and coordination of disaster operations and preparing Prefectural-level prevention

TABLE 20.3. Relevent National-Level Disaster management Actions in Japan

General Legislation

- 1880: Provision and Saving Act for Natural Disaster
- 1899: Disaster Preparation Funds Special Account Act
- 1947: Disaster Relief Act
- 1947: Fire Organization Act
- 1951: Act Concerning National Treasury Share of Expenses for Recovery Projects for Public Civil Engineering Facilities Damage due to Disasters
- 1961: Disaster Countermeasures Basic Act
- 1962: Act Concerning Special Financial Support to Deal with the Designated Disaster of Extreme Severity
- 1972: Act Concerning Special Financial Support for Promoting Group Relocation for Disaster Mitigation
- 1987: Act Concerning Dispatch of Japan Disaster Relief Team
- 1995: Partial Revision of Disaster Countermeasures Basic Act
- 1996: Act Regarding Special Measures to Weigh the Preservation of Rights and Profits of the Victims of Specified Disasters
- 1997: Act for Densely Inhabited Areas Improvement for Disaster Mitigation
- 1998: Act Concerning Support for Reconstructing Livelihoods of Disaster Victims
- 1998: Comprehensive National Development Act
- 2000: Housing Quality Assurance Act
- 2004: People Protection Law

Research-Related Initiatives

- 1880: Establishment of the Seismological Society of Japan
- 1925: Establishment of Earthquake Research Institute, Tokyo Imperial University
- 1951: Establishment of Kyoto University Disaster Prevention Research Institute
- 1963: Establishment of National Research Institute of Earth Sciences and Disaster Prevention
- 1969: Establishment of Coordinating Committee for Earthquake Prediction
- 1974: Establishment of Coordinating Committee for Prediction of Volcanic Eruption
- 1981: Basic Plan for Research and Development on Disaster Prevention (revised June 1995, June 1997, May 2000, December 2000)
- 1995: Establishment of Headquarters for Earthquake Research Promotion

Hazard-Specific Legislation

- 1897: Erosion Control Act
- 1897: Forest Act
- 1908: Flood Prevention Association Act
- 1911: Flood Control Expenditure Funds Special Accounts Act
- 1949: Flood Control Act
- 1952: Meteorological Service Act
- 1956: Seashore Act
- 1958: Landslide Prevention Act
- 1960: Soil Conservation and Flood Control Urgent Measures Act
- 1962: Act of Special Countermeasures for Heavy Snowfall Area
- 1964: River Act (1896 Act revised)
- 1966: Act for Earthquake Insurance
- 1969: Act Concerning Prevention of Steep Slope Collapse Disaster
- 1970: Marine Pollution Act
- 1975: Act on Prevention of Disaster in Petroleum Industrial Complexes and other Petroleum Facilities
- 1978: Act on Special Measures for Active Volcanoes (originally the 1973 Act Concerning Improvement of Refugees etc. in Areas of Active Volcanoes)

(Cont.)

TABLE 20.3. (*Continued*)

Hazard-Specific Legislation

- 1978: Large-Scale Earthquake Countermeasures Special Act (Basic Plan for Earthquake Disaster Prevention)
- 1980: Special Fiscal Measures Act for Urgent Improvement Project for Earthquake Countermeasures in Areas under Intensified Measures Against Earthquake Disaster
- 1995: Act for the Statement of Principles and Organization of the Great Hanshin-Awaji Earthquake Revival
- 1995: Earthquake Disaster Management Special Measures Act
- 1995: Partial Revision of Disaster Countermeasures Basic Act and Large-Scale Earthquake Countermeasures Special Act
- 1995: Act for Promotion of the Earthquake Proof Retrofit of Buildings
- 1998: Building Standard Law revised
- 1999: Special Measures of Nuclear Disaster Act
- 2000: Building Standard Law Enforcement Order revised
- 2000: Sediment Disaster Countermeasures for Sediment Disaster Prone Areas Act
- 2004: Law on Special Measures for the Tonankai and Nankai Earthquakes

National-Level Structures

- 1941: Establishment of Tsunami Warning Organization
- 1948: Establishment of Board of Inquiry for Prevention of Damage from Earthquakes
- 1952: Establishment of the National Fire Fighting Headquarters
- 1956: Establishment of Japan Meteorological Agency
- 1960: Establishment of the Ministry of Home Affairs Fire and Emergency Management Agency
- 1962: Establishment of Central Disaster Management Council
- 1963: Formulation of Basic Disaster Management Plan
- 1984: Establishment of Disaster Prevention Bureau in National Land Agency
- 1992: General principles relating to Countermeasures for Earthquakes directly below the Southern Kanto Region
- 1995: Amendment of Basic Disaster Management Plan
- 1997: Amendment of Basic Disaster Management Plan
- 1998: Amendment to Japanese Building Standard
- 1999: Amendment of Basic Plan for Earthquake Disaster Prevention
- 2000: Amendment of Basic Disaster Management Plan
- 2001: Earthquake Insurance system amended
- 2001: Establishment of Disaster Management Section in Cabinet Office in Connection with restructuring of Government ministries and agencies

Source: Bosner (2001), Cabinet Office (2005), Fire & Emergency Management Agency (2005), Palm (1998), Palm & Carroll (1998).

plans. Below this, municipal governments have responsibility to include specific disaster prevention operations on site and prepare a municipal plan. In practice, however, many decisions are deferred to higher levels in the hierarchy before action can be taken.

Another foundation enactment is the 1998 Comprehensive National Development Act which stipulates "making Japan a safe and comfortable place to live." This has been defined as improving the country's safety with regard to large-scale earthquakes and other natural disasters (Government of Japan, 2005). Specific objectives entail establishing a disaster-resilient transport and communications infrastructure; introducing public works design standards; promoting the assurance of earthquake-resistance capacity in buildings; establishing an earthquake watch network; promoting research into disasters and their prevention; assessing and publishing the degree of risk of local disasters and reflecting the information in local development and land use; providing disaster management manuals for local, corporate, and administrative bodies; and provisions for people requiring help in the event of disaster.

More recently, the People Protection Law, promulgated in 2004, obligates central government to develop a full security system for the nation which covers "the proper and prompt implementation of measures to protect people, using its own initiative and employing every available resource including its organization and functions" (Fire & Emergency Management Agency, 2005). It is unclear, however, how these legislative pillars and their planning accompaniments either bind or build upon the plethora of existing individual acts, national-level structures, national-level research initiatives (see Table 20.3) and other related national-level actions; or how it is being used to mold legislation and planning being pursued ahead of a series of specific anticipated future large earthquakes (Government of Japan, 2005; Higashida, 2005). It is also uncertain how recent debates about the use of Japan's Self-Defense Forces (SDF) will ultimately be used in a civil society context (see Nakamura, 2001; Schoff, 2004).

An additional contextual element is the Japanese risk management standard (JIS, 2001). In general, standards are self-regulatory generic system standards designed to help modify extremes of management behavior by providing information (Fernandez & Britton, 2004). A distinctive feature of the Japanese standard is a section on establishing disaster response procedures and preparation. The Japanese approach to risk is that it is a "top management" issue and hence there is little need for risk communication with its emphasis on feedback. Moreover, while the risk management approach has been useful as a research and practice tool by some Japanese researchers (Britton, 2004), and whereas the private sector demonstrates signs of exercising this standard, the government shows no knowledge of it (Fernandez, 2005).

Japanese research associated with the 1995 earthquake in Kobe (see Nakamura, 2000, 2001) concludes that the disaster revealed central and local government neglect in vital aspects of disaster management, where rivalry, competition, and failure to use designated focal agencies added to the stress of impact. In fact, Nakamura states that, "in Japanese public administration, successful disaster management rarely occurs" (2002, p. 23). Supporting his case with additional post-Kobe examples, he suggests that a lack of policy coordination is a perennial problem that neither organizational realignments nor establishment of new agencies has solved. While many lessons were learned (see Bosner, 2001, 2002; Eisner, 2000; Nakamura, 2000), many of which have resulted in greater central government centralization (such as the Prime Minister being able to order the Self-Defense Force to engage in rescue work if a request is not received from a stricken area within an hour), other issues have surfaced that the central government has yet to find suitable solutions for. For instance, Nakamura (2001) reports that the nation's economic downturn produced fiscal retrenchments at the local level that have significantly hit crisis management programs; and notes that public officials often consider disaster programs to be nuisances that interfere in routine administrative tasks.

A spate of widely publicized corporate transgressions from 2000 and into 2005, in sectors as diverse as the motor, food processing, amusement, power generation, and distribution industries, as well as unfathomable penalties meted out to whistleblowers, has resulted in public safety becoming a major political problem in which the populace look upon crisis management in a negative manner. This may help explain in part the findings of a study conducted in mid-January 2005 of 500 respondents from seven communities impacted by earthquakes in July 2003, and September and October 2004 wherein 60% of respondents had not taken any subsequent measures, and that on average 40% of respondents over the three earthquakes did not initiate strengthening measures on their dwellings (*Home quake measures still lax*, 2005). This relatively low level of personal action supports Palm's (1998) previous observation that the Japanese are more inclined to prefer government to take control on disaster-related issues, even if it does result in higher taxes. Likewise, Bloomberg reported that Japanese firms lag behind their overseas competitors to initiate business recovery preparations, apparently being lulled by the notion that a severe earthquake in Tokyo would destroy their competitors as well as them, rather than the reality that a prepared competitor is more likely to survive and be in a relatively good position to capture a greater share of business ("Morgan Stanley," 2005).

Two additional factors are raised with respect to the national-level system. The first is highlighted by a newspaper editorial in the Japan Times ("New Rules," 2005) wherein central government is reproached for developing a separate crisis management system for "new" threats (i.e., military, terrorist, or missile attack) rather than improving the existing natural hazard-based programs and restructuring existing organizational arrangements to create a comprehensive system. The editorial identifies some perennial issues associated with the Japanese bureaucracy (see also Chalmers, 1995, pp. 115–140). The first is a tendency toward compartmentalization that results in less than ideal interaction amongst relevant offices. The second is a proclivity to create a new organization when a new task has been identified rather than to incorporate the activity into an existing organization. A third is the tendency to focus on refining technical solutions and products rather than dealing with implementation processes. If new initiatives can be defined as technical, they can be developed in a relatively unfettered manner, even if this results in duplication of effort or jurisdictional overlap. The alternative, innovation through the establishment of new principles, would necessitate the creation of new norms or institutions (Eisenstadt, 1996) that would upset the complex and enduring social practices that put strict codes of behavior on relationships (Nakane, 1997). By opting to develop a separate system to cater for "new threats" (even though, as the editorial reminded its readers, the nation already has military emergency legislation), the national-level system maintains its incremental approach.

The second factor is Japan's proclivity to look to the United States, and in particular Federal Emergency Management Agency (FEMA), for inspiration even though structural configurations between the nations' focal agencies differ (Bosner, 2001, 2002); emergency services have different arrangements (in Japan they are national agencies); the nature of and relationship between central and local governments are not the same; power and authority relations are different; substantial differences exist in sociocultural behavior patterns (Nakamura, 2001); and at the same time FEMA itself is heading in new directions (Tierney, 2005a). The Japanese and Americans have had a formal research link for the social sciences since 1972 (the first meeting was held at the Disaster Research Center in Columbus, Ohio). This link was further cemented in the mid-1990s when U.S. President Clinton and Japan Prime Minister Hashimoto endorsed binational cooperative activities to improve earthquake disaster policies and programs (Palm, 1998), and lately top-level discussions suggest the United States is very keen for collaboration to continue on a wider crisis management front (Schoff, 2004). The U.S. Incident Command System (ICS) is also being investigated by Japanese social science academics who have government funding to create an accreditation system for standardized training and to prepare a human resources development curriculum for systematic learning (Sadohara, Shigekawa, Hayashi, & Chinoi, 2005). The project itself is part of a wider program of work looking at disaster prevention initiatives in the United States to ascertain what might be useful for Japan.

Such a course of action seems to be normal practice in Japan. For example, Sorensen's (2002) analysis of Japanese urban planning suggests that it is normal for academics to be instrumental in crafting practitioner-related actions based on overseas practices. He illustrates how the Japanese excelled in their ability to borrow, adapt, and to innovate technical aspects of planning, and to produce a systems based on best practice in the west, although its application fell short: the nation's planning scheme has not taken in hand the major issues (Sorensen, 2002, pp. 347–348). Sorensen also notes that public support for city planning was inhibited because of the narrow (academic) base from which it was conducted. Since the Kobe earthquake, however, attempts to remedy the latter issue have been made and the importance of voluntary activities in disaster reduction has been underscored in the Disaster Countermeasures Basic Act, which requires central and local public bodies to "endeavour to provide an environment conducive to the performance of voluntary disaster risk reduction activities" (Government of Japan, 2005, p. 3). Another issue associated with planning includes the issue of land-use management tools not being widely implemented for urban hazard management (Banba et al., 2004), while another issue associated with relying on the research community is that a single hazard focus remains dominant (Fernandez, 2005, p. 93).

NEW ZEALAND

For more than a decade New Zealand's disaster management system has been systematically moving from a conventional response-oriented arrangement to a comprehensive emergency management approach that links hazard analysis and impact assessment with land-use planning and resource management. Within an all-of-nation approach, the national-level system has been building platforms to develop a multiagency, all-hazard arrangement for circumventing, planning for and recovering from significant disaster. The intention is to introduce more robustness into New Zealand social systems when dealing with uncertainty by linking disaster management with sustainable hazard mitigation and sustainable development.

For decades, New Zealand followed the British model when it developed an Emergency Precautions Scheme (EPS) under the Emergency Precautions Act 1939. This scheme initially created structures to protect public for wartime events, and so by the end of the 1939–45 conflict most of the EPS organizations had disbanded. The concept remained, however, and in 1953 a Local Authorities Emergency Powers Act 1953 gave local government functions and powers to respond to natural hazards as well as war-like threats. A 1958 Review of Defence identified that defence planning would have to take into account the possibility of a direct attack with nuclear or non-nuclear weapons, and that a major role of the defence force would be to protect the civilian population. This led to the formation of the Ministry of Civil Defence in 1959 (Department of Internal Affairs, 1995), and the ensuing Civil Defence Act 1962 focused on protecting the public in the event of major disaster, a nuclear or other armed attack.

This orientation continued to be the basic building block until the 1990s when a number of reviews, reports, conferences, and workshops questioned the effectiveness of New Zealand's overall disaster management practices. A report by the Law Commission (1991) identified changes needed in executive powers to deal effectively with a national disaster, suggesting a review of relevant legislation. In like manner, in 1991 a major study of how utility lifelines would perform following a maximum credible earthquake in the Wellington region revealed a series of significant vulnerabilities that had not hitherto been considered (CAE, 1991). A 1992 review of civil defence found that reforms in the public sector that occurred since the passing of the Civil Defence Act 1983 (an update of the 1962 legislation) had "dislocated much of the current Act from modern realities" (Civil Defence Review Panel, 1992), and concluded that existing structures would not cope in a major civil disaster. Two years later, in 1994, the lessons of the Northridge (California) earthquake were the subject of local conferences, revealing inherent weaknesses in local emergency management systems and identified a need to concentrate on developing coordination between utilities and the emergency services.

The consistency of these messages started to be noticed by central government (Britton & Clark, 2000), and in late 1994, the Minister for Internal Affairs (who also Minister for Civil Defence) hosted a workshop to explore the performance of the emergency services sector and to generate ideas on improvements for the short and long term. The workshop proposed that a comprehensive "greenfields" review of emergency services be undertaken. Subsequently, in April 1995, encouraged by a conference in March 1995 that explored what impact a Kobe-type earthquake would have on Wellington (CAE, 1995), Cabinet appointed a Task Force to review the emergency preparation and response capabilities of the nation's emergency services, most of which are national-level instrumentalities. The review duly acknowledged a number of fundamental issues associated with the existing emergency management system, and noted the limited range of events the system was actually capable of effectively handling, and the narrow focus on preparation and response. At the same time, a number of concerns about the structure of the emergency response system were identified, including issues about cooperation between emergency services (issues about horizontal integration); problems of continuity management, especially if the level of management response may change (issues of vertical integration); the lack of disaster-relevant professional advice and management; and the need for elected authority to make declarations. Throughout its deliberations, the Task Force found there was general consensus of the need for change. Three factors in particular focused this need:

- The unrealistically high public expectations of assistance that was assumed would be provided.
- The reduced capacity of central and local government to respond following public sector reform.
- The need to improve the ability of the emergency services sector to adapt to changing circumstances, learn from overseas experience, and to better coordinate resources.

The Task Force accordingly recommended to the government a replacement national emergency management agency that would have policy as well as operational functions, and a structure to deal with disaster response that would integrate local and central government emergency service providers. The Task Force also recommended that the nation's emergency management system be more comprehensive in outlook and approach. It further suggested the sector move quicker and farther in areas of professional development for emergency managers; it also reinforced the existing view that accountability for declarations of disaster remains the task of elected officials at the most appropriate level of government. These recommendations were endorsed and extended by an Officials Committee established to comment on the report. Central government subsequently made five fundamental decisions:

- In 1996 a set of principles were approved as the basis for an overarching emergency management framework.
- Central government responsibility was redefined to include establishing the emergency management framework and identifying the principles, roles, and responsibilities of all agencies in the sector.
- In 1997 establishment of a new Ministry was approved and came into being July 1999.
- In 1998 the concept of local emergency management consortia (referred to as Emergency Management Groups) was approved based on the framework principles.
- In 2002 the Civil Defence Emergency Management Act was passed which redefined the duties of central and local governments and brought private sector utilities into the

emergency management strategic decision-making and operational contexts. The Act promoted sustainable management of hazards and risks in a way that contributes to the well-being and safety of the public and property.

The reforms called for a refocusing of attention and action onto the management of risk and the options available for reducing or managing different levels of potential impact. A key component of the New Zealand approach is the application of risk management principles (Britton, 2002), and recent legislation has implicitly, and often explicitly, called for a risk management application. In many cases private sector models for risk management have been modified to meet public sector needs, and while at times this has been difficult it has nevertheless proven useful because it has assisted in integrating risk management into everyday decision making. The framework for the national emergency management strategy is based on a risk management approach developed by Standards Australia and Standards New Zealand (Standards Australia, 1999). This nonmandatory Standard defines risk management as "the culture, practices, processes and structures that come together to optimize the management of potential opportunities and adverse effects." Together with a risk management approach for local governments (Standards New Zealand, 2000), the Standard has been promoted as the basis for developing a risk-based emergency management approach and for communicating the concepts of risk management to groups with emergency management responsibilities. The attempt to involve end-users is not restricted to emergency management practice: the New Zealand Foundation for Research, Science and Technology, a Crown entity that operates on behalf of the government to invest public funds in research, requires successful fund applicants to specifically identify and involve users of intended research outputs (FRST, 2003).

To ensure overall consistency, the 2002 Act requires central government's administering agency to develop a publicly notified national emergency management strategy that sets out goals, objectives, and measurable targets. The strategy is aligned to central government's vision of Resilient New Zealand (MCDEM, 2004). A consultation document widely distributed in August 2003 modified the final statement, which was published in March 2004 (see Table 20.4).

The redesign of New Zealand's devolved emergency management system needs to be put into the context of wider reform practices that have taken place since the early 1980s. Most sectors of the economy have been substantially deregulated, while social policy has changed to remove a perceived dependency on the State by many, toward a needs-based welfare system. Alongside these and other significant changes, many functions of the government have been significantly devolved and commercialized. This was described by some observers as an attempt to "get government out of business while bringing business into government" (May et al., 1996, p. 43). The New Zealand approach requires effort to understand how the natural and created (built) environments produce risk, and how to keep people and property out of the way of hazards that supports economic and social development on the one hand, and reduces social and economic risk on the other. The government's intention is that local authorities will identify hazards and the associated risks within their communities, and will consult communities about this. In this way, both local authorities and communities will know what can be expected, what local authorities are going to do, and what communities and individuals will have to do for themselves. What is important about the changes in New Zealand is that they were instigated in *anticipation* of a major disaster rather than being a reaction to a major event. Moreover, from the perspective of the national-level system, it was central government that took the lead by encouraging a wide-ranging review on how best to manage disasters.

TABLE 20.4. Main Strands of the New Zealand National Emergency Management Strategy

Principles	Goals and Objectives
1. Individual and community responsibility and self-reliance	1. *To increase community awareness, understanding and participation in civil defence emergency management (CDEM)* • Objective A: increase the level of community awareness of the risks from hazards • Objective B: improve community understanding and participation in CDEM • Objective C: encourage and enable community participation in determining acceptable levels of risk
2. A transparent and systematic approach to managing risks from hazards	2. *To reduce the risks from hazards in New Zealand* • Objective A: improve the coordination, promotion and accessibility of CDEM • Objective B: develop a comprehensive understanding of New Zealand's hazardscape • Objective C: encourage all CDEM stakeholders to reduce the risks from hazards to acceptable levels • Objective D: improve the coordination of government policy relevant to CDEM
3. Comprehensive and integrated hazard risk management	3. *To enhance New Zealand's capability to manage emergencies* • Objective A: promote continuing and coordinated professional development in CDEM • Objective B: enhance the ability of CDEM Groups to prepare for and manage emergencies • Objective C: enhance the ability of emergency services to prepare for and manage emergencies • Objective D: enhance the ability of lifeline utilities to prepare for and manage emergencies • Objective E: enhance the ability of government departments to prepare for and manage emergencies • Objective F: improve the ability of government to manage an event of national significance
4. Addressing the consequences of hazards	4. *To enhance New Zealand's capability to recover from disasters* • Objective A: implement effective recovery planning and activities for the physical impacts of disasters • Objective B: implement effective recovery planning and activities for the social and economic impacts of disasters
5. Making best use of information, expertise and structures	

Source: MCDEM (2004).

THE PHILIPPINES

The disaster management system of the Philippines originated from World War II and geared toward preparations for war. Under the auspices of Executive Order EO335 in 1941, President Manuel Quezon created the Civilian Emergency Administration to manage the population in case war in Europe moved to the Pacific. Under EO335 a hierarchical system was created whereby a National Emergency Commission set out arrangements for Provincial Emergency Committees which in turn supervised and controlled emergency committees at municipal and city levels. Almost forty years later, this framework was consolidated with the enactment of Presidential Decree PD1566 on June 11, 1978. PD1566 provides for a National Disaster Coordinating Council (NDCC) as the highest policy-making body on matters pertaining to disasters, advising the President. Chaired by the Secretary of Defence, NDCC is ostensibly a coordinating body. However, it does not have a regular budget and operates through member agencies and regional and local disaster coordinating councils. While membership is large, covering most of central government's 20 instrumentalities, the capacity of the agencies is limited, especially in the area of risk reduction. A decade after the Presidential decree, in 1988, a National Calamities and Disaster Preparedness Plan was prepared as a guide for action.

Completing the main national-level apparatus is the Office of Civil Defence (OCD) housed within the Department of National Defence, the intention of which is to coordinate the activities and functions of government, private institutions, and civic organizations. It maintains offices in each of the nation's 16 regions. While NDCC establishes priorities for allocation of funds, services, and disaster relief, subnational disaster coordinating is undertaken through OCD, which issues guidelines to lower-level committees. OCD is also the lead training agency, although programs are not compulsory for non-military disaster-designated personnel: since its first priority is to train Armed Forces of the Philippines (AFP) officers, little capacity remains to make available programs for local government personnel (World Bank, 2004).

In general, disaster management in the Philippines is seen as the responsibility of the central government, with most activities predicated upon a response-oriented practice ideology. Civil society organizations and the private sector have supported these efforts, and while they have primarily been directed to preparedness and response tasks, efforts have been undertaken to reduce risk (Luna, 2000; World Bank, 2004). While there have been some promising initiatives, nonresponse activities tend to be ad hoc, with little evidence of cumulative effect.

The disaster management system is guided by its definition of disaster, stated as "a situation usually catastrophic in nature, in which a number of persons are plunged into helplessness and suffering, and as a result may be in need of food, clothing, shelter, medical care and other basic necessities of life," and purports to support local level activities (NDCC, 2004). Guss and Pangan (2004) suggest this definition probably relates to the experience of disasters as frequent and powerful while acknowledging the country's lack of resources and infrastructure. However, while the assumption is that arrangements assist local levels, in reality the structure does the reverse: PD1566 perpetuates an unwieldy centralizing system. The arrangement comprises six levels encompassing almost 46,000 separate administrative units (Fig. 20.1), administered in a top-down manner. It is difficult to effectively operate, and there are few incentives for local level initiatives. For example, under NDCC provisions, while each operating level can "submit recommendations as necessary," all are required to adhere to guidelines established by the level above. Similarly, of the 1645 barangays (the basic political unit and primary implementing unit of government) in the Metro Manila area, only 220 have "some kind of disaster management organization" and 5 of the metropolitan area's 14 cities and three municipalities have operational disaster management bodies with legal support through approved ordinances (Castillo, 2005). It is widely acknowledge that the current legislation is outmoded and hinders activity (World Bank, 2004), while the government seems in no rush to affect changes. Since 2000, for example, at least two proposals for new legislation have been submitted, with the second bill stalled after being with the legislature for 2 years. Part of the current impasse appears to be the number of draft versions in circulation (there are at least 15 versions) and lack of access to them by interested parties.

The need for greater coordination is well recognized by almost all disaster-relevant agencies within the Philippines (Carlos, 2001). The type of coordination operators' state they need

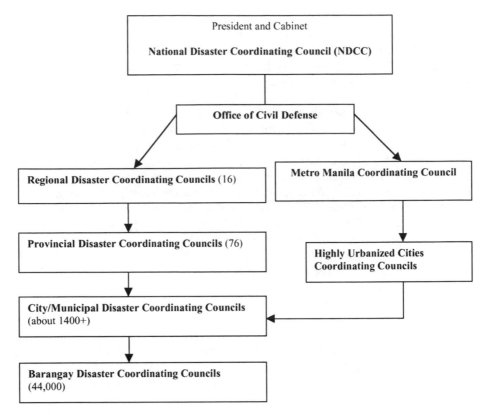

FIGURE 20.1. Institutional Arrangements for Disaster Management

is a proactive, participatory and enabling one and not the top-down oversight orientation they have. Greater organizational, management, and task synchronization are identified as prerequisites (ibid) that should extend across-the-board at all levels of the Philippines disaster management system. Related to this is the promotion of a risk reduction approach: many stakeholders have expressed concern that the current system is too ad hoc (World Bank, 2004), and lacks a strategic framework. Carlos (2001) asserts that the critical issues raised by key actors indicate that what is actually happening on the ground may not be what is stipulated in national-level disaster management initiatives and laws: she points out that the Philippine is continuously confronted with new disaster challenges and concerns which requires anticipatory measures and strategies rather than a reactive approach and a culture of concentrating on response. On this note, one encouraging sign is to note that the nation's disaster management system is highly dependent on donor and multilateral institutional assistance. A noticeable shift is being articulated, if not acted on, by the international community, which is becoming less supportive of repeatedly providing relief assistance and is realizing the value of integrating disaster risk management into development efforts. If this direction is maintained it is likely to force fundamental changes in the Filipino system.

This links to the main challenges facing the Philippines in the medium term, which remain reduction of poverty and continuing to overcoming institutional inertia in recognizing natural hazards as an obstacle for long-term sustainable development (World Bank, 2004), while dealing with practical problems of organization, finance, inefficiency, and incompetence (Bankoff, 2003, p. 90). The Philippines government has been embarking on a process of integrating disaster mitigation and sustainable development issues since 1991, within its Medium Term Philippine Development Plans, under the Development Sector Administration. Progress is slow, however: the most recent Medium-Term Philippine Development Plan 2004–2010 (NEDA, 2004) has statements acknowledging the damage natural disaster does to the nation but not how this vulnerability jeopardizes national economic goals, and offers no guideline for action. Local governments are required to integrate disaster management plans into local development plans, but few have done so. Notwithstanding these initial developments, however, the effectiveness of disaster management is still being seriously challenged (Bankoff & Hilhorst, 2004).

NEXT STEPS—WHERE WE MIGHT GO FROM HERE

The essence of this brief discussion on national systems is that central government has a special responsibility in relation to disaster management and that these roles are carried out in different ways that reflect cultural values and assumptions, including previous disaster experience. It has been repeatedly stated throughout this discussion that there is insufficient empirical data at the national systems level: the "void in the empirical data base" to which Drabek referred in 1986, nearly 20 years ago, is still there. Similarly, the issues identified by Tierney and her colleagues (2001) remain unexplored but still fundamental, namely: How do governmental structures and policies influence preparedness and response activities? Under what conditions and for what tasks does centralization work best? How do broader societal forces shed light on which hazard management activities are organized and the reasons why particular hazard adjustments are preferred over others? and Why do some approaches to loss reduction succeed in particular societal settings while failing in others and still others are not considered at all?

Added to this is the trend identified by Handmer (2000) concerning the increasing involvement of private enterprise in functions formerly provided by government. He suggests there is nothing inherent in aspects such as warning systems or disaster management to make them exempt from this general trend, and that in some nations, such as the United States, there have long been public/private sector partnerships to deal with flood and other weather warnings. Questions to be asked about this issue range from clarifying the responsibilities of governments to what mechanisms are needed to ensure effective service delivery, and whether these mechanisms are universal or specific to cultures or governance types. This leads to thinking about the implications of globalization in the context of national systems and disasters: this is an uncharted field.

Another area requiring assessment, which is a variation on an issue voiced by Tierney and associates above raised by practitioners Angus (2004) and Norton (2004), pertains to the appropriateness of centrist and dispersed models of accountability. Norton highlights the lack of central government trust in local capability and the tendency of central bureaucracies to turf silo, which he sees as an impediments in moving from the conventional response/reactive approach to the new environment of disaster risk management. How significant is this as an issue? What is the relationship between trust and control? Is lack of trust characteristic of some, or all governance types?

Hilhorst (2003) recognizes another fundamental issue by identifying the question of perception: the particular way a situation or an issue is perceived influences the manner in which responses are formulated. Her point is that the way a government and its officials see a disaster is not necessarily the same as a community and its citizens see the phenomenon. But, does the type of governance model play a role in how officials perceive and act on disaster?

Issues about trust and perception prompt further questions on the role the mass media has in national planning and response. Scanlon (2005), for instance, noted that governments have been known to censure and control media reporting of specific disaster episodes. He also pointed out there is no accepted definition about what is "news." Since the role of the media is potentially significant, in terms of reporting on and recording disasters, as well as framing public opinion and shaping governmental views, more effort should be directed to understanding the role of the media in the development of national disaster management policies.

Several other issues demand attention. For instance, how do the actions laid down by national-level systems during disaster response affect what takes place during later recovery activities? More specifically, how can central governmental assist long-term recovery by not impeding it in the initial stages of disaster? This leads to a wider issue about the need to undertake research on how central governments make decisions, prioritize risk, and balance risk management and disaster mitigation with other community needs. It also reintroduces an issue highlighted by earlier research, namely that disasters tend not to be politically salient until after they happen (Rossi, Wright, & Weber-Burdin, 1982; Wolensky, 1977; Wolensky & Miller, 1981). Hence, a question to be asked is has this situation changed after the decade-long IDNDR, its successor (ISDR) and events such as the December 2004 Indian Ocean earthquake and tsunami?

A final area to benefit from further study relates to understanding the differences between planning and responding for disaster in contested environments and where lack of consensus is a characteristic. Most of what we know about disasters and governance has been gleaned from nations that are not torn by internal conflict. Research needs to be conducted to determine what insights can be transferred to nations that are politically unstable, such as Kosovo, the Sudan, Sri Lanka, or in areas such as Iraq or Indonesia. What differences need to be taken into account? What criteria should be employed?

APPENDIX 1. Governmental Tasks Associated with Disaster Risk Managment

1. **Disaster management as a national-level issue**	Disasters are embedded in routine decisions and behavior and cannot be regarded only as low-probability–high consequence events that, with luck, may not occur. This shift in perspective requires national-level leadership, coordination, planning, and execution. Disasters have the potential to cause significant economic loss, social and psychological dislocation, and widespread physical injury and death, and are therefore not a specific sectoral issue, but a problem for entire communities and the nation.
2. **Developing national strategies**	Vulnerabilities change and it is essential to understand and address them as best we can. Nations are likely to face more and worse impacts in future. Developing appropriate countermeasures requires a systematic and coordinated approach. Central government, working with other groups, is the only sector that has a commission to develop nationwide strategies with power to bind, power to commit public resources and influence private resources.
3. **Regulatory requirements**	Sovereign governments typically comprise three distinct sets of offices, which together distinguish it from other sectors. The role of the *legislature* is to make the law; the *executive* is responsible in formulating proposals for new laws and for implementing the law; and the *judiciary* is responsible for interpreting the law and its application in specific cases. These functions provide the machinery through which government maintains community values. The level of importance a nation places on disaster management is reflected in wider community values; changes in those values are legitimated through governmental processes that enact, implement, and review regulatory functions.

(Cont.)

APPENDIX 1. (*Continued*)

4. National provision for public safety	A fundamental responsibility of central government is its authoritative exercise of power to provide for the safety and security of its citizens. This duty typically focuses on (1) providing a national defence system to protect sovereign soil from acts of aggression by hostile forces and (2) ensuring mechanisms to mitigate and manage the disruptive influences of natural, technological, and biological hazards. Differences exist among nations on how these two areas are resourced and structured.
5. Best use of scarce resources	To the extent that revenues used for disaster management are largely derived from public treasuries, government has a responsibility to ensure this resource is used wisely. This requires communities to adopt and implement risk reduction, hazard mitigation, and awareness measures. Governments are also potential disaster victims because they have investments in vulnerable infrastructures located in hazard-prone areas. Hence, it is important that they adopt measures to protect their own human, material, and financial investments. These measures should be commensurate with those required of the wider community.
6. Resilience	Government assumes a major responsibility for ensuring that disaster management is appropriately implemented. Effective disaster management reduces the likelihood of and impact from disasters. It also reduces the probability that members of the community who are not directly affected by the physical impact will be indirectly affected by the interruption of normal flows of goods and services. Hence, it is in government's interest to minimize community disruption, maintain essential goods and services, and ensure continuity of community by encouraging mechanisms that foster resilience.
7. Sustainability	It is wasteful not to develop sustainable hazard management programs: risk reduction and disaster prevention is likely to be cheaper than disaster recovery. Sustainable hazard management actions not only minimize damage, but also promotes a stable environment, provides incentives for investment and enterprise, as well as a sense that people can control their own economic destiny.
8. Risk management coordination	Government-sponsored risk management programs now attract increased attention by policymakers at the highest levels of government and the electorate. No matter what the source of risk to human life, safety, and well-being, electorates insist government reduce uncertainties associated with hazardous events, and design and enforce policies to mitigate their effects. Successful risk and disaster management is dependent upon strong cooperation and coordination among and within levels of government, volunteers, and the private sector. The most likely actor to achieve this is central government: it has a mandate to legislate requirements and promote community values within a public good context.
9. Economic management	Disasters destroy decades of human effort and investments, and threaten sustainable economic development by placing new demands on society for reconstruction and rehabilitation, and by diverting scarce resources away from planned activities that have been agreed to by the population. Disasters are costly in both immediate losses and in long-term consequences. They halt and in some cases, reverse economic progress. As the nation's economic manager, it is prudent for government to minimize circumstances that may disrupt markets.
10. Social equity	How governments choose to deal with both development and disaster issues has significant social, economic, cultural, and political implications. Many current approaches transfer risk to those who cannot object effectively, such as less powerful group or future generations. Government has a responsibility for considering these issues of social equity in its policies.

CHAPTER 21

Disaster and Crisis Management in Transitional Societies: Commonalities and Peculiarities[1]

BORIS N. PORFIRIEV

The dissolution of the Soviet Union in the 1990s had myriad social consequences, many of which were unintended. This chapter mainly discusses one such consequence: the effect of the disappearance of the Soviet Union and the reemergence of Russia on disaster planning and crisis management not only in Russia, but also in Eastern Europe societies that had been in the Soviet sphere of influence.

Our objective is threefold: (1) we describe the changes that occurred in organizations, policies, and operations associated with disaster planning and crisis managing; (2) we indicate the conditions, both general contextual and specifics ones, that are affecting the changes; and (3) we note consequences, both positive and negative, for the public and others who are affected by whatever disaster planning and crisis managing is in place at any given time. However, we do not treat changes, conditions, and consequences separately but instead discuss them together within 10 major propositions or generalizations that were produced by our analysis for this chapter.

HISTORICAL BACKGROUND

The change to more democratic systems, which had started to occur 20 years earlier in Eastern European nations as well as those in the former Soviet Union, dramatically changed the countries' existing political regimes including their institutional, legislative, and economic pillars. This tremendous and painful transition involves critical challenges to the resilience of newly established and emerging political and administrative institutions, and the values and norms of communities and society as a whole. We focus on what has and is going on during this transitional period with respect to disaster and crisis management in these systems undergoing major changes.

---

[1] Some of the ideas in this chapter were first advanced 4 years ago (see Porfiriev & Svedin, 2002). However, what is set forth here is an extensively revised, extended, rewritten, and updated version of those ideas.

However, this transition is occurring in governmental systems that have to bring together matters of security and safety, accelerating economic growth, and democratization, processes that sometime complement and at other times conflict with one another. These polities also have to deal with problems such as growing poverty, corruption and organized crime, and the decay of critical lifeline infrastructures, as well as excessive monopolization in the economic sphere. To these can be added well known global challenges such as climate change, international terrorism, and new kinds of natural and technological disasters with their own distinctive characteristics (for a discussion of the latter, see the chapters by Boin and 't Hart, and by Quarantelli, Lagadec, and Boin in this handbook). Adding to all these problematical issues have been the recent permutations and economic recessions in the 1990s in the central and Eastern European states and in the former Soviet Union. In short, the changes in disaster and crisis management have to be seen in the larger context of the many problems we have just enumerated, and that we discuss in more detail later.

Moreover, these challenges are associated with increasing risks and crises in vital societal and political domains, implying that the importance of disaster and crisis management in those societies in transition has increased significantly. In fact, there have been significant changes in national disaster management systems in such societies. As described later, these have increased the planning and response capabilities of such systems although many problems persist..

All the aforementioned complications and problems suggest that changes in crisis and disaster management systems in societies in transition may have to occur faster than is typical in highly developed social systems. If this is a correct assumption, it suggests that the top decision makers in societies in transition have to be even more sophisticated and skillful strategic risk managers than their counterparts in the West. Given that, there is a need for an in-depth investigation of the specific hazards that dominate the disaster scene of societies in transition, as well as research on their coping capabilities (which is determined primarily by the state of development of their national crisis management systems). This chapter can be seen as a first step toward that needed research.

From our perspective, one of the basic issues that needs to be studied is the following. The major political and economic transformations in the former socialist bloc have led their national disaster management systems toward an increasing ambiguity about the status of their disaster preparedness. This is paralleled by a growing vulnerability of the transitional societies because of a combination of traditional hazards and new risks. However, some important elements of national disaster management systems are strengthening.

Such an inconsistency most vividly manifests itself in what we label as "net effect of their social and economic vulnerability." Given the scarcity of worldwide data other than traditional numbers about lives lost and economic damage, in our assessment of the world regions vulnerable to natural hazards and calamities in the 1990s, we used certain indicators of such an effect. We recognize that there may be limitations in the data we use, but accepting that, Table 21.1 shows the results of our analysis.

Table 21.1 shows that in terms of economic vulnerability to disasters the transitional societies we are discussing were quite close to the more industrially developed nations in the 1990s. Moreover, according to our preliminary assessment for 2004, the V_e values for the two nation groups were practically equal and lower than those of the developing countries. Meanwhile, the transitional societies are almost twice as much socially vulnerable to disaster impact than the industrially developed nations, but more than four times more resilient than developing nations, leaving aside the least developed states. (For further details see Porfiriev, 2003.)

TABLE 21.1. The World Regions' Vulnerability to Disasters

World Regions	V_s	V_e
Industrially developed nations	0.19	0.98
Nations in transition	0.30	0.91
Developing nations	1.24	1.12
Least developed countries	7.50	2.50

V_s (social vulnerability index) and V_e (economic vulnerability index) are variations of the standard Gini coefficient we developed to measure the world regions' relative vulnerability to disasters. V_s shows the ratio between a region's percentage in the number of those killed by disaster agents in the world and its share in the world population, while V_e reveals the ratio between the region's share in the world economic damage provided by disasters and that of the region's percentage in the global GDP. Both indexes for the whole world are equal to 1.

THE RESEARCH DATA

First, we mention the research data used in this chapter. Then we advance certain generalizations or propositions that we derive from our analyses. What are important and interesting for both academic and practical exploration are fundamental research studies of these and other specific characteristics of the vulnerability of transitional societies to as well as their management of disasters. However, there are very few such studies. Among a few exceptions we can cite two series of books. One of these focused specifically on the former Soviet Union and contemporary Russia and was written in cooperation with and published by the Disaster Research Center (DRC) at the University of Delaware (Quarantelli & Mozgovaya, 1994; Porfiriev & Quarantelli, 1996). The other series was jointly prepared and published by the Swedish Crisis Management Research and Training Center (CRISMART) and currently covers key research issues on disaster and crisis preparedness and response in the three Baltic nations (Estonia, Latvia, and Lithuania), Poland, and Russia, along with the volumes on Romania and Ukraine in preparation (see Bynander & Chemilievski, 2005; Hansén & Stern, 2000; Porfiriev & Svedin, 2002; Stern & Newlove, 2004; Stern & Norstedt, 1999).

While not as numerous, extensive, and exhaustive as the research publications on and from industrially developed societies (see many of the chapters in this handbook), the aforementioned research publications do provide the opportunity for some generic considerations about crucial features of transitional disaster and crisis management. They are the major research data we use in our analyses in this chapter. Having mentioned this, two reservations should be noted. First, our descriptions and analyses are based mostly on the Russian experiences. Those of other societies in transition, especially the former Soviet Union republics and Eastern European countries, are only occasionally discussed. Second, the generalizations made are preliminary (partially because of the first limitation) and should be treated as hypotheses and propositions rather then solid and unequivocal conclusions.

HYPOTHESES AND PROPOSITIONS

Our analysis produced 10 hypotheses and propositions. The important elements in the proposition are first stated in an overall title, followed by a brief description and then an extended discussion usually providing specific examples and illustrations.

Institutional Erosion and Resource Constraint of Disaster and Crisis Management

This proposition assumes that as transitional societies move from one disaster policy and crisis management regime to another, the eroded institutional frameworks are excessively strained and there is a serious strain on resources. This creates for a society and its institutions an increasing vulnerability to the negative impacts of a disaster agent or crisis factor, which constrains the efficiency of preparedness and response.

The vast data available on transitional nations both within the former Soviet Union and Eastern Europe confirms major shifts in regimes in the late 1980s and further into the 2000s. They moved from exclusively centralized disaster and crisis planning and response to a more decentralized model. They also moved from an overdominant orientation toward wartime threats, with civil defense as the organic element of the Ministry of Defense being a key crisis actor, to peacetime preparations with civic or quasi-civilian institutions prevailing on a crisis management scene. For instance, in the Baltic States only Lithuania kept the defense ministry as the key governmental body responsible for comprehensive crisis policymaking including disaster management, while Estonia and Latvia as well as Poland vested this responsibility in the Ministry of the Interior. At the same time, practically all former Soviet Union republics including Russia share the governance of crisis and disaster situations and areas between the Ministry of Interior, the Federal Security Service, and the Ministry for Emergency Management and Disaster Response (EMERCOM in Russia). In all countries, war prevention, preparedness, and conduct of course remained the prerogative of the Ministry of Foreign Affairs and the Ministry of Defense, respectively (see Porfiriev, 2001b).

This major change is consistent with the more generic trend typical for both developing as well as established democracies in Europe in particular. However, a number of new and independent republics were created by the collapse of the Soviet Union. This led to conspicuous changes in the size of territories and populations, particularly in Russia, and, more important, in qualitative political, economic, and social permutations. Such an abrupt upheaval could not but lead to institutional erosion. Norms, rules, and values that had existed for decades in the former socialist bloc nations, in particular existing industrial and ethnic group relationships, were abolished or lost their binding character. These were replaced by alternative ways of proceeding that were often alien to the public conscience, or not replaced at all, creating societal anomie, frustration, and marginalization. In the specific area of disaster and crisis policy, some 10 to 15 years of existence of novel institutions such as a specific ministry or agency for emergency management and disaster response, proves that still a great deal of work is required to make them established and fully effective structures.

At the same time, radiation, ecological, and earthquake disasters in Chernobyl, Karabash, and Neftegorsk in Russia and the major floods in Central Europe, particularly in the Czech Republic in 2002 and Romania in 2005, vividly demonstrate a high degree of strain experienced by current institutional frameworks, particularly those associated with disaster mitigation and alleviation (Vorobiev, Akimov, & Sokolov, 2003). This leaves aside regional wars, armed conflicts, and terrorist attacks that brought major disturbances to the fragile structure of the emerging disaster and crisis management systems, especially in the former Soviet Union and Yugoslavia.

For instance, the Chernobyl disaster, which occurred at the beginning of the large-scale political and economic changes known as perestroika, considerably and negatively impacted the pace and pattern of economic development in Byelorussia, Russia, and Ukraine. Some economists believe that it served as the prime reason for a lasting economic slow down in the next decade. If true, this means the disaster's adverse impact on and excessive strain for national institutions was indirectly responsible for economic and social reforms.

In addition, the social security system that existed in the former Soviet Union had never considered and thus had not been prepared to handle the problem of multiyear caring of hundreds of thousand of disaster victims, especially workers involved in dangerous "clean up" efforts after disasters. The system had tackled, although not efficiently, such a problem in terms of caring for numerous war veterans, but not for people affected in peacetime crises. The relevant national legislation for social security of those as a specific community was missing, with the aid provided only on an individual basis and in lump sum payments. The emergence of thousands of Chernobyl clean-up and rescue workers who were disabled or in poor health left the existing inflexible institutional and legislative system under high pressure. The federal government of the collapsing Soviet Union and then Russia needed to, under conditions of uncertainty and shortage of time and funds, introduce new laws and regulations and to establish new agencies responsible for the long-term socioeconomic and medical aid to the affected rescuers. In turn, thousands and thousands of rescuers unsatisfied with the pace and amount of such aid as was provided organized a movement to protect their vital interests, which added to the strain on the institutional framework.

The aforementioned major earthquake and flood disasters in 1995–2005 in Central Europe and Russia also created an excessive burden on the developing national emergency management systems in the transitional economies. In this respect, an earthquake disaster in the Sakhalin Island in 1995 serves as an excellent example, with the remoteness of the region exacerbating a key problem in logistics and delivery of resources. This problem existed within the old regime's model of centralized crisis response (see Porfiriev, 1998, pp. 170–190). However, in Sakhalin this turned out to be much more complicated given the existence of a new national emergency management system (USEPE). Its weak points and peculiarities created delays in the preplanned and organized response, and led to wide use of ad hoc solutions and voluntary initiatives. The initial volunteer effort was performed mainly by the victims of the disaster themselves, and lasted over the first critical 36 hours of the response. To a small extent, the volunteers helped to fill the gap for getting a proper response, but could not improve its efficiency.

The response was further reduced by the severity of the quake's impact, which put the local response teams out of operation. It revealed one more dimension of societal vulnerability and suggested the need for improvement of organizational coordination between geographically neighboring response units and higher-level response units. Institutional vulnerability was also associated with crisis communication, in particular with the extent to which disaster response was dependent on well established and functioning communications, particularly by telephones. The system in place at the time was based on a primary local response with availability of backup resources further up in the organizational chain or further away geographically. The vulnerability of the system in terms of communication had tragic consequences as telephone lines were disrupted by the earthquake's impact.

Many other disaster cases and response to those in the countries in transition could be easily added to the above one to corroborate that the efficiency of the new regime disaster and crisis policy was constrained by an excessive burden on institutional entities and by the shortage of funds. This supports our institutional erosion hypothesis in that there is substantial evidence in the post-Soviet and Eastern European nations that disclose a regime shift from the old hierarchical and state-centric crisis management system to a new one. The latter tends to be more decentralized, oriented on mitigation and timely response and open to more non-state (public, private, and mixed) initiatives and solutions. The latest changes in the national disaster policy in Russia, instigated by the major administrative reform in 2004–2005, have involved moving the responsibility for disaster preparedness and planning from federal to regional authorities, and from the latter to municipalities. This is additional evidence of the trend.

However, how far this shift will progress and what are its implications for disaster vulnerability and crisis and emergency management significantly depends on institutional rigidity. This factor constitutes the essence of the next hypothesis. As a prelude to it, we think it is worth mentioning that in the other latest permutation within the national disaster management system in Russia there is an indication of a backward tendency toward centralization reestablishing its position. For instance, in 2002 the fire service was moved from the Ministry of Interior (in which it had existed for almost two centuries!) to EMERCOM, with the latter's personnel and response capacity increasing an order of magnitude. In addition, EMERCOM was also vested with responsibility for disaster recovery, primarily but not only in terms of reconstruction coordination and supervision. If the impact of terrorist attacks is further added, it would be possible to talk even about a regression to a centralized disaster model and crisis policy in transitional societies.

For the sake of fairness, however, one should mention that such a regression is typical not only in transitional but sometimes in industrially developed societies. It suffices to note that the United States response to the 9/11 terrorist attack led to the creation of the Department of Homeland Security (see the chapter by Waugh in this handbook). Or that Hurricane Katrina in 2005 vividly suggested to many, especially in government, the need for a more centralized and concerted response effort at the time of a major catastrophe (see the several articles expressing different views on this matter on the Social Science Research Council Web site at: http://understandingkatrina.ssrc.org).

Institutional Rigidity and Reduction of Disaster Policy and Crisis Management Efficiency

Implied here is a proposition that the transitional polity persistence of existing institutional structures and practices at the meso- and micro-levels of society and government creates conflict with the swift change occurring in the basic foundations at the macropolitical and macroeconomic levels. This precipitates increasing uncertainty and restricts the efficiency of disaster policy. In addition, those in transitional societies who use polities similar to Western regional institutions such as the European Union (EU) and the North Atlantic Treaty Organization (NATO) are likely to experience stress-inducing tension between their domestic norms and European/Western norms.

The basic idea in this proposition suggests that old institutional practices in society and in government persist, particularly at the micro- and meso-levels, despite the rest of the system's overall move toward change. This could even imply dramatic attempts to challenge or destabilize the new regime by proponents of the old regime in the crisis management structure, government, or society at large.

The case of the Chernobyl clean-up and rescue workers provides perhaps the most convincing and comprehensive example of the validity of such a proposition (see Shlikova, 2002). The struggle for better social security between these workers and at first the Soviet, and later the Russian government, was based on and mostly kept relying on the norms, values, and structures typical for the former Soviet social policy carried out by the national government. The poor efficiency of the "pure" state system in the social security area was then replaced by a mutant "privatized-public" system. This reveals the powerlessness of the national law and/or the weakness of the law enforcement system and is a policy failure.

Not surprisingly, absent an alternative system providing such services, especially during disasters, the administrative system continues to be not interested in or deeply concerned about the living conditions of the Chernobyl clean-up and rescue workers. Moreover, the national government has been gradually reducing the number and amount of privileges provided to these workers. This has been carried out through introducing regulations, which reduce the list of those eligible to use in particular the opportunities provided by the social security reform. Among other things, this implies the so-called monetization of privileges (i.e., replacing services by the payment of money). In addition, the benefits have been cut within the ongoing national administrative (governmental) reform by the shifting of responsibility, but not funds, from the federal and regional authorities to the more poorly funded municipal level.

Such a discrepancy in interests between old bureaucratic structures and clean-up and rescue workers in need created a conflict. This led to the instigation of self-protection initiatives by the workers, who organized action groups and even special nongovernmental organizations (NGOs) to regain their rights to receive social aid. National and particularly regional NGOs, which represent the elements of the new regime in crisis management geared more toward a decentralized system and a multitude of actors (including private actors), play an important role in the struggle between the federal government (macro-level) and to a less extent the regional authorities (meso-level) on the one hand, and on the other hand, those directly involved in the alleviation of the Chernobyl disaster (micro- and meso-levels).

The latest experiences in disaster response reveal a persistence of existing institutional structures and practices not only at the lower levels of society and government but also at the top level. In turn, this precipitates conflicts within macropolitical and macroeconomic levels. As an example, one could contrast the recovery from the disastrous floods in Yakutia in 1998 and 2001 to that in the Southern Russia in 2002 (Vorobiev, Akimov, & Sokolov, 2003). This comparison shows that tensions and conflicts between the Ministry for Construction and EMERCOM regarding both responsibilities and implementation issues did not subside over time. In turn, this adversely affected the pace and efficiency of recovery from the floods and increased the risk of a new crisis in the coming winter cold for the residents, who either moved into the newly built but inadequately protected houses or who were left homeless.

As to the part of the proposition concerning some of the transitional polities likely to experience stress-inducing tension between domestic and European/Western norms, the issue of industrial and environmental safety standards provides a good example. These are the battles between local communities and enterprises as well as the federal authorities, phenomena also widespread in Western societies. However, what is absent in the West is the disregard for standards by personnel at hazardous facilities who are more interested in keeping their jobs than in lives and health (a situation also well known in developing countries). Further, as some case studies show (Mozgovaya, 2002), at times local communities with large numbers of miners and their families fiercely oppose the federal and regional authorities trying to enforce stricter (Western-like) safety rules and regulations.

In addition, we could mention the case of the air disaster in Ukraine in 2001 when a civilian passenger aircraft heading from Israel to Russia was accidentally downed by a missile launched during military drills, or the sinking of the Kursk submarine in 2000 or the AS-28 bathyscaphe near-disaster in 2005 in Russia. These cases reveal serious failures by national authorities attempting to meet Western standards of disaster and crisis communication, primarily openness in contacting local communities in an attempt to obtain public trust. (We of course are aware that at times even in the West this effort may be more nominal than actual.)

In this respect, it is worth mentioning the "theatre crisis" and the "school seizure crisis," both provoked by major terrorist attacks in 2002 in Moscow and in 2004 in Beslan. There was a major dispute between Western-oriented citizens and experts in Russia (leaving aside emergency professionals, politicians, and the mass media in the West) and supporters of a hard line approach that showed the wide gap between advocates of rather different cultural standards. We should add to this the discrepancy in the coverage of the response to the terrorist attack, particularly its aftermath, by Western and Russian independent media and by official sources of information. An in-depth analysis of the mass media and crisis communication issues during those terrorist attacks also supports the next proposition, which involves the under-institutionalization issue.

Under-Institutionalization and Mass Media Structuring of Disaster and Crisis Policies

Involved here is the idea that as transitional societies move toward Western style democracy and a market economy, crisis management and disaster policy, to overcome existing under-institutionalization, will tend to be increasingly politicized. In parallel, the mass media will play an increasingly important role both in reporting crises (disasters) as well as being crisis management actors. This results in disasters being seen as they are shaped by the mass media and in their becoming a political issue. It also implies that a more open and extensive reporting by the media, together with a real or imagined shift in crisis and emergency management regime or socio-economic changes in general, might generate increased expectations by the public that the government should be able to better cope with a disaster.

Numerous experiences of the recent past and present provide abundant evidence of the mounting openness and mass media coverage of disasters and emergency and crisis management issues in transitional societies. This is particularly obvious when compared with what went on under the former socialist bloc. In earlier times the phrase "no victims, no destruction" captured the description of major disasters in the official media with no alternative independent data sources available. This leaves aside accidents at military sites and activities, which almost never were made public. Since the late 1980s, the press media and television have produced countless articles and comments on disasters using both domestic and international data sources. Widespread coverage of major floods in the Central European countries in 2002 and 2005 and of regional wars and armed conflicts in the former Yugoslavia and in former Soviet Union republics are but a few illustrations of the point.

Increasing coverage, however, does not mean full transparency in disaster reporting, for example, in Russia, the cases of the sinking of the Kursk submarine and the AS-28 bathyscaphe in 2000 and 2005, respectively as well as the previously mentioned terrorist attacks in Moscow and Beslan. The evidence is that the new disaster and crisis regime indeed is more open than in the times of the former Soviet Union and even about media coverage of the accidents at strategic military objectives. On the Kursk tragedy alone, five books along with hundreds of newspaper articles and TV comments were issued within a year—far beyond the number of writings about Chernobyl, the most publicized previous disaster in Russia.

What should be compared, however, is the media's complicated access to and distortion of some essential data concerning coping with the crisis that left significant room for media and public speculations on these disasters. A side effect of the new critical media reporting on disasters in Russia and other nations in transition is that, like in Western countries, they tend to fill in the blanks with whatever they can or see fit. This kind of reporting sometimes produces sensational stories that generate the risk of a second-order crisis (Cherkashin, 2001, pp. 36–44).

Some interesting observations in support of the crisis politicization and media structuring hypothesis also can be seen from findings about the Neftegorsk earthquake in Russia and the floods in Czech Republic and Romania. Such disaster issues were not a substantive part of either the old political regime at large and crisis management in particular or official media policy. However, various social actors, particularly citizen groups and NGOs, pushed these items further up on the political and media agenda.

In this, the "theatre crisis" in Moscow provides another good illustration. Three days of silence by the responsible agencies about the gas that was used by special antiterrorist teams left the media free to speculate about the nature of the combat and the chemical weapons used. In turn, those speculations, which spread both within and outside Russia, gave rise to suspicions of a political nature and increased political tensions. After the issuance of official statements, most of the public pressure lessened. The families of Ukrainian hostages, however, started a media campaign and their lawyers initiated suits against the Russian government, openly using this opportunity to put together this case with the aforementioned accident in 2001, when a Ukrainian missile accidentally hit a T-154 aircraft flying from Israel to Russia.

With regard the NGOs, worth mentioning is the case of Karabash (the Ural region in Russia considered by environmentalists as the most contaminated area in the world), where a local "green peace" organization started to picture ecological issues as a "new" type of threat (new in the sense of becoming recognized as a disaster). The emergence of NGOs and other private groups as active interest or influence groups that structure the disaster management agenda is a sign of the shift in the crisis regime, leaving the new context more open to the media and the public. In particular, adding to the influence of other groups and interests in addition to those of the federal, state, regional, or local governments and official media is the increasing influence of the new independent information sources.

At the same time, the mounting politicization of disaster and crisis events, especially those associated with compensations, property redistribution, and all-level authority elections, pushes in the opposite direction by reducing the number of such sources, primarily at the local and regional levels. Moreover, the politicizing of these sensitive issues in the mass media and in public forums can increase tension between different ethnic and social groups. For instance, this resulted from the speculations that developed about the gap in the amount of compensation (sometimes of a considerable magnitude) received by the neighboring communities located in the Chernobyl plume area in Byelorussia, Ukraine, and Russia, and what was given to the families of those killed in the Moscow and Beslan terrorist attacks.

Are there increased public expectations about the government's mounting ability to improve disaster management as a result of more open and extensive reporting by the media and a real or perceived shift in this management's regime or socioeconomic changes in general? Our observation is that the experiences of transitional societies seem mixed. People in general do not expect, or accept to the same degree as with other services, a decrease of a government's ability to cope with a crisis when the "old" way of doing things allows room for the "new" disaster or crisis policy. Available studies of the mass media in the former Soviet Union nations reveal that the developing critical scrutiny of disasters and emergency management does put pressure on decision-makers acting as crisis managers. The question of whether the mass media actually succeed in creating change is still unclear. Media reporting itself, however, creates expectations among the public with the further possibility of leading or not leading to a second-order crisis or crisis amplification (Kasperson et al., 1988).

From a different perspective, the persistence of the social security problem of the Chernobyl clean-up and rescue workers is not totally the result of gaps in disaster recovery programs. The problem is partially rooted in the unwillingness of some of the victims and those indirectly affected by the irradiation to waive their claims and receive social security instead of direct compensations from the government. Thus, the ongoing struggle between the clean-up and rescue workers and the government could be portrayed as a part of the new regime, meaning that issues such as compensation to disaster victims and their families in Russia (and other post-Soviet nations) can really be managed through lawsuits as in the West.

The aforementioned issue can be considered a reaction to a perceived failure by the state to provide the proper care for citizens who sacrificed their lives and health for their homeland. A "caring" government, solidarity and perception of those who sacrificed themselves for the nation as heroes, are values that were very entrenched in and associated with the old Soviet system. These traditional values still persist in many ways in the post-Soviet Russia transitional societies. There is therefore an emotional and open negative expression when the government is perceived or really fails to perform its expected duties.

The recent experience of transitional economies supports the assumption that the more lasting a crisis or disaster is, the less the public expects it to be managed efficiently. The case study of recovery from a creeping ecological disaster in Karabash shows that the local people perceived that the government was not responding to their environmental concerns (Mozogovaya, 2002). But there was a public expectation that the heavy dependency on the mono-production of copper, which gave birth to the town but resulted in a very high hazardous contamination, would be replaced or compensated in some way when the federal authorities decided to do something about the ownership of the plant and its future work. However, the authorities did not show any eagerness to take any responsibility to do something concrete to alleviate the environmental disaster. When in the late 1990s they understood that the government was not going to step in and intervene in the privatization of the plant, the plant workers and citizens organized action groups to protest the move (Mozgovaya, 2002).

In a sense, this new social movement was about experiencing the new goals and aims of the crisis management regime, with new identified problem areas and new processes for managing them. But at the same time, it was a perception of the very real and tangible lack of hands-on management of the problem. For the people concerned, very little changed in their living conditions and everyday priorities. The practical solution to the government's new way of looking at the plants' ecological impact was not by any means readily at hand (no other means of employment were available, for instance). Therefore the local people did not perceive the authorities as taking their part of the responsibility in this case. From this perspective the new regime can be viewed as not institutionalized enough, thus leaving some substantial implementation issues unresolved.

Institutional Overstrain and Zugzwang: An Impact on Disaster Preparedness and Response

The hypothesis here is that in transitional societies overstrained decision-making units increasingly experience institutional *zugzwang* (this word is a chess term describing a situation in which a player needs to make a move that will lead to a worsening of his (her) position). This will lead to poor detection (identification of threat) and a delayed prevention of or an inefficient response to a specific crisis occasion.In turn,the frequency and severity of these tend to escalate, thus transforming them into major disasters.In conjunction with mounting politicization, this also leads higher level emergency managers to focus on acute rather than creeping crises and disasters and on short-term political and economic implications at the expense of longer term social and environmental effects.

Much crisis and disaster research literature exists that highlights different types of gaps in disaster preparedness and failures in response. However, only a small portion of it considers institutional issues involved in such loopholes that are precipitated by specific transitional conditions of development of nations in Europe, Asia, and Latin America. Conceivably, the Russian disaster and crisis management context could provide the most convincing evidence of the above proposition.

First, this involves the vulnerability to disasters resulting from the legacy of centralized planning and an excessive militarized economy that existed in the former Soviet Union, and from the problems of transition from a totalitarian regime to a more democratic and market-oriented polity that is characteristic of Russia, the former Soviet republics, and Central European countries as well as China and Vietnam. For instance, our analysis of the 1995 Neftegorsk earthquake disaster showed that the increased vulnerability of communities was primarily due to the poor construction of residential buildings in late 1960s through the early 1970s. In contrast to the earthquake disaster in Armenia in 1986 and Turkey in 2001, this happened not only because construction companies were attempting to reduce costs so as to maximize their profits, but also from a tradition of sticking to "universal" design and construction standards that was typical for centrally planned economies in the Soviet Union. This approach assumed that a "universal" design was applicable to practically every construction site, in contrast to using a more flexible but more time-consuming and resource-intensive construction technologies that take into account the particular conditions of sites.

This loosening of industrial and occupational safety measures was further exacerbated by the recurrent social and economic hardships and political disturbances that surfaced in the transition to the new economic and political regime in Russia and other societies in transition in the 1990s. These conditions strongly added to the existing uncertainty that considerably complicated not only disaster preparedness and crisis prevention, but also socioeconomic policy in general, thus involving the development process into a continuing national systemic crisis. Almost every major disaster and/or crisis in transitional economies reveals significant adverse impacts of such systemic crisis on specific disaster development paths and crisis management efficiency.

For instance, the rescue efforts carried out in response to the Neftegorsk earthquake and Kursk submarine disasters were of limited efficiency because of the shortage or the absence of modern rescue equipment and rescue personnel. The key reason for this was that the EMER-COM and Defense Ministry budgets were limited if not cut back as a result of the deep and lasting economic slow down and increasing indebtedness in the 1990s. In addition, in 1995, when the Neftegorsk earthquake occurred, EMERCOM had to respond to more than 1500 other emergencies that also used much needed resources and personnel. In 2000, when the Kursk submarine sank, the Russian Defense Ministry had to use its scarce resources in responding to a number of other, fortunately less serious, military accidents as well as carrying out routine operations. Moreover, almost at the same time as the Kursk disaster, EMERCOM and other ministries had to cope with the terrorist attack and a major fire at a TV tower in Moscow.

These multiple and overlapping crises created external synchronicities and internal event overload, leading to competition for limited resources and thus significantly complicating the handling of disasters. Such conditions excessively strain the existing institutional framework, putting the national disaster management system in particular into a zugzwang position. This system, like those for management of social, economic, and political crises, have been forced to focus on crises that have already occurred, rather than trying to anticipate possible future ones. This means that some crises are not detected, are detected too late, or that responses are considerably delayed.

In the case of Russia, this problem is exacerbated further by the fact that its vast territory extends over 11 time zones, which has major negative implications for national disaster policy. The very large area involved results in a reduction of prevention/mitigation capability, contributing to increased vulnerability, crisis recurrence, and substantial costs. In the late 1990s, the latter amounted to 6% to 7% of the gross national product (Ragozin, 1999).

As previously noted, there tends to be a focus on the short-term social and economic issues involved in instant crises (e.g., sheltering, compensations, etc.) rather than on long-term social and environmental effects of creeping crises. Evidence for this comes, for example, from comparing the Neftegorsk earthquake disaster and the Kursk tragedy with the slowly moving Karabash ecological disaster and the long-lasting Chernobyl clean-up and rescue workers' crisis in Russia. Additional supporting data come from looking at the considerable strengthening of the national disaster and emergency management policy with EMERCOM as the lead organization, in contrast to the national environmental policy. In the 1990s, the latter was increasingly losing its position. The responsible federal body was first reduced from a ministry to a committee (agency). Then in 2000 the agency was further downgraded to a department within the federal Ministry for Natural Resources which is responsible for resource development rather than for conservation and the prevention of excessive exploitation.

The Bureaucratic-Politics of Disaster Response and Recovery

The point of this proposition is that transitional polities are likely to experience a high frequency and a high intensity of bureaucratic political behavior in both everyday routine times and in disaster and crisis situations.

Studies of political and financial crises and crisis management present good illustrations for this proposition, for example, the economic overheating in Estonia in 1997 (Stern & Nohrstedt, 1999), the major financial default in 1998 in transitional and some industrialized economies, as well as the smaller banking crises in Russia in 2000. They all involved considerable bureaucratic political behavior.

However, research studies of "classic" disasters also provide convincing data for the notion of a close relationship between crises and bureaucratic organizational politics. For instance, investigation of the mass media coverage of the Kursk submarine disaster clearly reveals the ambiguity in both the crisis response and crisis communication of the various social actors involved. In particular, comments on and explanations of the submarine's sinking varied from external impact (e.g., collision with or even attack by an alien submarine, or impact with a civilian Russian warship or a sea mine), to internal explosion of torpedoes because of some technical deficiency or human error. A similar gamut of stories was characteristic in the discussion of the opportunities for the survival of the crew and early rescuing. (For a detailed discussion see Cherkashin, 2001; Kouznetsov, 2005; Ustinov, 2005).

Apparently, these varying stories partly followed from the complexity and uncertainty of the disastrous accident as such, as well as the heterogeneity of the units involved both in the initial military exercise and the later rescue activity. To a not lesser extent they reflect underlying intragovernmental and intraorganizational tensions (Kouznetsov, 2005). However, regardless of which version is closer to the truth, an important observation becomes crystal clear: the extremely hectic conditions, with key crisis decisions being taken in an ad hoc way, provided much room for bureaucratic maneuvering and politicking by specific crisis actors. This amplified the adverse impact of the event by adding crisis communication issues to the earlier severe implications of a major technological accident, thus exacerbating the damage that occurred and escalating it to major disaster in the public perception, both in Russia and internationally.

A crucial question here is to what extent the transitional state of a society (Russia or any other) contributes to a bureaucratic–organizational and a bureaucratic–political behavior by the actors responding to a particular crisis and/or disaster. Admittedly, bureaucratic and political maneuvering was quite typical in the former Soviet Union but it also occurs in established democracies. There are often situations when responsible officials or institutions try to shift responsibility to some other crisis actors, especially to journalists, political opponents, and citizen groups. One might assume that especially in hierarchical institutional and social systems, such motivation explains the frequent organizational and political tendency to assign blame to parties other than themselves, and to seek in man-made disaster scapegoat culprits.

At least two factors are specifically associated with the predicament of transitional societies that are conducive to bureaucratic politics. One of these involves the impact produced by frequent replacement of top political leaders accompanied by significant reshuffling in their teams, which are typically composed of a specific mixture of both newcomers and "veterans" in administration. These high-level decision support makers use different, often opposing, principles and methods of disaster communication. This makes the dialogue between the crisis actors and especially with the mass media and the public very difficult. This is further complicated by the involvement of international political and media communities, which monitor and evaluate disaster response and rescue operations commanded by the new leaders. Such psychological pressure, along with organizational innovations, cannot help but encourage routine bureau–political maneuvering.

One additional factor is associated with the increased mass media involvement in disaster and crisis policy. The great number and activities of the new independent media information sources that seek more transparency of official reports on crises sometimes forces responsible officials and institutions to manipulatively seek an "exit strategy." To do this they often use holes and gaps provided by 'transitional' but not fully established legislation, and by competition between different social actors to justify specific (in)action or shift of responsibility.

Such behavior occurs not only during the trans-disaster phase (at the height of a crisis as such), but also in post-disaster situations. One can see bureaucratic tricks to attempt to postpone or even to denounce any official recognition of the conscription in the republics of the former Soviet Union of clean-up and rescue workers in the response to Chernobyl, and attempts to move the responsibility for social security and aid from the federal government to municipal authorities, the families of the rescuers, and NGOs. Similar behaviors could be cited from studies of recovery from disasters, particularly the compensation to the communities affected by the major floods in Central Europe and Russia in 2002 (Vorobiev, Akimov, & Sokolov, 2003).

These and other cases highlight some of the sophisticated bureau–organizational maneuvering in disasters. This indicates that the existing political–administrative system is relatively weak and likely to attempt to change emergent patterns of procedures, functions, and powers including that of interagency coordination in disaster response and recovery. At the same time, this illustrates that the new group syndrome at the policy regime level, where conflicts easily escalate into power struggles, is really a major characteristic for transitional polity.

Institutional Reflexive Change, Overlearning, and Disasters.

Our point here is that when transitional societies face disaster and/or crisis conditions, they tend toward reflexive institutional changes and volatility. Also, in transitional as opposed to established democracies, there is a greater chance that crises will generate "double loop" and/or "third order" learning processes (explained later), and by inference, a higher likelihood of overlearning the lessons of the last crisis for the next one.

Research studies show that in the last 15 years there have been significant institutional changes in national disaster policy in the former Soviet Union republics, and notably Russia. The very organization and development of EMERCOM in Russia and its analogues in the other members of the CIS, i.e., state agencies that did not previously exist in these countries, is good evidence for this point. To a great extent, these transformations reflect past experiences and lessons learned from them, with the earlier changes being the quickest and reflexive. For instance, in 1991–1993, the chief of EMERCOM was ordered by the president of Russia to step in and handle the conflict between Northern Ossetia and Ingushetia, although before (and afterwards) this was not a formal function of the agency. In the same period, the earlier independent hydrometeorological service was incorporated into EMERCOM but soon after was separated again and returned to its earlier status. Similar situations occurred in 2004, a decade after the start of the ongoing major administrative reform in Russia.

However, this and other examples indicate such transformations use a medium-term perspective rather than an after-every-event restructuring such as happened in Estonia or Poland (Bynander & Chemilievski, 2005; Stern & Nohrstedt, 1999). For instance, between 1994 and 2000 EMERCOM underwent serious but incremental reorganization, with disaster policy shifting from emergency response to specific events in the early 1990s, to emergency preparedness and more comprehensive response in the mid-1990s, and to disaster mitigation and risk reduction in the late 1990s to the early 2000s. The same process has been underway in the Interior Ministry, manifested in intraorganizational changes. There have been attempts to cope with the sharp increase in organized crime, involving but not limited to the creation of new kinds of special task forces (*spetsnaz*). Meanwhile, in the ministry dealing with crises such changes have been more frequent than in EMERCOM, being instigated by a more recurrent replacement of its top management, rather than just changes in the crime pattern alone.

This puts to the fore the institutional volatility issue that is part of the proposition mentioned earlier. An important factor is the role of personality and the decision-making framework created by and within the historical development and culture (including the political culture) of a given polity. The more modern nations that have replaced the former socialist bloc, particularly most of those of the former Soviet Union, are no longer totalitarian and authoritarian societies. Yet their political systems still preserve much of a hierarchical structure, with a high concentration of power in the hands of a head of multilevel authority. This creates conditions for relatively easy structural and functional changes and replacement of top management in a specific ministry or state organization. It is even more so in disaster and crisis policy areas, which according to the constitutions of the CIS members is the exclusive prerogative of the president. If he or she favors changes and personnel replacements, as did the first president of Russia, the present-day leaders in Byelorussia in the Ukraine, and the Central Asian nations, the changes will actually happen and make institutional volatility more organic and persistent.

The reflexive institutional changes in transitional societies when there are disasters also provide mixed evidence about overlearning from previous crises. While this learning was notable in some Baltic states, for example, Estonia and Latvia (Buss, Stern & Newlove, 2005;

Stern & Nohrstedt, 1999), in Russia and in the Ukraine at least one should have more reason to talk about underlearning. This implies drawing few if any lessons from earlier disasters.

A case study of the Chernobyl clean-up and rescue workers (Shlikova, 2002) illustrates the point. Despite the failure of the existing official institutions to provide adequate social security services to thousands of those workers in Russia, Byelorussia, and the Ukraine, that turned a radiation contamination disaster into a creeping and long-lasting sociopolitical crisis, almost nothing changed. This forced people to organize action groups and NGOs to protect their legitimate interests. The same was also done by the families of those killed in submarine disasters and terrorist attacks in 2000–2004. However, it should be noted that actions such as these in modern Russia and most of the CIS economies are few, thus showing that the development of civil society there is only at the earliest stage.

These and other recent experiences of recovering from disasters show that learning from crises may be more characteristic of citizens than of governmental institutions. If press reports are accurate, it might be argued that the response to Hurricane Andrew in 1992 and Hurricane Katrina in 2005 showed that the government did not learn much from the first experience. However, perhaps a transitional polity government will not have time or experience to allow its political and bureaucratic interests to become entrenched and fail to become more open or may see its practices and institutional arrangements as provisional and call for revisions in response to negative feedback from the public. This leads to a suggestion that in a risk society, historical, cultural, and other social core factors determine the pace of post-crisis reflexive change and learning from crises to a much larger extent than the very process of transition itself.

TRANSITIONAL VULNERABILITY, CRISIS DEVELOPMENT, AND DISASTER MANAGEMENT[2]

Research studies of disasters and disaster policy in the new democracies give us a basis for the identification of the common characteristics that affect the vulnerability of nations to and the severity of crises (Hansén & Stern, 2000). The most important political, institutional, and sociocultural features are uneven/unstable regulations, the shadow of authoritarianism, discrepancies and conflicts between public values and norms accompanied by intra- and intercommunity strain (including ethnic tensions), and changing mass media cultures. The most crucial economic characteristics involve resource constraints and infrastructural decay. We discuss these matters in the following sections.

Key Sociocultural and Politico-Institutional Changes in Transitional Societies

All transitional societies by definition have been evolving from state socialism toward various forms of liberal democratic states and societies. In addition, a number of the polities have made a transition from being an internal part of the Soviet Union, to national sovereignty as independent states. These profound changes in the sociopolitical order pose great challenges to the new democracies.

---

[2] This section builds upon and expands the conclusions of Hansen and Stern (2000) as well as the creative comments of Paul 't Hart.

First, the public values and norms long existing and rooted in the societies of the former Soviet Union republics were replaced by new ones. This resulted in a shift from a totalitarian and authoritarian state to deregulation and a liberal, people-oriented, public policy that provided for more community and individual freedoms including those of private property, entrepreneurship, and ability to move around. These were almost immediately shared by the younger generations much less experienced or having mostly negative experiences of living in the old political regime. However democratic and positive, though, these radical changes could not but conflict with those of giving priority to public and collective interests over individual preferences and willingness, nonmonetary over monetary values, and others. These dominated before and are deeply entrenched in the mass consciousness of older generations, who only two decades ago lived rather different lives but now have lost their social orientation and find themselves in conditions of social anomie.

Second, the old institutions and regulatory arrangements have been discarded or incorporated into a radically changed political and institutional context, with the de-legitimization of the existing regime in many cases having been so profound that large areas of legislation and legal practice were eliminated. Given the laissez-faire zeitgeist, often the plan-based or authoritarian structures have not been replaced promptly with the kinds of regulatory bodies common in the West, which could moderate and mitigate market failures of various kinds. Thus, a highly segmented and uneven process of legal and political reform has left lacunae and politicoeconomic disequilibria of various kinds.

Implications for Crisis Development and Disaster Vulnerability: Particular Role of Ethnic Tensions

The aforementioned transitional processes, which involve social norms and value conflicts and legislative and institutional gaps and imbalances, have major implications for dealing with both crises and disasters. In terms of crisis and disaster development, they often create a fertile environment for the incubation of new kinds of crises or catalyze existing latent crisis conditions into producing creeping and instant crises. Such conditions also mean increasing vulnerability to disaster impact or directly lead to the escalation of disasters.

For crisis and disaster policy, the transitional processes mentioned earlier have a number of implications. They imply that there will be increasing complexity and uncertainty in preparedness and response operations, persistent and pronounced shortage of resources in competition with profitable market segments of the economy, and a weak state only loosely interested in producing public benefits, including disaster protection. For example, the banking crises, which occurred in both Latvia and Estonia, paralleled in some respects what took place after waves of deregulation in Sweden and the United States in the 1980s and early 1990s, as well as the property redistribution in various industries and issues of social security including those privileges of rescuers in Russia. Similarly, the need to redefine the criteria for citizenship (which affected primarily Russian communities there) as part of the national restoration of Latvia and Estonia became a source of much domestic intra- and intercommunity ethnic strain and international controversy including tensions between these Baltic States and Russia. In addition, there were disastrous regional and ethnic conflicts in the latter, with the North Caucasus being the major "hot bed," the existing tensions in the modern Ukraine between the Russian-speaking southeastern part, Crimea region with a high percentage of the Muslim Tatar communities and the other parts (the bulk) of the country.

The above results in the exacerbation of the already high level of regional and ethnic tensions as a striking characteristic of many transitional polities. Dramatic population shifts following the dissolution of the Soviet Union contributed to making the rising tensions a thorny issue in many post-Soviet countries. The changing social, economic, and political status of both local ethnicities and what have become Russian expatriate communities pose major challenges in many transitional states. Particular national identities deemphasized (some would use stronger language) during the Soviet era have been heartily embraced by the newly independent nations. In some of these areas (Latvia, the Central Asian nations, to a lesser extent Georgia, and even in the Ukraine) this placed the status of Russian minorities in doubt.

Resource Scarcity and Infrastructural Decay as Disaster Vulnerability Factors and Crisis Management Constraints

The sociocultural and sociopolitical permutations in the transition of old regimes to more democratic societies are exacerbated by resource constraints and infrastructural obsoleteness. These both encourage crisis conditions and reduce the disaster mitigation potential of transitional polities.

Urbanization is placing increasing demands on the infrastructure of major cities at the same time as this infrastructure is aging and in need of major investments for maintenance and/or modernization. This is a global trend and is true irrespective of the level of industrialization or democratization of a nation, as can be seen in the examples of recent power blackouts in the United States, the United Kingdom, and Sweden as well as in Russia, Georgia, and Argentina. However, in many of the new democracies this problem is particularly acute, following from former Soviet practices regarding construction and urban planning that often failed to meet modern standards for safety and performance. A related problem has to do with infrastructural interdependence. In many of the transitional societies, infrastructure was developed as part of the larger Soviet or Soviet Bloc systems. For example, Estonia shares water and electric infrastructure with Russia, which may lead to conflicts.

To make matters worse, such structures have not been properly maintained, mostly because of the shortage of funds or, in more generic terms, resource constraints. Many of the new democracies are handicapped by severe shortage of resources. While infrastructure as well as institutions and legislation vitally need modernization, political and especially economic resources are already stretched very thin. Given these limitations, potentially avoidable crises occur when preventative investments might well have averted them. Deficiencies in preparedness are often revealed when crises occur and may be hard to remedy on an ad hoc basis when there are so few extra resource capabilities in the system (Cyert & March, 1963; Levinthal & March, 1981; Meyer, 1982).

Implications for Crisis and Disaster Management: Authoritarian Reflex and Development Strategy

A decreased disaster and crisis preparedness as a result of an imbalanced institutional framework and a resource-deficient economy is particularly evident when the kinds of crises new to the former socialist bloc nations (and not always to them alone) occur. These involve refugee crises in Estonia and Russia; the insolvency of banks and property redistribution crises in

Latvia, Russia, and other countries; as well as SARS and the bird flu epidemics in China, Romania, and a number of other transitional and developed economies.

At the same time, the aforementioned sociocultural and political changes and resource constraints loosen security and safety policies, weaken protective standards, and weaken an institutional framework and personnel training that are critical to efficient disaster management. Not surprisingly, this also precipitates inferior levels of preparedness and response to the kinds of disasters and crises that existed in old regimes, too. Those include, for instance, floods and earthquakes in China, the Czech Republic, Romania, and Russia, and technological accidents (a collapsed platform in Latvia and the explosion of a submarine in Russia). Added to this could be criminal justice and police management crises (robbery of weapons and the tragedy of peacekeepers in Estonia, a "police werewolves" scandal in Russia, the kidnapping of journalist and high level officials in the Ukraine and Byelorussia), and the failure of the public infrastructure in many places.

The implications of all this are that crisis and disaster vulnerability management is further exacerbated by the persistence of an authoritarian reflex typical in transitional societies. This is particularly strong in the Asian economies such as Turkmenia and Uzbekistan, and to lesser extent in China. Undoubtedly, the very exigencies of disasters and crises often call for quick and authoritative decisions and strong leadership, which often are not consistent with democratic values of openness, transparency, and public participation in the political process. Therefore, a certain degree of authoritarian reaction to disaster or crisis conditions can be found in many established democracies, for example, in provisions for declaring states of emergency and martial law, which curtail citizens' rights and concentrate power in the hands of crisis managers. But in the United States, as the latest hurricanes Katrina and Rita showed, there was a very strong reluctance to institute such severe measures, and almost none were ever implemented.

Similarly, in the new democracies, the citizenry (and political elitists) who have only recently succeeded in redistributing political power in a more democratic fashion and in securing civil and political rights in normal circumstances are very skeptical about relinquishing those rights in disaster situations. Nevertheless, during disasters and crises in transitional in contrast to established democracies, political and bureaucratic actors are more likely to resort to top-down models within hierarchical and centralized systems of emergency response ('t Hart, Rosenthal, & Kouzmin, 1993).

In this context, it is interesting to make a special note of the possible use of martial law, one of the most tangible and vivid manifestations of authoritarian reaction to crises. In Russia, this was not applied during the first (1994–1999) and the second (from 1999 and current) regional armed conflicts in Chechnya. Nor was martial law used in the catastrophic floods in Poland in 1997 and in Romania in 2005. However, the Chechnya case shows that the absence of martial law does not preclude very tough counterterrorist measures from being widely used.

These specific experiences show that a transitional crisis and disaster management policy does not necessarily imply an authoritarian reaction, and when it manifests itself in preparedness and/or response to disasters it looks controversial rather than unequivocally negative. What is more important is that such a reaction does not preclude learning from crises that sometimes could result even in reconsideration of the strategy that should be used.

In this respect, the case of China is of particular interest. The outbreak of the SARS epidemic in 2003 was considered by both local and international experts as a watershed in the developmental history of China. This crisis revealed institutional and policy constraints and loopholes precipitated by the vulnerability of local communities to novel kinds of crises and disasters. In turn, this could jeopardize if not suspend the dynamics of future economic growth.

The understanding of and concern about the epidemic by the national government resulted in a reconsideration of the existing socioeconomic policy. In fact, this policy was replaced by a more comprehensive and balanced long-term (*syaokan*) strategy for 2003–2025. This assumes reducing imbalances between humans and nature, economy and society, urban and rural areas, between the various regions in the country, and between domestic development and openness to the international community. Such an approach should provide for better preparedness and adaptation to major natural hazards and modern technology, and to reduce the risk of national systemic crises and threats to national security. (For more details see Mikheev, 2005, pp. 565–574).

The Changing Role of the Mass Media in Crisis Management and Disaster Policy

Even in many Western countries, the last few decades have been characterized by what some believe has been a qualitatively significant increase in the vigilance and power of the mass media in the political process (Blumer & Gurevitch, 1995; Edelman, 1988). This seems to be also occurring in the new democracies. In the past, old guard politicians in socialist countries could count on a docile and supportive mass media, but public officials in the new democracies are increasingly confronted with an aggressive, commercially oriented, and critical media, which takes its "watchdog" role very seriously. Strategies such as "covering up" errors or mistakes, which might have been effective under the old regime, have the potential to backfire dramatically if journalists manage to discover embarrassing information.

Recent disasters and crises experience in transitional societies show that despite the roadblocks to mass media operations that are much more serious than in established democracies, many officials and decision makers in the former have great awareness of how the contemporary Western media operates. In particular, they tend to use a more proactive, open communication strategy and more rigorous accountability measures. These, along with a set of sophisticated tools of media manipulation (invented or first introduced in the West, e.g., purchasing of newspaper companies), have been replacing the tough stance toward the press of the old regime. However ambiguous, such tendencies favor enhanced public communication skills on the part of officials involved in the management of various kinds of crises. In turn, this helps to avoid or reduce the risks of crises escalating into major disasters.

In addition to the helpful implication for disaster policy associated with mass media operations, however constrained in transitional societies, one more aspect should not be overlooked. This involves the "flip side" of the aforementioned institutional rigidity. Along with resource constraints this is a typical characteristic of transitional crisis policy significantly reducing its efficiency. However, in a certain respect, institutional rigidity could also be seen as a "healthy conservatism" preserving some of the legacy of old authoritarian regimes at the partial expense of democracy. At the same time, however, it could help to avoid some devastating effects of a major disaster. One could cite as an example the tough measures against hijacking of aircraft introduced in the times of the former Soviet Union by the special antiterrorist service. The latter are still present in Russia today, even though many believed they involved "anti-democratic policing" or were "excessive" in their operations. However, as the tragic events of September 11 in the United States and the bombing of two aircraft in Russia in 2004 showed, such rigid control seems reasonable not only for the new but also for established democracies. Contrary to some beliefs (see, e.g., Hansén & Stern, 2000, p. 351), established democracies are no less crisis prone than transitional societies.

These observations have two important ramifications for transitional disaster and crisis management. From a researcher (or scholarly) perspective these indicate that transitional polities, especially "crisis abundant" Russia, could be valuable social laboratories for studying real-time crises and crisis managing. From a practitioner's viewpoint these suggest keeping the institutional innovations within such a policy in pace not only with reforming national development strategies, but also with current world trends, which contribute to the vulnerability of communities and societies.

CONCLUDING REMARKS: PRELIMINARY FINDINGS AND A FUTURE RESEARCH AGENDA

Some of the key findings discussed in this chapter along with the results of ongoing research studies suggest a number of common characteristics in the crisis development and crisis management that exist in transitional societies. The most important political, institutional, and sociocultural features of transitional societies are uneven/unstable regulation and institutionalization, the shadow of authoritarianism, and discrepancies and conflicts between public values and norms that reflect the emerging status of a civil society in these countries. These are accompanied by intra- and intercommunity strain (including ethnic and regional tensions), changing mass media cultures and mass media structuring of and politicization of both disasters and crises, and disaster and crisis management policies. The most crucial economic characteristics involve resource constraints and/or inefficient allocation, and infrastructural decay that critically affect the transitional societies' vulnerability to disasters.

However important they may be, these findings require further investigation and testing. This calls for more in-depth social science research in the following areas or directions:

There is a need for studies of the social and economic changes precipitated by globalization and its implication for the vulnerabilities of transnational societies to crises and disasters.

Research needs to be conducted on how earlier and ongoing political and economic transformations and reforms impact the resilience of transitional nations to crises and disasters. Particular effort should be made to study permutations in disaster policies and the implication of those transformation and permutations for the coping capabilities of these countries.

There is also a need for studies of the two key issues associated with emerging and new kinds of hazards. These include first ascertaining the implications of global threats, that is, those that could originate anywhere in the world and affect communities in any transitional economy and its disaster and crisis policy efficiency (e.g., cyberterrorism, etc.). Second, what are the implications of the risks and hazards endemic to or primarily associated with transitional societies (e.g., dissolution of political regimes, mass and increasing obsoleteness of hazardous facilities, etc.). It might be worthwhile to study these possibilities with regard to the security of global and industrially developed communities.

Research is necessary on the specific experiences of particular groups or specific nations in transition with respect to disaster preparedness and response. This implies conducting a series of both case studies of recent and current crises, as well as comparative research. The latter should contrast the management and policy practices for different kinds of crises and disasters in transitional societies, as well as between those and industrially developed and developing economies.

CHAPTER 22

Terrorism as Disaster

William L. Waugh, Jr.

According to the old common wisdom, terrorists want an audience, but not a large number of dead (see Waugh, 1990). The reasoning is that, while attacks can demonstrate the power and commitment of the terrorists, the vulnerabilities of their targets, and the ineffectiveness of government authorities, large numbers of deaths can alienate political support. Grisly pictures of car and suicide bombings cause television viewers to weigh the objectives of the organizations against those human lives. Now, the old common wisdom itself has been a casualty of evolving terrorist motivations and technologies of war. Since the 1980s, terrorists have shown increasing willingness to kill many people, often innocent bystanders, without regard for the impact on public opinion and potential political support. Bombings of aircraft, public markets, schools, and other gathering places have increased the casualty lists. The general populace, rather than representatives of the state or socioeconomic elitists, has become the target of choice. As a result, the new common wisdom since the 1990s is that terrorists may wish to kill hundreds or thousands or even millions of people and may well have the wherewithal to do it. The shift to mass casualty and mass destruction attacks by some terrorist organizations has increased the potential for disaster and fundamentally changed the nature of the hazard. Moreover, as the scale of the attacks has increased, the psychological and social impacts of terrorism have certainly changed. Individuals and communities often surprisingly adjusted to the relatively localized violence that characterized terrorism during the early decades after World War II. The potential lethality and destructiveness of terrorism today makes it a hazard that cannot be ignored.

There are a number of reasons why terrorists have been willing to kill and/or injure large numbers of people. First, they frequently have their own financial and material sources and are not as dependent on outside support. Financial support from so-called "rogue" states, criminal activities (e.g., robberies, kidnappings, extortion, and drug smuggling), and wealthy benefactors reduces the need for outside fund raising, and thus reduces the need to appeal for broad popular support. Second, groups motivated by religious or political extremism or very broad international goals are less likely to draw support domestically or internationally than those seeking autonomy from central authorities or colonial powers. Many groups have little expectation of or need for broad popular support. Third, access to military weapons from assault rifles to sophisticated explosives, as well as capabilities to build such low-tech weapons as homemade fertilizer and fuel oil bombs, have increased the potential lethality of such groups. Little sophistication is needed to improvise a large explosive device. As a result, terrorists have created disasters on a scale that has required the same kinds of hazard management, disaster response, and long-term recovery that nations have had to provide for major earthquakes, typhoons, floods, industrial accidents, and other acts of nature and man.

The escalation of the potential lethality of terrorist attacks was evident in the first World Trade Center bombing in 1993 and the sarin gas attack in the Tokyo subway in 1994. In both cases, the scale of the disasters could have been much greater had the terrorists' devices functioned as intended. The attacks were relatively unsophisticated in terms of the technologies involved, but either could have caused hundreds or even thousands of casualties. The escalation of terrorist capabilities was clear in the bombings of the Khobar barracks in 1996, the U.S. embassies in Kenya and Tanzania in 1998, and the USS *Cole* in 2000. Those attacks were directed against targets that were assumed to be secure. Since then, the 9/11 attacks in New York and Arlington and bombings in Bali (Indonesia), Riyadh (Saudi Arabia), Istanbul (Turkey), Beslan (Russia), Madrid (Spain), Taba (Egypt), London, Netanya (Israel), and Sharm el Sheik (Egypt) have provided evidence that the risk of terrorist attack is increasing and from several quarters. While none of the attacks involved chemical, biological, or radiological devices or materials (so-called weapons of mass destruction [WMD]), they did involve large numbers of casualties and significant destruction. They also had and continue to have tremendous impact on the nations involved and have raised questions concerning the efficacy of government officials responsible for providing security. Perhaps more importantly, the increasing consequences and frequency of terrorist attacks, the two common measures of risk, have encouraged policymakers to respond. The potential costs of such attacks are so great that preventing them, rather than apprehending terrorists after their violence, has become the focus of government efforts (Heymann, 1998). No leader wants to have a major attack on his or her "watch" because public safety and security is a fundamental responsibility of government. The political costs of failure can be very high. Unfortunately, too little attention has been paid to the need to mitigate the effects of potential attacks, to lessen their physical, economic, and psychological impacts.

For the United States, the deaths of almost 3000 people in the airliners, collapsing towers, and damaged Pentagon on September 11, 2001, have had a profound effect on the nation's sense of security. The attacks led to the largest reorganization in the U.S. federal government since the creation of the Department of Defense in 1946 when the Department of Homeland Security was created in 2003. Massive investments in security programs have also meant major shifts in federal spending away from social and economic programs. Similarly, the attacks in Madrid in 2004 and London in 2005 have shaken public confidence in their governments' capacities to protect residents and visitors and encouraged increased investments in security technologies and programs. The political costs of failure were evident in the aftermath of the rail station bombings in Spain. Spanish officials responded poorly to the bombing, blaming a domestic group, and were voted out of office as a result. Around the world, terrorist violence has precipitated increased security measures to monitor public gathering places, to control national borders, and to protect sensitive facilities (such as airports, ports, and rail stations). The economic and sociopolitical costs of security are growing exponentially with little evident reduction in the risk of attack, although some potential targets are much better protected.

DISASTER AND TERRORISM

The association of disaster with terrorism is not new and the scale of recent attacks and the potential for future attacks have certainly focused official and public attention on the consequences of worst-case scenarios. In some measure, the historical association of disaster with war (Gilbert, 1998, pp. 12–13) may be how officials view the association between disaster and terrorism. Their major concern seems to be how people will react to external threats, rather than how people and communities might deal with such threats. Indeed, the disaster research community and many professional emergency managers tend to focus less on the specific nature of "weapons of mass destruction" than on developing capabilities to deal with those and similar hazards and the resilience to adapt and recover quickly. The shifting official focus from NBC (nuclear, biological, and chemical) weapons and materials to the current CBRNE (chemical, biological, radiological, nuclear, and explosive) weapons and materials has been seen as something of a policy "shell game" and the limited attention given to community preparedness and resilience has been a source of great frustration. It is encouraging, however, that the U.S. military is now interested in the importance of "civil security," the role of individuals and communities in reducing vulnerabilities to attack and developing measures to reduce their impact (Dory, 2003). Dealing with the disasters that might result from terrorist attacks is an increasing concern, but the focus of Department of Homeland Security policies and programs is still overwhelmingly on preventing such attacks. That same pattern appears common among other nations dealing with the threat of terrorism. Facilities and officials with high "target value" are secured and military and law enforcement authorities focus on apprehending terrorists before they act (see Alexander, Y. 2002).

The potential for terrorist-caused disasters is clear in Homeland Security planning. In 2004, the Homeland Security Council created 15 planning scenarios to aid in the development of preparedness programs (see Table 22.1). Twelve of the scenarios involve terrorist attacks and the dimensions of the disasters that are identified as important are the expected casualties (killed, injured, and hospitalized), damage to infrastructure (broadly defined), economic impact, and recovery time. The detonation of a nuclear device that might result in an extremely high casualty rate and total destruction of infrastructure within a half to a full mile radius is the worst case in the listing in terms of casualties and damage in the immediate area, economic costs, and recovery time. The projected casualties from the biological and chemical attack scenarios range from a few hundred to thousands with recovery in weeks to months. Interestingly, the casualty estimates from a pandemic influenza outbreak are 87,000 fatalities and 300,000 hospitalizations. Current estimations from the Centers for Disease Control and Prevention of fatalities from an influenza outbreak such as the catastrophic 1918 outbreak are from 2 million to 150 million, with 7.4 million being a "reasonable estimate" (McKenna, 2005). The potential for millions of deaths is one of the reasons why public health officials have argued that influenza is a much bigger threat than bioterrorism and, consequently, much more funding should be provided for programs to identify and respond to influenza outbreaks early. After Hurricane Katrina, it would also appear that estimations of casualties and costs for natural disasters should also be reassessed. The damage, economic costs and recovery time for the Hurricane Katrina disaster far exceeds the Homeland Security Council's hurricane scenario estimates.

Homeland Security policies have been designed and adopted and programs have largely been implemented with little assessment of risk (Reese, 2005). Plans are being made to deal with worst-case scenarios, rather than the most likely scenarios. While recent attacks have demonstrated that terrorists can cause mass casualties and mass destruction, tax response capabilities, and require long-term investments in recovery, not all are at equal risk of attack and, in fact, many are at very little risk. Not all potential targets are of sufficient symbolic value to attract terrorists. More importantly, not all terrorists have the wherewithal or even the desire to kill many or cause catastrophic destruction. A reasoned assessment

TABLE 22.1. Homeland Security Council's Fifteen Planning Scenarios

Scenario	Casualties	Infrastructure Damage	Economic Impact	Recovery Timeline
Nuclear detonation 10-kiloton improvised nuclear device	Can vary widely	Total within radius of 0.5 to 1.0 mile	Hundreds of billions of dollars	Years
Biological attack aerosol anthrax	13,000 fatalities and injuries	Minimal	Billions of dollars	Months
Biological disease outbreak pandemic influenza	87,000 fatalities, 300,000 hospitalized	None	$70 to $160 billion	Several months
Biological attack plague	2500 fatalities, 7000 injuries	None	Millions of dollars	Weeks
Chemical attack blistering agent effects	150 fatalities, 70,000 hospitalized	Minimal	$500 million	Weeks, but long-term
Chemical attack Toxic industrial chemicals	350 fatalities, 1,000 hospitalized	50% of structures in area	Billions of dollars	Months
Chemical attack nerve agent (in a building)	6,000 fatalities, 350 injuries	Minimal, but contamination	$300 million	3–4 months
Chemical attack chlorine tank explosion	17,500 fatalities, 10,000 severe injuries, 100,000 Hospitalized	In immediate area and metal corrosion	Millions of dollars	Weeks
Natural disaster major earthquake	1400 fatalities, 100,000 hospitalized	150,000 buildings destroyed, 1 million damaged	Hundreds of billions of dollars	Months to years
Natural disaster major hurricane	1000 fatalities, 5000 hospitalized	Buildings destroyed 100,000 buildings seriously damaged	Millions of dollars	Months
Radiological attack radiological dispersal devices	180 fatalities, 270 injuries, 20,000 detectable contaminations	Near explosion	Up to billions of dollars	Months to years
Explosives attack improvised Explosive device	100 fatalities, 450 hospitalizations	Near explosion	Local	Weeks to months
Biological attack food contamination	300 fatalities, 400 hospitalizations	None	Millions of dollars	Weeks
Biological attack foreign animal disease (foot and mouth disease)	None	None	Hundreds of millions of dollars	Months
Cyber attack	None directly	None	Millions of dollars	Weeks

Source: Homeland Security Council, Planning Scenarios: Executive Summaries, July 2004.

of risk might better identify potential targets, better prepare law enforcement and security officials and emergency responders, and help better target resources for the attacks that may come.

Terrorist acts do pose some unique problems for those targeted and those responsible for dealing with attacks and threatened attacks. Fortunately, the unnatural disasters resulting from terrorism are very similar to those resulting from natural phenomena, as well as human accidents and technological failures. In many respects, recent terrorist-sponsored disasters have been very similar to natural and other man-made catastrophes. The same first responders have to deal with the consequences of terrorist acts that have had to deal with structural collapses, fires, train wrecks, vehicle crashes, pandemics, and other large-scale disasters. The same second responders have to deal with the physical and psychological trauma, restoration of lifelines, and other activities to get individuals and communities functioning again. The same support agencies need to assist with short- and long-term recovery.

However, terrorist-sponsored disasters are different from other kinds of disaster in several ways. First, disasters caused by terrorists are not accidents or "acts of God." They are caused by people and they are caused on purpose. The images of dead and injured children recovered from the daycare center in the collapsed Murrah Federal Building in Oklahoma City in 1995 were all the more disturbing because the act that brought down the building was intentional and was committed by other Americans. Similarly, the fact that British citizens were involved in the July 2005 London subway bombings was met with disbelief by many Britons and has led to a reassessment of the terrorism threat in the United Kingdom

Second, disasters caused by terrorists are crime scenes. Consequently, responders to terrorist disasters should avoid, as much as possible, disturbing the crime scene in order to preserve evidence that may help law enforcement officers apprehend the terrorists. Protocols have been developed in the United States since the Oklahoma City bombing to minimize contamination of crime scenes by rescue workers and to lessen the likelihood that law enforcement officers will interfere with lifesaving action when they are securing the sites and preserving evidence. Third, disasters caused by terrorists normally involve a mix of responders very similar to that for a natural disaster, but generally involve law enforcement and military personnel in lead, rather than support, roles. Large-scale disaster responses frequently involve large numbers of governmental and nongovernmental agencies, as well as organized and spontaneous volunteers. In that regard, responding to natural disasters and terrorist disasters are very similar in that the resources of broad networks of public, nonprofit, and private organizations and individuals may be needed (Waugh, 2003b; Waugh & Sylves, 2002). While authorities dealing with terrorist incidences may be reluctant to use nongovernmental resources, particularly volunteers, they may be essential in very large events. The response to the Oklahoma City bombing involved dozens of organizations, from the American Red Cross to the Oklahoma Restaurant Association, and hundreds of individual volunteers (City of Oklahoma City, 1996). The response to the World Trade Center attack drew hundreds of organizations and many thousands of volunteers (see, e.g., Lowe & Fothergill, 2003; McEntire, Robinson, & Weber, 2003; Sutton, 2003). Similar intergovernmental, multiorganizational responses occur in other nations. For example, the responses to bombings in Istanbul in November 2003 were very similar to the response in Oklahoma City (Ural, 2005) as nongovernmental organizations (NGOs) assisted with the response and recovery efforts. Designing an effective response to terrorist disasters, in fact, is complicated by the lead roles of agencies unfamiliar with the networks that respond to large natural disasters and unused to communicating and collaborating closely with nongovernmental actors (Waugh, 2004a). The largest difference between the responses to terrorism-related disasters and other kinds of disasters is just that—the lead roles of agencies and officials responsible for capturing or killing the perpetrators rather than performing lifesaving roles and helping reduce the impact of the disaster on people and property.

Contamination, surge capacity to deal with mass casualties, need for close cooperation among agencies at all levels and among all agencies involved in the response, legal measures before the event to facilitate prevention and apprehension of terrorists, and heightened risk of panic and posttraumatic stress disorder (PTSD). The dependence upon local responders is a key element in the response (Pangi, 2003b) as it is during a mass casualty natural disaster. There is still some uncertainty concerning how the public will react to large scale terrorist attacks even after the 9/11 attack (Winslow, 1999), but better public education can reduce the impact of the violence (Pangi, 2003a) and facilitate recovery.

THE NATURE AND PURPOSE OF TERRORISM

Terrorism is difficult to discuss without some attention to its nature and forms. The threat of catastrophic terrorism was not new in 1993 when the World Trade Center (WTC) was bombed and certainly was not new in 2001 when hijacked aircraft hit the WTC towers. Hundreds of terrorist attacks occur every year (Waugh, 2003a) and terrorist violence has caused millions of deaths and countless physical and psychological injuries for millennia. Ancient armies massacred civilian populations to frighten and demoralize opposing armies. Medieval armies flung plague-ridden bodies over city walls and dropped animal carcasses into water supplies to frighten and sicken residents. Villagers were slaughtered and crops burned to discourage resistance to foreign and indigenous rulers. In short, terrorism is an ancient tactic of warfare and political conflict and it has remained a weapon in modern warfare and the politics. Terrorist violence has commonly been used by combatants on all sides in ancient and modern conflicts. The bombings of London, Dresden, Hiroshima, and Nagasaki during World War II were designed to demoralize enemy populations, officials, and armies. Since World War II, threats of violence have chased—indeed, continue to chase—civilian populations from their homes and put them at risk of attack, as well as at risk of famine, disease, and other threats to life. Such is the case in Darfur in the Sudan. Terrorism was used by Serbian forces in Bosnia-Herzegovina, by Saddam Hussein's forces against Kurds and dissident Iraqis, by Taliban and al-Qaeda forces against officials in the new Afghan regime, and by indigenous insurgents and their foreign supporters and by terrorist groups against officials in the new Iraqi regime. Clearly, terrorism is neither a new nor an uncommon tactic in war and lesser political conflicts. Nor are catastrophic acts of terrorism new.

Some distinctions do need to be made between terrorism, terrorist violence, and other forms of political violence. The cliché that "one man's terrorist is another man's freedom fighter" is important to remember. The term "terrorism" has tremendous political baggage and generally is applied only to one's enemies, but the use of terrorist violence is more widespread than that would suggest. Violent acts to induce terror have been used for thousands of years as a part of psychological warfare. Terrorist violence has also been used for criminal and other nonpolitical purposes. There are common elements in most definitions of terrorism:

1. The use or credible threat of extraordinary violence;
2. The presence of a purpose or goal;
3. The choice of targets for their symbolic value; and
4. The intent to influence a broader audience than the immediate victims (Waugh, 1982, 1990).

If violence has been used in the past, the terrorists may only have to threaten further violence in order to cause fear or terror. Terrorists may have political, economic, social, or cultural, for example, religious, goals. The focus here is on terrorism with political purposes, but economic, religious, and other purposes may also be present. Because terrorist groups are usually small, from a very few to a few thousand, they tend to focus their attacks on people, facilities, and other targets that will maximize their impact and minimize their losses. Attacks on judicial officials, elected leaders, business persons, and other high-profile individuals, including foreign tourists, can get the public's attention. Direct attacks on military and law enforcement personnel, for example, usually are too risky for groups with limited human and material resources. Nonetheless, terrorists may have the wherewithal to engage military and police forces when they have a large enough base of support. In military terms, the violence can escalate into guerrilla warfare or insurgency and even into civil war. U.S. military spokesmen, for example, distinguished early in the Iraq War between Iraqi insurgents and foreign terrorists although the distinction became somewhat blurred for officials and the media alike as the violence escalated. Defining the conflict as a civil war would acknowledge that the insurgents have sufficient popular support or at least acquiescence to wage war on the new Iraqi regime. In reality, the new regime and its supporters are fighting with remnants of the old regime (i.e., Baathists and other insurgents), foreign groups (at least one associated with al-Qaeda), and indigenous criminal groups. Terrorist tactics appear to be common among all the groups, including those using kidnappings for financial gain.

Second, terrorism can be used by governments as well as nongovernmental groups. State terrorism is common. Governments may use violence and/or the threat of violence to silence political dissent, remove opposition, and/or enforce policies. Violence may be used or threatened to intimidate racial and ethnic and religious groups. Vigilante terrorist groups may emerge to help officials enforce laws and to punish dissenters. Terrorist organizations may be independent of government influence, loosely connected to government officials, or even directly connected to government authorities and acting as their agents. Terrorist goals may be revolutionary in terms of seeking to overthrow a government or social system or subrevolutionary in terms, for example, of seeking change in a particular law or removal of a particular official. Terrorist organizations may have broad or limited goals, they may or may not attack human targets, and they may or may not have links to states or officials. The question is whether they intend and have the capabilities of causing mass destruction and/or mass casualties—that is, causing catastrophic effects (see, e.g., Waugh, 1982, 1990).

Third, terrorist intent is critical. In the 1940s and 1950s, the most common motivations were independence from colonial influence or separation of ethnic groups from established nations. Popular support, including international support, was a goal. During the 1960s and 1970s, the motivations often were connected to the Cold War with the groups acting as agents of or surrogates for the United States and its allies and the Soviet Union and its allies. During the 1980s and 1990s and into the 21st century, transnational groups and the motivations often were mixtures of political and religious goals. The so-called "new terrorists" are difficult to locate and apprehend because they have relatively small units acting with minimal or perhaps no central control. Terrorists with religious motivation do tend to be more willing to kill large numbers of people than secular terrorists (Hoffman, 1999, p. 21).

Fourth, some terrorist organizations have demonstrated their willingness to cause mass casualties and the available weaponry has become ever more lethal. Current focus on the threat of so-called WMD is somewhat misleading when military-style automatic weapons and explosives are readily available in many parts of the world, including the United States Hazardous chemical, biological, and radiological materials are available and some groups have the capabilities of building weapons with such materials. And, there is a risk that terrorist organizations or states will buy, steal, or replicate a biological or nuclear weapon developed during the Cold War. Nuclear proliferation and the security of nuclear weapons left over from the Cold War are also concerns. There are hundreds of international terrorist attacks every year and the most common weapons are explosive devices, often homemade (U.S. State Department, 2004, 2005). The potential for terrorists to get weapons capable of killing thousands or even millions exists, but there is much greater likelihood that they will use homemade bombs or purchased or stolen conventional explosives (Smithson & Levy, 2000). Following the 2001 attacks by international terrorists, there was a series of attacks involving anthrax, a biological agent, which are assumed to have been committed by a domestic terrorist or terrorists. But, the scale of the attacks was relatively small. Having the capability of creating biological weapons does not necessarily mean having the capability of delivering such weapons.

All of this is to say that terrorists may be states or small organizations or even individuals and their goals may be limited or very broad. They may avoid killing or injuring human beings or they may be willing to cause mass casualties and mass destruction. Clearly, some wish to cause catastrophic disasters and have the capabilities to carry out those intentions. The U.S. experience with the World Trade Center attacks in 1993 and 2001 and the Oklahoma City federal building bombing in 1995, the Japanese experience with the sarin attack in 1995, the Indonesian experience with the Bali bombing in 2002, the Russian experience with the hostage taking in the Moscow theater in 2002 and the Beslan school in 2004, the Spanish experience with the train station bombing in Madrid in 2004, and the British experience with the subway attacks in 2005 are testaments to the disastrous consequences of terrorist acts. Airliners full of passengers, hotels full of guests and staff, schools full of children and teachers, corporate facilities full of workers and customers, and marketplaces full of shoppers have often been targets of terrorists. The resultant disasters have required quick action by emergency responders, coordination of efforts by emergency managers, and long periods of recovery, not to mention recovery from the physical and psychological damage suffered by their victims. The potential that chemical plants might be bombed, dams or bridges might be bombed, water supplies might be poisoned, critical computer infrastructure might be disabled, virulent diseases might be spread among human or animal populations, or any number of other catastrophes might be perpetrated by terrorists gives impetus to efforts to prevent, mitigate the effects of, and prepare for such events. Thus far, terrorist disasters have been handled reasonably well with the resources at hand.

TERRORISM DISASTER RESPONSES

Aircraft bombings have killed hundreds at a time, often with no survivors. For Americans, there were major terrorist attacks before the bombing of the World Trade Center in 1993 and the Murrah Federal Building in Oklahoma City in 1995 that required substantial emergency responses, but those experiences were often used as the baselines for dealing with terrorist events until the 9/11 attacks.

The Oklahoma City Bombing.

When a 4,800 pound homemade bomb exploded at 9:02 A.M. on April 19, 1995, in a truck next to the Murrah Federal Building, the front of the structure collapsed and buildings in a

10-block radius were also damaged. The police, fire, and emergency medical response was quick and the Oklahoma City Fire Department became the lead for the disaster response. Later, law enforcement agencies set up their own perimeters to secure the site and to collect evidence. The bombing of the federal building caused a disaster that elicited a national response and federal, state, and local responders converged to rescue victims and search the collapsed facility. Emergency responders from surrounding states were drawn into the effort as the days progressed. Via the media, the nation lived through the bombing and its aftermath.

Because the event involved a federal crime (terrorism), a federal facility, and the deaths of federal officers, the FBI and other federal agencies had clear jurisdiction. Nonetheless, the search and rescue operation was managed by Oklahoma City fire personnel. Federal resources, including "federalized" Urban Search and Rescue Teams and a Disaster Mortuary Team, were brought in by the Federal Emergency Management Agency (FEMA). The response and recovery operations lasted 16 days. One hundred and sixty-eight people were killed, some in surrounding buildings or on the street. Firefighters from more than 75 Oklahoma municipalities and more than 35 departments from Texas, Kansas, Arkansas, and other states were involved. More than 1000 FEMA personnel and hundreds of personnel from other federal agencies were involved. The American Red Cross and numerous other nonprofit organizations, as well as private sector organizations, were involved (Oklahoma City, 1996; Waugh, 2000b). The scale of the disaster required considerable resources from all levels of government and from NGOs. But, the Oklahoma disaster was very small in comparison to the disaster caused by terrorists on 9/11.

The 9/11 Attacks

The collapse of the World Trade Center towers was one of the largest terrorist caused disasters in modern history. While the number of deaths and injuries were remarkably small given the numbers of people in the towers, the surrounding streets, and the subway system below the towers that morning, the psychological impact of the disaster was tremendous. The physical and economic impacts upon the city and the surrounding metropolitan area were catastrophic. This was the most costly disaster for FEMA, the U.S. Department of Housing and Urban Development, and the U.S. Department of Transportation (U.S. GAO, 2003, p. 19). While statistics cannot adequately capture the scale of the disaster, Tables 22.2 to 22.5 do document the economic impact of the disaster response. Table 22.2 indicates the funds authorized and

TABLE 22.2. The 9/11 Disaster: Initial Response Assistance
(as of June 30, 2003)

	Total Committed	Total Disbursed
Search and rescue operations	$22,000,000	$22,000,000
Debris removal	1,689,000,000	695,000,000
Emergency transportation	299,000,000	298,000,000
Temporary utility repairs	250,000,000	0
Testing and cleaning	53,000,000	42,000,000
Other response services	232,000,000	114,000,000
Total	$2,554,000,000	$1,170,000,000

Source: USGAO, Federal Disaster Assistance, October 2003.

TABLE 22.3. Compensation for Disaster-Related Costs and Losses (as of June 30, 2003)

	Total Committed	Total Disbursed
Assistance for state, city, and other organizations	$3,319,000,000	$1,593,000,000
Assistance to individuals and families	807,000,000	546,000,000
Assistance for businesses	683,000,000	510,000,000
Total	$4,809,000,000	$2.649,000,000

Source: USGAO, Federal Disaster Assistance, October 2003.

disbursed for the initial disaster response in New York City and the surrounding area. The search and rescue operations cost $22 million and debris removal cost $695 million. Almost 2 years after the collapse of the World Trade Center towers, the total federal expenditures for response totaled $1.17 billion. As Table 22.3 shows, $2.649 billion was provided as assistance to state, city, and other organizations, to individuals and families, and to businesses.

As Table 22.4 shows, more than $5.5 billion was committed to rebuild the transportation system in lower Manhattan, repair utilities, and support short-term capital projects. The rebuilding of the transit system has been slow and only $54 million of the committed $5 billion were disbursed as of June 2003. Reconstruction continues in and around the old World Trade Center site. Lastly, Table 22.5 shows the commitment of $5.5 billion in funds and tax benefits for economic revitalization. By June 2003, $173 million in funds had been disbursed, and presumably the tax benefits had had some impact. Two items to note are the differences in funds committed and funds spent and the provision of tax benefits. Expenditures can stretch out for years as recovery projects are implemented. In addition to the losses covered by federal programs, the uninsured and insured losses were in the billions of dollars. It took 9 months to clear the debris and approximately 18,000 businesses were affected. Many businesses in lower Manhattan failed. It was a catastrophic disaster by any measure. The total amount of money committed to the New York City recovery through FEMA, the U.S. Department of Housing and Urban Development, and the U.S. Department of Transportation was in excess of $18 billion. The amount does not include Small Business Administration and other disaster assistance grants. FEMA activated 20 of its 28 Urban Search and Rescue Task Forces—almost 1300 members and 80 dogs (U.S. GAO, 2003, p. 24). Thousands of volunteers were used for search and rescue, support for emergency responders, and other critical tasks.

TABLE 22.4. Infrastructure Restoration and Improvement (as of June 30, 2003)

	Total Committed	Total Disbursed
Rebuilding and improving lower Manhattan transportation system	$5,006,000,000	$54,000,000
Permanent utility infrastructure repairs	500,000,000	0
Short-term capital projects	68,000,000	0
Total	$5,574,000,000	$54,000,000

Source: USGAO, Federal Disaster Assistance, October 2003.

TABLE 22.5. Economic Revitalization Efforts (as of June 30, 2003)

	Total Committed	Total Disbursed
Tax benefits—Liberty Zone	$5,029,000,000	—[a]
Job creation and retention grants	320,000,000	130,000,000
Small firm attraction and Retention grants	155,000,000	31,000,000
Other planning efforts	40,000,000	12,000,000
Total	$5,544,000,000	$173,000,000

Source: USGAO, Federal Disaster Assistance, October 2003.
[a] Tax benefits not disbursed as grants.

It should also be noted that the crash of TWA Flight 800 off Long Island in 1996 lead to the passage of the Aviation Disaster Family Assistance Act of 1996. Because the crash was initially presumed to be the result of a terrorist bomb, the lead agency was the F.B.I. rather than the National Transportation Safety Board (NTSB). Normally the NTSB would have investigated the crash and local authorities would have dealt with the victims and their families. The crash was deemed a crime scene and the F.B.I. acted to preserve evidence, including evidence associated with the victims' remains. There was little sensitivity to grieving families; a very slow process of identifying and releasing remains; and poor communication with families, airline officials, and local public officials. As a result of the public outcry, the Family Assistance Act was passed to ensure that the needs of victims and their families were met in aviation disasters. The Act specifies roles for the airlines, the American Red Cross, and other agencies and the airline industry has developed procedures to deal with such disasters.

HOMELAND SECURITY AND WEAPONS OF MASS DESTRUCTION

Since the 9/11 attacks, the U.S. government has focused its efforts on preventing further terrorist attacks and, to a lesser extent, on preparing for large-scale, mass casualty disasters. Homeland Security Presidential Directive 8 (HSPD-8) outlines the need for a "national preparedness goal" and a coordinated set of programs to encourage preparedness. Central to that effort have been the adoption of the National Response Plan, replacing the Federal Response Plan that guided the 9/11 response and previous natural disaster responses. Federal, state, and local agencies are being required to adopt a standardized structure, the National Incident Management System, to facilitate coordination during emergencies. The Department of Homeland Security provided guidance for the development of capabilities to deal with a range of national emergencies (U.S. Department of Homeland Security, 2005) and the Homeland Security Council in the White House developed a series of disaster scenarios to illustrate the range of threats that need to be address. There are four chemical scenarios, four biological scenarios (including one involving the plague), one disease scenario involving an influenza pandemic, one hurricane scenario, one earthquake scenario, one radiological scenario involving a "dirty bomb," one improvised explosive device scenario, one improvised nuclear device scenario, and one cyberterrorism scenario. The primary attention is given to large-scale chemical, biological, radiological, nuclear, and explosive (CBRNE) events. The scenarios have been criticized for focusing on worst-case scenarios, rather than the most likely kinds of events, and focusing too little on natural disasters. That problem is manifest in the planning scenarios the Homeland Security Council developed for preparedness activities (see Table 22.1).

Problems with the responses to the four Florida hurricanes in 2004 have raised questions about the capabilities of DHS to deal effectively with non-terrorism-related disasters in which federal authorities are not in charge, but expected to communicate openly with the public, NGOs, and their state and local counterparts. That may be part of the reason why FEMA's responsibilities were refocused on disaster response during the DHS reorganization in the summer of 2005. A Congressional Budget Office report (CBO, 2005) on fiscal year 2005 and proposed fiscal year 2006 funding describes disaster relief as a "non-Homeland Security" function. What the reorganization will mean for the increasing number of state and local agencies with combined Homeland Security and emergency management responsibilities is uncertain. The report also indicates that DHS funding only accounts for $27.6 billion of the $49.1 billion that U.S. federal agencies will spend on homeland security in fiscal year 2005. The Department of Defense (DOD) will spend $8.6 billion in fiscal year 2005 and the president has asked for $9.6 billion for DOD in 2006. The additional funding likely reflects the expectation of an expanded role, even a lead role, for DOD in large-scale terrorist attacks within U.S. borders and that raises questions concerning legal restrictions on military support for civilian officials (Graham, 2005).

Few terrorist organizations have the capabilities necessary to create large nuclear or biological weapons, but more may be able to buy or steal what they cannot make themselves. If such weapons are acquired by groups willing to use them, the potential for catastrophic disaster would be vastly increased. Still, there is a greater likelihood of attacks involving much less sophisticated weaponry, such as the bombs used in the Oklahoma City and first World Trade Center bombings or vehicles carrying hazardous materials like liquefied natural gas or conventional "dirty bombs" designed to spread radiological or chemical material. The amount of military weaponry that might be available to domestic and international terrorists in the United States is also a serious problem. Tons of military-grade explosives, hundreds of assault rifles, and countless other munitions are missing from police and military facilities in the United States

Fortunately, capabilities developing to deal with pandemics may be used to deal with bioterrorist attacks, capabilities developed to deal with large-scale hazardous materials spills and accidents can be used to deal with chemical and nuclear terrorist attacks, and capabilities developed to deal with nuclear accidents can be use to deal with attacks involving nuclear materials. Preparedness, response, and recovery programs developed for natural and technological disasters can be adapted to deal with terrorist disasters (Waugh, 1990, 2001). The "all-hazards" approach that has been used in emergency management for the past two decades is predicated on the development of such adaptable capabilities (Waugh, 2005) and the "dual use" concept promoted by state and local emergency managers as Homeland Security programs were developed is based upon the necessity of adaptable programs.

While the focus of Homeland Security efforts has been on the prevention of terrorist attacks, there are also opportunities to mitigate the effects of attacks that cannot be prevented. Mitigation programs are currently underway to strengthen buildings so that they can absorb bomb blasts without collapsing, designing and redesigning buildings so that terrorists will have less opportunity to gain access, reprogramming activities to reduce access to sensitive areas of facilities, and so on (see, e.g., Waugh, 2001). Linking prevention activities to emergency response activities is also suggested in areas such as mass transit where systems may be vulnerable to attack (Waugh, 2004b).

THE CHALLENGES OF TERRORIST
DISASTERS

Many questions remain concerning how to deal effectively with natural and technological disasters. How to provide effective alerts and warnings, how to educate the public about hazards and appropriate protective actions, how to encourage adequate emergency preparedness at the individual and community levels, and how to design and manage effective evacuation programs are a few of the many questions that have not been completely answered. Many questions have been answered, such as why people may not choose to evacuate when authorities ask them to do so. The question that arose in the months after the 9/11 attacks and as the nation's Homeland Security programs were being put into place was how much knowledge gained over a half century of dealing with natural and technological disasters is transferable to terrorist disasters. The emergency management professional community and the disaster research community have generally argued that much of what we know about dealing with natural and technological hazards and disasters is applicable to Homeland Security. Nonetheless, relatively little has been transferred. For example, the weight of social science research supports the conclusion that panic is rare in disasters, particularly when people are given sufficient information to determine what they should do. That is also true in disasters involving nuclear and biological material, in chemical accidents and spills, and in pandemics. There was no panic at Chernobyl in 1986 during the world's worst nuclear accident (see, e.g., Medvedev, 1990). There was no panic in the Tokyo subway in 1995 during the Aum Shinrikyo sarin attack (see, e.g., Murakami, 2000). There are also remarkable stories of heroism and calm from the World Trade Center collapses. Panic appears to be far more common in circumstances where information concerning appropriate protective action is poor or nonexistent or people are literally trapped in buildings or ships or other structures. Experience and research strongly support the need to provide as much information as possible during emergencies, rather than withhold information for fear of causing panic. Unfortunately, Homeland Security and law enforcement decision makers appear disinclined to provide information when it is needed in an emergency.

The coordination of federal, state, and local Homeland Security programs has also been problematic as three TOPOFF (Top Official) exercises have demonstrated. While there are still coordination problems when federal, state, and local emergency management agencies work together, some of the cultural and organizational differences have been worked out over the years. The frequency of natural and technological disasters does provide plenty of opportunity to test and correct systems and to become familiar with the capabilities and priorities of other agencies. The infrequency of terrorist incidences limits opportunities to learn how to improve capabilities, although greater funding of Homeland Security programs may encourage more training and exercising. In fact, funding shifts may well mean a loss of federal, state, and local capabilities to deal with more common natural and technological hazards and disasters.

CONCLUSIONS: TERRORISTS AND
DISASTER

Terrorist disasters can closely resemble natural and other man-made disasters. The 9/11 World Trade Center disaster involved airliner crashes, high-rise fires, structural collapses, hazardous materials events, as well as numerous lesser emergencies. The scale certainly was greater than for other terrorist events, but less than that of the 1906 San Francisco earthquake or the next great "urban" quake in California. The organizational effort following the World Trade

Center attacks required extraordinary coordination and communication (much of which was ineffective), but, in many respects, the disaster itself created familiar imperatives.

There are differences between terrorist disasters and other kinds of disasters. However, the range of possibilities makes it extremely difficult to identify potential targets, let alone protect them. The next terrorist disaster could take many forms—from a dam collapse to a biological attack to a nuclear blast. The attackers may be al-Qaeda operatives or American militia members or they may be from any number of other international or domestic extremist groups. The attacker may be another lone bomber or a lone biochemist with anthrax or ricin or hoof and mouth virus. The point is simply that the range of possibilities is so great that a broad approach is necessary to ensure that law enforcement, military, and emergency response personnel have a range of capabilities, therefore a more generic "all-hazards" program would be more adaptable to circumstances than a terrorism-focused program (Waugh, 1984, 2005).

FUTURE RESEARCH AGENDA

The literature on terrorism, terrorists, terrorist weapons, antiterrorism measures, and counterterrorism policies and programs is large and growing. Much is known about terrorist motivations, organizations, weaponry, and tactics and much is known about anti- and counterterrorism measures. The persistent issues have been related to the relationship between terrorists' political objectives and their choice of targets and to the effectiveness of anti- and counterterrorism policies and programs. It has also been common to focus on the instruments of terrorist violence, rather than on the human targets. Military studies have tended to focus on the lethality of weapons and measures to preempt or prevent attacks through improved intelligence gathering. Nuclear proliferation and the potential for chemical and biological agents to be lost, stolen, or sold to terrorists are the major concerns. Security studies typically focus on risk and vulnerability assessments and the "hardening" of facilities, including security "layering." Law enforcement studies tend to focus on prevention and the apprehension of the terrorists. The problem of terrorism is, in fact, many problems, but there is a need to find a broader perspective that will facilitate the development of a comprehensive strategy to deal with the hazard of terrorism. The "all-hazards" model is a logical vehicle for doing so.

The study of anti- and counterterrorism policies and programs in the United States has been seriously hampered by the secretiveness of the Department of Homeland Security. Access to officials and offices has been severely limited. Even analysts from the Government Accountability Office and Congressional Research Service, the agencies that provide information to members of Congress and other policymakers, complain that Homeland Security officials do not respond to their inquiries and do not provide requested information. Academic researchers generally are even less successful in gaining access to people or data within the Department. The lack of transparency in decision making and lack of openness in dealing with the public and its representatives may protect the Department from critics, but it also reduces trust in Homeland Security leaders and programs and denies the Department the benefits of outside review. The creation of the Department of Homeland Security was the largest federal reorganization in almost 60 years and academic researchers are anxious to see how the constituent programs and personnel are being integrated. The creation of the Department also consolidated many, but not all, of the federal programs that deal with the internal and external threats from terrorism. The operation of the new department needs careful analysis and access by academic and government analysts would provide useful information to Homeland Security decision makers, as well as to researchers, policymakers outside the department, and the public.

Future research efforts should focus on at least the following general topics:

1. A better understanding of terrorism and why individuals and groups choose to use violence to achieve political ends is critical, if the risks of violence are to be addressed in the long term. To counter the choice to use violence authorities need to address the precipitants of terrorism, including poverty and religious intolerance, and to provide alternatives.

2. More effective organization of anti- and counterterrorism programs is a fundamental need. Intergovernmental coordination to deal with terrorism and other potential disasters has been problematic. Coordination is awkward in a federal system like the United States because of the division of powers. National authorities generally have greater resources, but cannot always bring them to bear during terrorist incidences. Local authorities may well have more experience dealing with bombings, hostage cases, and other terrorist-type events than their federal counterparts, but too often lack sufficient resources to deal with threats and attacks. Local authorities typically have much more experience dealing with disasters and can bring essential skills in hazard mitigation, preparedness, response, and recovery to counterterrorism programs.

3. Better coordination of multiorganizational operations is a critical need. Incident command systems (ICS) were developed to coordinate large fire responses. That type of hierarchical command structure seems to work in those kinds of environments, but have serious limitations in other kinds of disasters and with other kinds of organizations. Unity of command may not be practicable in many complex emergencies, such as pandemics or even large-scale terrorist incidences. Unified command with a more consensus-based decision process may be much more effective. Similarly, the National Incident Management System (NIMS) which is supposed to use ICS principles to structure a national response to large-scale disasters and terrorist incidences may be seriously flawed because it may run counter to the system of shared governance in the United States and may interfere with local first response. Certainly newly centralized decision processes delayed deployment of National Guard troops and first responder volunteers during the Hurricane Katrina disaster. Reliance on officials in Washington to make critical decisions that could have been made at the local or state level is a serious flaw in the system. The disconnection between local needs and the national response is a reflection of the centralization problem, as well.

4. The integration of law enforcement and military personnel into disaster response is problematic. Law enforcement officers have interfered with lifesaving activities in major disasters, including terrorism-related disasters, in the past because of their priority of preserving evidence. The Katrina experience demonstrated the value of military participation in catastrophic disaster responses, particularly in security and in search and rescue operations, but military personnel are not trained to deal with victims more broadly. Research is needed on how to prepare law enforcement and military personnel better for disaster relief operations and how to prepare local officials to interact effectively with those personnel. A starting place might be a better understanding of legal, political, and social roles.

5. The development of intersector collaboration has been very slow. Most of the nation's infrastructure is in the private sector and there has been limited success in encouraging preparedness efforts by businesses. Incentives need to be developed to encourage private investment in emergency planning, business continuity planning, and other

preparedness activities. Research is needed on issues such as how to create a market for emergency preparedness.

6. The exercise of federal jurisdiction in events involving terrorism raises issues that have been dealt with in other kinds of large-scale disasters. In emergency management, the solution has been to build local and regional capacities to deal with disasters until state and federal resources are available. Investments in training and equipment for local first responders have been a priority. Prepositioning critical resources, such as medical supplies and pharmaceuticals, has also been a priority. The implementation of The National Guard Civil Support Teams to deal with radiological events is one of the measures that has been enacted since 9/11. More research, including policy and program evaluations, would help target resources where they are needed to build local first responder capabilities and where the risk of attack is greatest.

7. The human dimensions of terrorism-related disasters have been far from adequately explored. Research on how people perceive the hazards posed by terrorism, how they interpret the risks, what they know about potential terrorist acts, how they make decisions concerning protective action, and how authorities can influence the public to take appropriate action, including preparation for potential attacks, are some of the questions that need to be answered. The presumption on the parts of officials and the media that the public is likely to panic needs to be dispelled. The disaster literature answers many of these questions in relation to natural and technological disasters, but, evidently, validation may be necessary for the research to be accepted by Homeland Security officials and the media.

8. Effective risk communication is also a serious issue that needs more study. What kind of information does the public need to make decisions concerning evacuation, sheltering in place, and other protective action? How much can be delivered via public education programs and how much can be delivered via alert and warning messages? How much information is needed by the public—certainly large segments of the public want to access such information via the Internet. Disaster research shows that information needs differ, but that adequate, accurate information is essential if authorities wish the public to respond appropriately. The public has to trust those providing the information in order for it to be accepted.

9. Psychological impact is the raison d'être for terrorism. Terrorism is violence for effect, but what influences that effect? What variables affect how people perceive and respond to terrorism? How can the effects of terrorism be mitigated? Are there differences in how people perceive threats and attacks and are the impacts of biological and nuclear threats and attacks greater than the impacts of other kinds of terrorism?

10. If terrorism is different from other kinds of disasters, how is it different and what do the differences mean for recovery? How can societies ensure that individuals, families, and communities recover quickly from terrorist-related disasters?

11. To the extent that terrorist acts may cause catastrophic disasters, much more research needs to be done on long-term recovery issues. The Homeland Security Council's scenarios include the explosion of nuclear and chemical devices which could cause long-term contamination in major cities, displacing thousands of residents. How can large numbers of evacuees be resettled if their communities cannot be quickly cleaned up? Homeland Security and emergency management officials have struggled with issues such as mass decontamination and mass burials, but issues related to long-term housing and employment of evacuees have certainly become major concerns since Hurricanes Katrina and Rita.

12. Surge capacity issues have also been major concerns. The capacities of hospitals and the medical system as a whole to deal with large numbers of casualties are important, but much more research needs to be done on the capacities of local emergency response and emergency management agencies, the National Guard, and the multitude of nongovernmental disaster relief organizations during major disasters. NGOs, from local community groups to national faith-based organizations, represent that nation's capacity to deal with large-scale disasters and more research needs to be done on how to integrate them into disaster operations better.

There are many other questions that need to be answered and research that needs to be conducted to inform policies to deal with the threat and the actuality of terrorist attacks. Fortunately, much is known about managing hazards and dealing with large-scale disasters that is applicable to terrorist events. More open communication among Homeland Security officials, emergency management officials, terrorism and counterterrorism researchers, and disaster researchers would help identify research needs better and improve policies and programs to deal with the risk posed by terrorism.

CHAPTER 23

Recent Developments in U.S. Homeland Security Policies and Their Implications for the Management of Extreme Events[1]

KATHLEEN J. TIERNEY

SUMMARY

The terrorist attacks of September 11, 2001 have resulted in profound changes in the U.S. policy system. The federal government has responded to the events of 9/11 and to the ongoing terrorist threat by passing new laws, creating the Department of Homeland Security, issuing presidential directives, developing new preparedness and crisis management programs, and reorganizing and redirecting existing programs. Among the effects of these actions are a decrease in emphasis on preparedness and response for natural and technological disasters; an increase in the role of law enforcement agencies and the military in the management of domestic emergencies, accompanied by a decline in the importance and influence of the emergency management profession; and an increase in the importance of "special purpose" initiatives that have the potential for interfering with efforts to develop comprehensive, integrated, all-hazards approaches to managing extreme events.

---

[1] *Author's note:* This paper was originally written for the First International Conference on Urban Disaster Reduction, which was held in Kobe, Japan in January of 2005. Among the key arguments made in the paper was that homeland security policies implemented since the terrorist attacks of September 11, 2001 have been detrimental to U.S. disaster response capabilities. That was before Hurricane Katrina, an event that demonstrated that the U.S. intergovernmental system is incapable of managing catastrophic disaster events. Rather than requesting a complete rewrite of the paper, the editors have elected to publish it in its original form. However, additional comments related to Katrina and other recent developments have been added in brackets at appropriate places in the text.

INTRODUCTION

Under certain conditions, disasters can serve as "focusing events" that lead to the development of new legislation, policies, and practices (Birkland, 1997; Rubin & Renda-Tenali, 2000). In the United States, disasters that have led directly or indirectly to significant policy changes include the 1984 Bhopal, India chemical disaster, which influenced the passage of Title III of the Superfund Amendment and Reauthorization Act in 1986; the 1989 Exxon Valdez oil spill, to which the 1990 Oil Pollution Act was a partial response; and earthquakes in California, including the 1933 Long Beach event, which led to the passage of the Field Act.

The September 11 disaster has had far-reaching effects spanning a wide range of policy domains, including policies on waging war and adherence to the laws of war; policies toward international bodies such as the United Nations; policies on civil liberties, privacy, and surveillance; immigration law, border security, and the rights of noncitizens. With respect to laws, policies, and procedures affecting domestic preparedness, response, and "consequence management" for extreme events of all types, September 11 was the ultimate focusing event. While other U.S. disasters have led to significant institutional realignments and new laws and policies, none has brought about changes of comparable scope and scale. This chapter discusses and contrasts new crisis-relevant policy and programmatic initiatives with pre-9/11 arrangements, and assesses the likely consequences of these changes.

THE POST-SEPTEMBER 11 POLICY LANDSCAPE

The Department of Homeland Security

The creation of the Department of Homeland Security (DHS) was perhaps the most visible policy response to the events of September 11. The government reorganization that accompanied the formation of DHS was the largest in U.S. history since President Truman created the Department of Defense in 1947, incorporating all or part of 22 federal agencies, 40 different federal entities, and approximately 180,000 employees.

The reorganization merged together agencies (or parts of agencies) with very diverse organizational structures, missions, and cultures, and, importantly, diverse ideas about the management of domestic threats and emergencies. In the emergency management arena, the overall effect of the reorganization has been to expand the role of defense- and law enforcement-oriented agencies concerned exclusively with terrorism while curtailing the role and decreasing the prestige of entities with all-hazards emergency management responsibilities. The Federal Emergency Management Agency (FEMA), which was formerly an independent agency within the executive branch of government whose director had de facto cabinet status, was incorporated into DHS as lead agency for emergency preparedness and response. FEMA, which is the only agency within DHS that is charged specifically with reducing the losses associated with non-terrorism-related disasters, has lost significant visibility and financial and human resources in the reorganization. As a small agency within a massive bureaucracy, its activities are now overshadowed by much larger and better-funded entities within DHS. Indicative of this shift, much of the responsibility, authority, and budget for preparedness for terrorism events, which might logically have been assigned to FEMA, are now channeled to the Office for Domestic Preparedness (ODP), an entity that was transferred into DHS from the Department of Justice. ODP has taken on many and varied responsibilities, including overseeing preparedness assessments on a city-by-city basis, training, planning, exercises, and the provision of grants to local agencies. ODP manages a number of important DHS programs, including the Urban Area Security Initiative, the Homeland Security Grant Program, and the Metropolitan Medical Response System, which was transferred from FEMA. Unlike FEMA's director, the director of ODP is confirmed by the United States Senate, which is yet another indication of the relative importance of this office.

Since ODP had its origins in the Department of Justice, it is not surprising that it defines domestic preparedness primarily in terms of law enforcement functions. For example, ODP's "Preparedness Guidelines for Homeland Security" (DHS 2003) give priority to police and other public safety agencies. One effect of ODP involvement has been to institutionalize a system of terrorism prevention and management that is largely separate from the existing emergency management system. Another has been to increase direct "top-down" oversight of local preparedness activities on a scale that had not existed prior to 9/11.

The decline in FEMA's prestige and influence in the wake of 9/11 has caused great concern among U.S. emergency management experts. Testifying before the U.S. Congress in March, 2004, former FEMA director James Lee Witt warned that the nation's ability to respond to disasters of all types has been weakened by some post-September 11 agency realignments. In written testimony regarding the loss of cabinet status for the FEMA director and the current position of FEMA within DHS, Witt stated that "I assure you that we could not have been as responsive and effective during disasters as we were during my tenure as FEMA director, had there been layers of federal bureaucracy between myself and the White House" (Witt, 2004). [In the aftermath of Hurricane Katrina, questions have again arisen regarding whether FEMA's poor performance during the catastrophe was related to its status within the DHS bureaucracy. Other questions have centered on whether FEMA and other DHS officials have the qualifications to perform their job-related duties.]

As a consequence of the increased flow of resources into law enforcement agencies and counterterrorism programs from ODP and other sources, preparedness for natural and technological disasters has assumed far less importance on the public policy agenda. Moreover, as agencies based on command-and-control principles assume greater importance in local preparedness efforts, the influence of organizations that focus on hazards other than terrorism and that operate in a broadly inclusive fashion and on the basis of coordination, rather than control, has waned.

At the same time, questions exist regarding the power and influence of DHS vis-à-vis other more-established federal entities, including the Pentagon and the Department of Justice. These tensions were evident in the summer of 2004, when Attorney General John Ashcroft, rather than Homeland Security Secretary Tom Ridge, released information indicating a heightened terrorism threat against major financial institutions.

Mirroring shifts at the federal government level, law enforcement agencies are increasingly assuming influential positions in homeland preparedness at the local government level, in some cases supplanting local emergency management organizations. Some emergency management professionals have criticized this trend as potentially weakening community crisis management programs, rather than strengthening them. Jerome Hauer of George Washington University, the former director of the New York City Mayor's Office of Emergency Management, has been publicly critical of the manner in which the city has reorganized its crisis management functions in the wake of 9/11. In an opinion piece in the *New York Times*, Hauer faulted New York's current mayor, Michael Bloomberg, for increasingly placing authority for managing emergencies in the hands of the police department—an agency that according to Hauer has historically been weak with respect to interagency coordination and disaster preparedness—while diminishing the role of the more inclusive Office of Emergency Management (Hauer, 2004).

Presidential Homeland Security Directives and Resulting Actions

Direct presidential action is also transforming the U.S. crisis management policy system, most notably through a series of homeland security presidential directives (HSPDs) that have been issued since 9/11. The two directives that are most relevant for extreme event management are HSPD-5, "Management of Domestic Incidents," and HSPD-8, "National Preparedness." The stated aim of HSPD-5 was to improve the nation's capacity to respond to domestic disasters by creating a single, comprehensive incident management system. To this end, HSPD-5 mandated the development of a "concept of operations" for disasters that would incorporate all levels of government as well as crisis and consequence management functions within one unifying management framework. The Secretary of Homeland Security was given responsibility for implementing HSPD-5 by developing a National Response Plan (NRP) and a National Incident Management System (NIMS). Under this directive, all federal agencies were required to adopt NIMS and to make its adoption a requirement for other governmental entities receiving federal assistance. HSPD-8, "National Preparedness," gives the Secretary of Homeland Security broad authority in establishing a "national preparedness goal" and implementing programs to improve "prevention, response, and recovery" operations.[2] Although the directive explicitly calls for actions that address all hazards within a risk-based framework, its major focus is on preparedness for terrorism-related events. Similarly, while HSPD-8 is intended to address issues related to preparedness, a broad term that is generally conceptualized as an integrative and comprehensive process, the directive is mainly concerned with training and equipping emergency response agencies.

In calling for the development of a new national response plan, HSPD-5 seemingly ignored the fact that the United States already had a plan for coordinating the federal response to major disasters. The existing Federal Response Plan, which had been developed in the late 1980s and adopted in the early 1990s, had proven effective for coordinating federal resources in a number of major national emergencies, including the 9/11 attacks. At the time the new plan was mandated, the United States had an internationally recognized emergency management structure in place that was compatible with its system of "shared governance." While the NRP did not supplant that framework, it did make several important modifications. Under the NRP, the primary responsibility for managing domestic crises now rests with the Secretary of Homeland Security. The plan also contains language strongly suggesting that the federal government will in the future assume more responsibility for directly managing some crises, which significantly modifies "shared governance" policies that assign disaster management responsibility first to local authorities in affected jurisdictional areas. [The NRP was officially released in December of 2004. Katrina provided the first test of its use in a very large-scale disaster event. Questions remain about the extent to which responding entities, including DHS itself, understood their roles and responsibilities under the plan. Future research will reveal the extent to which new plans and procedures created confusion, rather than intergovernmental, cohesion, during the response to Hurricane Katrina.]

---

[2] Interestingly, HSPD-8 defines "prevention" as "activities undertaken by the first responder community during the early stages of an incident to reduce the likelihood or consequences of threatened or actual terrorist acts." The directive does not discuss the concept of mitigation.

In mandating NIMS, the plan also institutionalizes the Incident Command System (ICS) as the preferred organizational structure for managing disasters for all levels of government and within all organizations that play (or wish to play) a role in disaster response activities. While numerous U.S. jurisdictions and organizations already use ICS, this directive may nevertheless have problematic consequences. Some critics fault ICS for overly emphasizing command-and-control principles; they also question the wisdom of mandating one particular management framework for the many and diverse organizations that respond to disasters. Emergency management policy expert William Waugh observes that ICS "was created utilizing management concepts and theories that are now more than 30 years old" (Waugh, 1999) and that current management theory places much less emphasis on the command-and-control philosophy on which ICS is based. Waugh also notes that ICS is far more compatible, both structurally and culturally, with command-oriented organizations like police and fire departments than with the structures and cultures of the many other types of agencies and groups that play key roles in responding to disasters but that do not operate according to hierarchical principles. In his view and that of other critics, top-down management models like ICS (and now NIMS) are particularly ill suited to the distinctive challenges disasters present, which call for flexibility, improvisation, collaborative decision-making, and organizational adaptability. The danger is that in mandating a single, standardized management approach that is familiar mainly to command-and-control agencies, the NRP will stifle the capacity to improvise and will exclude many entities and groups that can make critical contributions during extreme events.

More broadly, the push toward universal adoption of NIMS and ICS reflects the highly questionable assumption that once a consistent management structure is adopted, preparedness and response effectiveness will automatically improve. Such an assumption ignores the numerous other factors that contribute to effective disaster management, such as ongoing contacts among crisis-relevant agencies during non-disaster times, common understandings of community vulnerability and the likely consequences of extreme events, realistic training and exercises, and sound public education programs. [Hurricane Katrina revealed significant strategic weaknesses in the nation's approach to extreme events—weaknesses that go far beyond issues that NIMS and ICS can address. Katrina allowed for days of warning, and it was common knowledge within scientific and governmental circles that the impacts of a Category 4 storm striking the Gulf region would be catastrophic. It was also well understood that up to 300,000 poor residents would have extreme difficulty evacuating from the city of New Orleans. The Katrina response revealed massive and almost inconceivable failures in strategic planning.]

The growing emphasis on terrorism readiness and ICS principles has led to a concomitant emphasis on "first responder" agencies and personnel. In current homeland security parlance, the term "first responder" refers to uniformed personnel (fire, police, and emergency services personnel) that arrive at the scene of a disaster. Missing from this discourse is a recognition that, as numerous studies indicate, ordinary citizens are the true "first responders" in all disasters. For example, in HSPD-8, a mere two sentences are devoted to the topic of citizen participation in preparedness activities. New policies and programs may thus leave vast reserves of talent and capability untapped in future extreme events. [Following Katrina, responding agencies treated stranded disaster victims in New Orleans as a problem population requiring strict policing, and there was little evidence of any efforts to engage the public in constructive ways in the emergency response. That the mass media also characterized victims as engaging in criminal behavior and even capital crimes further reinforced the notion that the disaster-stricken area needed to be under strict law enforcement and military control.]

REINFORCING PRE-SEPTEMBER 11 TRENDS:
MILITARIZATION AND STOVEPIPES

Some trends that were already under way during the 1990s were greatly accelerated by the events of September 11. One such trend involves an extension of military authority in domestic emergencies. Since the end of the Cold War, military and intelligence institutions had been increasingly seeking new responsibilities in areas such as environmental monitoring and disaster management (Global Disaster Information Network, 1997). With the advent of the war on terror, and with enormous increases in available funding, the domestic missions of defense- and intelligence-related agencies have further expanded. With respect to defense activities, for example, prior to September 11, there was no U.S. military entity with a specific mission to coordinate military operations within U.S. borders. In 2002, the U.S. Northern Command (NORTHCOM) was created with the express mission of engaging in homeland defense. Although its responsibilities in the homeland defense area are quite broad, NORTHCOM's public communications also stress that it operates according to U.S. laws governing the provision of military assistance to civil authorities (MACA), which require that military entities operating within the United States do so only in support of decisions made by civil authorities. Nonetheless, the creation of NORTHCOM does represent a major policy shift regarding the role of the military in U.S. domestic affairs.

At the same time, terrorism-related concerns have led President's Bush administration to reevaluate U.S. laws such as the Posse Comitatus Act (PCA), which bars the military from carrying out domestic law enforcement functions. New interpretations of the PCA allow considerable latitude in the use of the military within the United States, not only in situations involving terrorism, but for a wide range of other purposes. Indeed, the domestic use of military resources in crises (and potential crises) of all types is becoming increasingly routine. For example, the military is involved in ongoing efforts to enhance border security, troops were used extensively to provide security for the 2002 Winter Olympics in Salt Lake City, military assets were employed in the hunt for the Washington area sniper, and the military played a major and highly visible role in the response to the 2004 Florida hurricanes. (Whether it was necessary to deploy troops to guard Home Depot stores and disaster assistance centers is another matter).

In the aftermath of the 9/11 attacks, the military is widely seen as having superior skills and technologies that can enhance the effectiveness of domestic crisis management—including the management of disasters. Its expertise is being called upon in areas such as the design and conduct of terrorism drills in U.S. communities, gaming and simulation, and surveillance. Former military officers are sought out by civil authorities and public safety agencies charged with homeland security responsibilities—again presumably for their superior knowledge and training—and military entities are being given responsibility for assessing domestic crisis preparedness programs (Healy, 2003). Homeland security terminology now includes the concept of the "domestic battlespace," a term that is applied both to terrorism-related emergencies and to disasters.

Federal and state military assets have long played a role in responding to disasters and other domestic crises, but with the recognition that the military would become involved only if "tasked" to do so under existing laws and policies. However, the position taken by the Bush administration—that the United States is now at war with terrorism and will be for the foreseeable future—has the potential for drastically expanding military participation within the nation's borders in a variety of activities that formerly were considered the domain of civil authorities, including emergency management. This shift raises questions regarding the extent to which military culture, doctrine, and modes of operation are consistent with the crisis-related needs and requirements of a diverse civil society. War and domestic emergencies are not analogous, and new domestic military missions that conflate disaster response with battlefield operations could ultimately be detrimental to both. [In the aftermath of Hurricane Katrina, the military is once again being framed in political discourse as the only institution capable of managing major disasters. Calls for a greater militarization of disaster response, such as those made by President Bush, have generated extreme controversy. For example, many U.S. governors have rejected proposals for an expanded military role in disasters.]

The post-9/11 environment has also been marked by the acceleration of a second trend: the involvement of "special purpose" entities in crisis and consequence management activities. Such entities include Joint Terrorism Task Forces and Urban Area Security Initiative programs (UASI), which focus specifically on terrorism-related risks from a law enforcement perspective, and Metropolitan Medical Response Systems (MMRS), which were established to enhance the emergency response capacity of public health systems, particularly with respect to incidents involving weapons of mass destruction (WMDs). All three of these programs predated 9/11, but their importance, as well as their budgets, have grown as a consequence of the new war on terrorism.

This trend toward "special purpose" preparedness can also be seen in the proliferation of centers for public health preparedness in schools of public health across the nation. Again, some investment had been made in addressing public health needs related to terrorism and WMD prior to 9/11, but in the aftermath of the attacks, virtually every school of public health of any significance has launched initiatives in the homeland security area. While some centers have been funded by means of competitive grants from federal agencies, others have received funding through special legislative "earmarks." As a consequence of this rapid expansion, needed public health education and preparedness efforts are often poorly coordinated and isolated from broader community preparedness activities.

These programs and forms of funding were initiated in order to address serious gaps in response capability, notably challenges associated with intergovernmental collaboration on law enforcement issues and with inadequate public health emergency response resources. However, such initiatives also have other unintended consequences. They encourage collaboration and integration within sectors (e.g., law enforcement and public health), rather than across the diverse sectors that must be involved in responding to crises. They also promote specialized planning for particular types of emergencies. In other words, both in structure and in function, these increasingly influential entities contravene widely accepted principles of emergency management, which emphasize the importance of developing comprehensive, integrated preparedness and response networks and of all-hazards preparedness activities, rather than hazard-specific ones.

Many post-9/11 investigations have highlighted problems associated with "stovepiping," or the tendency for organizations and agencies to closely guard information, carry out their own specialized activities in isolation from one another, and resist efforts to encourage cross-agency collaboration. Indeed, DHS itself was created in order to overcome stovepipes, better integrate disparate agencies and programs, and improve information-sharing and cooperation. It is ironic, then, that some homeland security initiatives appear to be creating new stovepipes and reinforcing existing organizational and institutional barriers. For example, while diverse law enforcement agencies at different governmental levels may be making progress in working together on terrorism-related issues, the law enforcement sector itself may have little incentive to take an active role in broader cross-sectoral preparedness efforts. Rather than promoting comprehensive preparedness for all potential threats—including disasters and terrorism—special-purpose initiatives encourage organizations to interact and plan within their own separate spheres and to focus on particular kinds of threats. Large infusions of funds into specialized programs only exacerbate the problem.

CONCLUSION

It is far too soon to speculate on longer-term impacts of new initiatives adopted in the wake of the tragic events of September 11. We may yet see a day when the United States declares victory in the war on terrorism and homeland security becomes less important on the national policy agenda. Or some future catastrophic disaster may bring about a reordering of national priorities. At this point, however, such possibilities seem remote. What does seem clear is that post-September 11 policies will very likely result in permanent and fundamental changes in the nation's approach to preparing for and responding to extreme events, including earthquakes and other disasters. Whether those changes reduce the vulnerability and enhance the resilience of the nation and its communities in the face of terrorism and other threats is a question that can only be addressed through future research.

[The Hurricane Katrina tragedy vividly illustrates the nation's lack of preparedness for catastrophic disaster events. Sadly, it is also now clear that failures to respond to Katrina will be matched or even exceeded by additional failures in the areas of short- and long-term recovery. The large death toll and the devastation wrought by Katrina were avoidable, but responsible parties were incapable of effective action. As of this writing, it is unclear whether Katrina will serve as a window of opportunity for advocates of disaster loss reduction, whether the disaster will further increase the role of military and law enforcement agencies in future disasters, and whether the Gulf Region will find the resources it needs to recover from Katrina in ways that enhance sustainability and resilience.]

CHAPTER 24

Unwelcome Irritant or Useful Ally? The Mass Media in Emergencies

JOSEPH SCANLON

When the crew of a derailed Canadian Pacific Railway (CPR) freight train at Minot, North Dakota spotted anhydrous ammonia leaking from damaged tank cars, they immediately dialed 9-1-1. As a result of that call, the Minot fire department:

- Called the local TV stations;
- Called the local radio stations; and
- Put a warning message on cable television.

None of these actions alerted residents of Tierracita Vallejo, the area closest to the wreck. The leaking ammonia led to one death, 11 serious injuries, and 322 other injuries.

Because the incident occurred at night, neither of the local TV stations was broadcasting and two of the three radio stations were carrying remote programming. Though a staff member was at the third radio station, he did not answer the phone. The messages on cable did not reach those at risk because the derailment cut power to the area closest to the wreck. In any case, many viewers get television reception via satellite. Even sirens did not help: the ones in Minot could not be heard in the area affected (Operations Group Factual Report, U.S. National Transportation Safety Board, June 11, 2002).

In contrast, when Eastern Canada was hit by a severe ice storm in January, 1998, a radio station in Canada's capital, Ottawa, devoted its entire broadcast schedule to that storm. Not only did it provide live coverage of all news conferences by regional officials, but it also accepted and broadcast calls from local residents about what was going well and what was not. The general running the military response assigned soldiers to monitor that station, and ensured that any concerns were dealt with. After the emergency was over, he visited the station to thank it for its public service (Scanlon, 1998a, 1998b).

Although the media can play an effective role in disasters, as in the Canadian ice storm, Minot indicates that they are not always available when needed. The media may be critical for effective warning. They can act as a link between the public and officials and be the single most important source of public information. They can provide an outlet for the aggrieved and, on some occasions, become the glue that binds society. But there are limits: if officials are to make effective use of the media in a disaster they must understand how media function, and it is increasingly important to recognize that radio and television are not the sole means of

413

high-speed mass communications. Cell phones and the World Wide Web have augmented the way information is transmitted.

This chapter examines the role of the media before, during, and after emergency incidents. It shows that the media can perform an extremely valuable function during a disaster and that media participation is crucial to effective warning. But it also shows that there are concerns about the way the media may distort what is happening, partly because they focus on official sources and ignore the role of individuals. In addition, it looks at the role of some of the newer media which may not be as new as they appear, but emphasize that there will be high-speed communication in the wake of a dramatic event, whether via the older mass media—radio, television, and daily newspapers—or by the newer media—cell phones and Web sites—or by the longest surviving form of mass communication, interpersonal communication by word of mouth. Finally, it suggests that research is needed to compare what happened to what the media report; in short, why the media select what they do for their stories.

MEDIA RESPONSE TO DISASTERS

Media find crises and disasters engrossing, especially—in the case of television—if there are dramatic visuals, which carry more impact than the simple factual statements. It was the visuals that led to the extensive coverage of the initial assault and stand-off at Waco. It was the visual of a plane hitting the World Trade Center and the images of both towers collapsing that intensified 9/11 as a media event. The availability of personal videos made television broadcasts about the December 26, 2004, tsunami even more compelling.. But even before television, some word pictures such as the end of the Hindenburg held audience attention, and disasters have been media themes ever since there were newspapers.

When disaster strikes, the media learn about it, report what they hear, try to obtain more information, use their files to add background to their stories, and dispatch news crews. Often—as happened in Ottawa during the ice storm—media outlets will devote all of their air time or most space available to that single story (Scanlon & Alldred, 1982), and draft anyone at hand to gather material to fill in information. When two teenagers killed 13 fellow students, wounded 13 others, and then shot themselves at Columbine High School in Colorado, KCNC-TV in Denver used every staff member available for 13 hours of nonstop coverage: "Well over 150 newsroom regulars and extras pitched in to make the extensive coverage possible. Off-duty employees came . . . without being summoned and took up posts . . ." (Rotbart, 1999, p. 24).

The media also use technical resources and ingenuity to gather information. When Mount St. Helen's erupted, NBC took a helicopter into the crater and persuaded a geologist to view and comment on the resulting tape. At Three Mile Island, staff from the Philadelphia *Inquirer* copied the license plates of all vehicles in the parking lot, traced the owners, and started phoning them. Many were hostile but 50 agreed to interviews (Sandman & Paden, 1979, p. 48).

Most U.S. daily newspapers belong to the cooperative agency, the Associated Press (AP), and share all their news with AP. The electronic media have similar arrangements. For this reason, visuals filmed by one media outlet soon appear around the world. When major stories break, there is also widespread cooperation among reporters. In the wake of Three Miles Island journalists shared everything they had: "We got drawings and pierced together events. . . . We went out and got books on nuclear energy and compared them and discussed how a reactor works" (Sandman & Paden, 1979, p. 16). It was the same in Dallas on the day John Kennedy was assassinated: "Every one who picked up a bit or piece passed it on. I know no one who held anything out. Nobody thought about an exclusive. It didn't seem important" (Wicker, 1996, p. 28).

Even when formal or informal cooperation does not exist, the media monitor each other and take what they hear and see and read from their rivals and report it. Any single report—true or false—is soon copied and published everywhere, and as the Barseback incident in Sweden illustrates, false reports may be circulated. A single inaccurate report by one journalist led to worldwide coverage of "panic" after a radio drama about a nuclear reactor (Rosengren, Arvidson, & Struesson, 1974, p. 6).

CONVERGENCE

The media not only cover dramatic events, but they do so in a large-scale way. After a 1985 air crash involving the 101st Airborne in the isolated Newfoundland community of Gander, 325 media personnel arrived within 24 hours. Within 48 hours there were several thousand media in Lockerbie, Scotland after the 1988 crash of Pam Am 103. There were media-created helicopter traffic jams over Coalinga, California after the 1983 earthquake and a media city with its own mayor and Saturday entertainment in 1993 near the Branch Davidian compound at Waco. John Hansen handled media relations after the bombing at Oklahoma City: "... we ... nicknamed the media area "satellite city" as there was almost a two square block area of nothing but satellite trucks and live trucks lined up side by side ... " (Hansen, 1998, pp. 56–57).

This massive response and incessant demand for information creates enormous pressures on officials.

Officials in smaller communities are usually on first-name terms with the reporters for local radio and television and the local newspaper. They believe—usually correctly—that they can count on their cooperation when incidents occur. On several occasions, the Royal Canadian Mounted Police (RCMP) kept a local reporter briefed on a local incident and let that reporter deal with outside media. However, in a major incident, local officials are overwhelmed. There will be reporters not just from major U.S. television stations such as NBC, ABC, CBS, CNN, Fox, but also from major newspapers such as the *Los Angeles Times, The New York Times,* and the *Washington Post.* There will be reporters from the major news magazines—*Time, Newsweek, US News and World Report.* And there will be foreign journalists from broadcasters such as the BBC and magazines such as *Paris Match.* Many of these journalists are likely to be much more experienced with disasters than are the officials. All have their own deadlines and their own priorities. When Florence was hit by severe flooding, the Italian journalists were concerned about the impact of the flood on local residents, and the British about the impact on Florence's art (Alexander, p. 24).

In 1957, Charles Fritz and J.H. Mathewson labeled the massive response to incidents as "convergence" and identified three types: personal—the physical movement of persons on foot, by automobile or other vehicles; materiel—the physical movement of supplies and equipment; and informational—the movement or transmission of messages (Fritz & Mathewson, 1957). They stated that convergence causes problems: "[In Lockerbie] massive congestion to the public telephone network ... brought normal telecommunications almost to a standstill" (McIntosh, 1989).

Fritz and Mathewson blamed convergence on the media, arguing early reports are not specific enough to satisfy the needs and curiosity of those hearing them. They suggest a temporary media blackout would reduce convergence (Fritz & Mathewson, 1957, p. 75).

This conclusion was largely accepted for nearly 40 years; but it is flawed. In a study of a tire fire in Southern Ontario in February, 1990, 14 million used rubber tires burned for 18 days. There were hundreds of responders: 12 police detachments and three police forces,

26 fire departments, 27 federal government agencies, and 60 voluntary agencies. None came as a result of news reports. In fact, initial media reports were quite limited (Scanlon & Prawzick, 1991). Similarly, in 1975, when a downtown office building filled with gas and exploded in North Bay, Ontario, there was no news coverage until 19 minutes after the explosion. In those 19 minutes, news spread by word of mouth so quickly that 80% of those interviewed by students belonging to Carleton University's Emergency Communications Research Unit (ECRU) reported they had first learned by word of mouth. Only 20% first learned through radio or television: "... somewhere between 3,000 and 4,000 persons were at the site within the first hour . . . 45 per cent said they went from simple curiosity. . . . Only a small percentage— eight per cent—said they went because their jobs took them there" (Scanlon & Taylor, 1975).

MEDIA MYTHS

Nevertheless, the massive coverage of untoward events does have a major impact. As E.L. Quarantelli has pointed out, practically everyone is willing to express opinions about what will happen in disasters, yet most in Western society have limited experience with such events.

> ... we think a strong case can be made that what average citizens and officials expect about disasters, what they come to know on ongoing disasters, and what they learned from disasters that have occurred, are primarily if not exclusively learned from mass media accounts. (Quarantelli, 1991c, p. 2)

What are those images? They are that officials must be careful about issuing warnings because of the danger of panic. They are that victims of disasters will be dazed and confused, perhaps in shock, and must be cared for by others. They are that in the wake of disaster, antisocial behavior is to be expected and there must be precautions against looting. They are that public accommodation will be required for those forced from their homes in case of an evacuation. They are in short a view that victims of disaster on the whole will not cope but that efficient emergency organizations will take care of their needs and protect them.

In fact, panic is rarely an issue in emergencies; it is so rare it is difficult to study. Instead of being dazed, confused, and shocked, the injured and uninjured survivors of widespread destructive incidents usually do most if not all of the initial search and rescue. They, not emergency services personnel, take victims to medical centers. Looting in the wake of disasters is not only rare, but crime rates also normally fall because people—even criminals—are preoccupied with other things. And though there may be some need for public shelter, usually about 95% of evacuees find their own accommodation.

The fact that so many individuals act on their own makes coverage of disasters difficult to impossible. The media do not have the time or space to focus on all these individual acts—and for the most part are unaware of them and their importance—so they portray the event as one that is being managed by emergency agencies such as the police, the fire department, and the medical agencies. This leads to what Quarantelli calls the "command post" view of disaster, meaning that since journalists do not know the important role of survivors and are unaware how of how limited a role emergency personnel play in early response, they will assume that emergency officials know what is going on. Their reports will reflect the official view of what has happened and is happening at the moment.

Because of this, the media tend to ignore nontraditional activities such as search and rescue, conducted mainly by volunteers working in emergent groups. Wenger and Quarantelli found, for example, that only 8.6% of newspaper articles and 8.4% of electronic media reports on disaster mention search and rescue. When it *was* mentioned, those stories inevitably relied to some extent on nontraditional sources. In other words, to cover search and rescue activity, reporters would have been forced to use nontraditional sources. Because such sources were often missed, an important activity was given slight attention (Wenger & Quarantelli, 1989, p. 62).

One problem caused by journalists is that in the early stages of a disaster—when no one knows what is happening—they will demand specific information about damage and destruction and casualties. This is what their editors want and what they are taught to get by journalism instructors and in studying journalism texts. One of the most respected journalism educators, Curtis MacDougall, said no reporter covering a disaster can overlook casualties (dead and injured), property damage, cause of the disaster, and rescue and relief work (including the numbers involved) (MacDougall, 1982, pp. 320–321). Even if they accept that detailed information may not be available immediately, most journalism texts assume that eventually there *will* be specific information. Scholars disagree. Janet Kitz, author of *Shattered City*, a book on the catastrophic 1917 Halifax explosion, wrote:

> I am frequently asked how many people died in the explosion. I have come across so many different figures; for example, 1,635 or 1,963. No list I have seen has ever included all the people I know to have died. I believe the figure was higher than 2000. (Kitz, 1989, p. 15)

The December 26, 2004 Sumatra tsunami illustrates the accuracy of her comment. The figures for the total number who died were at first far too low overall but far too high for the European dead. It is now evident that there will never be close to an accurate count of the dead. Even if the death toll could be calculated with precision, it would be hard to calculate the injury toll because many victims decline to go for medical help for what they see as minor injuries. Even those who do are often not recorded accurately. In disasters, record keeping is one of the first casualties (Scanlon, 1996).

EFFECT OF NEW REPORTS

News reports that portray the dazed and confused victims and express fears about looting lead to public misunderstanding about disasters. As Wenger, James, and Faupel (1980) found, people tend to believe the myths about individual behavior in disaster because these myths are so frequently reported by the mass media. Fortunately, whatever people think about disaster, they behave differently. They may think people panic but they don't panic. They may think victims will be dazed, confused, and in shock but they act very rationally. They may think looting will be a problem but much looting doesn't occur.

However, although individuals are not apparently swayed by the myths, that is less true of emergency agencies. Unlike individuals, organizations sometimes act as if the myths were correct. There is a tendency to hold back warnings for fear of panic and to order evacuations even after danger has passed because officials think victims can't cope. There is a tendency to use resources to prevent looting that might be better used elsewhere. Radio stations have held back warnings—even when these were officially requested—for fear of causing panic. Television journalists have encouraged people to alter their behavior so visuals will match the myths. At Three Mile Island, they advised people to get off the streets because that confirmed their view of public fright (Sandman & Paden, p. 58). They also played down reports for fear of panic: "At Three Mile Island, reporters faced a pressure that was new to science reporting.... Overly alarming coverage could have spread panic; overly reassuring coverage could have risked lives" (Stephens & Edison, 1982, p. 199). The same concern showed up after 9/11: "There is no point in allowing this thing to appear worse than it is, it is already horrendous, and we don't need to make it worse by misstating numbers and we want you to keep that in mind" (CNN anchor Aaron Brown). And: "Tom as you point out we try not to exaggerate ... and yet in many ways it's hard not to exaggerate just the things we have been seeing and the things we are told." (NBC reporter Pat Dawson talking to Tom Brokaw [Reynolds & Barnett, p. 698]). The fact is that people find it easier to cope with the truth, with clear factual accounts of what is known. It is lack of clarity and confusion that makes persons uneasy.

AUDIENCE

The mass media can have enormous audiences. The 2005 Academy Awards attracted an estimated 42.1 million viewers in the United States alone. There are also huge audiences for top-rated shows such as "American Idol," "CSI," and "Survivor." Given this and the massive attention the media devote to disasters, it would seem that they would be the ideal way to inform the public. That is not always the case, for four reasons.

First, even those huge audiences represent only slightly more than 10% of the population and the audiences for major news programs are much less. Each weekday evening, for example, about 20 million Americans tune in to watch the evening news on NBC, ABC, or CBS. That's about 10% of the population. The other 90% won't see a story even if it is on all three networks. Of course, some people watch CNN or other 24-hour news networks but those audiences are much smaller. Even "Larry King Live" draws only a million viewers, one eighth as many as NBC or ABC news.

Second, those large media audiences are often specific segments of the public. The mass media make money by selling advertising. To do that they must be able to show advertisers that their audiences are the ones advertisers want to reach. That means they wish to attract audiences of interest to specific advertisers. Let's suppose a college or university decides to start providing special classes for retired persons. There would be little point in placing an advertisement on a radio station that plays the latest hits for a young audience. It must find an outlet that reaches retired persons who may be interested in continuing education.

Those trying to plan effective warnings and public information must understand local media and local media audiences. They must know which media outlets cater to the young and which serve a more mature audience. They must be aware that some television programs are targeted for specific audiences: for example, daytime programming may be aimed at women working at home, Saturday morning programming at children. And they must know how to tailor a message issued at specific times. For example, a warning message shown while cartoons are running would have to be capable of getting children to alert their parents. When *Sesame Street* developed educational broadcasts on coping with hurricanes, it designed its programs to get children to start asking parents about the family's plans for evacuation. Most important, they must realize that large audiences may be useful to advertisers, but unless they include the persons who need to be reached they are not of value for effective warnings.

Besides age—older people tend to have different listening and viewing habits than younger people—a number of factors affect the nature of an audience. One is occupation. Some persons, for example, farmers in tractors and delivery persons, can listen to the radio as they work. Others cannot. Another is time of day. Radio draws a larger audience in the morning, television in the evening. A third is language. In Canada, one fifth of the population speaks French at home. In the United States, the foreign born population is now 12% of the total and half of those persons speak Spanish as a first language. Even those who are fluent in English may turn to their first language during emergencies.

A third problem is that the mass media, especially network media, tend to paint a broad picture—"Flooding has become more severe in North Carolina," "There's another snow emergency in Wyoming." These statements may be sufficient for a general news audience but they do little to inform persons in a specific community whether they should evacuate because of the flood threat or cancel a trip because of the snow emergency. They also tend to trigger inquiries from those who are unsure of precisely what areas are affected. This confusion can become a major problem for agencies trying to identify those who are missing in the wake of a catastrophe. Canada's Department of Foreign Affairs accepted calls from persons who thought a relative might have been in the World Trade Center. Many who called did not know the difference between New York State and New York City and would report the persons they were concerned about were in Buffalo, which is obviously a long way from the World Trade Center.

Officials need to encourage both the networks and, more important, local media to be as specific as possible about areas affected and not affected. A useful report might say, for example, that a plane hit one wing of the Pentagon in Arlington, Virginia but that neighboring buildings were not impacted and no buildings in the District of Columbia were affected.

A fourth reason why the media are not always an asset is that some media do not carry news reports even in a community struck by disaster. Wenger and Quarantelli found that while newspapers and television provided extensive coverage of disaster—83.3% of television stations preempted regular programming—many radio stations ignored even local disasters: "A total of 18.6 per cent of the radio stations [examined for the study] did not cover the disaster in their community at all. Thirty per cent of the stations . . . never pre-empted local programming, and 28.3 percent did not increase their normal time allocated for news" (Wenger & Quarantelli, 1989, p. 39).

When a train derailed and spilled some chemicals in Petawawa, Ontario on a Sunday morning, the local radio station did not interrupt its regular religious programming (Scanlon, Prawzick, Osborne, Medcalf, & Cote, 1985). As news of what was happening spread by word of mouth, local residents began listening to an Ottawa radio station that *was* providing information about the derailment.

WARNINGS AND RUMOR CONTROL

As the incident in Minot indicates, the media are crucial to an effective warning. Quarantelli concluded that this is "without doubt, the clearest and most consistent role [of mass media] in a disaster . . . (Quarantelli, 1991c, p. 23). However, to be effective, warnings must be specific about the threat, about who is affected, and about what to do. Most important, they must come from all possible sources at the same time. That is because when persons receive a warning, they check with another source to see if it is credible. Perry and Green found that at Mount St. Helens, 80% of those who received a warning tried to confirm it (Perry & Greene, 1983, p. 66).

"Technically any single communication channel cannot meet the information demands . . . , a mix of channels should be used to send messages . . . the news media need to be systematically incorporated into this mix (Perry & Lindell, 1989, p. 62)."

If interpersonal sources come first, people turn to the media (Kanihan & Gale, 2003, p. 89). If the media provide the first information, people will turn elsewhere. A study of how persons learned about two hurricanes showed that more than 60% first saw warnings on television, 17 and 25% heard first on radio (Ledingham & Masel Walters, 1989, p. 43).

In contrast, on 9/11, when persons were informed by word of mouth, they turned immediately to the mass media, especially television.

When a train derailed and spilled chemicals in Mississauga, just west of Toronto, Peel Regional Police Force made its warnings effective by following all the rules for effective warning. They not only announced that there had been a train derailment, that some cars were leaking chlorine *and* that there had been propane explosions and could be more, but also went door to door to make sure those directly affected were so advised. And they were very clear about what residents should do—leave! Persons were told to use their own vehicles or accept a ride on a Mississauga Transit bus. (Buses with police were coming along each street.) The warnings were reinforced by loud hailers alerting residents to the threat and the evacuation order.

In addition, instead of telling the media *when* they had ordered an evacuation, Peel Police told the media when they were *about* to do so—and provided maps so television could show precisely what area was to be evacuated next. Many residents received the evacuation message first over radio or television. Some heard first via a phone call from someone who had heard or seen a news report (Scanlon & Padgham, 1980). They were gone or at least ready to go when police arrived at their door. In contrast, after the ammonia spill in Minot, in the absence of information on radio 9-1-1, the police station was swamped with phone calls. Many had heard the train crash or the sirens or, perhaps, had smelled ammonia. They called to find out what was going on. Since there was nothing on local radio or TV, they had to search for some other source of information.

EMERGENCY INFORMATION

The mass media can also play a vital role in keeping people informed after disaster strikes. During a snow emergency, CFPL in London, Ontario turned its entire programming over to information related to the emergency. A study by Singer and Green showed that the station served as an intermediary between officials and the public. The station would take phone calls from the public and relay any questions to officials. It would then broadcast the answer so that all could hear. Similarly, when ice jams blocked the river and water poured over the dikes in Peace River, Alberta, everyone turned to local radio for information: 100% of a sample reported that was how they kept informed. Many said the only time they were really worried was when the local station temporarily went off the air. It had been evacuated and had to reestablish above the flood plain (Scanlon, Osborne, & McClellan, 1996). The mayor had arranged for it to relocate at the telephone building on high ground. It was off the air for only 20 minutes.

Sometimes, even more dramatic ways have been found to maintain media service. In the wake of Hurricane David, a British destroyer used its own telecommunications facilities to broadcast to the Island of Dominica. After Cyclone Tracy devastated Darwin, Australia on Christmas Eve, 1974, the Director of Australia's Natural Disasters Organization ordered one of the first relief flights to bring in 2000 battery-powered transistor radios so he could reach Darwin's residents (Stretton, p. 61).

Many communities have a number of stations—some larger cities may have as many as 15 or 20—so it is useful to know which ones are most likely to provide information in a disaster. [There is evidence people drop their normal listening and viewing habits and will lock onto the station or stations providing the information they want.] If even one survives, its presence is an asset. When a severe windstorm hit Nova Scotia, there was a rumor that the ferry between North Sydney and Port aux Basques, Newfoundland, had sunk. The mayor asked the one station still on the air to send a reporter in a mobile unit to interview the ferry captain. The captain said that the voyage had been rough but his ship was fine (Scanlon, 1977). That stopped the rumor. The mayor was aware of what was being reported. An efficient media relations operation will monitor what is being reported and—if there are errors—take steps to correct those as quickly as possible. Because the media are devoting so much time and space to the single incident, it is usually possible to have corrections reported faster than at any other time.

Media outlets may have plans for covering major incidents, though even that is rare, but they usually do not have plans about how they will continue to operate in destructive incidents. Yet the media need power. They need the ability to get staff to work and to move staff when transportation is disrupted. They also need to know that the Federal Communications Commission allows stations to maintain their daytime programming signals and remain on the air during crises and to do so without seeking advance permission (National Association of Broadcasters, p. 19).

Wenger and Quarantelli found that most media outlets do not do such planning and those that do are not very successful at it. They found that when planning was done, it was generally inadequate, outdated, untested, and in any case could not be located. (Wenger & Quarantelli, 1989, p. 33).

When a power blackout hit New York City on November 9, 1965, *The New York Times* had to scramble to find a way to print at least part of a newspaper. As those on staff tried to determine the seriousness of the problem, some wandered around the newsroom with matches; others went to nearby stores to buy candles or to nearby Roman Catholic churches to borrow some. Eventually the paper made a deal with the *Newark News* in neighboring New Jersey to publish an abbreviated version of the *Times* and supply vital copy. For example, the stock listings in that issue were not produced by the *Times* staff but borrowed from the ones already set in type for the *News*.

On 9/11 the *Wall Street Journal* was ready for an emergency. The *Journal* had a backup facility with equipment installed and the decision to get it up and running was made as soon as the first plane hit the first tower. The facility has been outfitted in the 18 months prior to 9/11 and editors had done two test runs to make sure it worked. "The South Brunswick offices seemed from another world—a comfortable, modern, suburban campus with expansive green lawns. The two "emergency" newsrooms were ready to go (Baker, 2001, p. 13)."

The move was handled so well that the *Journal* managed to deliver to its subscribers all but 180,000 of its normal 1.8 million copies.

MEDIA, VICTIMS, AND RELATIVES

One action that often arouses criticism is the way journalists treat victims and their relatives. When Pam Am 103 went missing over Lockerbie, Scotland, journalists waiting for information were cordoned off near the first class lounge at New York's Kennedy Airport. Seeing them, a woman asked what the fuss was about. An official said a Pam Am plane had crashed. She asked for the flight number. He replied, "1-0-3." She collapsed on the floor, screaming, "Not my baby. Not my baby." While her husband tried to shield her, photographers and television crews recorded her grief. "All I remember is losing control. . . . I felt like I was being raped by the media. I felt violated. I felt exploited. And there was no one there to protect me" (Deppa,

Russell, Hayes, & Flocke, 1994, p. 29). When she finally left Kennedy airport, she noticed something on her taxi's front seat: She asked the driver if she could see it. It was the *Daily News* and on the front page was her photo on the floor of the airport. "I was actually appalled," she said. "I just couldn't believe it." (Deppa, Russell, Hayes, & Flocke, 1994, p. 33).

That type of incident explains why Everett Parker of the United Church of Christ was so critical of the mass media at the Committee on Disasters and the Mass Media: "Day in and day out, we see reporters bullying statements out of stricken people; they take pride in their ability to do so.... It is dehumanizing to stick a camera and a microphone in the face of an injured or bereaved person and demand a statement" (Parker, 1980, p. 238).

Yet the media are *not* as guilty Parker charges. The widespread perception that in the wake of incidents the media act as ghouls, harassing victims and the relatives of victims and showing no sensitivity is misleading. Both anecdotal and research data suggests some victims and relatives welcome a chance to talk to reporters. After the 1985 Gander air crash that took the lives of 248 U.S. soldiers, an officer was assigned to media relations at the soldiers' home base, Fort Campbell, Kentucky. He told the media that the military intended to protect the privacy of the soldiers' families. To his surprise, a number of families wanted to speak to the media. Most agencies now make it clear to victims and victims' families that they will protect their privacy if that is what they want but they will also facilitate access to the media if that is their wish.

Though they may feel uneasy when they make the approach, reporters often discover they are made welcome by relatives of those who died. These relatives are anxious to talk to someone and the reporter is anxious to listen. When the Broadcast Standards Committee of the United Kingdom interviewed 210 victims of violence and disaster, including 54 who had been interviewed by reporters, three quarters said they were not offended. That was especially true of those in a disaster. Most who complained were upset with newspapers, especially tabloid reporters, but not with broadcast journalists. Survivors said they were prepared to talk if stories had a purpose, for example, "exposed the human frailties and negligence that had contributed to major disasters and so help to minimize the danger of such disasters happening again" (Shearer, 1991).

In the wake of the Kennedy assassination, it was television that bound Americans together. Television also provided a shared public platform during the aftermath of the terrorist attacks on 9/11:

> During the month following the attacks, these three magazines [*Time, Newsweek* and *U.S. News & World Report*] told a cohesive story of the tragedy and its aftermath, a story that moved from shock and fear to inspiration and pride. They did so by using testimony from readers and mourners across the country, as well as from victims and witnesses of the attacks. These actors participated, along with the journalists themselves, in the performance of a ritual with symbolic visual representations of candles, portraits of the dead and the American flag.... Overall, this coverage corresponded with the stages of a funeral ceremony. In that sense, it provided evidence that journalism plays an important role in—and can in certain circumstances be a form of—civil religion. (Kitch, 2003, p. 222)

By writing about victims as individuals, the media "humanizes" events.[1] During the Viet Nam war, *Life* magazine ran the photo of every service person killed in a single week. After 9/11, day after day *The New York Times* ran photos and brief articles about those who died, material later incorporated into a book (*The New York Times*, 2003). This "humanization" can lead to a

---

[1] I am indebted to a former researcher, David Tait, for this idea. Tait is now a member of faculty at Carleton University.

distorted impression. Noting that "human interest" stories are staple items in disaster coverage, Wenger, James, and Faupel suggests they tend to focus on the most impacted:

> Such stories detail the plight of the individual who has been "wiped out" by the disaster, who has lost their family, or suffered great misfortune. However, these atypical cases are often presented as if they were typical. ... (Wenger, James, & Faupel, 1980, p. 40)

Another aspect of humanization is the attempt to link an event to the perceived audience. Journalists call this searching for a "local angle." Events are more likely to be reported if they occur close to the place of publication and if nationals are involved. (That leads to bizarre headlines such as; "10,000 dead in mudslide, no Americans involved.".) When Gladys and Kurt Engel Lang reviewed the 139 disasters illustrating front pages from *The New York Times* up to that point, they found that of the 18 really big stories ... those for which coverage ran over four different pages—five occurred within the New York area. Since only 7 of the 139 disasters were in the New York area, it seems evident that the local ones get special treatment in the *Times* (Lang & Lang, 1980, pp. 217–272). This was evident everywhere in the wake of the Sumatra tsunami. In Sweden, Norway, the Netherlands, the United Kingdom, the United States, and Canada, the media focused on nationals.

SPECIALIZED AUDIENCES

As mentioned, one problem with the mass media—radio, television, and print—is that they are, in fact, mass media with mass audiences. It is impossible, except in a general way, to know whether they are reaching the specific audiences officials want. There are other effective ways to communicate, some very simple, others taking advantage of new technology.

When disasters occur in small communities or in specific areas of larger communities, one of the best ways of sharing information is a public meeting. If such a meeting is well advertised, most persons will attend and will therefore hear the same information at the same time, get to ask questions about anything that is not clear, and get answers. They will hear the questions asked by others and the answers they receive. They will not get information second or third hand. Such meetings are the ideal way to put down any false information or rumors. When a flash flood occurred in the rural Pemberton Valley of British Columbia, the province placed fliers in the mail boxes of all local residents announcing a public meeting, during which they reviewed exactly what was being done and kept answering questions until everyone was satisfied (Scanlon, Conlin et al., 1984).

Sometimes the most effective way to reach specific groups in a community is by identifying the leaders of those groups, whether in religious or social organizations or perhaps leaders in the business community. This may be especially important for reaching immigrant populations. Sometimes it is also possible to reach those who do not speak English through their children who do speak English and can be approached through the schools. Teachers may be aware of which families have language problems and which parents may be seen by others as leaders in a specific community. Coroners have learned that when sudden death occurs it is important to have knowledgeable contacts in the community so that ethnic sensitivities will not be inadvertently offended. Emergency planners need to do the same.

When an incident occurs, it is common to make special arrangements for next of kin. After the Swissair crash in Nova Scotia, the Canadian Admiral in charge—the plane crashed into the ocean—decided to be as transparent as possible. He visited the Lord Nelson Hotel, where most relatives were staying, and met with the families every day, told them what was going on, and what would be released. No information was given to media before families were informed. When United States Navy underwater cameras secured pictures of the tangled wreckage, the tapes were shown first to the families, then, with their support, made public. The families were also kept informed on a daily basis by the medical examiner and individual families were notified when a family member was identified. The Swissair response team set up a Web site, and posted information on that Web site, including visuals such as the underwater photos as soon as they had been shown to the families. Families could update themselves by logging onto the Web and there was a readily available public record of everything that had been released.

Similarly, on 9/11 when many trans-Atlantic flights were diverted to Canada's Atlantic Provinces, the authorities realized stranded travelers would want to contact relatives by phone and by e-mail. In Gander, the telephone company installed a bank of phones outside its offices (the weather was excellent) and managed to bring in and install an extra telephone tower so that there would be sufficient capacity for cell phones. Shelters made certain that there was access to the Web. A group of executives from the Rockefeller Foundation actually ran their affairs working on line from a school in the village of Lewisporte. Because the travelers were in schools, churches, camps, and other facilities in several different locations, Gander also used its town Web site to provide information as quickly as it could. For example, it posted information about each departing flight so those waiting could see what was happening (Scanlon, 2002a).

Another way to deal with communication in crises is to establish call centers where members of the public can call to clear up their own personal concerns. These proved extremely effective in Ottawa Carleton during the 1998 ice storm. Every phone call to the region was answered and those answering were briefed hourly to make sure they had the latest information. In addition, those handling the calls noted the questions they were being asked. If it appeared a particular question was being asked continually, the information requested was covered at one of the twice-daily news conferences. The same sort of approach was taken in the Toronto area during the SARS outbreak. Some agencies establish call centers for the media, hoping, in this way, they can make certain the media are well informed. These call centers do not provide new information but they do guarantee that media personnel are up-to-date on what has been said (Scanlon, 1998b). These are now standard when the Centers for Disease Control in Atlanta deal with health emergencies.

NEWER MEDIA

There is a perception that mass communication began with the advent of radio and television. It actually started long ago. Daniel Dafoe in his novel *A Journal of the Plague Year* reports, no doubt quite accurately, how news of the plague reached London:

> We had no such things as printed News Papers in those days to spread Rumours and Reports of Things; and to improve them by the Invention of Men, as I have lived to see practis'd since. But such things as these were gathered by Letters of Merchants and others, who corresponded abroad, and from them was handed about by Word of Mouth only; so that things did not spread instantly over the whole Nation, as they do now. (Dafoe, 1969, p. 1)

The flow of news, however, speeded up with the telegraph and telephone. When a French munitions ship exploded in the harbor of Halifax, Nova Scotia, on December 6, 1917, the news spread across that province just as fast as news of the Kennedy assassination spread across the United States nearly half a century later. This occurred because of the efficiency of the railway telegraph system—which linked every town on the railway—and because of the existence of rural "party line" telephones, which allowed everyone on a line to listen in on someone else's call. The "party line" was in effect a rural broadcasting system.

Incidentally, research on diffusion of news shows that news of truly major events—including ones of local importance—travels quickly and accurately and that much of it travels by word of mouth. For example, in Port Alice, a small mill town on the west coast of Vancouver Island, word of a threatening mudslide raced through the town even though Port Alice has no local radio yet alone TV. Similarly, news of rioting in Detroit spread extremely quickly by word of mouth despite a media blackout (Singer, Osborn, and Geschwender, p. 44).

Of course, the newer means of communication are also playing a role in the way information is shared:

- When a British Midlands aircraft crashed and blocked the M-1 auto route North of London, one vehicle in the subsequent traffic jam was an NHK Japan television satellite unit. It immediately uplifted visuals and sent them to Tokyo. The news thus reached Asia before it spread in England.
- On 9/11, when passengers on a hijacked aircraft used their cell phones, they learned that other aircraft had also been hijacked and had been used as missiles to attack the World Trade Center. On the basis of that information, they managed to force their plane to crash into a field instead of its target.
- In 2005, when the tsunami struck Indonesia, Sri Lanka, India, and Thailand, there were almost immediately reports humming around the world on the World Wide Web. There were also comments on the warning system or lack of it and on the problems in specific areas. Some of those affected used mobile phones to call Europe. Several foreign ministers got first word of the catastrophe by phone calls from Thailand and they got those calls before their embassy knew what was happening and well before the story broke on BBC News or CNN.

Today many Web sites known as blogs are targeted for specific communities and specific parts of communities. There is, for example, even a guide to blogs for New York City organized by subway line and stop. This map shows two blogs—"Sam's L.J." and "Tangled in the Web"—at the Old Town stop on Staten Island. If there was an emergency in that area it would be wise for someone to monitor those blogs in order to make sure any information posted was accurate—or quickly corrected—and to see whether there was information on the blog that had been missed.

Another modern communications system that needs to be included in emergency plans is the Amber Alert. At present, it is used for missing persons, especially children. But it could be equally important if there is a need to warn motorists of a toxic threat or that they may have been exposed to a toxic threat. In past incidents, persons transporting contaminated victims have become disoriented as they themselves began to breathe in the toxic fumes.

And the potential keeps growing. Tom Clancy's novel, *The Bear and the Dragon*, portrays a Chinese attack on Russia being picked up in detail on UAV (unmanned aerial vehicle) drones, relayed by satellite to Washington, and then released onto the World Wide Web so that Chinese could see what was happening on their individual laptops. It is not a far-fetched idea. In fact, it was suggested recently that similar drones could be used by America's enemies for biological or chemical terrorism. Anyone at any time can log on to his or her home computer and watch the incredible number of earthquakes that are continually occurring off North America's West Coast. Most are relatively minor but if the big one hits it will be possible to have watched it on a laptop. The day this section was written, there were three minor earthquakes in the San

Francisco area. That information can be accessed within seconds; so there is no way it can be concealed from the media.

Despite all these developments and the fact many incidents affect those far removed from the impact area, news of some events is still slow to spread. The incident at Chernobyl on April 26, 1986, for example, even though it led to 31 deaths, 150 hospitalized with radiation sickness, and an evacuation of 130,000 persons, was not known world wide until scientists in Sweden and Finland began to notice unusual levels of radioactivity. Even then there was skepticism. The Swedes, for example, evacuated one of their own nuclear plants before they realized something must have happened elsewhere (Scanlon, 2001, p. 1). Eventually, most of Europe and North America recorded increased radiation, especially if elements from Chernobyl passed while it was raining.

DISCUSSION

If the mass media are to be useful before, during, and after a disaster, it is important that officials understand what media exist, what audiences they serve, when they are broadcasting, and how they can be reached. (This includes knowing how to reach off-duty personnel with the authority and the knowledge required to get a radio or television station on the air when it is normally not broadcasting.) It is especially important to know if some local media provide ethnic programming or broadcast in a language other than English. And it is important to know where there are concentrations of ethnic groups or language groups so a sensible decision can be made as to whether particular media are important in issuing a warning or providing public information in the wake of a disaster. Finally, it would be wise to have someone ascertain whether local media have backup power and the other resources they need to continue to operate in an emergency.

It is far more likely that the desired cooperation will be given if contacts with the various media are made well before incidents occur and if material is prepared and tested before it is needed. It would make little sense to have an announcement in Spanish read by someone who was not well liked in the Spanish-speaking part of the community. It would be far better still if there was a sustained effort to involve all media in disaster education so that the media and their audiences are aware of threats and what to do if those threats materialize. One of the tragedies of the recent tsunami was that coastal water receded before the tsunami struck but very few recognized the significance of this warning sign. Perhaps the best way to develop such education programs is to schedule them on a seasonal basis, especially where the threats come on a seasonal basis. In other words, hurricane-related education would best be started just before the beginning of the annual hurricane season.

Such an education program should start by making sure that various audiences, including school children, are taught about the community's disaster history, about the threats that face that community, and about the appropriate response to each threat. (Different threats may call for a different response: going to the basement for shelter might make sense for a tornado; it would not for a flood.) At the same time, the public and the media should be taught about human behavior in disaster and made aware of the myths that exist. This is especially important for the media because it might reduce the probability of faulty reports. Tied to such public and media education must be an explanation of why in the early stages of a widespread destructive incident, no one in emergency agencies will know precisely what is happening. Emergency response initially involves catch-up because rationale decisions cannot be made without adequate information—and gathering that information takes time, especially if roads are blocked with debris and telephone and radio systems are down or overloaded.

Of course, if officials are going to make contact with specific groups they need to know not only how to reach those groups but also what is the appropriate way to make contact. They also need to be sensitive to things that might be acceptable to one group but unacceptable to another. And they need to know if a group is cohesive or split into segments. (Early in my research career I asked a person who spoke a particular language to make contact with a source, unaware that the country those two came from consisted of two distinct and antagonistic groups.) As part of the preparation, it is essential that census data be reviewed to ascertain what language and ethnic groups exist in a community and how things are changing over time.

It is also becoming increasingly important that some members of any emergency response team have sophisticated computer skills. These will be needed to monitor the various Web sites including relevant blogs, to post information on the Web, and to make certain errors are promptly corrected no matter where these occur. Such skills are also essential if a community is to keep its own Web site up-to-date and expand it if an incident merits that.

MEDIA SPECIALISTS

It makes sense even for a small community to have someone involved in emergency planning who understands how media operate. This might well be someone from local media, ideally someone nominated by the media community. In larger communities, there needs to be a public information specialist who can advise officials on dealing with media. A media specialist should develop policies and procedures for special media relations problems and explain those to the persons who will have to implement them. For example, persons in shelters should be guaranteed privacy but arrangements should also be made so that anyone willing to talk to the media can do so. Similarly, plans need to be put in place to deal with relatives of those who are killed or seriously injured in an incident. There must be some place for them to stay and some arrangements to guarantee them privacy.

Perhaps the specialist can also consult with the person running the call center about the way inquiries are to be answered. If a call center is created, inevitably some journalists will pose as ordinary citizens and ask questions about what is going on. The answers from the call center staff need to be the same as the ones being given to the media. Call center staff also need training and ideally some experience at answering public inquiries. Experience shows that some persons are not at ease in such a position.

In Ottawa Carleton during the January, 1998 ice storm call center staff noted the kind of questions that were being asked and advised those at the Emergency Operations Centre (EOC) about these. They then discussed what sort of information needed to be made available to the public. At the same time, those in the EOC were receiving reports about problems in the community. The result was that the twice daily news conferences dealt with issues that people were concerned about:

- January 9 to 3 P.M. The Regional Fire Coordinator urges people to use extreme caution when either trying to heat or light their homes. We have already lost three homes in Ottawa-Carleton due to accidents with fireplaces and other heat sources. Never use a barbecue inside a building. Do not substitute one fuel for another as this can cause problems.

- January 10 to 3 P.M. Regional officials are advising that even without power, there is no present danger of frozen buried water pipes.... HOWEVER, if your home is without power and heat, and if the temperature inside the building goes down to zero or lower, you must start your water immediately to protect your plumbing from freezing.
- January 11 to 10 A.M. Hypothermia, food safety, and carbon monoxide poisoning remain the prime concerns of the Medical Officer of Health. We had three cases of carbon monoxide poisoning overnight due to fumes penetrating the house from the garage where a generator was running. The only reason these people survived was because of a detector. **Please do not run generators from inside buildings that are attached to living quarters.**

It is important that whatever happens and no matter how many outside media arrive to cover an incident, local officials remember that, when the incident is over, they will still have to deal with local media. And it is the local media that will write the editorials and host the hot line shows that may determine how the public feels about the way the emergency was handled. In Peel Region, during the Mississauga evacuation, the police provided special help for local media, even helping a weekly newspaper to move equipment so it could continue to publish.

When there is no proper planning, the job of dealing with the media is often passed off onto someone who has no media relations experience and is not well informed about what is going on—or is given to the mayor of head of council, because those persons are used to dealing with the media. Neither decision is necessarily a good one. The media can be an important asset in an emergency. They can assist with public education. They can make a warning effective. They can keep people informed throughout a crisis. But they can also create pressures that make officials feel uncomfortable and can perpetuate myths and spread rumors. That is why dealing with the media requires someone trained for that role, someone who is comfortable in front of a camera and microphone.

In today's sophisticated world, dealing with the media also requires a fair amount of knowledge about a community as well as significant technical skills. Unless someone understands the composition of the community—especially its ethnic and language makeup—messages may fail to reach significant groups. Unless someone understands how information is transmitted and consumed over the Internet and how such things as blogs work, inaccurate information will remain uncorrected. The media can be a useful ally in disasters but they can also be an unwelcome irritant. Which it is may be determined by how much preparation has gone into media relations planning.

SUMMARY AND CONCLUSIONS

The media can clearly be a major asset before, during, and after emergencies. They are crucial in fact for effective warning, for warnings must come from all possible channels at the same time. They are often the main way those in an impacted community learn what is happening, especially if they are forced to leave their homes. They are the single best way to get out public information to a mass audience and can be crucial if rumors are to be stopped. Yet they are also the main purveyors of disaster myths because they focus on emergency agencies and officials and ignore the role played by individuals. Yet in most destructive incidents, the initial response is by individuals and not by emergency personnel.

Although there is now a fair amount of literature about the role of the media in disaster, there is little research comparing what actually happens in a disaster to what the media report.

There have been attempts to analyze media content, for example, to see if myths are present, but such research has a serious weakness. One cannot establish whether media are accurate in what they report without knowledge of what has happened. What is badly needed is a study of what the media report during an incident tied to a study of what actually happened or, perhaps, as a starting point, an attempt to document what the media reports and check to see its accuracy. The few general studies that have been done in this area tend to show that the average news report contains factual errors and that many of those inaccurate statements are not tied to any source. It might also be helpful if it were possible to arrange to do participant observation study to observe how a reporter covering a disaster operates. There is also still room for case studies of media operations. The decision of the New Orleans television stations to relocate before Katrina stuck was a superb chance to see how the media performed in a major catastrophe.

CHAPTER 25

The Popular Culture of Disaster: Exploring a New Dimension of Disaster Research

GARY R. WEBB

In January of 2002, just 4 months after the tragic terrorist attacks on the World Trade Center in New York, the President of the United States delivered the annual State of the Union address. That speech contained chilling words about life in the post-9/11 era. Specifically, the President (2002) said, "The last time I spoke here, I expressed the hope that life would return to normal. In some ways, it has. In others, it never will."

Is it possible for a single event to permanently alter social life? And, if so, how has that event changed things? Does everybody perceive those changes in the same way? Is there agreement or disagreement on the desirability of those changes?

These questions point to an important, but not always appreciated, point about disasters—that they have a significant cultural dimension. Looking across the landscape of popular culture, disasters are everywhere. Television news media flock to the scenes of major disasters and provide around the clock coverage of human suffering. Film producers make millions of dollars on special effects-laden tales of man against nature. Investigative television shows look into the causes of a single disaster or attempt to rank the devastating impacts of numerous events. Cable networks allow those interested to keep continual tabs on weather developments and offer viewers periodic recollections of past storms. And apocalyptic video games give people the chance to save an entire city from complete and utter ruin.

Following catastrophic events, survivors and responders also engage in a wide range of cultural production. They tell jokes and share stories about the events. Buildings are spray-painted with graffiti to convey messages of hope, humor, or frustration. New rituals are enacted to provide order and meaning to their lives, including those surrounding the handling of the dead. Makeshift memorials are created to allow survivors the opportunity to share their emotions and remember those they lost. And poems and songs are written in efforts to make sense of what happened.

Clearly, disasters are important cultural events. But should social scientists spend their time studying movies, graffiti, and jokes? The assumption of this chapter is that they absolutely should study these things. Over the past 50 years, we have learned a great deal about the structural aspects of disasters, but our knowledge of their cultural dimensions is far less developed and somewhat scattered.

Thus, the primary objective of this chapter is to make a case for exploring the cultural dimensions of disasters. In discussing what will be called the popular culture of disaster, this chapter reviews a range of studies from different disciplines, all of which deal in some way with culture. The chapter is organized into five sections: (1) a review of the structural bias in disaster research, (2) a discussion of the cultural strain of disaster research, (3) a conceptualization of the popular culture of disaster and a review of relevant studies, (4) a rationale for studying the topic, and (5) a discussion of future research possibilities in the area.

THE STRUCTURAL BIAS OF DISASTER RESEARCH

Social scientists in the United States first began systematically studying disasters in the 1950s (Quarantelli, 1987a, 1994). Findings from their studies have been summarized at various times over the past 50 years (Drabek, 1986; Fritz, 1961a; Kreps, 1984; Quarantelli & Dynes, 1977; Tierney, Lindell, & Perry, 2001). In sum, researchers argue that various conventional images of disasters—including chaos, panic, looting, and social breakdown—are stereotypes and myths (Fischer, 1998a; Quarantelli, 1960). Instead, empirical studies consistently demonstrate that human societies are remarkably resilient in response to large-scale crises.

In studying the social aspects of disasters, researchers have assumed that such events provide real-world laboratories for examining basic social processes (Fritz, 1961a). Specifically, they have explored the relationship between social structure and disaster (Kreps, 1989c). And in that equation they have for the most part treated social structure as a dependent variable—that is, they have examined the impacts of disasters on social arrangements. Dynes (1970), for example, developed a typology to capture the various ways in which organizations alter their structures and tasks to meet heightened demands created by disasters. Similarly, but at a different level of analysis, Kreps and Bosworth (1993) have documented the impacts of disasters on role systems.

The structural bias of disaster research makes sense when one considers the intellectual climate in which the field emerged. During the 1950s, structural functionalism dominated the discipline of sociology in the United States (Turner, 1986). That approach views society as a system in which various parts must work in concert to ensure the successful performance and survival of the larger system. According to this model, a disruption to one part has ripple effects throughout the entire system. Disasters, then, represent a type of disruption that has potentially debilitating effects on the social system. Reflecting on the pervasive influence of functionalism at the time, Fritz (1961a, p. 655) defined disasters as, "... an event, concentrated in time and space, in which a society ... incurs such losses ... that the social structure is disrupted and the fulfillment of all or some of the essential functions of the society is prevented." This definition, which views society as a system of interrelated and interdependent parts, is clearly derived from structural functionalism, and it continues to guide a substantial amount of research in the field today.

In recent years, disaster researchers have increasingly turned toward conflict and political economic perspectives to guide their work (Stallings, 2002c; Tierney, 1989), but even these studies tend to emphasize structure over culture. However, instead of treating social structure as a dependent variable, researchers are beginning to view social structure as a causal force—that is, an independent variable—behind disasters. They point out that organizations

play a significant role in creating disasters (Tierney, 1999) and that race, class, and gender stratification places some people at greater risk than others (Enarson & Morrow, 1998; Fothergill
& Peek, 2004; Fothergill, Maestas, & Darlington, 1999).

Beyond the intellectual influences on disaster research, there are other factors that may
help explain the structural bias of the field. Because the military funded the earliest studies, the
area has had a strong applied orientation from the beginning. Early on that meant producing
research that would improve the military's understanding of what might happen in the event
of an enemy attack (Fritz, 1961a). Today, that means conducting research that helps various
local, state, and federal agencies better respond to disasters. While this applied orientation
is important and valuable, some critics contend that it has impeded theoretical development
and resulted in a managerial bias—that is, a primary concern with improving the efficiency of
response agencies (Bolin and Stanford, 1998).

On the basis of this discussion, it is clear that important intellectual and applied influences
have shaped the field of disaster research. Those influences have combined to produce a
structural bias, which has been both productive and limiting. On the positive side, we have
learned a great deal about social system responses to disasters—namely, that those responses
are organized, not chaotic. However, our understanding of the cultural dimensions of disasters
is far less developed.

THE CULTURAL STRAIN OF DISASTER RESEARCH

Within the discipline of sociology, culture is beginning to occupy a more prominent position
(Bonnell & Hunt, 1999). For example, rather than focusing on Durkheim's (1984) structural
analysis in *The Division of Labor in Society*, scholars are paying much more attention to the
role of culture and rituals highlighted in *The Elementary Forms of Religious Life* (1995). Neo-
Marxists, such as Habermas (1975), argue that social change comes about not just from changes
in the economic base but also from the cultural life world. And Weber's (1958) *Protestant Ethic
and the Spirit of Capitalism*, which showed the powerful role of cultural beliefs in shaping
human history, continues to be popular.

Various subfields in sociology have also taken cultural turns recently. For example, scholars in the field of social movements focused for years on organizational structures, resources,
and political opportunities, but now they are more likely to emphasize symbols, cultural
framing, and collective identity in their analyses of protest (Johnston & Klandermans, 1995;
McAdam, McCarthy, & Zald, 1996; Tarrow, 1998). Similarly, sociologists who study organizations now talk about "organizational impression management" and other cultural dynamics
(Giacalone & Rosenfeld, 1989).

While the field of disaster research has not fully made a cultural turn, it is moving in
that direction. And there is a historical basis for that move. Indeed, there is an important,
but to some extent ignored, cultural strain of disaster research. As Nigg (1994) points out,
symbolic interactionism exerted a strong influence on the field's development. That perspective
characterizes society as fluid and emergent, and it emphasizes the importance of symbols,
meanings, and the definition of the situation. Given that symbolic interactionism has its roots
at the University of Chicago and that the first field studies of disaster were conducted by
researchers there, it is not surprising that this perspective has influenced the field.

Unlike the functionalist perspective, which emphasizes social structure, the symbolic
interactionist view recognizes the importance of culture. Reflecting that concern, Fritz (1952,

p. 2), a pioneer of disaster research, wrote in an unpublished paper, "The folklore ... of every society reflects the powerful role that disasters have played in the life of the people." He goes on to point out that in every society disasters have provided one of the most dominant themes in art, music, folk tales, and other cultural products. Thirty years later Quarantelli (1985, p. 32), a member of the first disaster field teams at Chicago, similarly observed, "... that another major source of beliefs about disasters is derived from popular culture." He then described popular culture as including television programs, films, novels, comic books, and other cultural products disseminated through the mass media.

Thus, although the field of disaster research has a strong structural bias, it also has a noticeable cultural strain running through it. And in recent years, a number of scholars have been adding to it. For example, a recent special issue of the *International Journal of Mass Emergencies and Disasters* was devoted to the popular culture of disaster (Webb, Wachtendorf, & Eyre, 2000). In addition, several books focusing on the cultural dimensions of disasters have been published in the last few years (Biel, 2001; Browne & Neal, 2001; Hoffman & Oliver-Smith, 2002; Webb & Quarantelli, 2006).

There is clearly something of a cultural turn occurring in disaster research. As the field makes that turn, it is important to get some grasp on what has already been done and develop conceptual tools to guide future research in this burgeoning area. Thus, the next section offers a conceptual view of the popular culture of disaster and reviews relevant empirical studies that have been published over the past few years.

CONCEPTUALIZING THE POPULAR CULTURE OF DISASTER

While most people are likely to have some sense of what the popular culture of disaster is, the boundaries of the new area are still somewhat unclear. For research purposes, though, it is important to develop some guiding ideas as to what should be considered under this topic. Because disaster themes are prevalent across a diffuse range of cultural products, it is difficult to frame specific research questions without at least a generic definition of the popular culture of disaster. To develop that definition both deductive and inductive approaches can be taken. In the former case, one would start by spelling out even in general terms what the popular culture of disaster is and then researchers would go out and conduct studies that fit into that framework. In the latter case, one would develop the concept on the basis of various studies that have already been done. Ultimately, perhaps the best way of getting a better grasp on the concept is to employ both deduction and induction.

Thus, from a deductive approach, we could begin developing an inventory of cultural products with disaster themes and delineating some specific dimensions along which those items vary. As Quarantelli observed in an e-mail message in 1998 (cited in Webb et al., 2000), the popular culture of disaster includes—but is certainly not limited to—such things as disaster jokes and humor, board games and puzzles with disaster themes, folk legends and beliefs about disasters, disaster calendars, songs and poems created at times of disasters, disaster predictions (e.g., the Iben Browning earthquake prediction) and reactions to them, disaster novels and films (including spoofs of the latter), disaster anniversary newspaper issues, Great Flood myths, on-site graffiti, memorial services of certain kinds, cartoons and comic strips with disaster themes, and disaster apparel (e.g., t-shirts, hats, and buttons).

While this type of inventory is an important preliminary step in defining the topic, the next step is to formulate a systematic definition. At a very general level, for example, we can distinguish between material (e.g., books and movies) and non-material (e.g., jokes and myths) products. We can also distinguish between the cultural products of disaster survivors (e.g., graffiti), and those things that are produced by mainstream cultural workers. Similarly, we can distinguish between those cultural items produced in the immediate aftermath of a disaster event and those that are produced, distributed, and consumed via more traditional means (e.g., disaster movies). Therefore, a formal definition of the popular culture of disaster must capture the following four dimensions: (1) a characterization of the product itself, (2) the identity of its producer(s), (3) the timing of its production, and (4) the means by which it is distributed and consumed.

An inductive approach to conceptualizing the popular culture of disaster begins with empirical observations. Based on that approach, it is necessary to survey the studies that have already been done on the topic. While the existing studies on the topic are varied and scattered, it is possible to separate them into at least two broad camps. One camp consists of those studies that assess the impacts of disaster events on some aspect of culture—that is, like the earlier work on social structure, they treat culture as a dependent variable. The other camp approaches culture as an independent variable, examining the role of cultural beliefs and practices in contributing to or exacerbating disasters.

Numerous studies in recent years have focused on the cultural impacts of disasters. For example, researchers have studied the emergence of humor in the wake of disasters (Couch & Wade, 2003) and its use as a coping strategy among emergency workers (Moran, 1990). They have assessed the impacts of disasters on collective memory (Bos, Ullberg, & Hart, 2005) and the emergence and meaning of post-disaster memorials (Eyre, 2006; Imai, 2002). Research has been conducted on the varieties of graffiti that often appear in disaster-stricken communities (Hagen, Ender, Tiemann, & Hagen, 1999). It has also looked at the role of women's quilting groups in making sense of disasters (Enarson, 2000b). And several studies have documented the broader cultural impacts of recent terrorist attacks (Abrams, Albright, & Panofsky, 2004; Stein, 1999; Turkel, 2002).

In addition to research on the impacts of disasters on culture, a growing body of work focuses on the ways in which culture puts people at risk. For example, research suggests that disaster movies perpetuate various myths that alter people's perceptions of risk and understanding of protective measures they should take (Bahk & Neuwirth, 2000; Mitchell, Thomas, Hill, & Cutter, 2000; Quarantelli, 1985). Research has also pointed out how cultural and religious beliefs sometimes impede communities from taking proactive steps to prevent future disasters (Schmuck, 2000). Importantly, several recent studies argue that cultures that exist in bureaucratic organizations produce mistakes and disasters (Adams & Balfour, 1998; Hopkins, 1999; Richardson, 1993; Vaughan, 1999). These organizations often value profit over safety, misperceive risk, and produce "fantasy documents" that give the public the sometimes misleading impression that things are under control (Clarke, 1999). Even "high reliability organizations" that are purported to have deeply entrenched safety cultures have serious shortcomings (Sagan, 1993).

Based on this discussion, it is clear that disasters have an important cultural dimension. Disasters impact culture, and culture contributes to disasters. It is also clear from this discussion that the field of disaster research has begun to take a cultural turn. While other fields of study have gone much further down that path, disaster research is building momentum. And, as the studies reviewed here demonstrate, the cultural path is worth pursuing. The next section provides a rationale for paying closer attention to the cultural side of disasters.

RATIONALE FOR STUDYING THE POPULAR CULTURE OF DISASTER

In terms of a rationale for studying the popular culture of disaster, there are important conceptual and applied reasons for this type of research. At a conceptual level, work in this area should sharpen our understanding of popular culture more generally and inform ongoing debates about the role of elitists and locals in the production of culture. In an applied sense, popular images of disaster are likely to shape people's knowledge about disasters and how they respond to them—not just members of the public but also those working in emergency management, law enforcement, and other governmental agencies. Thus, it seems worthwhile for those who study disasters to gain a thorough and systematic understanding of how disasters are interpreted in a variety of contexts.

The conceptual value of studying the popular culture of disaster may not be obvious to some, but it is substantial. In the broader areas of social and cultural theory, the concept of popular culture is treated in two vastly different ways (Mukerji & Schudson, 1991; Storey, 1998; Traube, 1996). Some theorists, on the one hand, consider popular culture to be synonymous with mass culture, and they view it in very negative terms. Drawing on the concept of hegemony (Gramsci, 1971) and the idea of a culture industry (Horkheimer & Adorno, 1996), they view popular culture as something that is produced by society's elitists to control and appease the masses. Control is exerted by influencing people's understanding of public issues, shaping the tastes and preferences of consumers, and silencing genuine political debate (Habermas, 1994; Mills, 1963). Appeasement is accomplished by using entertainment to divert people's attention away from important social problems and political concerns. In light of this rather cynical view, theorists in this tradition regard popular culture as a major threat to participatory democracy.

Some theorists, on the other hand, view popular culture as something that is produced by common people for themselves (Williams, 1983). This view, which emerged relatively recently, represents a major paradigm shift in the field of cultural studies. McGuigan (1992, p. 4), for example, refers to this new approach as cultural populism, defined as "the intellectual assumption, made by some students of popular culture, that the symbolic experiences and practices of ordinary people are more important analytically than Culture with a capital C." From the perspective of cultural populists, culture is produced from the bottom-up not top-down. While "mass society" models emphasize elite ideological control, populists view culture as something that is locally produced and empowering.

Since its inception disaster research has contributed to our understanding of basic theoretical issues (Fritz, 1961a; Kreps, 1985). In light of the two divergent views on popular culture summarized here, there is an opportunity for disaster researchers to contribute to an important and long-standing theoretical debate. While studies of the popular culture of disaster may not resolve the debate, they will certainly shed light on it.

On the one hand, for example, research on disaster movies affirms the cynical view of popular culture. These movies, which are very popular and generate millions of dollars, are produced by powerful and wealthy elitists who have vested interests in the status quo. And they often perpetuate harmful stereotypes about race, class, and gender. On the other hand, survivor-produced culture is very different and affirms the populist model. Disaster survivors often use graffiti, for example, to convey messages of hope and humor or express grievances about the official response. Unlike disaster movies, which are preplanned, carefully produced, and strategically distributed, graffiti is emergent, spontaneous, ephemeral, and publicly displayed.

Based on these examples, the popular culture of disaster can be interpreted from both mass society and populist perspectives.

There are also important applied reasons for studying the popular culture of disaster. Whether one is concerned with disaster preparedness, response, recovery, or mitigation, the role of culture must be understood. In some instances, such as in the case of "disaster subcultures," culture serves as a source of resilience for local communities (Wenger & Weller, 1973). However, in other situations culture contributes to disasters.

Arguably, the greatest impediment to effective disaster response in the United States is the perpetuation of disaster myths, even among those in the emergency management profession (Fischer, 1998a; Wenger, James, & Faupel, 1985). These myths suggest that disasters create chaos, panic, looting, and other antisocial behavior—that is, complete social breakdown. Of course, 50 years of social science research demonstrates that the opposite occurs in the wake of disaster—crime rates go down, solidarity increases, and pro-social behavior prevails. If communities are actually resilient under stress, why do so many people, including public officials, believe they are so fragile and susceptible to collapse?

Tierney (2003) argues that disaster myths have survived because powerful institutional interests benefit from them. In particular, the military–industrial complex, law enforcement agencies, and the growing information technology industry all stand to profit from the erroneous beliefs that civil society is vulnerable, that individuals faced with crisis are irrational and need to be controlled, and that the most effective way to respond to a disaster is by establishing a strong hierarchy of command and control. Tierney's assessment of the situation is particularly astute in light of recent changes at the national level in the area of emergency management. With the creation of the Department of Homeland Security (DHS) after 9/11 and the placement of the Federal Emergency Management Agency (FEMA) within it, critics feared that the move would undermine FEMA's autonomy and weaken its ability to respond to disasters in a timely and effective manner. Those fears proved valid in 2005 when Hurricane Katrina struck the Gulf Coast and left residents of New Orleans stranded on rooftops for days before the federal response reached adequate levels.

Culture is also an important factor in disaster preparedness. For example, research has long suggested that disaster warnings need to be clear and consistent, come from a credible source, provide clear instructions, and reach a diverse audience (Tierney et al., 2001). Yet, in response to the attacks of 9/11, one of the most devastating disasters in U.S. history, the federal government developed a warning system that is seriously flawed (Aguirre, 2004). Rather than clarifying the nature of the terrorist threat and providing citizens specific instructions to make themselves less vulnerable, the color-coded alert system has created substantial confusion and ambiguity.

Mitigation is another area in which culture plays a significant role. At the most general level, consider the competing and potentially contradictory values of safety and profit in capitalist societies. In making decisions about safety federal, state, and local governments make trade-offs in determining which measures are feasible and which are too costly. While some politicians may place a little more emphasis on safety, profit is a highly cherished value in capitalist societies. For communities to become safer, then, a change of values will have to occur. Thus, Mileti (1999) advocates a cultural shift in which sustainability, not merely profit, but becomes a guiding value. In a recent article about the 9/11 attacks, Mitchell (2003) identify another threat to disaster mitigation: terrorism. He describes a cultural shift after 9/11 in which preparedness and response to terrorism became top policy priorities at the national level, overshadowing mitigation for natural hazards. The consequences of this shift became apparent to everyone when Hurricane Katrina struck the Gulf Coast.

Based on this discussion, a case can easily be made for studying the popular culture of disaster. Conceptually, disaster researchers have an opportunity to contribute to important debates about the role of culture in society. And in an applied sense, research in this area provides insights that can be used to improve disaster preparedness, response, recovery, and mitigation. The next section discusses some possible areas of future research.

FUTURE RESEARCH ON THE POPULAR CULTURE OF DISASTER

Having discussed what the popular culture of disaster is and having provided a rationale for studying it, this section of the chapter suggests some possible directions for future research. As the field develops, it will surely benefit from studies on a diverse range of topics conducted by scholars from various disciplines. While there are numerous directions the field could go, this section will discuss five potentially fruitful areas of investigation. Specifically, future research should address: (1) prominent cultural symbols and their preservation, (2) the rhetoric or framing of disaster, (3) the persistence of disaster myths, (4) the production of culture in consensus and conflict events, and (5) the impact of cultural representations on disaster research.

Every society has prominent symbols in which great pride is taken because they embody core values and commemorate notable accomplishments. Capital buildings, monuments, skyscrapers, museums, and other cultural artifacts are highly valued and deeply cherished assets, but they are vulnerable. Tornadoes, hurricanes, and earthquakes are capable of destroying them. And, as the attacks on the World Trade Center revealed, they can become targets for terrorists. Despite the prominence and vulnerability of these cultural objects, very little social science research has been conducted in this area (Quarantelli, 2002). In the humanities, some important applied reports have been published on how to preserve books, photographs, and other collections (Norris, 1998; Ruzicka, 2002b). Social science research could further shed light on how to protect and preserve important cultural symbols by studying, for example, disaster preparedness levels among museums, libraries, and other repositories. In their studies, researchers could identify various factors associated with higher or lower levels of preparedness. Certainly, there is still a need for research on emergency management organizations, police and fire departments, and other response agencies, but we also need studies of those organizations that exist to protect and preserve important elements of culture.

When disasters occur, people interpret them in different ways. Some people view disasters as the result of divine intervention. Others regard them as failures of government. And still others see them strictly as natural phenomena. Given this diversity of views, it is clear that disasters are social constructs (Larabee, 2003; Stallings, 1995). The post-disaster time period is a contested terrain in which various groups (victims, the media, and public officials) attempt to make sense of the event. In some cases, there is agreement on what happened, and in other cases there is conflict and disagreement. As Dove and Khan (1995) suggest, the way a disaster is socially constructed matters. If an event is defined as unforeseeable or beyond human control, it is not likely that corrective measures will be taken to prevent future occurrences. Thus, future research should place a much greater emphasis on the rhetoric and framing of disasters.

Disaster myths persist despite 50 years of social science research. The myths suggest that disasters produce social breakdown, while research consistently points to the resilience of human societies. For years, researchers have argued that the most effective response to disaster is one that is decentralized, flexible, and based on realistic assumptions of human behavior under stress. Yet, as Dynes (1993) points out, many public officials subscribe to a "command and control" ideology that promotes the centralization of authority, implements rigid structures, and makes inaccurate assumptions about how people respond to disasters. As discussed previously, Tierney (2003) argues that the perpetuation of disaster myths benefits certain powerful groups in society. It was also discussed previously that these myths have led to significant changes at the federal level with FEMA becoming a part of DHS. Clearly, disaster myths, an aspect of the popular culture of disaster, matter. Thus, it is time for researchers to take a fresh look at an old topic—namely, the sources, content, and consequences of disaster myths.

For many years, researchers have made a distinction between consensus and conflict events (Quarantelli & Dynes, 1977). On the one hand, natural and technological disasters are considered consensus events because there is general agreement that the impacts are undesirable and a response is necessary. On the other hand, wars, riots, and terrorism are considered conflict events because they create disunity. Importantly, some researchers argue that technological disasters are in fact conflict events because they have negative, corrosive impacts on communities (Couch & Kroll-Smith, 1985; Cuthbertson & Nigg, 1987; Erikson, 1976; Freudenburg, 1997; Picou, Marshall, & Gill, 2004). Thus, there is an important question to be asked: Do natural disasters, technological crises, wars, and terrorism produce similar cultural responses or do they differ in important ways? While some researchers argue that the response to the 9/11 terrorist attacks resembled a natural disaster in the immediate aftermath (Webb, 2002), others suggest that the longer-term impacts may be quite different (Marshall, Picou, & Gill, 2003). There is clearly a need for more research on the social and cultural impacts of various types of disaster events.

While it is important for researchers to examine how the popular culture of disaster has impacted society, they should also reflect on how it has impacted their own area of study. It has been established that disasters are social constructs—that is, the media, politicians, victims, and other groups decide what is and is not a disaster. With the emergence of national media conglomerates and the loss of many local outlets, the disasters typically covered today are those with national and international implications. Events that are smaller in scale with primarily local impacts simply do not get covered. The important question is: Do disaster researchers primarily study those larger events that are defined as disasters by the media? These questions are not abstract; rather, they are empirical. In every field of study, it is necessary to periodically reflect on what has been studied and what has been neglected. Disaster research is no exception.

Having described several possible areas for future research, something should be said about research methodology. In conducting studies on the topics described here and others, researchers have at their disposal a wide range of data sources and methodological techniques. As Phillips (2002) describes, disaster research has historically relied a great deal on qualitative research strategies, including observations, interviews, and document analysis. Because these approaches yield thick and rich descriptions of social reality and allow the researcher to better understand the worldviews of those being studied, they are essential to the study of the popular culture of disaster. However, as Bahk and Neuwirth (2000) demonstrate in their study of the impact of disaster movies on risk perception, quantitative methods can also be effectively employed to study the cultural dimensions of disaster.

As research in this area continues to grow, researchers should also consider the time dimension. For decades, disaster researchers have conducted "quick response" studies, in which they enter the field as soon as possible after an event occurs (Michaels, 2003). This is a useful strategy because it enables researchers to gather important data that might perish or disappear quickly. Given the emergent and ephemeral nature of some disaster culture products, this type of research will continue to be important for the field. However, longitudinal research is also needed. As described earlier, the attacks of 9/11 have certainly impacted American culture, and they have resulted in significant policy changes at the national level in a variety of areas, including emergency management. It is possible that those changes will endure, or they may be reversed at some point. Longitudinal research is valuable because it enables researchers to track changes over time.

In studying the popular culture of disaster, researchers must embrace a cross-cultural perspective. Although globalization has resulted in some degree of cultural leveling or ho-mogenization, there is still a great amount of cultural diversity across the globe. Both non-material culture—that is, beliefs and values—and material culture—that is, tangible products— vary from society to society. Moreover, technological capabilities differ across societies. In developed societies, for example, the widespread use of cellular telephones, the inter-net, and electronic communications impacts the way in which culture is produced and the speed at which it is disseminated. Thus, the cultural impacts of disasters would be different in developed countries compared to other societies. The broader field of disaster research has been biased toward studying developed Western nations, but there is an opportunity here to correct that bias. By focusing explicitly on the cultural dimensions of disasters, re-searchers will find it necessary to think about their subject in a comparative, cross-cultural perspective.

This section of the chapter suggested some possible directions for future research on the popular culture of disaster and discussed some important methodological considerations. There are many ways in which the area may develop, so at this early stage it would be most beneficial if researchers proceeded with an open mind, adopting a flexible rather than rigid view of the topic. While we have already learned a fair amount about the cultural dimensions of disasters, there is still much work to be done.

CONCLUSION

Disaster movies, graffiti, and myths may seem trivial and inconsequential, but they are not. Rather, they are essential elements of cultural life. Culture shapes the way people view the world, how they live, what they value, and what they do. It is ubiquitous and pervasive. Therefore, it is impossible to study any aspect of social life without also studying the influence of culture.

The primary objective of this chapter has been to make a case for studying the popular culture of disaster. Social scientists have learned a great deal about human response to disaster over the past 50 years, particularly in terms of social structure. They have shown, for example, that societies are resilient to disasters in large part because elements of the social structure (e.g., organizations) become flexible and adaptive in responding to extreme events. They have also revealed ways in which stratification within the social structure (e.g., race, class, and gender) makes some groups more vulnerable to disasters than others.

However, researchers know far less about the cultural dimensions of disasters. There has always been a cultural strain running through the field, but it is less developed than the structural side. In an effort to promote further work on culture and disaster, this chapter provided some thoughts on what the popular culture of disaster is, a conceptual and applied rationale for pursuing the topic, and some suggested research directions.

In concluding this chapter, an important point needs to be made. To call for more research on the cultural dimensions of disasters is not to say that research on their structural aspects should be abandoned. Indeed, recent disasters, including the 2004 tsunami in Asia and Hurricane Katrina in 2005, have made it abundantly clear that much remains to be learned about effective organizational response to disasters and social vulnerability to them. The central point of this chapter is that the field of disaster research will greatly benefit from an approach that pays adequate attention to both social structure and culture.

CHAPTER 26

Remembering: Community Commemoration After Disaster

ANNE EYRE

Those who cannot remember the past are condemned to repeat it.
——George Santayana (1863–1952)

On August 21 2005, Prince Charles led national commemorations in Britain marking the defeat of Japan in World War II 60 years earlier. A series of events on this day and over the previous months highlighted the value and significance of communities remembering the war, not only for the past, but also for the future. Like other forms of mass fatality incidents, including disasters, these events and their marking have become an important part of the history and identity of past and present communities, not only in Britain, but throughout the world. An indication of the function of commemoration both in relation to war and other events is reflected in a comment made that day by the British Armed Forces Minister Adam Ingram, who stated that these events had encouraged veterans to talk about their wartime experience, some for the first time, and pass on their own family's story to younger generations giving them the opportunity to keep these memories alive (BBC News, August 21, 2005).

This chapter explores key issues associated with the nature, meaning, and purpose of community remembrance following disaster. First the historical roots of the study of death rituals within anthropology, sociology, and psychology are reviewed. This is followed by a discussion of traditional and changing expressions of grief and remembering after disaster, from spontaneous to more organized displays. The symbolic and social meaning of activities associated with body recovery, identification, and disposal are briefly examined, along with analyses that suggest that religion and rituals might reflect both community consensus and conflict. The political nature and role of remembrance activities is highlighted in a review of the development of official memorials service and other anniversary events. Finally, the involvement of communities in the establishment of permanent memorials is discussed as an example of a move towards the increasing empowerment of those affected by disaster. It is suggested that in the future, opportunities for individuals and communities to take control of their own recovery might be enhanced through greater control over the organization and ownership of remembrance activities, including through use of the Internet and the work of disaster action groups.

POST-DISASTER RITUALS: ANTHROPOLOGICAL AND SOCIOLOGICAL ROOTS

The study of communal remembering is linked to the studies of the social recognition of death and associated rituals which generally can be traced back to anthropological and sociological roots at the beginning of the twentieth century. Ethnographers such as Arnold Van Gennep (1960) became interested in the general patterns of ritual in societies celebrating changes in social status and position. The rites of passage he discussed included those marking the physical and symbolic transition from being alive to being dead, these states being both biologically and socially defined.

The sociologist Emile Durkheim (1915) developed the study of collective ritual in relation to their integrative effects and the ways in which they bind communities together. For him, and later sociologists such as Parsons (1971) and Bellah (1975), religious rituals were an expression and affirmation of collective ideals; thereby they functioned to reflect, sustain, and legitimize the social and moral order of society. Such Functionalist approaches to ritual are relevant to our study of post-disaster rituals in so far as they reflect and endorse a sense of family and community, expressing and reinforcing a shared sense of meaning and understanding, even if that sense of order and meaning has been temporarily suspended at a time of shock and loss. Following disaster, when a fundamental sense of order and security can feel threatened, the potential value of such rituals in reestablishing feelings of control, belonging, and social solidarity within and beyond one's immediate community is understandable.

These anthropological and sociological approaches to the study of ritual as symbolic actions make an important link for disaster researchers between the physical or biological status of death and the social. They highlight that in considering the nature and meaning of disaster rituals, we need to look at their deeper significance and purpose, and the transition they mark between one state of individual and social being and another. They suggest that disaster rituals might also be as much about social and political identity and change as about individual expressions of loss, change, and status. As we will see, commemorative activities after collective tragedy are indeed often accompanied by social and political commentaries on a broader change of state and status for a family, community, or society, for example, from being "innocent" to tarnished, broken or damaged; from being "safe" and resilient to "unsafe" and vulnerable. They can suggest and echo a sense of things never feeling or being quite the same again.

RITUALS, GRIEF AND MOURNING

The anthropologist Paul Rosenblatt links the social function of death rituals with the psychological importance of grieving when he suggests that proper grieving involves engaging in certain rituals and being able to think, feel and do certain things (1997, p. 43). A further context for the study of post-disaster rituals is thus provided by studies of grief, mourning and bereavement, including those emanating from the fields of psychology, counselling and psychoanalysis. The notion of "grief work" engendered in these disciplines follows from the classic study of mourning and melancholia pursued in 1917 by Sigmund Freud (1984). The notion of mourning as a process has been developed in relation to identified stages or phases of grieving, as reflected in the series of mourning "tasks" outlined by writers such as William Worden (1982). More recently, as our understanding of trauma has increased, researchers in this field have also reinforced the significance of social support for those who are traumatized, including the value of social responses to death, grief, and mourning embodied in rituals. The significance of social acceptance and support in either helping or hindering psychological recovery is illustrated in the works of writers such as Judith Herman as we shall see later.

By extension, the lack of ritual and collective expression following death has often been regarded as an impediment to successful grieving and recovery. In 1965 Gorer suggested that the apparent lack of ritual in contemporary Western societies made grieving more difficult. In contrast to this, some have suggested more recently that British society has become stricken with "mourning sickness," addicted to showy displays of empathy because it is a lonely and unhappy society (West, 2004, p. 7). What both approaches recognize, however, as reinforced by Rosenblatt, is that grief is fundamentally a social process: "Many Westerners think of grieving as an individual action, and much of grief therapy is individually focussed. Yet the mourning rituals of many societies are complex, elaborate, spread out over months or years, and generally require collective participation" (1997, p. 43).

Building on a range of disciplinary backgrounds, therefore, the study of ritual and remembrance following disaster can be more fully enhanced by drawing on from both individualistic and collective intellectual perspectives. Indeed within disaster studies the sociologist Kai Erikson has made a valuable connection between psychological, anthropological, and social approaches in his writings on the human experience of modern disaster. From his analyses of communities afflicted by collective tragedy, he has highlighted two types of disaster trauma, namely individual trauma ("a blow to the psyche that breaks through one's defences so suddenly and with such force that one cannot respond effectively") and community trauma ("a blow to the tissues of social life that damages the bonds linking people together and impairs the prevailing sense of community" [1994, p. 233]). Rob Gordon has developed this analysis of the effects of emergencies on social fabric and the practical implications for recovery strategies (2004).

The study of post-disaster rituals that follows draws on this approach in acknowledging both personal and communal elements of disaster impacts and responses. The meaning of "disaster" as applied in this chapter embraces a wide range of events, causes and consequences, from "natural" disasters such as the Asian tsunami (2004), to humanly caused incidents of multiple deaths, including terrorist acts. They include incidents that, according to some definitions or agency protocols might not be considered "disasters" as such, but in relation to agency responses and the extent to which they are "major incidents" either operationally or in terms of their extensive communal impact, are relevant to our analysis here. They all share in common the fact that they involve trauma and communal expressions of grief and mourning.

SPONTANEOUS EXPRESSIONS OF GRIEF

Despite Gorer's lamentations forty years ago about the decline of ritual, within Western societies such as Britain symbolic expressions of grief following sudden death appear to be increasing rather than diminishing. According to West, "today's three Cs are not, as one minister of education said, "culture, creativity and community," but rather, as Theodore Dalrymple has put it, "compassion, caring and crying in public" (2004, p. 1). Spontaneous expressions of grief are now the rule rather than the exception following sudden, tragic death in, for example, fatal road crashes, acts of murder and disasters.

Today, with advances in technology and the growth in immediate media interest through "twenty-four hour news," disasters become headline stories and publicly owned virtually as they happen or very soon after. In many instances, following the first news stories, people start to gravitate toward disaster-stricken communities and places to express their shock and grief. Flowers, candles, toys, and other mementoes are often left at such disaster sites and associated focal points as these forms of convergence become management challenges for those tasked with organizing disaster response and recovery. Personalized tributes may take the form of poignant messages left with such memorabilia and, as disaster response becomes more formalized, facilities may be provided for visitors to contribute through organized books of condolence.

An example of such spontaneous outpourings of grief was the response in the first week following the Hillsborough Disaster of 1989. Following the deaths of 96 Liverpool fans at the Hillsborough Stadium in Sheffield, England, more than a million people visited Anfield, Liverpool's home ground, to lay flowers and place written tributes. On the day after the disaster the media reported how some visitors had left flowers at Liverpool's famous "Shankly Gates." Soon the club had to open the gates and admit the thousand of visitors who started queuing to leave their own tributes at the ground. This ritual continued during the following week of official morning in the City. Of the first week I wrote:

> By five o'clock the Kop end of the ground, where home supporters always stand, had become a shrine bedecked with flowers. The visitors continued to arrive from all over the country over the next seven days of official mourning, queuing for hours in silent solemnity. The field of flowers gradually grew towards the centre of the pitch, whilst the concrete steps behind the goal were transformed into a carpet of scarves, pictures and personal messages. Scarves were also hung on the metal barriers, many of which became dedicated to the fans that stood behind them week after week. School friends penned the names of their lost classmates on the walls outside the stadium. These messages expressed personal and communal grief as much, if not more, than any of the official ceremonies could have. For many people, visiting Anfield—Liverpool's home ground—brought their grief to the surface. (Eyre, 1989, p. 12)

CONNECTEDNESS IN LIFE AND DEATH

Analyzing the social impact of this community tragedy, Walter makes the point that the communal grief at Anfield seemed different from the fragmented grief following the major train and plane accidents that had happened in Britain in the preceding 12 months, incidents that between them had claimed more than 300 lives. With each of these, Walter states, most of those who had died were strangers to one another. The grief, he suggests, was the same, but how could it be shared? What Anfield showed was that "where there is connectedness in life, there is connectedness in death—even in the late twentieth century" (1990, p. 70). Walter noted that the City of Liverpool has both a uniquely strong sense of communal identity and an identity symbolised by football, so "a footballing tragedy attacks the city's very heart" (1990, p. 69).

The aftermath of Hillsborough was not the first time such large-scale spontaneous grief was witnessed and broadcasted via the media in Britain and in a way that reflected the connectedness within a community's life and death. More than 20 years earlier, in 1966, the disaster in a small village called Aberfan had prompted a similar response. On October 21st, the last day before the half-term holiday, a waste coal tip suddenly slid down the side of a mountain overshadowing the small mining community in South Wales and engulfing the village school and all within the vicinity. 144 people perished, including virtually a generation of its schoolchildren. The sense of national and even international grief was huge, as demonstrated in the convergence of gifts, money and flowers sent to the community and in the continuing media interest in the plight of the village's survivors. Of the initial response Miller wrote,

"Flowers were sent from all over the world and the Director of Parks and Cemeteries laid them out in a giant cross on the hillside, 130 feet high with arms 40 feet across" (1974, p. 29).

At Aberfan, as elsewhere, the extent of tragedy is often symbolically expressed in the number and status of official visitors to the scene within the first few days. In South Wales this included a visit by the Queen and other dignitaries. In 1996 at Dunblane, a small Scottish town where the shooting of 16 children and their teacher in a primary school caused widespread national shock and revulsion, the Prime Minister and leader of the Opposition appeared together in the community within days of the tragedy, a symbolic gesture made all the more meaningful by its proximity to political elections. Sometimes, however, the attendance (or not) of a national dignitary can cause upset in communities where relationships within or with outsiders are already fractious. In Liverpool following Hillsborough, the Prime Minister Mrs. Thatcher was not a welcome figure given preexisting tensions between local and national governments in the years prior to the disaster.

Emergency managers responding in the initial days and weeks of an incident often find themselves involved in organizing the itinerary, security and media management of such visitations, including public statements of shock and sympathy as well as visits to the injured in hospital. There can be a feeling that such time and energies might be better used in dealing with the more important tasks associated with dealing with other aspects of the disaster. Yet such symbolic appearances are important because they demonstrate the political dimension of disasters, not least through their being an opportunity to display political leadership, the demonstrative sincerity of pubic officials and their social solidarity and support for the vulnerable and victimized.

SEARCHING AND IDENTIFYING: A PHYSICAL AND EMOTIONAL ACTIVITY

Bereavement writers have identified searching behavior as a characteristic reaction to the feelings of numbness associated with sudden loss. In his classic study of bereavement, Parkes (1972) identified patterns of "yearning and searching" in behavior such as calling out to the dead one or misidentifying someone in the street. Only once the reality of the loss is accepted, it is argued, can the bereaved begin to move gradually through grief to recovery.

In the aftermath of disasters, where there may be large numbers of people missing and there are difficulties in identifying for certain who has been killed, searching behavior is also a physical activity. In these initial days and weeks of shock, disbelief, and denial, searching becomes an understandable activity and one that becomes also the preoccupation of the authorities managing the incident.

In the aftermath of the terrorist attacks of September 11, 2001, for example, many thousands of tons of rubble were removed in the search initially for survivors and later to recover and remove the dead. In the days after the disaster walls around the city were covered in posters and photographs of those missing. These were expressions initially of hope and ultimately remembrance. Friends and families gathered at these and at help centres set up in New York in the hope of tracing their loved ones. For very many, the search for a surviving loved one increasingly became a search for information, for reassurance that they did not suffer and for a body to prove that they had really gone.

In the days and weeks after the Asian tsunami struck on December 26, 2004, similar scenes were broadcast through the media of survivors and bereaved relatives scanning photographs outside makeshift mortuaries. As with September 11, one of the features of mass fatality events such as these is the extensive period of time it takes to complete search and recovery tasks as well as the painstakingly slow process of identification. More than 20 international teams have been involved in trying to identify victims and send their body's home. In August, 2005, officials in Thailand stated that it could take 3 years to identify everyone killed in Thailand during the tsunami (BBC News, August 22, 2005). The possibility of identification following mass fatality incidents and the return of bodies or body parts to loved ones is now not only more possible, owing to the development of sophisticated identification techniques such as DNA, but also increasingly expected by those bereaved and those responding to disaster.

BODY RECOVERY AND MANAGEMENT: REPERSONALIZING THE DEAD

The need to find, identify, name, and officially dispose of the dead is in part a symbolic activity, the mark of a civilized society that seeks through great effort to ensure individual treatment of each body. Blanshan and Quarantelli (1981) have discussed this symbolic element in the process of handling victims in terms of "a person-to-object-to-person transformation of the dead" (1981, p. 275). The overall process of body recovery, transportation, clean-up, identification, and disposal goes beyond a purely practical approach to dealing with the dead. The fact that the living wish to treat the dead as persons feeds the expectation that safety, rescue, and relief personnel will at least locate, if not retrieve, dead bodies as quickly as possible. The overall process of body recovery and management thus reflects a process of "personalization," the turning of dead bodies into "respected, although dead persons." Society insists that disaster victims be treated as "persons, not bodies" (1981, p. 275).

Recent guidelines on the management of dead bodies in disaster situations issued by the Pan American Health Organization (PAHO) reinforce this by recognizing and including these sociocultural and psychological considerations into what traditionally have been regarded as predominantly and technical operational activities. They emphasize the significance of body recovery and return for ritual and the proper disposition of bodies, stating that the inability to perform rituals condemns a family to "a second death": the symbolic death of their loved one for "the lack of a tomb that perpetuates his or her name and confers social worth to the deceased and his or her inclusion in the generational continuity of a family" (PAHO, 2004, p. 85).

In line with this, PAHO recommends against the use of common or mass graves. They go so far as to suggest that mass burial or the use of mass cremation is both unnecessary and a violation of the human rights of surviving family members (2004, p. 171). In some circumstances, however, such recommendations are clearly ignored; the response of the authorities following the Asian tsunami of 2004 is but one illustration of this. In this case, differing cultural beliefs and practices about the right approach to death and disposal has caused additional upset to some bereaved families, particularly where they are then also denied the chance for an inquest and repatriation.

RELIGION, RITUAL AND REMEMBRANCE

Initial spontaneous expressions of grief are often accompanied by increased attendance at religious places in the immediate aftermath of communal tragedy. Even in traditionally secular societies and among nonpracticing individuals, latent religious beliefs can become important and overt at such times. Following the sinking of the Estonia ferry in 1994 with the loss of over 800 lives, mourning prayers were said on Swedish radio. In what was commonly thought of as one of the most secular societies in Europe, the government immediately declared an official mourning period and, by the first evening, more than 500 churches had opened for prayers and for people to enter, sit, and reflect and light candles. The Swedish Archbishop was interviewed on national television, which also broadcast the official mourning service live. Reflecting on this, Pettersson (1996) suggested that at such times, implicit religious sentiments in society became latent and explicit.

In some cases, religious communities can combine their spiritual roles following disaster with practical ones relating to relief efforts. One example of this was a candlelight vigil held in a London church 2 weeks after the tsunami, to which people of all religions and cultures were invited. As well as offering prayers, and the opportunity to light a candle, attendees were invited to drop off donations of money, dried and tinned food, medicines such as paracetamol, and toiletries to be delivered to stricken communities in Sri Lanka. Similarly, donations of aid were coordinated through other places of worship, including one Buddhist temple where piles of donations reached almost to the first floor (BBC News, January 8, 2005).

It also appears that places of worship can become a focus for solace and silent reflection, whether spiritual or not, in communities directly affected by tragedy. Some might regard the quiet solace of such places as a form of sanctuary away from the prying eyes of the media and other convergers that make up the multitude of emergency responders to an area, many of whom will respect the sacred space of a church or cathedral and its symbolic significance as a focal point of community sentiment and grieving. Indeed local churches became such a central reference point after both the tragedies at Dunblane and Soham, England (where two schoolgirls were abducted and murdered; this was declared a major investigation and was regarded as a national event since the girls were missing for a number of weeks and the search became an ongoing national news story throughout this time). The focus on the churches at the center of these two communities helpfully detracted some attention away from the schools involved in both these events.

In terms of a Functionalist analysis, the unifying role of commemorative reflection at religious places of worship is apparent here. Perhaps this is an example of the sort of the "honeymoon" period often referred to post-disaster, when usual communal conflicts are temporarily suspended. An example of putting usual lines of social division aside was the opening of St Anne's Cathedral, Belfast (traditionally a religiously divided community) for commemorative activities in memory of those who died in the Asian tsunami 10 days earlier. Describing its purpose, the Presbyterian Moderator Ken Newell stated that it offered "a sacred space where people can stop and think." He added that such a crisis puts the suffering of others high on our agenda by "shifting people two or three centimetres towards holding other parts of the world in our hearts" (BBC News, January 5, 2005).

Social analysts focussing on the more divisive nature of society however, might be more likely to focus on the potentially conflictual role of political and religious ideologies and symbolism, both before and after disaster. In the aftermath of the London bombing incidents in July 2005, the link between terrorism and Muslim extremists led to fears of a backlash against Muslims worshipping at local mosques. Following reports of attacks to mosques in various parts of the country, Church leaders pledged to stand by Muslim colleagues, saying terrorism affects all communities. The political dimension of these incidents and their aftermath was reinforced in a letter to written to mosques by Sir Iqbal Sacranie, head of the Muslim Council of Britain, who said that unscrupulous elements of society, including in the media, were already using the London attacks as a means to undermine the position of Muslims in

British society. At the same time, the ongoing aftermath of the threats from terrorism and the recognition that innocent members of the community might be vulnerable to attack has enhanced cooperation and unity between multifaith leaders. Following the July attacks, the Home Secretary Charles Clarke met Sir Iqbal and other faith leaders to devise a plan to protect Muslims or other minorities in the wake of a bomb attack. The plan involves close liaison between Muslims and other faiths, principally churches and Jewish communities (BBC News, July 11, 2005).

Where religious differences preexist in communities, these can be reflected in disagreements and conflicts focussing on the organization, content, and symbolism associated with post-tragedy rituals and commemoration. In Littleton, Colorado, following a tragedy where two schoolchildren opened fire and killed a number of their peers at Columbine High School in 1999, disagreements about the appropriate ways of commemorating the event reflected denominational divides. Conflict erupted over issues including the question of whether a memorial garden of trees should include trees for the perpetrators themselves. Later the families of the two dead students sued the school for failing to install ceramic tiles, which the families designed as memorials to their murdered children. The families claimed Columbine High School officials asked them to create the tiles, but then refused to install them because of their religious themes (Jones, 1999).

REMEMBERING IN SILENCE

An increasingly popular way of ritually commemorating disaster is through observing periods of planned silence, a tradition which is centuries old. According to West (2004), France lays claim to inaugurating this tradition to honor its fallen heroes in the nineteenth century, but it gained wider cultural currency the following century. Example of ceremonial silence include those throughout the United States to mourn the sinking of the *Titanic* at noon on April 16, 1912. West recounts how soon afterwards, the two-minute silence to remember those who had died in the World War I was introduced in 1919. For most of the twentieth century in Britain, the minute's silence was observed on sporting occasions, normally to remember the death of a national figure or someone connected to the club. Meanwhile the two minute silence was reserved to honor those who had died fighting for their country (2004, p. 19).

West is critical of the apparent increase in both the number and lengths of periods of silence that have become part of the ritual commemoration following collective as well as significant single cases of sudden death. Such episodes are certainly frequent and extensive. On New Year's Eve 2004, two minutes' silence was observed just before midnight as a mark of respect to those who died in the Asian tsunami. Five days later thousands of people across Europe stopped what they were doing again to remember the victims. This included countries such as Sweden which by then was known to have lost 52 of its citizens, with a further 2000 missing. Typical of such periods of silence, in many European cities public transport stopped, flags were flown at half mast, and radio and television stations paused programs for the midday tribute. The three-minute silence was observed in places "ranging from the Monaco palace to Norwegian oil platforms." (BBC News, January 5, 2005). In some societies such as Sri Lanka, additional commemorations and silences were held one month on.

Two months later, a five-minute silence was held in Madrid at midday on March 11, in memory of the train bombings a year earlier in which 191 people were killed. A few days after this, leaders of nations across the continent led people in a further three-minute silence for the victims. This had been proposed by the Irish Prime Minister Bertie Ahern, president of the European Council, who called on all EU states to show solidarity with Spain. The demonstration took place at a time when there were calls across the continent for greater cooperation between countries in fighting terrorism. In this way the opportunity for commemorative acts to be appropriated for political use is evident.

On July 14, 2005, one week after Europe had again witnessed a series of terrorist attacks, a two-minute silence in memory of those killed and injured was once more held across Europe and other parts of the world. This included British and Australian tourists who joined local people in Bali for a candlelit ceremony at Kuta, scene of the terrorist attacks in 2002, and people in the three U.S. states directly affected by the September 11 attacks who also observed the silence. In Afghanistan too, soldiers from the multinational force paid silent tribute, with British, Afghan, and American flags in Kabul flying at half mast. Following the developing trend, there are likely to be periods of silence again at the official memorial service for "7/7," at the opening of the inquest and at significant anniversaries.

CONSPICUOUS COMPASSION OR
COLLECTIVE COMFORT?

West sees this extension in silences as symptomatic of the "conspicuous compassion inflation" he feels all are compelled to participate in, a compassion that is suffering from inflation, with individuals and organizations "seeking to prove how much more they care by elongating the silences" (2004, p. 20). This, he suggests, is a reaction to the minute's silence being practised so frequently: "It is as if by extending these periods, there is competition to prove who is more empathetic" (ibid).

Others, however, see different meanings being conveyed in the language of silence. The day after the London silence, the leader in *The Times* newspaper gave a vivid description of what it described as a "moving display of public unity" and suggested that the bombers had failed in their plans to divide the community and the country: "A nation was united in grief, determination and common humanity." The emphasis was very much on the strength of "collective comfort," of a "shared vision" and of a "common future" (*The Times*, July 15, 2005).

It is not merely the demonstration of compassion that West deplores, but the sense of compulsion to participate in it. Those deviating from the observance are likely to be vilified, to feel the anger of the crowd. Thus West criticizes the cultural phenomenon he sees as feeding on mob mentality and the desire for conformity: "It betrays the hallmarks of a society not 'in touch with its emotions' but one that is intolerant of dissent" (2004, p. 22). While others might not go as far as West in suggesting this is close to being a form of fascism, there have been other critics of such imposed silences. The Conservative Party vice-chairman, Roger Gale, described the European three-minute silence after the tsunami, as "the worst kind of gesture politics," adding that the U.K. public did not need a "state-imposed" silence to express their feelings. (BBC News, January 5, 2005). The Member of Parliament's disdain seemed not just to be about the imposition but also about its timing, it being the wrong initiative at the wrong time: "There will, certainly, come a time when a proper memorial service and silence of an appropriate length might be held but that time is not now." Further, he was quoted as saying that some self-styled world leaders—including the prime minister—had shown very little leadership when it had been needed in the preceding days. Once again, commemoration became linked with political opportunism.

MAKING IT OFFICIAL: FORMAL
MEMORIAL SERVICES

The political role and context for remembrance is perhaps most explicitly illustrated in the organization and conduct of official memorial services, particularly those that are regarded as national events. Formal memorial services often follow some time after the initial aftermath of communal tragedies, allowing for a more extended period of planning and organization. Their location, formality, and content symbolize the sense, scale, and significance of communal loss. In England, for example, official memorial services take place in local cathedrals or parish churches, with events marking disasters of national significance being held in London and attended by key national dignitaries.

In the United Kingdom the government has become increasingly invoked in formally organizing official memorial services. As civil emergency management in Britain generally has become more formally organized, guidelines for dealing with disasters have been developed and refined by the Government (Cabinet Office, 2003) and other organizations. These include references to memorial events and other post-impact services. In part this reflects a broader cultural shift over the last 20 years or so in favor of increased recognition of the needs and rights of the bereaved and survivors and their wish for participation in commemorative acts and rituals.

This is not unique to Britain; in the United States, for example, the Family Assistance Act (1996) has gone so far as to legally require airline companies to complete plans and, in the event of a disaster, to organize memorial services as part of their emergency management function. These additional memorial services in the first few days and weeks after disaster might be more privately focussed opportunities for families than official government-led services; however, they can add to the range of both private and public sets of rituals that follow in the wake of disaster.

In Britain in 2005, a new Disaster Response Unit has been established within the Department of Culture, Media and Sport. Though rather inappropriately named, this Department was originally tasked with preparing for Princess Diana's funeral and has since played a role in arranging for commemorative services following the Bali and September 11 terrorist attacks as well as the official memorial service at St. Paul's Cathedral in London after the 2004 tsunami.

Cabinet Office guidelines highlight the purpose of such official memorial services and planning implications, stating that a memorial service provides an opportunity for those affected to share their grief with others. They also emphasize how it often has an important national as well as local role and is likely to receive extensive media coverage. For these reasons they suggest it is important to consider the organization and structure carefully, covering such aspects as "timing, invitations, representation and conduct" (Cabinet Office, 2003, paragraph 4.59).

As well as the list of official invitees, decisions made about issues such as where dignitaries sit in relation to the bereaved and survivors have symbolic meaning and political consequences. The presence or lack of representation by figures such as senior politicians or members of a royal family might potentially cause resentment and further distress given the significance attached to participation. This is especially so given the charged emotional atmosphere of such events. At the same time, where numbers of attendees are restricted, extended family members and survivors can often be left feeling aggrieved and excluded, particularly where the invitation of dignitaries is prioritized over direct victims left to observe on the streets outside or on television. It is understandable that they can be left asking who and what the commemoration is really for.

ANNIVERSARY EVENTS

In the same way as formal memorial services conducted shortly after a tragedy fulfill both psychological and social functions, so do anniversary events. They mark the passage of social and chronological time as well as the impetus and long journey toward community rehabilitation and recovery.

Despite the Latin origins of the term, "anniversary" events have now started to extend to ritual displays marking the first week, the first month, and even 6 months' time lag following disaster. This is partly a media-driven activity, but at times it can also reflect the cultural and religious significance of dates. In line with Buddhist tradition, which says that the dead should be honored 100 days after their passing, ceremonies were held for 3 days along Thailand's west coast to mark 100 days after the tsunami hit that part of the region(BBC News, April 4, 2005).

Tom Forrest suggests disaster anniversaries entail an interactive process in which people share personal experiences. Public officials, he says, make "decorative comments" while the press and electronic media "reconstruct the disaster experience" by recording current thoughts and reflections. Disaster anniversary, he concludes, is a process of "collective remembering" (Forrest 1993, p. 448).

The first anniversary after disaster is often particularly significant, well attended and marked by the mass media and wider community. Indeed, even during the first few days following the Ladbroke Grove rail disaster in London in 1999, a television crew began filming pictures to use in a special coverage to be broadcast on the first anniversary. On that day a series of memorial services took place at key sites, including the car park next to the crash site, at Paddington rail station (close to the accident site) and at Reading Minster (the focal point of a local town which one of the fated trains passed through).

Similarly the first and subsequent anniversaries of the tragedies following the September 11 attacks on the United States received much national and international coverage. In Britain, the loss of U.K. citizens was marked on the first anniversary by an elaborate service at Westminster Abbey attended by a number of senior royals and other national leaders. Families were consulted and included in both the planning and conduct of the service, including the symbolic lighting of candles for the dead. Beyond Westminster, a further array of dedicated services reflected the extensive impact of the disaster on communities such as national sporting teams, the airline industry and financial sectors.

While Spain and other countries united to remember the victims of the bombings on the first anniversary in March, 2005, some survivors boycotted the events, complaining of political interference. The Association of Madrid Bombing Victims protested that that pain of victims and relatives had been used as a political football. According to Graff (2005), Pilar Manjón, president of the Association of 3/11 Victims who lost her son in the bombing, had implored parliament some months before "not to use the pain of the victims for party ends."

Commenting that many of the victims have steered clear of the public ceremonies on the anniversary, Graff stated the reproach was apt, since the parliamentary investigating commission had spent months discussing the dramatic political aftermath of the bombings rather than the police and intelligence failures that allowed them to happen. On March 14, three days after the attacks, the Popular Party had lost a general election it had been expected to win. It subsequently blamed the Socialist victors for exploiting the atrocities, widely seen by Spaniards as the terrorists' retribution for the former government's support of the Iraq war. Graff reports that the Socialists' response was to suggest that the Popular Party undermined its own credibility by insisting the attacks were the work of the Basque separatist terrorist group ETA (Graff). According to Manjón, the commission "focussed on what happened between 11 March and 14 March. Nothing could be further from the interests of the victims" (BBC News, March 15, 2004).

By way of illustrating the commemoration of significant anniversaries, on September 25, 2004, a memorial service to mark the tenth anniversary of the Estonian ferry disaster was held in Dartford, Kent. This town had been linked with the Estonian capital, Tallinn, since 1992, and originally held a service immediately after the accident, in which 852 people died. The Estonian ambassador joined official representatives from the Foreign Office for the service of remembrance in the town. A candle was lit for each person that died and arranged around a ship's anchor, reflecting the original memorial in Tallinn.

Commenting on the honor felt by the town in hosting the memorial service, Council leader Kenneth Leadbeater said: "It will give us the opportunity to empathise with our friends and offer them our support on this sombre occasion" (BBC News, September 25, 2004).

REMEMBERING FOREVER: PERMANENT MEMORIALS

The importance of remembering the past is illustrated post-disaster in the erection and maintenance of permanent reminders of tragic events. War cemeteries are a classic example of this of course, but in other smaller scale events forms of permanent memorial serve similar functions—personal and collective remembrance as well as social testimony to events of the past. Disaster trust funds are sometimes used to finance permanent memorials. In Britain Charity Law dictates specific use of such money, including its use "for the benefit of the community." While some memorials are dedicated to other social functions, such as the building of a community hall, for example, others are more specifically dedicated in memory of those who perished.

At Aberfan, as elsewhere, the actual site of the disaster has been turned into a garden of remembrance reflecting the original layout of the school's classrooms. In sociological terms, such areas are "sacred" spaces, that is to say they are set apart as being of special significance and regarded as worthy of particular respect. Failure to respect such space and inappropriate use of a disaster site can lead to anger and outrage, as was the case at the site of the gas explosion in Bhopal, India which it was mooted might be the setting for a theme park some years after the factory explosion there which claimed many thousands of lives.

Reflecting sensitivity as well as the need for practical considerations surrounding permanent memorials, the trustee of the Bradford City Fire Disaster Fund wrote the following about his Committee's deliberations in deciding how to mark the mass death of many football fans at a fire in Bradford City's football stadium in 1985. He personally would have liked some kind of a garden which could be used as a place of peace for those who suffered. But the committee realized this had complications and would need to be maintained. The committee concluded that whatever shape their memorial took, it was important that it commemorated the generosity of people contributing to the fund. So in the end they agreed on a memorial plaque to be held in the safety of the cathedral. Suddards describes it as "a thing of beauty" that those affected by the disaster may come and see "in peace, quiet and privacy" (Suddards, Price, & Picarda, 1987).

Advances in technology and increasing use of the Internet have resulted in the development of virtual memorials following disaster in recent years. After tragedies such as the Columbine School shootings (1999) and the murder of two Cambridgeshire schoolgirls in Soham (2002), much use was made of this vehicle as a tool of commemoration and for the expression of grief. As discussed later, the use of the Internet to carry sites such as "We are Not Afraid" (http://www.werenotafraid.com/), with political messages of defiance to terrorists perpetrating mass atrocities has also evolved. This site also includes a page remembering the victims of the four attacks in London on July 7 with pictures and obituaries for those who died. Similarly, following the tsunami, a number of commemorative sites have been established by those directly affected. This includes Tsunami Stories, a site set up by and for survivors and the bereaved to give them a chance to tell their stories and share their pictures and messages (http://www.tsunamistories.net/).

COMMUNITY CONTROL AND CONSULTATION

These developments in commemoration are significant not only in terms of representing a changing form of remembrance, but also insofar as they also give control over the nature, design, and focus of commemoration to those directly affected by disaster.

It is increasingly recognized that the bereaved and survivors are key stakeholders to be consulted in planning the design and development of permanent memorials commemorating disaster. Of course, the greater the number of consultees, the greater the potential for disagreement and dissent and there are likely to be restrictions on what might be practical and feasible in the design, cost and location of a permanent memorial. Not only this, there can be huge symbolic and political significance attached to actual disaster sites, as illustrated in the long-running battle between architect Daniel Libeskind and leaseholder, Larry Silverstein over plans to rebuild on the foundations of the obliterated twin towers in New York.

A good example of community engagement in the planning of a permanent memorial is the consultation framework established in Canberra following the Australian bushfires in January 2003 which destroyed lives, homes, pets, and possessions. The notion of a permanent memorial was recognized as acknowledging a significant event in the history of the region and marking a milestone in people's lives. Consequently, a Bushfire Consultation Advisory Committee comprising community and government members was established to provide guidance on the project and assist in the consultation process with the broader community. In June 2004 a community consultation discussion paper was circulated and feedback invited as the basis for the development of a design brief for a memorial.

In January 2005, the winning design was announced. It will consist of two sites in Deek's Forest Park, with the opening planned for the third anniversary of the bushfires on January 18, 2006. Site 1 is marked by a gateway made from the community's salvaged bricks and will be framed by a grove of casuarinas. The area also contains red glass inserts to represent glowing embers. The second site, which focuses on the recovery rather than the event, includes an amphitheatre with a bubbling spring and columns containing details of photographs provided by the people of Canberra.

Residents involved in this consultation process had stressed that they wanted the memorial to be simple and natural—a quiet place to reflect and find peace (Gorman, 2005). Reflecting the value placed on community engagement and participation, the winning designers stated: "Contributions by the community will form an integral part of the final memorial which will gain its "heart" from community involvement and from the ongoing use of the setting" (artsACT, 2005).

As with the Bushfire example, permanent memorials may focus on the importance of looking forward as well as back to an event. "Remembering for the future" is a theme, for example, captured at the memorial dedicated to those killed at the Oklahoma City bombing in 1995. A National Memorial Institute for the Prevention of Terrorism is among the activities developed here. Also illustrative of a forward-looking approach, the regeneration and renewal of the centre of the City of Manchester, which was blighted by a terrorist bomb in 1992, was symbolically marked by the reopening of the City Centre on November 24, 1999. A parade of 50 drummers and flame-carriers led a procession before gathering in the square for street theatre and a fireworks display. Commenting on the revamped city and its new facilities, City council leader Richard Leese said the people of Manchester had waited for more than 3 years to regain their city centre, and nothing would keep them away from their city (BBC News, November 24, 1999).

REMEMBERING AS RECOVERY

The sorts of post-disaster ritual and symbolism discussed in this chapter are examples of ways in which individuals and communities may work toward recovery from the traumatic effects of disasters. Of relevance to the themes discussed here is the work of Judith Herman, who writes about the political context of trauma and comments on recovery requiring remembrance and mourning: "Restoring a sense of social community requires a public forum where victims can speak their truth and their suffering can be formally acknowledged" (1997, p. 242).

As Herman's quote suggests, recovery requires a sense of social community in which people feel supported in looking back and looking forward. She refers to events such as the Truth and Reconciliation Commission in South Africa, but her writing has implications for other types of post-disaster situations and remembrance. As family reactions to Commissions into the terrorist events on September 11 and March 3 and other post-disaster inquiries illustrate, it is important to stress that moving forward from disaster physically and symbolically is about more than acknowledging suffering and giving survivors an opportunity to tell their story through commemorative rituals. It is also about establishing legal and political processes to address objectively, openly and honestly the causes of events and the accountability of all involved. This is a necessary condition for the learning of lessons and mitigation of future risks. The passing of legislation on corporate responsibility in the United Kingdom in 2005, aimed at enhancing measures for addressing corporate killing, is an encouraging sign but there is more work to be done.

REMEMBERING: THE FUTURE

Despite the predictions of some commentators in the past, post-disaster ritual and remembrance remains vibrant in societies across the world. The forces of globalization are changing both the ways in which people experience disaster and the ways in which they respond to them. The growth in world travel means most disasters have an international dimension such that communities of more than one country are involved in grief and mourning rituals in the aftermath. The development of the media's coverage of disaster, as well as bringing about an increased sense of vulnerability, awareness and exposure to the traumatic impact of disasters, has led to increased participation in acts of remembrance and commemoration. The rise in access to and use of the internet has increased the capacity of people to communicate globally and is empowering individuals and communities—physical and virtual—to influence post-disaster agendas and activities. Commemorative and campaigning Web sites can be vehicles for this.

The trend in future-focussed commemorative activities is likely to persist. Today bereaved families and disaster action groups use windows of opportunity provided by public interest in inquests, investigations, and anniversaries to attract media interest and government attention to their plight, interests, and causes. Survivors create their own websites to assist them in telling their stories, uniting with others who have been through similar experiences and thereby taking control of their own recovery. More broadly there may be societal implications in terms of the potential for family support and victim-led action groups to use their experiences to campaign for changes to those conditions of society which might generate, prevent or mitigate the effects of disasters.

This chapter has highlighted that although expressions change over time and culture, some common aims and functions can be observed in post disaster rituals and remembrance. They are an important part of grief and mourning, helping to mark the transitions of time and status for individuals and communities. For those who are bereaved and/or survivors, remembering can be a focus for staying stuck or for moving towards a new normal. They can reflect and represent the connectedness between the living and the dead, and symbolize an important continuity between the past, present, and future. Collectively, they can generate social solidarity and unity while at the very same time reflecting and reinforcing political conflict and division.

Remembering is an inherently political activity, which can be manipulated for the purposes of socially constructing a community's past and the design of its future. However, the trend in some areas toward greater consultation and ownership within affected communities of post-disaster rituals and memorials, suggests this will remain a vibrant area for research and activity as disaster management and recovery evolves in the years ahead.

Future studies might focus on the dynamic relationship between the forces of religion secularization and modernity in relation to the changing nature of rituals after disaster and particularly on the impact of political contexts where religious ideologies are seen as playing a part in uniting or dividing communities in disaster and its consequences. There is also scope for comparative analysis of disaster management protocols, rituals, and commemorative processes across different types of societies and in relation to different types of disaster, such as those regarded as "natural" and those that are technological, and humanly caused, including those caused by deliberate acts of violence. Finally, research might explore further the potential or actual impact of human rights agendas on post-disaster ritual and response, including the extent to which victims are being empowered by evolving approaches to emergency management focusing on the right to basic standards of care, before, during, and after disaster strikes.

CHAPTER 27

Research Applications in the Classroom

BRENDA D. PHILLIPS

If disaster research is helping to spawn a new discipline as some suggest (Mileti, 1999; Phillips, 2005), then its work remains incomplete. For a new discipline to emerge, take shape, and become recognized as a substantive field of knowledge, research must infuse the writings and materials used in the classroom. The presumed benefits of doing so include legitimacy and acceptance within the academy (Phillips, 2005); professionalization that generates promotions, higher salaries, and social prestige (Neal, 1993); and more effective emergency management practice. As one practitioner illustrates, "Decision makers must rely on sound conceptual understanding of the community, established research findings, and data that have to be collected with systematic methods" (Rossman, 1993, p. 132).

However, despite considerable growth of emergency management (EM), hazards, risk analysis, and antiterrorism programs around the world (especially within the United States), few empirically based, scholarly textbooks exist. Publishers have not produced adequate research anthologies either, particularly at the undergraduate levels. It is equally questionable how extensively research has penetrated related disciplines and classes such as geography, sociology, and political science except as topical seminars. This chapter thus reviews the challenges and barriers to research applications in the classroom, examines select case examples from around the world of how research is being used, identifies and describes the contributions of efforts driving research applications in the classroom, and specifies necessary actions to change the situation. Thus, despite the pessimistic scenario outlined here, opportunities exist to further research applications in the classroom.

CURRENT RESEARCH APPLICATIONS IN THE CLASSROOM

Generally, research in the U.S. classroom is used in a variety of ways. At the undergraduate level, traditional approaches rely on empirical content summarized and translated into general textbooks. For the field of emergency management, textbooks options remain slim and/or dated, although a new version of the popular *Emergency Management: Principles and Practices* published by the International City Manager's Association (Waugh and Tierney, 2006) is underway. Revisions to this book are being made primarily by active disaster researchers albeit with overview by an advisory board composed of both academics and practitioners.

A more common way to integrate research into the emergency management classroom stems from faculty lectures. However, because so many students come from the practitioner community, some degree of skepticism must be overcome in order for students to accept lecture content (Dawson, 1993):

> That's not what I've always heard." Because it was not what we had always heard. We assumed the panic, looting and mass confusion were common place in disasters. Fortunately we have "seen the light."

The apparent predisposition of EM students to eschew research exists in emergency management practice as well. Mileti (1999, p. 328) surveyed 28 practitioners and "none reported receiving findings from academic journals," preferring e-mail and the Internet instead. Advanced undergraduate classes may incorporate research as required readings; however, an undergraduate-level compendium of articles remains unavailable. This unfortunate situation might result in a surprising economic benefit to a willing publisher given the rapid growth of EM programs in the United States.

Generally, graduate level programs typically rely on original research, particularly at the advanced master's and doctoral levels. Based on discussions with EM colleagues and observation at conference panels (in the United States and internationally), however, it is evident that many EM faculty attempt to meet both academic norms and practitioner needs by incorporating both research and technical guidance into graduate-level classrooms. This practice is probably appropriate given that a minority of students will progress into doctoral programs while the majority will return to or seek careers in the field.

REVIEW OF RELEVANT SYLLABI

Syllabi collections represent one starting point to examine the filtration of research writings into relevant classrooms. For the purposes of this limited inquiry, one set of voluntarily donated syllabi can be accessed at the U.S. Federal Emergency Management Agency (FEMA) Higher Education Project Web site (http://training.fema.gov/EMIWeb/edu—click on Education and Training tab). It should not be assumed, however, that these syllabi reflect the perspectives of FEMA; rather, they represent the perspectives of those faculty members willing to share their work with others. Further, these syllabi emanate primarily from emergency management-type programs and do not reflect how disaster research is (or is not) under use in discipline-specific classes. As such, they are not necessarily representative of the field but do offer a starting point for discussion. Syllabi date back to 1997 but do provide some insights into how research has been (or not been) used.

Any examination of available syllabi suggests several tentative conclusions given the delimitations just mentioned. First, it is clear that many EM educators are not using research extensively in the emergency management classroom. Faculty members at research-oriented universities appear most likely to use peer-reviewed articles than faculty at community colleges, in undergraduate programs, or at teaching-oriented institutions. Second, it is evident that a sufficient body of knowledge does not exist across the areas of inquiry or, at times, in appropriate contexts (Cole, personal communication, 2005). To illustrate, consider that the warning and response phase has been studied extensively while a topic like recovery remains underexamined (Mileti, 1999).

The most frequently occurring source for empirical, scientific scholarship remains embedded in review-type textbooks in which the research is summarized by a book or chapter author under topical headings. For the most part, it appears that emergency management students are simply not reading published research reports, particularly at the undergraduate level. Rather, technical reports and Internet links represent the lead favorite reading assignment. Graduate programs are more likely to include original research readings although edited volumes appear to be preferred over full research articles. For both undergraduate and graduate levels, the available books remain dated, with most in use published prior to September 11, 2001. It appears that the majority of the research articles in use explicate some practical or policy implications. In short, applied research is favored over basic research. Further examination is warranted on this topic, with controls for type of institution, level of the degree program, focus of the degree program, and student market.

THE CHALLENGES

What might explain the failure to integrate disaster research across all EM programs? Until pedagogical research is initiated in this emerging discipline, we must conjecture on the conditions that limit research applications. First, based on my classroom experience and discussion with colleagues, scientific articles often exceed student comprehension. For example, imagine a first-year student attempting to read through the traditional format for an article let alone attempting to grasp statistical analyses, something that even graduate students grapple with. Second, because of the institutional demands for peer-reviewed work from its professoriate, many publications are simply not user-friendly for undergraduate programs. Although doing so may threaten tenure or promotion, research faculty need to write scholarly based articles in trade journals, newsletters, anthologies, and electronic sources. Many senior research faculty members already know this dilemma, having worked many double-days to write works usable for both scholars and practitioners. A promising trend of late has come from senior faculty, near or at retirement, starting to write books suitable for use in the advanced undergraduate or graduate classroom.

Third, publishers have not fully recognized the burgeoning worldwide market; they must do so and develop materials for use at undergraduate and graduate levels particularly a full range of textbooks suitable at least for the four phases so common in U.S. classrooms: mitigation, preparedness, response, and recovery (Singh, 2004). And, although some edited books exist, most scholarly books work more effectively at the doctoral level. Translation of those exceptional works (e.g., see Perry & Quarantelli, 2005; Quarantelli, 1998) into classroom-friendly materials is essential, in part so that graduate students can understand the importance of conceptualization before launching research inquiries. Who will take the lead among academics and publishers to do so? Who will compile a compendium of understandable, scholarly materials suitable for the undergraduate level?

Fourth, a broader but significant barrier stems from an apparent lack of consensus among EM educators. Although implicit curricula are developing for general EM programs within the United States, a lack of consensus over what to call the degree as well as over course content still exists (Phillips, 2005). For example, is it emergency management, disaster management, homeland security, or something else? Is the field primarily public sector work or is there room in the academy for the private or nonprofit sectors? Although business contingency programs have emerged, only one institution—Hesston College in Kansas—has taken on the challenge of developing a nonprofit focus. Such development problems have beleaguered the field for decades, although such issues are not unknown to emerging fields when disciplines emerge (Neal, 2005). Lack of a clear conceptualization hinders research; without clear conceptual definitions, publishers lack direction. The absence of an agreed-upon canon also may impede research applications (Phillips, 2005), particularly because of the "proliferation of claims" over what constitutes a canon (Haydon, 2004). The presumed conceptual canon of the "four phases" does appear to transfer fairly well across cultures (Morrissey, 2004); although the specific phase names may vary, the general idea of mitigation, preparedness, response, and recovery phases reappear worldwide (in New Zealand, for example, they are called the four R's: reduction, readiness, response, recovery). However, despite considerable angst over how to conceptualize and thus measure "disaster," only limited discussion over phase conceptualization has occurred (Neal, 1997).

Fifth, across the existing U.S. programs, few EM programs require courses in research methods. An EM research methods textbook does not exist at the undergraduate level either—so how can we expect students to read, understand, interpret, and appreciate research? To date, only one edited volume has been published suitable for use at the graduate level, although it is a general compendium rather than a "cookbook" of how to do research (Stallings, 2003). This glaring gap in EM curricula runs counter to accreditation standards which expect "an understanding of the subject matter, literature, theory and methodology of the discipline; Research, scholarly activity and/or advanced professional training" (Southern Association of Colleges and Schools, 2003). In short, we lack teaching resources to inculcate research methods in a meaningful way or to meet basic accreditation standards.

Sixth, considering the rapid growth of EM programs in the United States, professional development opportunities for faculty members need to be created. Given that faculty positions go unfilled, sometimes for years, and that EM programs appropriately rely on a mix of both academic and practitioner qualified faculty, efforts to disseminate disaster studies might be expanded. Allowing an emerging discipline to progress without adequate faculty preparation lessens EM's internal academic legitimacy and undermines reputations of both programs and graduates.

Perhaps we should not be surprised by the lack of research integration across the EM programs. Knowledge transfer problems between researchers and practitioners have always been a challenge (Fothergill, 2000; Mileti, 1999). Four factors appear to influence knowledge transfer between these communities. First, cultural influences on jargon and academic communication styles impede knowledge transfer. Communication, as the foundation of cultural transmission, serves as the key to breaking barriers between the professions. Second, institutions demand that researchers "focus on pure rather than practical research" to earn tenure and promotion (Mileti, 1999, pp. 329–330). Third, linkages between researchers and practitioners (such as workshops) remain insufficient. Fourth, a lack of interaction between the two groups stymies knowledge transfer. Educational programs can serve as a pivotal transfer mechanism (Neal, 1993). Given the preliminary findings of this chapter, though, generating that transfer still requires considerable effort.

SOLUTIONS AND APPROACHES

The Roles of Research Centers and Research Associations

Historically, research centers have played an important role in getting research out, though more can and should be done. The Natural Hazards Research and Applications Center (NHRAIC) at the University of Colorado-Boulder has clearly taken the lead in generating, promoting and disseminating research (http://www.colorado.edu/hazards). NHRAIC's Quick Response Report series remains popular among some EM programs, with its reports easily accessible and/or downloadable for classroom use.

More could be done to promote the use of Web sites at other institutions and organizations, including online purchases or free access. In a noteworthy step, the International Research Committee on Disasters recently made most of their back inventory of the *International Journal of Mass Emergencies and Disasters* available free of charge to the public (http://www.ijmed.org). To access the past 3 years (a rolling time period), one must become a member, although rates remain affordable with reduced costs available for students and persons in developing nations.

To date, publications can be downloaded or otherwise accessed at several key institutions:

- Millersville University, Center for Disaster Reduction and Education (http://muweb.millersville.edu/~CDRE/). See also *Contemporary Disaster Review* (http://muweb.millersville.edu/~cdr/) which features a new section on EM pedagogy.
- Texas A&M University, Hazards Reduction and Recovery Center (http://hrrc.tamu.edu/research/index.shtml).
- University of Delaware, Disaster Research Center (http://www.udel.edu/DRC).
- University of Colorado, Natural Hazards Research and Applications Information Center, (http://www.colorado.edu/hazards).
- Oklahomo State University, Center for the Study of Disasters and Extreme Events.

PROMISING NATIONAL INITIATIVES

Several efforts spanning the last decade (some longer) suggest brighter futures for integrating research into the classroom. These efforts include the National Science Foundation's approach to funding engineering research centers, FEMA's Higher Education Project, grants funded to write books, and a joint academic-practitioner review of the literature called the "Second Assessment."

National Science Foundation

The National Science Foundation (NSF) has been supporting an Engineering Research Center (ERC) funding initiative since the 1980s. Key centers now integrate engineering with the social sciences, which can facilitate mainstreaming information into management programs that are typically social science based. NSF emphasis on the broader societal impacts of such research has been influential in making multidisciplinary research useful in the classroom. Part of that emphasis includes the transfer of research findings by involving students, creating new classes, and reinvigorating existing courses with newly produced research. Specific recommendations from NSF to partner with emergency management programs could improve that transfer.

Funded Books

Specific initiatives funded by various foundations and organizations have also produced research-influenced books usable in the classroom. The Public Entity Risk Institute partnered with UC-Boulder's NHRAIC to produce *Holistic Disaster Recovery*, a practical guide written by a collective of academics and practitioners and made available free of charge (http://www.colorado.edu/hazards/holistic_recovery). The Heinz Center convened a group of experts to tackle challenges related to coastal disasters, though the product serves as a broader, useful, readable introduction to social vulnerability (Heinz Center, 2002, www.heinzctr.org). These initiatives have resulted in usable classroom products, an effort that should merit continuation and expansion by funders.

Second Assessment and Applications

Perhaps most useful to educators, the "Second Assessment" of disaster research led by the University of Colorado's Natural Hazards Research and Applications Information Center, produced a set of research-based, state-of-the-knowledge books usable at the advanced undergraduate and graduate levels. The National Academies has facilitated access by placing each book online or available for purchase (downloadable PDF or hard cover) by chapter or by volume. The lead book, *Disasters by Design* (Mileti, 1999, http://books.nap.edu/catalog/5782.html), reviews general findings in an introductory manner with a readable format. Additional volumes offer detailed content on preparedness and response (Tierney, Lindell, & Perry, 2001, http://books.nap.edu/catalog/9834.html), geographic perspectives on hazards (Cutter, 2001, http://books.nap.edu/catalog/10132.html), and land-use planning (Burby, 1998, http://books.nap.edu/catalog/5785.html).

FEMA

FEMA's Higher Education Project has provided contracts to develop courses, generate video streamed lectures, write textbooks, and bring educators together in an annual conference. Several recent college courses, notably "Social Vulnerability to Disaster" have emphasized intensive scholarship, extensive bibliographies, and reliance on a strong academic team. Most recently, FEMA contracted with North Dakota State University to assess the books "most commonly prescribed by educators" for emergency management graduate students. In order, the top five include:

- *Disasters by Design* (Mileti, 1999)
- *At Risk* (Wisner et al., 2004)
- *Disaster and Democracy* (Rutherford, 1999)
- *Disasters, Collective Behavior and Social Organization* (Dynes & Tierney, 1994)
- *What Is a Disaster?* (Perry & Quarantelli, 2005).

SELECTED SYLLABI REVIEW

Based on the review of syllabi from the FEMA Higher Education web site I solicited syllabi from faculty most likely to use research in the classroom. This section first reviews syllabi in EM or natural hazards management programs, followed by an illustration from a discipline-specific case. Recent trends to either internationalize the U.S. curriculum or grow international programs are then discussed.

EM Type Programs

First, it is clear that the Second Assessment has made a considerable difference in disseminating research into courses in emergency management and natural hazards management programs. For example, use of these scholarly books is evident in courses at Texas A&M University. In Dr. Michael Lindell's "Organizational and Community Response to Disaster," virtually all of the second assessment books are used either fully or in part, supplemented by additional scholarly works. Students must serve as a weekly discussion leader by generating research-based discussion questions. A term paper option challenges students to craft 20-page research proposals or case analyses complete with scholarly citations. Lindell's approach reorganizes scholarly readings into topics suitable for emergency management: disaster impacts; hazard vulnerability, agents, and analysis; disaster preparedness and response; hazard mitigation and insurance. A complementary course, "Disaster Recovery and Hazard Mitigation" does likewise, with readings tied to the management process: hazard analysis and vulnerability, sustainability, household and business mitigation and recovery, the adoption and implementation process, socioeconomic and political influences, hazard insurance, and both structural and land-use mitigation.

At the University of North Texas, Dr. David McEntire's senior undergraduate capstone course employs *Disaster by Design* along with NHRAIC Quick Response Reports and journal articles from *Disaster Prevention and Management*, *Natural Hazards Review*, the *International Journal of Mass Emergencies and Disasters,* and *Public Administration Review*. A specific course such as Response and Recovery relies on a mix of scholarly and practical materials. The same journals reappear in this syllabus; several emphasize hazards likely to occur in a regional area. McEntire partners these scholarly items with the Texas Department of Emergency Management agency's Disaster Recovery Manual. The UNT program's perspective is that students must comprehend the theory and assumptions behind their actions. Relying on the literature "permits critical thinking in the classroom" and allows students to see the bigger picture (quote from McEntire, personal communication, 2005; see also Drabek, 2003b; Phillips, 2004).

Dr. David Neal, Director of the Center for the Study of Disasters and Extreme Events at Oklahoma State University, has taught disaster research and emergency management classes since 1979 and emphasizes the value of research in every class. His efforts draw from research on the myths of disaster behavior and how they have infiltrated planning and response assumptions. Recognizing that research does not always resonate well with the practitioner community, he then brings in perspectives from practitioners who have "seen the light" (Dawson, 1993). Neal ties the value of research to the growing professionalism of the field, where we need to make "disaster management decisions based on well-grounded research rather than on biased, selective ones." The inspiration for his approach came partly from former colleague Tom Joslin, who was a career FEMA employee. Joslin, despite his practitioner background, advocated against teaching a "rules and regulations" approach because these policies are subject to continual change. Joslin, according to Neal, said that knowing the ideas and inspiration behind the regulations was more important, and that emergency management was about "the people, the victims, not the bureaucracy."

DISCIPLINE-SPECIFIC USE OF RESEARCH: THE CASE OF SOCIOLOGY

The longest-established institution generating discipline-specific research in this field is the Disaster Research Center (DRC), now at the University of Delaware (originally at The Ohio

State University). Faculty associated with DRC share a legacy of disseminating research through the classroom. For example, Dr. Joanne Nigg's "Social Impact of Disaster" course launches with a consideration of "how the term disaster developed as a theoretical concept" followed by an examination of the causes and impacts of various types of disasters, a comparison of loss reduction approaches (preparedness and mitigation), and an overview of the disaster recovery process. Using the four phases, Dr. Nigg requires students to read only empirical work. Students must also complete a term paper based on sociological research.

DRC's newest faculty member, Dr. Tricia Wachtendorf, follows strongly in the DRC sociology tradition in her "Disasters and Society" course, emphasizing that "disasters are actually social events, not merely physical ones." Wachtendorf expects students to achieve certain course objectives, including one tied to research. Students must demonstrate skills in research methodologies to study disasters and research various aspects of a particular disaster as part of a student team. From the more than 50 syllabi that I reviewed for this chapter, Wachtendorf appears to be the only faculty member to require that students read scholarly articles on how to do research (e.g., Stallings, 2003).

DRC's legacy continues in the classroom of Dr. Gary Webb at Oklahoma State University. He continues in the DRC myth debunking tradition, then engages students in a "detailed review of sociological research" at the individual, organizational, and community levels. Of all the syllabi reviewed for this chapter, Webb's course is distinguishable as the most intensively focused in sociological knowledge, deeply grounded in a wide variety of sociological and disaster-oriented journals, and linked to the conceptual and theoretical substance of the discipline.

In my own political science research methods courses, I use a traditional approach but incorporate disaster research examples for students in the emergency management program. In various sections, I connect content to EM practitioner skills. Doing so satisfies graduate-level accreditation standards for methods content, builds student skills to understand methods terminology, and links research skills to practice. In the qualitative section, for example, we discuss how interview, document analysis, and observation skills could facilitate hazard analysis. I require students to interview a long-term resident to learn about prior disasters and to research local archives. In the quantitative section, students access and analyze local census data and then generate descriptive statistics to illustrate their data. Students read peer-reviewed articles by hazards researchers and identify the parts of a scientific article, review and critique the methodology, and assess the findings for theoretical, practical and policy relevance. To this day, I rely on E.L. Quarantelli's (the co-founder of DRC) lecture notes from the graduate seminar I took from him.

Dr. Henry Fischer's (a graduate of DRC) undergraduate course "Sociology of Disaster" at Millersville University of Pennsylvania relies on *Disasters by Design* in conjunction with Fischer's own research-based *Response to Disaster*. Students apply the course content by choosing from a wide variety of very creative components integrating research with practical application: a disaster film critique vis-à-vis sociological knowledge, a Web site with disaster information, a disaster plan critique, a hazards assessment, content analysis of media coverage, an annotated bibliography of a disaster researcher's work or a disaster journal, a disaster agent primer, and shadowing a disaster mentor—either a practitioner or a researcher (Fischer, personal communication, 2005).

It is worthwhile to pause and consider the impact of the widespread media images from Hurricane Katrina. Despite the efforts of many social scientists to exercise caution in assuming that looting, panic, and role abandonment were occurring across New Orleans, the media unfortunately perpetuated what is currently turning out to be yet another gross misrepresentation of sociobehavioral response to disaster. And, despite articles to the contrary in media such as *The New York Times* and the *Chronicle of Higher Education*, it is likely that many television viewers will retain these misperceptions. In the aftermath of Katrina, educators around the world will have to work doubly hard to counter these images by not only using pre-Katrina research but the media retractions and new research as well. A new Web site "Understanding Katrina" may contribute to this effort (http://understandingkatrina.ssrc.org, accessed October 10, 2005). Beyond the individual response to Katrina, organizations may face the same challenges. Though a limited body of research exists on "blame" it may be worthwhile to examine that work when talking about organizational response (FEMA and the Red Cross) in classes (Phillips & Ephraim, 1992).

INTERNATIONALIZING THE U.S. CURRICULUM

One limitation noticeable in most American syllabi is an overemphasis on the U.S. context. However, Dr. Carla Prater's (Texas A&M University) syllabi demonstrate how a course can be broadened through international readings (Prater, personal communication, 2005). Students in her graduate disaster seminar read *At Risk* (Wisner, Blaikie, Cannon, & Davis, 2004) and *Confronting Catastrophe* (Alexander, 2000). As another example, the "Disaster Recovery" course I teach at Oklahoma State University relies on guidance documents produced by the New Zealand Ministry of Civil Defence and Emergency Management (MCDEM), an effort that MCDEM produced from a review of the literature and consultation with the academic community (MCDEM, 2005a, 2005b; Norman, 2004). For a further review regarding the value of internationalizing the EM curriculum, see McEntire (2001a). Given the ways in which the United States has assisted in international disasters (e.g., the Indian Ocean tsunami) and given that disasters do not respect political boundaries, further globalization of the EM curriculum seems warranted. Providing a comparative perspective also generates richer and deeper insights and may serve to inspire applications of lessons learned from abroad. An overemphasis on the U.S. context will only serve to limit the growth of the field, let alone the development of intellectual capitol necessary to apply research and practice disaster management across national and cultural borders (Phillips, 2005).

INTERNATIONAL INITIATIVES

Internationally, a strong research emphasis can be found in several institutions. For example, in the United Kingdom, Coventry University's Risk and Emergency Management Program uses research through faculty lectures particularly in their Level 3 (final year) undergraduate module. Undergraduates are also expected to look at original research for their dissertation, which is then used in the classroom (Cole, personal communication, 2005). A familiar problem stems from "such a little body of knowledge with regard to UK emergency management, that sometimes we have to go out and do it in order to teach about it" (Cole, personal communication, 2005).

Auckland University of Technology's Bachelor of Studies in Paramedic program also expects students to be able to read, critique, and apply original research. Faculty members report that professional first responders need to communicate effectively with physicians and nurses. This means that paramedics must be able to understand the context of a medical decision and offer their perspective. In addition, paramedics often make spot decisions in life-threatening situations. Understanding an empirical basis for that research makes them more effective practitioners and motivates them to contribute to paramedic research (Costa, 2005).

Falkiner (2005) reviewed undergraduate courses across 38 of the largest Canadian universities. From a sample of 100 courses, she concluded that geography dominated the social science offerings. An emphasis on the physical nature of natural hazards has apparently influenced the growth of these types of courses. She suggest that the "findings are rather disappointing, with relative few schools offering any undergraduate courses in planning." Only seven sociology courses were identified albeit offered infrequently. Within the United States, larger universities appeared to be among the last to develop courses and programs, a pattern that may be repeating itself as Canadian programs develop.

The University of the West Indies (UWI) is among the Caribbean institutions that has benefited from infusion projects. The United Nations Disaster Relief Office (UNDRO), the Pan American Health Organization (PAHO), and the League of Red Cross Societies supported the Pan-Caribbean Disaster Preparedness and Prevention Project (PCDPPP) which then transformed into the Caribbean Disaster Emergency Response Agency (CDERA). The original PCDPPP encouraged a "coordinated approach to disaster research" at the UWI campuses, particularly interdisciplinary research. Researchers then infused undergraduate courses at the Mona campus and launched an interdisciplinary disaster research study group on campus (Morrissey, 2004). In response to a 1993 earthquake, the Office of Domestic Preparedness in Jamaica offered a teacher training program to transform textbooks and school content. Teachers in the certificate, diploma, and bachelor programs at UWI must complete a "classroom based research study" (Morrissey, 2004).

India's value for higher education has resulted in emerging efforts to establish natural disaster education courses and programs, primarily in geography, geomorphology, and climatology at undergraduate levels (Singh, 2004). Students are required to conduct field surveys to "train students in primary data collection and analysis." Field research uses both structured and unstructured interview guides, resulting in data that are collected, analyzed, and subsequently mapped (Singh, 2004). Massive events have also prompted the Administrative Staff College of India to disseminate lessons learned to government and nongovernmental officials. Various institutes have also participated in gathering data and organizing training courses, including the National Environmental Engineering Research Institute and the National Civil Defence College. Indira Gandhi National Open University offers distance learning courses on disaster preparation (Singh, 2004).

INTERNATIONAL INITIATIVES FROM THE PRACTITIONER SECTOR

Beyond universities, other initiatives have proven useful in developing EM programs tied to research. For example, the New Zealand Ministry of Civil Defence and Emergency Management has convened groups of international and domestic faculties on the subject of emergency management education several times during the past several years. Their efforts have served to facilitate interaction, build linkages across programs and countries, and generate exchange of research materials. Ministry personnel have visited with researchers and educators in other nations, bringing new ideas and contacts back as resources to their nation. As another example, the recent U.S. National Science Foundation research competition on the Indian Ocean tsunami required involvement of non-U.S. researchers, an effort that is resulting in ties between

American, Thai, and Indian institutions fostering research exchanges and expansion of educational programs particularly in tsunami-impacted nations.

The Natural Hazards Project at the Organization of American States (OAS) launched the "Hemispheric Eduplan" nearly a decade ago to encourage the development of academic programming across the Americas and the Caribbean. To date, their efforts have brought scholars together in Hemispheric-wide workshops, conferences, and exchanges and established "technical secretariat" offices to support the Eduplan at various universities. As one consequence of the relationships fostered by the technical secretariats, I was awarded a Rotary International Teachers Abroad Award to teach at the University of Costa Rica. Students came primarily from the practitioner community to attend classes where I taught and disseminated social vulnerability research. This novel OAS effort has generated even more practical applications from research exchanges, including development of a Disaster Resistant Universities initiative as well as cross-interdisciplinary exchanges of research content used in classes. For example, research from the University of Bogota, Colombia on structural mitigation is used in emergency management classes at Oklahoma State University.

CONCLUSION

A number of needs exist in order to more fully integrate research into the emergency management program. The foremost need stems from the lack of existing textbooks, anthologies, and other usable materials especially at the undergraduate level. A related problem is that research is not necessarily available for undergraduate consumption, nor is research always integrated or recognized in some of the available undergraduate textbooks. Several steps could address these problems. *Publishers* must recognize that a new market exists, one that can be connected to a rich history of existing studies already verified through the peer review process. Another solution could stem from *online databases* of articles and critical readings that faculty can tailor to their specific courses. *Journal* editors could add sections to their publications that address pedagogical issues, or could even consider short pieces by established scholars on topics suitable for classroom use. Publishers and journals could make these pieces easily accessible through Web sites. Disaster *researchers* in particular should actively publicize their own works. EM professional *associations* should promote research across their publications and within their membership ranks.

Foundations and other funding organizations, as well as key research centers, could develop and contribute to online archives by funding and videotaping lectures on substantive topics and the research process as well as policy and practical applications of their work. Currently available technologies make this a relatively easy process, including Microsoft Producer, Camtasia, and distance education tools like Blackboard and WebCT. An early example of this can be found on the FEMA Higher Education web site, featuring disaster mini-lectures by Dr. Henry W. Fischer of Millersville University.

Organizations and agencies that fund research might require efforts such as those established by the National Science Foundation: infusion of research findings into new and existing courses with stronger ties to emergency management education programs. Institutions like those cited earlier should continue to model best practices for research applications into the classroom; however, they should strive to influence classroom content more visibly and assertively. Institutions and authors not currently integrating research into classes and textbooks are failing not only accreditation standards but their students and those they will seek to serve.

Perhaps most appropriate, research useful to the teaching of disaster studies must be conducted, within discipline-specific (e.g., sociology, political science, geography) and inter-disciplinary classrooms (e.g., emergency management). Such a research agenda might include:

- Compilation and careful assessment of syllabi and course handouts using a rigorous sampling, with controls for historic events such as September 11 and Hurricane Katrina.
- Examination of pedagogical choices and their impact. For example:
  - The "myth debunking" approach used by many social scientists as an initial course entry point, with particular attention paid to how this may be more difficult due to the incorrect media images so widespread after Hurricane Katrina.
  - Effective teaching strategies to disseminate the research literature from the perspective of both teachers and students.
  - The traditional classroom vis-à-vis nontraditional formats including expedited and/or online programs (Neal, 2004; Phillips, 2004).
- Further consideration of the impediments faced by disaster researchers when attempting to disseminate their research (Fothergill, 2000; Mileti, 1999) but with a focus on the classroom environment.
- Longitudinal analyses of the careers of disaster researchers in both disciplinary and interdisciplinary settings.
- Identification of the key conditions that result in the use of research in the classroom.
- Review of accreditation standards vis-à-vis the content of courses, particularly in emergency management programs.
- Examination of the key conditions that influence textbook publishers to adopt or decline manuscripts using empirical works.
- Examination of the growth of EM programs (Neal, 2000), particularly since September 11, and the extent to which they use research in the classroom. A further line of inquiry might consider administrative location and its impact on research use.
- Review of faculty curriculum vitae, especially those faculty working in emergency management and homeland security programs, as an indicator of knowledge of, participation in and use of research. A comparison between these instructors vis-à-vis those offering discipline-specific courses might prove insightful.
- Identification of the ways in which faculty collaborate and exchange ideas for the purposes of teaching disaster studies, including review of new technologies: Internet conferencing, course Web sites, virtual classrooms and more (Phillips, 2005).
- Systematic, longitudinal student outcomes assessment studies focusing on acquisition and application of disaster research to the student's place of employment (Phillips, 2005).

CHAPTER 28

From Research to Praxis: The Relevance of Disaster Research for Emergency Management[1]

Richard A. Rotanz

The field of emergency management is "the discipline and profession of applying science, technology, planning, and management to deal with extreme events that can injure or kill large numbers of people, do extensive damage to property, and disrupt community life. When such events do occur and cause extensive harm, they are called disasters" (Hoetmer, 1991). This definition eloquently defines emergency management clearly explains what a disaster is, and exemplifies how academia and research provides conceptual and practical tools for emergency managers. Researchers tell us who we are; what we do; how and why we do the things we do; as well as provide guidance and advise as to where we should be going.

Emergency management, similar to the disciplines of fire fighting, medicine, political science, sociology, mental health, and others, relies on researchers to observe, evaluate, and provide referents and reports offering recommendations; reflect on how and what we have done; and to help us define, recognize, and understand the multitude of issues we face in the field of emergency management. This chapter describes the value of such research and provides examples of past and current topics that have significantly contributed to our understanding of emergency management. The chapter attempts to provide *some* answers regarding the relevance and benefit of disaster research to emergency management and planning and how we should conduct operations in events such as the hurricanes that impacted the United States in 2004 and 2005, the 2004 Indian Ocean tsunami, the massive power outage of 2003, and the terrorist attacks on the World Trade Center on September 11, 2001. Is research actually helping us in this process? Do we as emergency managers heed the findings and conclusions of such arduous work? How does this research impact emergency managers and other decision makers

---

[1] *Editors' Note:* This chapter was written by Commissioner Rotanz, an emergency manager with extensive experience in the field. In his years as an emergency manager, Rotanz has used and values the cumulative body of knowledge generated by disaster researchers. Rotanz provides a general overview regarding the role and importance of disaster research for practitioners and makes a compelling case calling for increased communication, coordination, and integration of experiences and knowledge generated by practitioners, researchers, and scholars in the field of disaster research.

during crisis situations? How can one take advantage of this precious resource called disaster research?

PRESENT RESOURCES

Emergency managers need clearinghouse centers of definitive research regarding threat and consequence management from natural, technological, and terrorist agents. The study of planning constructs, communication, response operations, media relations, recovery, and mitigation activities are but a few research areas and resources that are currently available in these centers. Gaining access to such centers is a simple process and information can be obtained either by a direct visit, through mailings, by phone, or through the Internet. Internet access in some portals allows interactive access to some databases that allow for robust search capabilities for text versions of abstract or complete documents.

Two of the many large and prestigious centers that I have encountered when venturing out as a student of emergency management are the Disaster Research Center (DRC) at the University of Delaware and the Natural Hazards Research and Applications Information Center (NHRAIC), led by Havidán Rodríguez and Kathleen Tierney, respectively. These centers provide some of the most extensive collections of research and public policy documents relating to emergency management, disasters, and the social sciences. The library at the NHRAIC can be accessed through their online program HazLit, a database index providing access to the Center's full collection of papers. The Disaster Research Center has a similar computer interface allowing and extensive search of their database based on their 42 years of dedicated disaster research.

To complement these two entities, there are also a large number of centers (based in academic, state, federal, and international organizations and institutions) that conduct an array of research projects, studies, and conferences. A link found in the NHRAIC website, for example, provides an up-to-date listing of academic organizations in alphabetical order beginning with the Benfield Hazard Research Center up through to the World Institute for Disaster Risk Management, while other links provide listings of domestic organizations ranging from the American Society on Veterinary Disaster Medicine to the Western States Seismic Policy Council.

Finally, the Federal Emergency Management Agency (FEMA) Emergency Management Institute (EMI) located in Emmitsburg, Maryland serves as the federal government's center for the development of courses and curriculum in emergency management. As stated on its Web site, "Through its courses and programs, EMI serves as the national focal point for the development and delivery of emergency management training to enhance the capabilities of federal, state, local, and tribal government officials, volunteer organizations, and the public and private sectors to minimize the impact of disasters on the American public" (http://www.training.fema.gov/ emiweb/). During the past 10 years, EMI has developed numerous college programs and has provided assistance in the development of theses programs throughout the country. Today, more than 100 colleges and universities provide certificate and degree programs ranging from an associate's degree up through the Ph.D. level in emergency management and related areas. Some recent examples include the George Washington University (located in Washington, DC), with its newly developed doctoral degree program; North Dakota State University, with a doctoral program in emergency management; and Adelphi University (located in Long Island, New York), with a new graduate certificate program.

CURRENT APPLICATION

It would require a separate book to describe what has been accomplished in the field of disaster research, how it is being applied, and what is needed for further analysis. My personal experience as an emergency manager is that collaboration with academic institutions can serve to establish important and productive relationships between researchers and practitioners. The following sections provide a general overview of how past and present research has guided me in defining events; how I have come to conceptualize and perform *planning* functions; how we can recognize and interact with the various forms of *organizational behavior* that will be expected during a response to disasters; *communications;* types of *improvisation*; and the functions of an emergency operation center (EOC).

DEFINITIONS—REFERENTS

It is important for any discipline to have standardized terminology and jargon. For example, the term emergency should imply a specific, but familiar state of condition. Lagadec (1993) defines emergencies as classical incidents that are "well understood; are clearly defined; require a limited amount of "actors" or "emergency response providers"; participating organizations that are familiar with each other; roles and responsibilities are clear-cut; there is a present authoritative structure; the event is manageable; and the condition is brought under control quickly." Hoetmer (1991) defines emergencies as "routine" adverse events that do not have community-wide impact or do not require extraordinary use of resources or procedures to bring conditions back to normal." In other words, events are managed by local emergency response personnel. Hoetmer (1991) elaborates on his definition of disaster stressing the need to incorporate the term "catastrophic" in his definition. A catastrophic disaster is one that affects the entire nation and requires extraordinary resources and skills for recovery. E.L. Quarantelli (1981) expands on the definition of the term disaster by including various dimensions such as predictability, frequency, controllability, the speed of onset, the length of forewarning, and the duration of its impact. These characteristics allow emergency managers to conceptualize more effectively mitigation efforts, planning, preparation, and response to complex events.

These terms have allowed us to catalog events and to establish response patterns for emergency organizations. Most metropolitan areas in the United States have developed matrices based on the intensity of a hazard event matched with the required resources involving numerous agencies and disparate jurisdictions. Cities such as New York and Salt Lake City have established several levels of response (e.g., 1, 2, and 3), with level 3 involving the greatest deployment of resources as well as the active involvement of the media and political leaders and other public officials. In January of 2005, the Department of Homeland Security (DHS) issued the National Response Plan aligning all federal, state, and local agencies into an all-hazards approach for the management of domestic incidents. The plan includes a glossary with the intention of standardizing the way we define and think about our operations, functions, and situations. The term "catastrophic incident" is defined as any natural or manmade incident, including terrorism, that results in extraordinary levels of mass casualties, damage, or disruption, severely affecting the population, infrastructure, environment, economy, national morale, and/or government functions. A catastrophic event could result in sustained national impacts over a prolonged period of time and it exceeds the resources normally available to state, local, tribal, and private-sector authorities in the impacted area. Further, it significantly disrupts government operations and emergency services to such an extent that national security could be threatened.

Although the use of terms such as emergency, disaster, and catastrophe are slowly becoming standardized and understood, one concept that is widely abused is "crisis." Crisis, unlike the previous concepts, illustrates a lack of stability and the uneasiness of a situation and odes not necessarily focus on the degree of response that is required. Fink (1986) provides several stages of a crisis, beginning with the **prodomal** stage, the warning or symptomatic period; the **acute**, or "its' happening now" stage; the **chronic** stage, the point in the time-line that we recognize our successes or our failures; and the **resolution** stage, perceived as the time of restoration. Further, Rosenthal, Boin, and Comfort (2001) discuss various dimension of crisis, including discontinuity, threat, opportunity, change, uncertainty, disturbing regularity, isolation, the surprise, urgency, time pressure, and exhaustion. These factors help emergency managers better understand the circumstances that lead to a crisis situation, the dilemmas and coping mechanisms that emerge, and the strategies that allow us to mitigate the existing crisis.

Lagadec (1993) provides emergency managers with a most practical definition of crisis indicating that it is "a situation in which a range of organizations, struggling with critical problems and subjected to strong external pressure and bitter internal tension, find themselves thrust into the limelight, abruptly and for an extended period; they are also brought into conflict with one another... this occurs in the context of a mass media society (i.e. "live") and the event is sure to make headlines on the radio and television and in the written press for a long time." These definitions are but a few of the multitude of terms that emergency managers, governments, and businesses must recognize. It is important to note that each state in the United States had previously developed definitions for the above terms. As a case in point, the term disaster relates not only to the size of the event, but also to the requirements for federal funding and material assistance along with a laundry list of probable causes.

PLANNING PRINCIPLES

One of the most important functions of emergency management is planning. Research has taught us that for effective response and recovery operations, all members of any emergency response organizational network (ERON) need realistic, flexible, and uncomplicated planning documents to provide knowledge, guidance, and reference points during times of disaster. Dynes, Quarantelli, and Kreps (1981) provide several emergency planning principles that I have found very useful as the Deputy Director in the New York City (NYC) Office of Emergency Management (OEM), and presently as Commissioner of Emergency Management in Long Island. Briefly, the eight planning principles demonstrate that planning is a continuous process; it attempts to reduce the unknowns; it should evoke appropriate action; the planning document should be based on what is likely to happen; the process is based on knowledge; it must focus on principles; it should be partly an educational activity; and it must overcome resistance and encourage participation and cooperation. These principles should keep emergency managers focused on the planning document as well as prepare them for a variety of issues and complexities that arise during the process.

I have also discovered, through a number of research documents, that disaster demands are divided into agent- and response-generated demands. Agent-generated demands are those that are specific to the agent and directly affect planning and response strategies regarding which types of *warnings* are appropriate; specific *pre-impact preparations*; what skills and equipment will be needed for *search and rescue;* how to care for the *injured and deceased*; identify anticipated *welfare demands* when differentiating, for example, between those impacted by a disease outbreak relative to the needs of those evacuated and sheltered; *restoration of essential community services,* such as the restoration of electrical power from utility disruptions or the rebuilding of a bridge destroyed from a flash flood; *protection against continuing threats;* and *community order.* These agent-generated demands can be used as guiding principles in anticipating how each disaster agent will challenge us.

Response-generated demands are more general and basic involving communications, continuing assessment of emergency situations, mobilization and utilization of human and material resources, coordination (the most important of all agent and response-generated demands), and control and authority. This typology of demands has led to successful development of planning documents for response strategies throughout the emergency management field. For example, during my tenure with the NYC OEM we worked on the development of a biological hazard annex. An elaborate "warning" system was put in place in the form of a robust syndromic surveillance system produced through OEM and the NYC Department of Health; pre-impact preparations were established in the form of identified points of dispensing emergency pharmaceuticals; and all other agent and response-generated demands were incorporated into planning efforts. It is noteworthy that one common error planning personnel often commit is an assumption that during the writing of plans, everyone understands each others' jargon or definitions. To plan for the multitudes of missions that are anticipated during disasters, and during incident action planning for emerging conditions, all responding agencies and nongovernment organizations must "be on the same page" and in agreement; thus, communication and coordination are essential.

Previous research has linked the response-generated demands to four basic and important concepts: domain, tasks, activities, and human and material resources. *Domain* refers to which organization has responsibility for which disaster-generated demands. *Tasks* define how the domain of the organization is to be performed while *activities* refer to the actual implementation of these tasks. Finally, *human and material resources* are the workers and tools that are required to perform the "activities" in order to accomplish the "tasks" relating to the organization's domain.

ORGANIZATIONAL BEHAVIOR

What I have found to be an important construct of planning is the awareness of organizational behavior during disasters. A typology, developed by researchers at the Disaster Research Center, has allowed me to conceptually categorize each government and nongovernment organization into one of four possible forms of organizational structures and disaster-related tasks. The first category, Type I or *established,* are organizations that perform routine tasks and maintain their basic organizational structure during disasters. Examples of Type I organizations include fire departments, law enforcement, Emergency Medical Services (EMS), and hospitals; these organizations routinely respond to a variety of emergencies and disasters. Type II or *expanding* organizations engage in routine tasks during a disaster but are required to expand their "everyday" but limited staff and activate volunteers. Examples of Type II organizations may include the Salvation Army, the American Red Cross, Community Emergency Response Teams (CERT), and state militia, such as the National Guard. *Extending* organizations (Type III) are those who do not generally perform routine tasks in response to emergencies or disasters but have been part of established planning and preparedness initiatives; however, they maintain their organizational structure while performing tasks and activities during an emergency or disaster type of environment. Construction companies and government agencies that perform debris removal or assist in recovery efforts given their specialized equipment and related skills are common examples of Type III organizations. Finally, Type IV, *emergent groups,* are those with no formal disaster-related tasks or structure but they emerge as small groups or en masse and respond to the areas that have been impacted. These groups will fulfill tasks during disasters that municipalities are not able to accomplish or are simply not available to do so, especially when they are overwhelmed or have been destroyed by the hazard agent. Such tasks and activities can take the form of ad hoc search and rescuers or feeding or caring for the victims. These groups can be useful to responding organizations given their manpower and talent, but if not managed and supervised properly, their efforts and desire to "just do something" can impede the response or they could be placed in harms way. During the few weeks following the attacks on the World Trade Center (September 11, 2001), thousands of civilians converged on the site with the intent to help, while thousands more came to seek family members or watch the rescue events unfold. This compelled NYC's OEM to rapidly credential thousands of essential responders, a form of improvisation briefly described in the following sections.

COMMUNICATION

Communication is the most important function during the planning and preparation phases in order to generate effective response and recovery efforts during and following disasters. It is not only which technology we use to communicate but the form or methods used to communicate. How do we communicate preparedness and planning strategies? What critical assets do we transport and to where do we transport them? What is the status of our fuel, power, and water supplies? What is our situation with human service issues, casualties, and fatalities? Communication is essential to provide accurate and reliable answers to these questions. Quarantelli (1988a) provides us with five forms of communication: (1) intraorganizational; (2) interorganizational; (3) information flow from organizations to the general public; (4) information flows from the public to different organizations; and (5) information flows from within different systems of organizations. These forms of communication help emergency managers understand and improve the communication process.

COOPERATIVE EFFORTS AND
SAMPLED RESULTS

One of the most important outcomes in establishing robust relationships with academic institutions is the collaboration and cooperative efforts that emerge before, during, and after a disaster. As mentioned earlier, I have reached out to the Disaster Research Center and to the Emergency Management Institute in Maryland. This outreach has resulted in face-to-face meetings and interactions on an array of topics as well as the sharing of research material and my experiences as a practitioner.

During the attacks on the World Trade Center (2001), DRC researchers responded to a makeshift office on Manhattan's West Side to initiate credentialing and to gather real-time data and information. Tricia Wachtendorf and James Kendra were the first, among others, who gathered vital information during the response phase, resulting in excellent reports not only for social scientists but for emergency managers as well. A report that I found very enlightening, and has helped in our emergency planning, was written by Wachtendorf (2004) and pertains to improvisation. She presents an analysis of three forms of improvisation—*reproductive, adaptive,* and*creative*—identified during the response to the 2001 WTC event. The first form of improvisation presented, *reproductive*, depicts the re-creation of New York City's EOC at Pier 92, 3 miles north of Ground Zero. The NYC OEM was formerly housed on the 23rd floor of WTC 7, the last building to collapse during that fateful Tuesday, resulting in the loss of the City's EOC.

Adaptive improvisation was exemplified during the mass credentialing of essential personnel at the impact site of the WTC as well as the development of special three-man teams from the New York Fire Department (NYFD) and the New York Police Department (NYPD) to respond to the hundreds of alarms regarding the anthrax attacks that took place between September and December 2001. Finally, *creative improvisation* is reflected in the recovery of human remains and the complexities surrounding the ensuing criminal investigations and debris removal operations.

REACHING OUT: FROM PRAXIS
TO RESEARCH

As a practitioner, my interest in the field of disaster research emerged as questions continued to be generated regarding the strategies needed in order to maintain stability and continuity of our society during and after a catastrophic event. My interests focused on how the functionality of emergency operations centers could provide an adequate response in a cooperative environment.

My personal experiences in managing an EOC show that, when properly managed and staffed, it can be a facility that can provide an adequate environment for the coordination of response functions during major complex events, such as disasters; it can also serve to maintain the continuity of critical services.

My involvement with disaster researchers has led me to write and elaborate on articles and reports that affect our field. For example, I recently stepped up to the plate and presented an article which elaborated on Quarantelli's (1979) six functions of the EOCs by modifying and adding new components to his list. I argued that, in order for EOCs to operate properly, they must perform the following functions: (1) coordination; (2) surveillance management; (3) establish levels of activations; (4) information management; (5) planning; (6) operations and missions management; (7) policy making and legal issues; (8) public information; (9) facility environment; and (10) host visitors.

WHAT NOW?

Collaboration is critical to foster interactions between researchers and practitioners. We can learn from each other and can contribute to the enhancement of this partnership while incorporating the public and private and nonprofit sectors. We must learn from each other what are the functions that we perform, the questions that need to be asked and answered, how we can aid each other in finding these answers, and how we can learn and take advantage of our mistakes and best practices.

Those of us who are responsible for educating and preparing our social networks on how to properly mitigate, respond, and recover from disasters, need to better understand how to communicate risk to the public, businesses, and our governments. For example, is there a better "warning" system than color coding terrorist threats (e.g., Homeland Security Threat Advisory Level) or should this scheme be applied to all hazards? Can legal researchers with legislators formulate standardized sets of law and rights, allowing doctors, medics, and many regulated practices to function across political boundaries during disasters?

Industries in the technology arena must establish a relationship with first responders and emergency management agencies to provide a platform where, for example, a fire fighter can express their technological needs instead of being provided with items that simply do not work or do not apply to their field. What educational courses should be taught in elementary through high school levels to achieve a needed paradigm shift in how our society perceives, prepares, and responds to the inevitable impact of disasters? As a young boy growing up in the 1950s, I was instructed to hide under my school desk when the warning of a potential attack occurred. Smokey the Bear warned me not to play with fire while Donald Duck showed me how to stop, drop, and roll if one's clothes caught fire. What are our children being taught today regarding hurricanes, disease outbreaks, or terrorism? Are we too afraid to teach them about such horrors?

We have seen so many disastrous events since the great flood and the epic of Noah's preparation as well as the fateful results of complacency. The cliché of "those who ignore the past are condemned to repeat it" remains valid today, but there is no excuse for such arrogance and ignorance. How can researchers in motivational theory solve such dilemmas with today's technology and massive forms of communication to bring us all "onto the same page?"

But let's start here, in our university offices and from our emergency operation centers, and "pick up the phone." A simple introduction of each other will lead to a long-term relationship that will enhance our emergency planning and preparedness initiatives that will result in the protection and survival of our communities during disaster or catastrophic situations. There are a multitude of examples regarding how the findings of research are being applied through technology in history. Just in weaponry, medicine, transportation, and communication, we have seen massive leaps in the past 50 years. We should become part of this trend more so than we currently are. Let's raise the raise bar and move forward in closing the gap between research and praxis, for we have so much to lose if we choose not to act, but so much to gain if we choose to collaborate.

CHAPTER 29

Communicating Risk and Uncertainty: Science, Technology, and Disasters at the Crossroads[1]

HAVIDÁN RODRÍGUEZ, WALTER DÍAZ,
JENNIFFER M. SANTOS, AND BENIGNO E. AGUIRRE

It is estimated that about 80% of all disasters are directly tied to weather events; thus forecasting weather has become a very important scientific, economic, and political endeavor. With the development of new and enhanced technology, weather forecasting skills have improved significantly both in the United States and internationally (National Research Council [NRC], 1999, 2003). However, weather forecasting is a probabilistic science and many uncertainties still remain (see National Science Foundation [NSF], 2002). Indeed, despite significant improvements in our ability to predict the weather in the short and long-term, recent experiences with natural hazards show that we continue to confront important challenges regarding lead times, false alarm rates, the accuracy and reliability of the information that is being communicated, and in our ability to elicit the appropriate response from the local, state, and federal governments as well as the general public, as the case of Hurricane Katrina (2005) clearly demonstrated.

We argue that with continued improvements in weather monitoring, detection, and mass communication technology, the social and organizational features of integrated warning systems become paramount as key factors in saving lives and reducing damages to property. Therefore, there is a need to continue to expand our knowledge regarding how individuals, communities, and organizations perceive and react to weather forecasts and warnings. This knowledge must be integrated with other technical information on weather forecasts already available so as to make weather information more useful to society (NRC, 1999).

This chapter explores the role of science, technology, and the media in the communication of warnings, risk, and disaster information. We also focus on how researchers can communicate

[1] This work was supported primarily by the Engineering Research Centers Program of the National Science Foundation under NSF Award Number 0313747. We also want to acknowledge the anonymous reviewers for their comments and recommendations. Any opinions, findings, and conclusions or recommendations expressed in this material are those of the authors and do not necessarily reflect those of the NSF.

the importance, value, and contributions of hazard and disaster research to the end-user community, including emergency management organizations and the general public. Further, we provide a critical analysis on the importance and potential contributions of interdisciplinary research in the disaster field. We emphasize the need to develop an integrated model to communicate risk and warnings, which takes into account new and emerging technologies, the role of the media, and the changing socioeconomic and demographic characteristics of the general population. Because of space limitations, these issues are discussed primarily in the context of the United States (for an extensive and quite comprehensive bibliography on communicating risk and warnings to the public, both at the national and international level, see Bandy, Johnson Peek, & Sutton, 2004).

The Partnership for Public Warning (2003, p. i) indicates that "public warning empowers people at risk to take actions to reduce losses from natural hazards, accidents and acts of terrorism . . . [it] save lives, reduces fear, and speeds recovery." They also argue that the success of public warnings is measured "by the actions people take." Moreover, the NRC's Panel on the Human Dimensions of Seasonal-to-Interannual Climate Variability points out that the eventual value of improved weather forecasts "will depend on how people and organizations deal with the new kind of information. Are they likely to pay attention to it? Will they understand what the climate models mean for them? Will they trust the messengers?" (1999, p. 16). Even if the public understands weather forecasts, their trust in the reliability and accuracy of these forecasts and in the sources that provide such information may significantly impact their behavior and response (Lindell & Perry, 2004; Mileti, 1999; NRC, 2003; Perry & Greene, 1982). For example, public confidence and trust in the sources that provide such information (e.g., weather forecasts and warnings) has an impact on their perception of risk (Slovic, 1993; Slovic, Flynn, & Layman, 1991). Slovic (2000, p. 410) points out that "the limited effectiveness of risk-communication efforts can be attributed to the lack of trust . . . if trust is lacking, no form or process of communication will be satisfactory." However, trust in institutions is a function of many factors among which minority status and power are readily identifiable (Pérez-Lugo, 2001; Perry & Greene, 1982). Furthermore, mass media accounts conveying inaccurate, biased or sensationalistic information may easily undermine that trust (Fischer, 1994; Nigg, 1987; Quarantelli, 1987b; Pérez-Lugo, 2001; Wenger, Dyke, Sebok, & Neff, 1980).

In order for weather forecasts and warnings to be useful to individuals and communities, they must be understood, must meet their needs, and must provide accurate and reliable information as well as sufficient lead time to allow them to take appropriate action. In this context, up-to-date, continuous, and reliable communication is essential. Previous research has shown that one of the most significant problems with weather forecasts is how the information is presented and communicated to end-user communities (e.g., government agencies, emergency management organizations, industry, and to the general population; see Fischer, 1994; Mileti, 1999; NRC, 1999, 2003). It is noteworthy, however, that even forecasts of severe weather events that attempt to solve these problems may fail to elicit appropriate protective action given that an individual's response to forecasts and warnings is often influenced by factors that have little to do with the technical features of weather forecasts, such as the individual's social class, education, gender, race, ethnicity, cultural background, and previous experiences with weather events.

Access to weather forecasts and warnings, the type of technologies used to access weather information and perceptions (e.g., trust, confidence, and usefulness) regarding weather forecasts and warnings also vary according to race/ethnicity, levels of education, and income (Perry & Greene, 1982; NRC, 1999; Slovic, 2000; Weber & Hsee, 1998). Weather forecast information delivery systems are primarily oriented "to the educated, the affluent, the cultural majority, and the people in power . . . and they are . . . least effective in reaching the elderly, cultural minority groups, people with low incomes, and those without power" (NRC, 1999, p. 86) (For an extensive discussion on the intersection of race/ethnicity, social class and disasters, see the chapter by Bolin in this handbook). Further, although the perception of personal risk is a function of individuals' previous experiences with a given weather hazard, their views about the certainty of its impact, how close they are to it, and how severe they think the impact is likely to be (see Blanchard-Boehm, 1998), there also appears to be a relationship between perceived risk and ethnicity, although this evidence is contradictory. On the one hand, Perry and Greene (1982) suggest that minorities, when compared to majority individuals, have, on average, lower levels of perceived personal risk. On the other hand, more recent research (Slovic, 2000) shows that people of color (and women) are more likely to report a higher degree of perceived health risks to a number of hazards and activities relative to their white counterparts. Slovic points out that women and non-white men "see the world as more dangerous because in many ways they are more vulnerable ... they benefit less from many of its technologies and institutions, and ... they have less power and control over what happens in their communities and their lives" (2000, p. 402).

We should also note that although a hazard event can be devastating for a particular society or for a particular group of individuals, its effects are mediated by cultural, social, demographic, economic, and political factors. Some of these factors can ameliorate or exacerbate the effects of a hazard. Furthermore, political and public policy choices, such as whether or not to strengthen and enforce land-use and building codes, will work either to mitigate or exacerbate the hazards' effects, depending on the actual set of choices made. The decision by the United States federal government to not adequately fund improvements in the New Orleans levee system is a particularly striking example of the consequences of inadequate policy making (see U.S. Army Corps of Engineers, 2005). However, it is equally important to note that strategies that individuals, groups, and communities develop to deal with stressful events may result in increased resilience and, therefore, will work in the direction of reducing the hazard's negative consequences. The primacy of these social factors led Quarantelli (2005a) to contend that hazard events (e.g., earthquakes, tornadoes, floods, tsunamis, terrorist attacks, etc.) may result in disasters, not because of the event itself but because of the activities and actions taken (or not taken) at the governmental, community, and individual level.

COMMUNICATING RISK AND WARNINGS

An extraordinary amount of federal and state funding has been allocated to the advancement of science and technology. Financial support to improve weather forecasts, enhance prediction of hazard-related events, and increase lead times has been an institutional practice of governments at different levels. The prevailing assumption behind this spending is that reducing the levels of error or uncertainty in determining if, when, and where an extreme event, such as a tornado, will strike will lead to a reduction in the number of deaths or injuries and property damage as a consequence of improved sensing and prediction. However, this is not necessarily the case.

Although significant improvements in tornado warning systems have been alluded to as one of the important variables in the reduction of tornado-related deaths (see Balluz, Schieve, Holmes, Kiezak, & Malilay, 2000; Mileti, 1999), the research literature also suggests that inadequate warnings and warning systems are one of the primary factors contributing to the number of deaths and injuries caused by hazard events such as tornadoes (see Balluz et al., 2000). Therefore, improving weather forecasts and increasing lead times is only part of the equation in determining the population's preparedness and response to natural hazards.

Moreover, effective and reliable warning systems are only one component that may impact how individuals or communities prepare and respond to such warnings.

Communication is an extremely important component in contributing to or in averting a disaster situation. As Lindell and Perry point out, "one important function of risk communication is, explicitly or implicitly, to promote appropriate protective behavior by those to whom the information is directed" (2004, p. 3). The primary goal of communicating this information to the general population or to a particular community is to protect those who are at risk of being impacted by an impending hazard, with the aim of reducing the loss of life and the number of injuries. Researchers have argued that a disaster is a result of a crisis in the communication process or a result of a communication breakdown (see Gilbert, 1998). This process is commonly said to consist of the following stages: hearing, understanding, believing, confirming, and responding to the hazard warning (see Blanchard-Boehm, 1997; Mileti & Sorenson, 1990). Clearly, any breakdown in the process will most likely result in delayed or incorrect responses to the hazard warning (Blanchard-Boehm, 1998; Lindell & Perry, 2004; Mileti, 1999).

However, human behavior depends on a multitude of demographic, social, cultural, economic, and psychological factors. We know that individuals respond to warnings if they perceive that there is a serious threat to themselves, their families, or their property. Nevertheless, there are a number of other factors that will impact if, how, and when individuals respond to these warnings such as credibility of the information providers, perceived accuracy and reliability of the warning message, the role that the government and affiliated agencies are playing in the warning process, and the content of the messages and the frequency with which the population receives the same (see Blanchard-Boen, 1998; Lindell & Perry, 2004; Mileti & Sorenson, 1990; Nigg, 1995b, to name but a few). Also, the clarity of the message, its consistency, the presence and "respectability" of officials who are providing the warning, the accuracy of past warnings, and the frequency of the hazard will have a significant impact on the credibility of the message and on individual response to the same (Fischer, 1994; Lombardi, 2002; Mileti, 1999). Moreover, adoption of the recommended line of action in severe weather forecasts is a function of many factors including whether potential victims perceive that protection is in fact possible and can be undertaken, which in turn is a function of how much time is available, whether family members are accounted for, and the presence of prior emergency plans. It is also a function of the presence of a belief among those threatened that protective action can significantly reduce the negative consequences of the severe weather event and that the officially recommended actions, in fact, are superior to alternative lines of action taken by kin, neighbors, or advanced by conventional wisdom (Lindell & Perry, 2004; Perry & Greene, 1982).

The adoption of a recommended action also appears to be correlated with race and ethnicity, with the resulting implication that minorities will be less likely to adopt the recommended actions in cases of severe weather events relative to their majority counterparts. This issue is further complicated given that, despite the fact that minorities are more likely to report higher levels of perceived risk (Slovic, 2000), they are less likely to receive the warnings that would allow them to take protective action, and may have limited access to protective resources. For example, preliminary research on response to tornado warnings has shown that African Americans were less likely to report having received warnings when compared to their white counterparts (Paul, Brock, Csiki, & Emerson, 2003; also see Lindell & Perry, 2004). Previous research also shows that minority groups are more likely to be impacted by hazards and disasters, to sustain a greater amount of damage, and to have greater difficulty in recovering from these events relative to their Anglo counterparts (Dash, Peacock, & Morrow, 1997; Peacock & Girard, 1997; Steinberg, 2000). Therefore, having a minority status may be a "risk factor" that contributes to this group's vulnerability to natural hazards and other events (see Cutter et al., 2003).

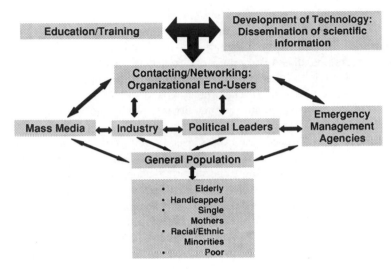

FIGURE 29.1. A model for communicating hazard risk and warnings. This is a modified model based on Nigg's (1995b) Components of an Integrated Warning System.

A MODEL FOR THE COMMUNICATION
OF RISK

The above discussion suggests that to generate scientific knowledge, communicate it to the general population in an effective manner, and, therefore, enhance its levels of preparedness and response to a particular hazard, we need to develop an integrated research approach combined with an effective communication model. Figure 29.1 presents a model for communicating hazard risk that accounts for the development of technology, dissemination of scientific knowledge, and education and training of end-users based on Nigg's (1995b) article on the components of a warning system.

The aforementioned model is a result of the integration of scientific knowledge generated by social and physical scientists and engineers regarding hazards and disasters and their impacts on society. This knowledge or scientific information needs to be disseminated to the end-user community using multiple communication sources in a way that is accessible and can be understood by this diverse community. Nevertheless, in order for this information to be useful and to have a significant impact on individual and community response, it must meet the following criteria:

- It must reach the intended end-users or the population at risk in a comprehensible and useful form.
- It must be perceived by them as relevant to their situation (i.e., individuals need to be made aware and recognize the hazard risk and potential outcomes such as the loss of life and damage to property).
- The end-users must have the capacity and the necessary resources to use this information in ways that will allow them to better prepare, respond to, and recover from a hazard or disaster situation.

The model presented in Figure 29.1 is dynamic, multidirectional, and highly dependent on frequent communication and coordination among and between end-user groups (see Nigg,

1995b), through both formal and informal networks. This model also highlights the role and importance of many actors in the risk communication process, including the general public, public officials and government agencies, emergency management personnel, the media, educational institutions and programs, and the private industry. The model reflects the importance of public-private partnerships in the communication of hazard risk. As stated by the Partnership for Public Warning (2005, p. 1), warnings and the communication of this information is a "public responsibility—shared by local, state and federal governments—that relies upon private sector technologies and infrastructure." They further argue that "developing an effective national alert and warning capability requires coordination, cooperation and consensus among the key stakeholders—both public and private."

The communication model in Figure 29.1 also requires the development of multi- or inter-disciplinary research efforts aimed at understanding and disseminating scientific knowledge that will impact society in a useful manner. Disaster losses result from the interaction between physical environments (i.e., hazardous events), the built environment (e.g., infrastructure such as roads, bridges, and buildings), and the social environment (i.e., the social, cultural, demographic, economic, and political characteristics of communities) (see Mileti, 1999). Therefore, to understand the full consequences of hazards and disasters (ranging from communication of risk; risk perception; mitigation and preparedness; behavior and response during an actual event; recovery efforts; and short- and long-term reconstruction strategies) and their societal impact, we have to develop a multi- or interdisciplinary framework.

The interaction between scientists (including engineers and social and physical scientists) and the end-users is indispensable if we are to develop a model that is effective in communicating hazard risk. For example, the NRC's Panel on the Human Dimensions of Seasonal-to-Interannual Climate Variability (1999) points out that the usefulness and utility of climate forecasts can be enhanced by systematically bringing together science and the needs of the end-users. Consequently, end-users will find information that is relevant to their needs, while forecasters can be clear as to what information they need and should provide (NRC, 1999, p. 36). This practice is generally contrary to academic customs in which researchers write for other academics while paying little attention to the needs of practitioners and other end-users (Quarantelli, 1991; Tierney, Lindell, & Perry, 2001). While providing training and education to end-users must be a priority if the proposed communication model is to be successful, researchers must be encouraged to keep in mind the needs of the end-user community. We should also note that public education regarding hazards is an on-going and long-term process that "primes people for response in some future warning" (Mileti, Nathe, Gori, Greene, & Lemersal, 2004, p. 2). Further, this type of hazard education needs to be "people centered" and take into account their socioeconomic and demographic characteristics (for a more detailed discussion on public hazard education, see Mileti et al., 2004).

It is important to highlight that this model (Figure 29.1) includes the general public and communities as integral and active components of the communication process and not as passive bystanders. Researchers, government, and industry must fully comprehend that "warning systems succeed or fail depending on community involvement" (International Strategy for Disaster Reduction [ISDR], 2005, p. 1) thus communities must be active participants in the communication process. We should note that not only do individuals actively participate in this process by seeking to confirm the information that they receive but, just as importantly, by choosing between different and, often, competing sources and technologies to obtain weather, hazard, and disaster information (Lindell & Perry, 2004; Pérez-Lugo, 2001). Further, they will interpret this information according to their unique experiences and perceptions on hazards and disasters. Therefore, attention must be paid to both the needs and preferences for information displayed by different segments of the end-user community and to how the information will be interpreted if we are to effectively communicate with individuals and communities.

THE MASS MEDIA AND THE
COMMUNICATION OF RISK AND WARNINGS

There are a variety of sources from which end-users may obtain information regarding hazards and extreme weather conditions or disasters. Among these, the mass media (e.g., television, newspapers, radio, etc.) plays an extremely important role in the communication of hazard and disaster related news and information (King, 2004; Mileti, 1999; Nigg, 1995b; Paul et al., 2003; Pérez-Lugo, 2001; Wijkman & Timberlake, 1988). The media is one of the most important sources of disaster information (Fischer, 1994) and it significantly influences or shapes how the population and the government views, perceives, and responds to hazards and disasters. Dynes (1998, p. 114) even contends that the media define disasters (for a comprehensive overview of the media and disasters, see the chapter by Scanlon in this handbook).

The opinions or views of individuals or groups who are perceived by the general population to be "experts" (in this case the media) play a central or defining role in the construction of risk. As Wildavsky (1979) states, the perception of risk is reflected by the media's coverage of these events. In the context of the United States, Fischer points out that given that Americans rely on the media for disaster information it follows that their beliefs about them will also be a function of the media (1994, p. 23). However, research on the mass media and disasters has often portrayed the media as conveying inaccurate, biased, and exaggerated information, focusing on human loss and physical destruction (Fischer, 1994; King, 2004; Nigg, 1987; Pérez-Lugo, 2001; Quarantelli, 1987b; Wenger et al., 1980). In relation to the negative effects that the media may have on our understanding of hazards and disasters and, therefore, on how we prepare and respond to these events, Mileti (1999) has indicated that the media often convey erroneous information about disasters, thus leading to both decision makers and the general public to draw the wrong conclusions about them. These issues became quite apparent during the aftermath of Hurricane Katrina with widespread rumors, fostered by the mass media, focusing on extensive looting, thousands dead, babies being raped in the Superdome in New Orleans, and criminal activity running rampant; in essence, "a state of chaos and anarchy" (Dynes & Rodriguez, 2005). Of course, it is now apparent that these events were largely exaggerated, based on rumors and incorrect or inaccurate information, sometimes promulgated by elected officials and widely disseminated by the mass media. Nevertheless, the media's portrayal of these events had a significant impact on the public's perception and response to this disaster.

The role and the power of the media in disaster situations are irrefutable. Platt (1999), citing information on what the National Academy of Public Administration has called the "CNN Syndrome," argues that the overwhelming interest of the news media in disasters now means that most disasters are viewed as national or international disasters and, therefore, local responders are thrown into a limelight that may detract from their ability to correctly manage the situation by unnecessarily politicizing it. Platt adds that this may even lead to unnecessary federal disaster declarations.

Further, media coverage does not necessarily focus on the geographic areas or the communities that have been the hardest hit by natural or technological hazards or those that are more vulnerable to these types of events (Steinberg, 2000). Therefore, governmental assistance (e.g., evacuation, shelters, and recovery and reconstruction efforts) may not reach the groups in greatest need but those that receive the greatest news media coverage. It is then logical to assume that the media plays an important role in defining disaster events and may even impact or drive government and community disaster policies and response to such events. On a more positive note, Mileti (1999, p. 225) argues that the news media can potentially play an important and positive role in communicating reliable and accurate information to the general public by disseminating warnings, providing information about affected areas to responders, and giving reassurance to victims.

TECHNOLOGY AND THE COMMUNICATION OF RISK AND WARNINGS

In our discussion, we must also consider the role that the new, or the not so new, and emerging technology has played and continues to play in the dissemination of disaster or hazard-related information and its impact on individual and community behavior and response to disasters. For example, the Internet has become a primary source of weather-related information for a large proportion of the United States population and for the international community as well. Although little is known about the general public's use of weather information (NRC, 1999), The Weather Channel® (2005a, 2005b) claims that 20 million unique individuals access its Internet pages every month and that its cable programming is viewed in 87 million households in the United States alone. AccuWeather™ (2005) claims 4.5 million unique visitors and 60 million page views per month. Further, Adya, Bahl, and Qiu (2002) report that weather forecasts accounted for approximately 500,000 (or 15%) out of 3.25 million notifications sent by a wireless Internet access provider over a 6-day period in August 2000. Other research confirms the primacy of weather as an Internet interest. The Pew Research Center for the People and the Press (2002) reported that, in 1998, with 41% of U.S. adults using the Internet, weather information was the "most popular online news attraction," given that 64% of Internet news consumers sought out weather information.

Practically all, if not all, major news organizations, the National Hurricane Center, the National Weather Service, and the Federal Emergency Management Agency (FEMA), among others, provide continuous and up-to-date weather or disaster information on the Internet and the evidence shows that an increasing number of individuals are accessing the Internet to obtain weather related information. Technological innovations, including weather radar and satellites, geographic information systems (GIS), global positioning systems (GPS), remote sensing, the Internet, wireless connections, e-mail, the development of cellular phones resulting in extensive communication and information networks, text messaging, personal digital assistants (PDAs) and other handheld electronic devices, and fax machines, among others, have transformed the way we communicate and consume weather and disaster information.

Adya et al. (2002) indicate, for example, that access to the Internet through wireless hand-held devices is gaining popularity. In a sample of 72 emergency managers in the State of Oklahoma, Rodríguez, Díaz, and Donner (2005) found that the primary sources used to access weather information by this group of respondents were: the Internet (93%), television (88%), radio (64%), cell phones (28%), and palm pilots and other handheld technology (7%), among others (respondents were allowed to choose all the sources from which they obtained weather-related information). This technology has radically altered the way we collect, process, analyze, utilize, and disseminate information. The media and the ever expanding communication networks have transformed hazards and disasters from local to national and even international events. At least one observer, Mileti (1999, p. 241), argues that these technological developments hold promise for sustainable hazard mitigation efforts because they improve the dissemination of information and reduce the gap between researchers and practitioners. Furthermore, the ascendancy of the Internet reinforces the view of end-users as active players in the communication process, as individuals generally cannot passively receive information through the Internet, rather they must actively seek it out.

Although the general population has greater access to weather information (including severe weather forecasts and warnings) from which to choose, and multiple channels through which they may obtain it, this can also generate problems for consumers of said information. This situation arises if they are receiving information from multiple sources that is inconsistent, contradictory, or incorrect, thus creating confusion and diminishing both its credibility and the population's trust in the sources of weather information and the information that they provide. This, in turn, may have a detrimental impact on individual behavior and response to warnings and to other types of weather-related announcements and messages (for a particularly compelling discussion of these issues in Puerto Rico, see Pérez-Lugo, 2001). Moreover, despite all the technological innovations in the communication field, there are still communities (primarily poor, rural, and minority communities) that do not receive warning messages (see King, 2004; Paul et al., 2003) because they do not have access to the necessary resources (including adequate technology), technological failures or malfunctions, and their lack of visibility to public officials and the mass media, among others. Nevertheless, given the important transformations in telecommunications and information systems and the potential advantages and problems that they may generate, it is time that we rethink and re-conceptualize warning systems and their impact on organizational and individual disaster preparedness and response in such a manner as to explicitly incorporate all of these factors into both our theoretical models and into the real world warning systems that follow from them.

Further, there are a variety of issues that emerge with the creation and development of new technologies. What is the intended use and applicability of emerging technology? What are the major advantages and disadvantages of such systems, particularly as they relate to extreme weather forecasts, warnings, and disasters? Who has the necessary resources to access such technology? How effective, accurate, and reliable is this technology in providing or communicating weather related information and emergency warnings? What type of education and/or training has been provided to end-users to enhance their use and management of the new technology and thus minimize errors and the dissemination of inaccurate or incorrect information to the general public? How has this technology increased our resilience as well as our vulnerability to natural or human-induced hazards?

We must also ask ourselves, how effective is this communication technology at responding to different types of hazards? Different hazards have somewhat different characteristics that are known to impact warning systems. Some events (e.g., hurricanes) are slow-onset hazards that can be followed for an extended period of time, allowing emergency management organizations and the population to track the same and initiate preparedness and response strategies. Tornadoes, on the other hand, are quick-onset events providing very little lead time, so that warnings may be issued only minutes before they strike. Our ability to develop technology and warning systems that take into account these climatological differences and effectively communicate information to emergency management agencies and the general population in an expedient manner is extremely important.

Increasingly, emergency management organizations are developing communication strategies aimed at automatically informing their constituents of impending emergencies. Just recently (October 2005), the Delaware Emergency Management Agency (DEMA) began testing a new emergency warning or alert system for the state, the Delaware Emergency Notification

System (DENS). This system would be able to send out about 3000 calls every 10 minutes to homes and business to provide a warning of an impending emergency. DEMA will be able to activate this system for localized or statewide emergencies and will provide information to the corresponding communities. It is expected that everyone who has a listed telephone number will have immediate access and will be informed of an impending emergency. Individuals or businesses with unlisted numbers will have to register for the service. It is also noteworthy that the State of Oklahoma (among other states) has developed or is currently developing similar warning systems, called "reverse 911."

Despite the spread of such "warning" systems, there are, however, a variety of questions that merit our attention. For example, given the high costs of developing and implementing such technology, will all local communities, particularly minority and poor communities, have the necessary resources to implement these emerging systems? Also, for those communities that are implementing the "reverse 911" systems, how will households that do not have telephone services be warned of an impending threat or danger? How will low-income, migrant, or minority groups, which have higher levels of poverty than the general population and may lack access to telephone services, receive these warnings? Ultimately, we need to know whether the new technologies improve information flows throughout the population or if they merely magnify the informational advantages that the "haves" already enjoy over the "have-nots" (Bimber, 2003), therefore, increasing the "digital divide" and accentuating existing inequalities. This is not an inconsequential issue, as we discuss in the following segment.

Data from the October 2003 United States' Current Population Survey (CPS) show that 68% of households in the United States have a computer, that 60% connect to the Internet from home, and that 34% of the population (61% of Internet users) have used the Internet to obtain "news, weather or sports information." However, there are also strong class and race biases in access to and use of the Internet. For example, in the lowest income quintile, only 37% of households report owning a computer and just 27% report connecting to the Internet, while for the second quintile the corresponding figures are 56% and 45%, respectively. However, for the fourth quintile, 88% of households own at least one computer and 84% connect to the Internet, while for the highest quintile the figures are, 95% and 93%, respectively. Further, similar biases are observed with respect to race and access to broadband Internet connections at home. These are critical issues which warrant our immediate attention in order to generate strategies aimed at effectively communicating risk, warnings, and disaster information to the population at large generally and to minority communities specifically (see Figure 29.1).

CONCLUDING REMARKS: NEXT STEPS AND FUTURE RESEARCH CONSIDERATIONS

It is important for us to emphasize that the payoffs of increasing technological sophistication (and improving lead time), for example, may be reaching a point of diminishing returns in which morbidity will not come down and in fact may increase in the absence of socially based programs to educate the public and facilitate their understanding of weather related information. In this context, the end-user community must be able to provide inputs and feedback to the technical or scientific community that generates this type of information. The science community must, therefore, be receptive and must encourage feedback from the user communities. However, these efforts also require the integration of the knowledge and contributions generated by social science into the technological scientific effort.

Risk and disasters are socially constructed phenomenon, which are influenced by social and cultural norms, prejudices, and values. Therefore, warnings, hazards, and disasters must be studied and understood within the societal context in which they occur. If we continue to emphasize the study and development of technology, while ignoring the social forces that shape individual and community behavior and response to hazards generally and warnings specifically, then we may have "improved" technology without understanding the complexities of human dynamics. Leading researchers in the disaster field have argued that improving local management and decision-making processes will be more critical or important than the majority of future technological innovations (Mileti, 1999, p. 7). Nevertheless, we argue that we should continue to promote the development of new technology but we also need to focus on the social forces that shape organizational, community, and individual behavior and response to hazards generally and warnings specifically. As indicated by Slovic (2000), in his analysis of risk and risk perception, these issues go beyond science and are "deeply rooted in the social and political fabric of our society" (2000, p. 402).

More accurate and reliable weather forecasts and warning systems may lead to improved disaster mitigation, preparedness, and response initiatives. However, improving weather forecasts and increasing lead times is only part of the equation in determining the ultimate effectiveness of organizational and individual preparedness and response to hazards, for it may be that continued increases in lead time of severe weather warnings may fail to protect people given that the associated warning and communication systems do not address the problems of subjectivity and the diverse socioeconomic, cultural, and political factors that may impact human behavior and response to severe weather events and other types of hazards and disasters, as shown by the aftermath of the 2004 Indian Ocean Tsunami (see Rodriguez et al., 2005) and, more recently, Hurricane Katrina. If we are able to link the knowledge and expertise of the social sciences with the technology and other scientific developments generated by engineers and other scientists and communicate the same in an effective manner to the private and public sectors, as well as to the general public, then we will contribute to the growth and development of disaster research and the corresponding communication process.

We must emphasize, however, that although improved communication processes are needed, significant changes also need to occur in the existing scientific paradigms in order to incorporate the needs and problems that the end-user communities confront. Scientists, particularly those focusing on the development of new technology (but not excluding social scientists), must realize that the needs of the end-user communities must be taken into account and integrated, from the very beginning, into the scientific and technical process, including the design and development of warning and communication systems.

As discussed in this chapter, we must reiterate that to develop effective risk communication models, the demographic, social, economic, and cultural characteristics of the population must be taken into account. Who is our audience? What are their characteristics? From what sources do they obtain disaster or weather-related information? Do they have access to the major or most important media outlets that provide information on hazards, disasters, and warnings? What media outlets do they access most frequently? Do they perceive that the media provides accurate, reliable, and up-to-date information? These are important questions that need to be addressed in order to obtain a better understanding of disaster warnings, the mass media, and the population's perceptions and their preparedness and response to disasters. Moreover, the communication process and related models must be modified and adapted to reflect the changing socioeconomic, demographic, and cultural characteristics of the population. For example, the United States is characterized by a growing elderly population. Consequently, the proportion of the population with chronic illnesses and disabilities (e.g., cancer, cardiovascular diseases, and diabetes) will continue to increase. Even if we incorrectly assume that this population has widespread access to the mass media and warnings, will they be able to respond to warning messages or a disaster situation without the assistance of family or community members or from emergency management organizations? These factors must be taken into account in the development of organizational emergency and disaster planning and management policies and in the communication process.

The United States has also experienced a significant increase in the number of female-headed households. These households have lower levels of education and economic resources and thus have higher levels of poverty relative to their male counterparts. Consequently, important issues and problems during a disaster event will emerge for this important sub-group of the U.S. population. Although important research focusing on gender and disasters has been conducted (see Enarson & Meyreles, 2004; Enarson & Morrow, 1998b; Morrow & Enarson, 1996; Peacock, Morrow, & Gladwin, 1997), it is still a slowly emerging subfield that merits the attention of the disaster research community (for a more extensive discussion on this issue, see the chapter by Enarson, Fothergill, and Peek in this handbook).

In a detailed historical analysis of "natural" disasters in America, Steinberg (2000) argues that racial and ethnic minorities (particularly African Americans) have been disproportionately impacted by these events (also see Peacock & Girard, 1997). He further argues, however, that the impact of disasters on these groups has been largely ignored and neglected, adding that "race has had a filtering effect on the collective memory of disaster" (2000, p. 79). In this particular context, it is important to note that, for the most part, disaster researchers have excluded or have "failed to measure" ethnicity in their research (Lindell & Perry, 2004, p. 163; see also the chapter by Bolin in this handbook). To compound matters, in the United States, the minority population has continued to increase and the Latino/a population has become the largest minority group on the mainland; the migration flows from Latin America and Asia will continue to be an important component of population growth for the United States. We also know that, generally, these immigrant groups tend to be at an economic disadvantage when compared to the general U.S. population, experiencing higher levels of unemployment and poverty.

The somewhat limited disaster research literature, which makes reference to racial and ethnic minorities, shows that these groups experience higher levels of vulnerability to natural hazards (Curson, 1989; Dash et al., 1997; Peacock & Girard, 1997). As Curson points out "the poor, the disadvantaged and the marginal generally suffer most, whether the disaster is an epidemic, famine, earthquake, flood or war" (1989, p. 10; also see Wisner, Cannon, Davis, & Blaikie, 2004). These groups are more likely to be minorities, to reside in hazard-prone areas and, given their limited economic resources, will have greater difficulties in recovering from disasters. The aftermath of Hurricane Katrina is a grim reminder of the devastating impacts and consequences that disasters can have on predominantly minority communities in the United States.

Preliminary findings, emerging from field research carried out by the Disaster Research Center (DRC) at the University of Delaware during the aftermath of Hurricane Katrina, show the differential impacts of disasters on minority groups; these problems are further exacerbated if these groups are undocumented immigrants in the United States. These preliminary results show how class, race/ethnicity, gender, and immigration status intersect to increase the vulnerability of minority groups to disasters. Further, variations in terms of previous experiences with hazards, personal life experiences, individual skills, education, cultural beliefs, assimilation into the dominant culture, and the period of time residing in the United States, suggests that minority groups experience and respond to disasters in ways that are quite different from the dominant groups, and are more likely to suffer the differential and disproportionate effects of disasters. As reported by Latino/a evacuees in the aftermath of Hurricane Katrina, one of the primary barriers they encountered was their relative lack of access to official warnings regarding this event and their inability to understand what limited information was available to them because of language barriers. Given these critical issues, we must also consider how the culture of minority groups and recent immigrants, including their primary language, social values, and attitudes, among others, which are distinctly different from those traditionally encountered in the United States, impact how they prepare and respond to disasters and how disaster outcomes, consequences, and recovery vary among these groups.

It seems to us that the warning and risk communication models and processes developed about two decades ago need to be reevaluated given the aforementioned demographic and technological changes that have occurred in the United States. Also, theoretical and methodological approaches to the study of disasters need to be reexamined and further developed in order to incorporate these demographic, cultural, and technological transformations that are impacting national and international communities. These changing factors will impact risk communication and disaster preparedness and response for the unforeseeable future. Thus, we must concentrate our research efforts in understanding how to effectively communicate warnings to this population through diverse mechanisms (print or visual media, radio, community and other informal communication networks) that they have access to, in ways that are understood and are culturally relevant, and through sources that are perceived as reliable and trustworthy. This is extremely important, particularly if one of our goals is to generate individual and community disaster preparedness and response behavior that will minimize the loss of life and property among these racially and ethnically diverse communities.

Finally, given the continuous transformation of communication systems and other technological innovations and processes, these must be further studied to determine their effectiveness in transmitting warning messages and disaster-related information. Extensive research initiatives are also needed focusing on who has access to these new and evolving technologies; how individuals and communities access weather and disaster information; how these systems are used to disseminate information or communicate emergency warnings; and their impact on disaster preparedness and response at the individual, community, and national level.

CHAPTER 30

Crisis Management in the Twenty-First Century: "Unthinkable" Events in "Inconceivable" Contexts

Patrick Lagadec

"Unbelievable," "unthinkable," "inconceivable": the twenty-first century opens a new era in the field of risk and crisis management. Many of the major recent crises, including the unconventional 9/11 terrorist attacks; the swift worldwide contamination by the bovine spongiform encephalopathy (BSE, "mad cow disease"), SARS virus, or avian flu; continental blackouts occurring within a few seconds, continent-wide effects of a tsunami in unstable geopolitical zones; and Hurricane Katrina seem to differ fundamentally from the seminal cases that gave birth to disaster research in the 1950s and the 1960s (specific floods, hurricanes, earthquakes) and the crisis management studies in the 1980s (e.g., the Tylenol tampering). The trend seems to be accelerating, so that crises today are increasingly global, intertwined, and "non-textbook" events.

The contents of the established crisis tool kit, including risk analysis models, crisis management tools, textbook techniques, organizational checklists, and communication rules, all seem meritorious. This is rightly so, because the lessons of the past still have their place. Failure to take them into consideration can ensnare any attempt at crisis management into the increasing complexities of the emerging world crisis, with potentially disastrous results. However, rear view mirror management is no solution; the discipline must move forward. As observed by astute military strategists, the warning is clear. Do not prepare to fight the last war.

This chapter aims to clarify the issue, identify the traps, and outline some creative lines of response and initiative.

When the discipline of crisis management was developed some two decades ago, long after disasters had become widely studied, it was basically the art of dealing with a specific breakdown and/or severe potential turbulence in a complex system. The aim was to prevent unmanageable cascading and debilitating effects. However, one condition was taken as a given: the triggering event was generally identifiable, and occurring in relatively stable and delineated contexts. However, although a great deal has been achieved by the work of many (Fink, 1986;

Heath, 1998; Irvine, 1987; Lagadec, 1993; Regester, 1989; Ten Berge, 1990) we must now go far beyond.

At the beginning of the twenty-first century, the global situation is infinitely more complex, blurred, and unstable (Lagadec & Guilhou, 2002). In every domain there seems to be a deep schism with the past types of crises, be it in the field of environment, global climate, public health, technological risks, social dynamics, international relations, or violence. The ingredients of these fractures include radical surprises, potential global domino effects, real time dynamics, and the destruction of ultimate references (e.g., destruction of the species barrier in the BSE crisis or the fact that individuals and communities choose death rather than life). What happened on 9/11 casts a very long and pervasive shadow, but it is far from being the only challenge. It is just the keystone of a global mutation in our emerging world, where crises must be anticipated, prepared for, prevented as far as possible and emergency situations tackled.

There is obviously a continuum from "old" to "new" type of crises and complex mix of various types of crises (see the chapter by Quarantelli, Lagadec, and Boin in this handbook). But it is crucial today to insist on the specifics of emerging challenges so as to be sure they are effectively acknowledged and tackled.

In brief, two dynamic elements have combined to create a new crisis universe. First, the agents are increasingly serious, with qualitative jumps in severity, speed, frequency, complexity, and so forth. Second, and much more importantly, specific events occur in extremely unstable, interlinked, and sensitive contexts. They can trigger fuzzy domino processes and dramatic vortex. The "butterfly effect" is no longer a merely theoretical discussion. These changes have required response to switch from single agent comprehension and management to holistic approaches and policies. The challenge is how to simultaneously maintain and develop our capacity to handle single agent disasters and to be able to face the unknowns of a complex world prone to wander on the brink of chaos (Cooper & Coxe, 2005).

Our responsibility accordingly is to rethink our tools, organizations, mindset, culture, and training processes. The stakes are incredibly high. The difficulties are more severe than ever. And the crucial point is not so much to focus on what could be worse, but rather to recognize our reluctance to accept what still remains alien to our culture. On this point, Quarantelli (1998) rightly stressed the importance of a new paradigm for disaster research, far beyond mere reformist adjustments. The same qualitative jump is required from managers, experts, political leaders, and journalists. These issues cannot be simply stimulating theoretical challenges.

Because of the sensitivity and profound fears triggered by the issue, any attempt at risk management must satisfy two fundamental requirements.

First, there is a need for honest and focused open-mindedness. General Foch saw into the heart of the problem saying "gunfire kills, outdated ideas also." Being a war behind is a natural trap, as it is always very comfortable to base any policy on past experience. People tend to base their approach to risk on the deeply believed, much repeated and safe affirmation that there is "nothing new under the sun" (Ecclesiasticus, 1:8-10). The problem with this mindset is that it excludes open questioning and can lead straight into bitter disasters, such as in 1914, when we marched into the industrial era with the agrarian mindset of the previous age (Lagadec, 2000). The type of strategic errors made at that time are too easily repeated, as illustrated by the maxim that in 1914 we were caught totally unprepared, but that in 1940, we were fully prepared, however, for the World War I.

Second, there is a need for courage. Officials or academics regularly and strenuously underline that the mere mention of anything that could represent a new challenge is a reprehensible and pathological manifestation of pessimism. However, optimism cannot be founded on blindness, evasion, and defection. Optimism demands open and questioning minds, personal involvement, and a determined spirit of initiative. For instance, when was the last time you participated in an unconventional rehearsal exercise in your organization (beyond a fire drill)? If you are among the very few who did, what role did you play? What have you learned? If you have never participated in such exercises, why not? I have repeatedly asked mayors, CEOs, cabinet ministers, and their inner circles these same questions. The answer is regularly: "No time," "Not at this level!" "Never, except if you give me the script of the good answers in advance." Now, everyone, and especially at the highest levels, must accept the challenge.

The aim of this chapter is to consider crisis management in this new global context. Three areas are discussed.

First, the new frontiers of our shared safety and the challenges we must now address, that is, the field of emerging crises, go far beyond usual typologies.

Second, the mental blocks and resistances are so dominant in the field that would certainly lead us from one fiasco to another if not recognized as such. These explain why they are so naturally predictable. If this in-depth examination is systematically avoided, there is no real possibility to find any promising outcomes.

Third, positive and creative dynamics must be generated if the challenges of our time are to be met. To a certain extent, this is our historic responsibility.

There is no doubt that these issues are inherently difficult and that our knowledge is still fragile, which inevitably limits suggestions and discussions. However, there is sufficient information to justify and give priority to urgent in-depth analysis of the situation and more importantly, to try and push this examination way beyond the normal boundaries. Proof comes too late, as illustrated by the story of "Minerva's owl" which begins its flight only in the gathering dusk. Of course patience and wisdom are essential to avoid illusion and traps. However, the urgency of these stakes is a total priority. Asking forever for more data, models, statistics, proofs, definitions, and taxonomies must not be an excuse for inaction. We have sufficient signals to measure both this urgency and the crucial need for bold analysis, beyond conventional frameworks (Boin & Lagadec, 2000; Dror, Lagadec, Porfiriev, & Quarantellli, 2001; Quarantelli, 1996d). As the hero of Camus' novel *La Peste* (1947) says to the official who wants to know if it "really" is the plague before he takes action: "This is not a question of vocabulary, it is a question of time."

Quite evidently, the terms inconceivable and unthinkable in this context mean inconceivable and unthinkable only for those who refuse or are unable to take a fresh approach to the emerging issues, and consequently fail to rise to the challenge. As Hegel once said, if reality is inconceivable, then we must invent inconceivable paradigms. Using airplanes to attack the World Trade Center was not inconceivable or unthinkable for everyone, including some atypical officials.

My own position is that unconventional questioning must neither result only from circumstance, nor be left as the preserve of terrorists. If we do not change our approach, repeated failure and fiasco are inevitable. More constructively, the severe turbulence in our complex and unstable world must be turned around and used as opportunities for the basis of a new policy. We must have a positive approach, based on honest and focused open mindedness, creativity, and determination. There is no time to waste.

PARADIGM SHIFT

New Frontiers: Risks, Vulnerabilities, and Emerging Crises

What happened on 9/11 was a watershed in the experience of and approach to risks. The underlying paradigm has shifted from local to global. This shift is clearly illustrated by actions in the United States on Homeland Security, in particular in the many discussions concerning protection of critical infrastructures. This debate emerged as early as 1997–98 with the establishment by President Clinton of the President's Commission on Critical Infrastructure Protection (1998), which pushed forward some new key words: "proliferation," "integration," "connection," "interdependence," "interlinkage," "combination," "constellation of threats," "need for partnerships," and clarified the challenge: "unprecedented" national vulnerabilities.

The 9/11 Commission Report underlined the gap between the threats on one side and the mindsets and available competences on the other. The key failures were identified to be in "imagination" and in "policy" (National Commission, 2004, p. 339). When the vision is a war behind, when technical tools replace policy, you are bound to be trapped.

However, terrorism is not the only issue that requires global safety security policy and "outside the box" crisis management. What happened on 9/11 is certainly the most spectacular, but certainly not the only incident, which has projected the world into a new and profoundly unstable orbit as far as crises are concerned. Other terrorist attacks perpetrated worldwide show that terrorism will be with us for a long time. Consider the SARS episode in 2003, which occurred as a result of the powerful interaction between an unknown virus and jet powered travel (Lagadec & Rosenthal, 2003); the power failure that affected the northeast area of the United States and Canada on August 14, 2003; the blackout that plunged Italy into darkness a few weeks later on 28 September 28, 2003; the 15,000 fatal victims of the heat-wave episode in France during August 4–14, 2003; and, as recently revealed, 20,000 heat victims in Italy during the same period; the tragedy of the large scale AZF fertilizer plant explosion in Toulouse, France on September 21, 2001; the large-scale computer meltdown such as the one which occurred at Heathrow airport on June 4, 2004; the BSE ("mad cow disease") crisis (Phillips, Bridgeman, & Ferguson-Smith, 2001) which stopped the illusion of a protective barrier between species; and most recently, on December 26, 2004 the tsunami tidal wave in Asia.

It is not any specific uncertainty or singular event, but the general trend, which seems to have propelled mankind into a disconcerting universe, that has disrupted the global conditions of risk assessment and crisis management. Even with no actual event, the mere plausibility of largely open scenarios has transformed the conditions of risk governance in our times.

GENERIC CHALLENGES

Following a major event, the usual line of action is to list the various risks and to clarify practical responses for each category. However, the new complexities are such that a different and more strategic approach is needed. The generic problems linked to the new unstable state of the world and the new risk frontiers must be elicited. Fundamentally, these in-depth challenges outclass our paradigms, organizations, and tools. The following eight "fault lines" can be considered.

Discontinuity

Our intellectual baggage has been designed for a stable and linear world with only limited and marginal uncertainty, where events and the contexts in which they occur can be clearly compartmentalized. But this is not the world most of today's crises emerge in. Threats and challenges now occur in a context of instability and poorly defined frontiers. In these situations, averages and statistical regularities and historical trends provide neither an adequate, nor even relevant basis to tackle the problem. Technically, we are equipped to treat massive phenomena involving swarms of points, which can be modeled and plotted. However, in modern crises the situation may hang on one single outlier point, which becomes the swing point. Our intellectual tradition is ill suited to deal with sudden mutations and nonlinear qualitative jumps. We have trained ourselves to ignore differences that are manifestly outside the analysis of variance.

Now we must confront phenomena outside accepted scales. The problems and difficulties have shifted from the edges, where they could be conveniently forgotten, to the core. For example, insurance mechanisms for covering damage used to work quite adequately. Today, the types of threats that loom mean that the entire paradigm base of insurance policy must be reviewed. What happened on 9/11 resulted in 34 billion dollars of insured damages, the most costly event ever in the history of insurance. Reinsurers paid about two thirds of that amount. Then most of them, if not stopping, drastically limited their coverage of this risk. That directly affected the insurance industry in most Organization for Economic Co-Operation and Development (OECD) countries, calling for new programs to be established (Kunreuther & Heal, 2003; Kunreuther & Michel-Kerjan, 2004). We used to work in stable, known contexts with a few difficulties and irregularities at the margins. But now the inconceivable has entered the field of our daily range of certainties; the improbable wild outliers have moved from the periphery (where they could be conveniently forgotten) to center stage.

Ignorance

The accepted practice in any difficult situation is first to consult expert opinion, then to make an informed decision, and then "communicate." Now, the expert finds himself sidetracked in the validation of these models. Whether the crisis is mad cow disease, SARS or the material resistance of the Twin Towers, in each case expert opinion has been at a loss to provide answers within the tiny decision time scale available. The traditional position of the expert, as one who delivers reference knowledge, has been usurped. The first message experts transmit to the relevant authorities must, from now on, underline the limits of current knowledge. Similarly, while policymakers become encircled in their desire to provide assurance, barriers disintegrate almost visibly around them. This is especially the case in food safety, or any issue in health risk. Experimental science cannot affirm something that does not exist. The same deliberately constructed indeterminism is also naturally evident in terrorism.

Massive Domino Effects, High-Speed Contagion, Erratic Effects

Over time, we have mastered the art of dealing with cleanly defined accidents and emergencies. Our societies are not armed to cope with ultrarapid, geographically dispersed contagion on a massive scale. It is quite probable that the source of any threat can now be geographically very far removed from the point of impact, and the effects of propagation can be startling. This was the case with SARS, where the unknown virus spread at literally jet speed from Hong Kong to Toronto via the transport communication hubs of the planet, from hospital to hospital; for example, when the specialized staff worked in several hospitals, all the key lines of defense are rapidly taken out. This was also the case for anthrax. The problem was not four specific contaminated letters, but contagion in the sorting systems. Here the network actually becomes part of the strategy of the attack. Indeed, the attacks were not physically oriented against the networks but these people use the diffusion capacity of our own networks and turn it against us. The network becomes the weapon (Michel-Kerjan, 2003).

Submerged Information and the Larsen Media Effect

Information sources are now almost infinite. Information concerning the phenomenon is distributed worldwide, and the complexity of the organizations seems to shatter the echo into penetrating fragments. News travels almost instantaneously around the global media networks and most particularly when the information is very uncertain and unsettling. Emotion has become a central factor of any reality, because emotion is the essential nerve of the media. The Larsen effect, the electroacoustic phenomenon of feedback between microphone and amplifier resulting in maximum sound output, quickly overwhelms any attempt at reasoned information. Excellent classic media communication is possible, but how can any decision maker cope when the whole context of an event is overwhelming? Structurally speaking, the media networks still seek and recycle any event that best suits their working tools and so favor camera-ready disasters. These are simple stories, binary formulae that combine maximum emotion with overt simplification, particularly when the complexity of the situation threatens the entire data treatment system.

The Citizen on the Front Line

The 9/11 Commission specifically highlighted the fact that the traditional model of "State intervenes, citizen receives aid" has attained its limit. Empowerment has become a vital necessity. In this vein, inquiries conducted after the severe 1998 ice storms in Quebec led to the conclusion that each citizen should ensure him- or herself a certain subsistence autonomy. Three days autonomy for each citizen and family at all periods of the year, particularly in terms of energy needs. This decision was taken in order to allow the authorities to deal with vital networks without having to concentrate on all fronts and from every angle of the shattered fragments of this particular problem.

The Global Dynamics of the Destruction of Known Phenomena, Loss of Orientation, Loss of References Points

Each of the identified phenomena intermeshes as it occurs. The result is that the solid base of our knowledge, our hold on the natural world is at best subject to uncertainty, at worst positively wrong or even destroyed. For example, there was the loss of the certainty that the species barrier was the ultimate protective wall between man and diseases rampant in other species. Similarly, there was the loss of the very characteristics defining temperate climate. Another example would be that of an aggressor attacking in the certain knowledge that he will lose his own life, a strategy that totally destroys the foundations of the techniques of negotiation, namely that you can negotiate only with someone who values his or her own life. Considering a death sentence for a kamikaze is clearly nonsense. The context is now entirely new, all previous approaches, commentary, and postures have been turned upside down. The principle of the new unconventional events is that they all seem to apply the principle of Sun Tzu, where the best warfare strategy is to attack the enemy's plans.

Governance, Not Communication

These episodes are essentially crises as defined by the ancient Greeks, namely, they are fundamental moments of truth. The hardest thing to grasp is their meaning. Business-as-usual management is no longer adequate. The problem must be seen and tackled from a multiplicity of fresh angles, new choices identified, and the logic of the actors involved redrawn. None of this falls under what was traditionally accepted to be management technique and expertise. This highlights the extent to which "good crisis management techniques," the tried and tested "recipes for crisis communication," are severely limited.

From Rationality to Wager?

Perhaps the most destabilizing factor lies in how emerging crises confront us with situations which at the beginning of which nobody can know for sure whether ultimately they will be classed as minor, critical, extremely severe or a non-event. AIDS was no great concern in the early days of the pandemic, and yet it has become a historic threat of monumental proportions limiting the social and economic development of countries or even continent (e.g., Africa). Conversely, when BSE emerged, some specialists predicted a global disaster. In reality, the mortality from the disease can be counted in hundreds in the United Kingdom and single figures in France, and not in the millions of deaths some predicted. Again, with the SARS pandemic in 2003, the threat was worse than the reality. At the time, no one could assess the gravity of the problem. For example, the Director of the U.S. Centers for Disease Control and Prevention, the world-leading center of expertise in the field, stated to the media that the death toll could rise to 16 million if it developed into a pandemic. Overestimation was certainly not the problem for the 2003 European heat wave. The initial alert estimated 50 deaths; the final count was nearly 15,000 in France. In the case of terrorism, the issue achieves a state of paroxysm as to what can or cannot be excluded. Responses run into problems of either under-provision of measures of protection or, on the contrary, massive over-provision. Or again there is the real risk of not even being able to define what is over-reaction or under-reaction, until it is too late. The swing point can occur at any moment, anywhere, from any event or news of an event whether founded or not.

Our rules of governance easily run aground in this new universe. The risk is avoidance strategies, waiting paralysis. There is also the danger of repeated U-turns in risk policy, which are rightly perceived as incomprehensible and which, in any case, are always a stroke behind. The ultimate trap is when fear becomes the driver of governance, which can lead to all manner of distasteful actions under the cover of "safety/security," and where any dissension becomes labeled as treason. In that vein, terrorism can extend the reach of its empire without any actual attack. It merely has to play on the capacity of the system to close in on itself. Sun Tzu is still right: "To subjugate the enemy's army without doing battle is the highest of excellence." Other risks also dramatically reinforce the feeling that society has lost some of its reference points. Thus the cycle of denial—dazed—manipulation is fed by fear.

To counter this lethal process we need both new systems of intelligence and of governance. These systems are still embryonic; they must be developed. The first step is trying to understand what could possibly block or slow the necessary reinvention of the machinery of action.

THE TRAP: FEAR AND PARALYSIS

Fierce Resistance

Our emergency culture is primarily equipped to grasp specific, limited problems, and solve them with specific responses. A crisis manager copes well as long as "a crisis" can be defined as a somewhat delicate situation requiring specifically adapted materials, plans, checklists, and organizational tools and rules. Here, the manager just has to request a list of the likely risks and crises. Using this information, he or she can delegate the task of preparing response plans and response data sheets and can recommend the implementation of practices to ensure that all the prepared responses and response equipment are in good working order. The crisis once neatly packaged, complete with set responses is domesticated, controlled, and can be "rubber-stamped" as acceptable.

It is far more difficult to try to bend the mindset of individuals and groups to work on the essentials of the crises. Any event outside normal experience presents extraordinary challenges, which by definition do not come with a prepared set of desirable responses. When it comes to preparing for unconventional events, most organizations still try to tackle the problem with some media training. However, it is very disturbing to observe that any attempt within any organization to go beyond this approach and to develop a crisis culture, whether conducted by external specialists or internal managers, systematically meets with ferocious resistance or determined inertia.

Experience repeatedly highlights the following observations with sickening regularity:

- When a "what if?" type question is asked on hypothetical issues of safety not normally examined, the reaction is always instantaneous, brutal, and final: "We are here to tackle problems, not to create new ones." "Sorry, but I am pragmatic, we are solution people here, not theoreticians."
- When the options are considered, the problems become evident. In suggesting that normal lines of defense could be bypassed, that "insurmountable" barriers might be crossed, the credibility of the initiator of the discussion is fundamentally at stake: "For goodness sake, we are optimists here!"
- Suggesting to someone lower down in the line management that a simulation could and should be organized is quickly rejected out of hand: "I am afraid that here we don't play at involving top management, top management would never accept it here. In any case, we never check who is actually qualified to intervene among the top managers who are on duty."
- Suggesting that during a simulation that, perhaps, it might be worth introducing an unconventional complication outside the usual rituals always leads to the horrified response: "Certainly not, it would destroy the exercise!"
- Suggesting to a major multinational group, that an in-depth study could be conducted on major vulnerabilities leads to instant refusal on the grounds that "No, all we need is a plan, and some media training for some of our directors."

- Suggesting that a president or minister/secretary could be included in an exercise, to give a little of their time to the problem of unconventional crises usually elicits sighs and concern: "We do not bother that level with this type of issue; anyway they simply don't have the time. Prepare a clear information sheet and they might just drop in."
- Suggesting an unusual and major innovation after a difficult event, for example an experience exchange, an initiative to be conducted with others, elicits the response: "Listen, we managed to get out of this one, let's not make things any more complicated."
- Suggesting that certain partnerships could be considered is the crowning lesson on the fact that the economic context is ferociously competitive and that any information sharing could prejudice the share of markets, budgets, and territory. Interestingly, this attitude is very similar in both the public and private sectors. Everywhere competition for territory is bitter, fundamental, and identity defining.
- Suggesting to an excellent management team that it might be good to reflect on the new frontiers of risk that affect that company usually elicits the response: "Impossible, our teams are engaged in calculations, have models to follow which are in their normal line of work. They would not tolerate overt questioning of their systems."
- Suggesting to multinational institutions that they could include issues of governance in highly unstable conditions on the agenda will likely lead to the response: "No, we are organizing a meeting with technical experts who will present specific scenarios. The rest is off the agenda." "We cannot include or decide anything if it has not been requested by all of our members, which is not the case at the moment."

There are an infinite number of specific examples. Over the last decades, as I have been working on this issue of unconventional fault lines, I have repeatedly faced such reactions. Others are reported to me on a monthly basis. Everyone would easily list reactions of this kind. Fortunately, there are remarkable exceptions, and these should inspire us. But, regrettably, even in the most advanced countries and corporations, they too often remain exceptions whereas they should develop into decisive programs.

The important trend is the homogeneity of the retreat: No questions, no anticipation beyond the bounds of known experience, no inclusion of the higher tiers of management, no simulations on events that might fall outside the normal rituals, no audacious partnerships. The field is wide open for crises.

It is crucial to measure the depth of this resistance. An example: In May 1989, speaking on the topic of "new risks" at a conference organized by a major international organization in Ottawa, the general who passed me the microphone had time to whisper under his breath: "Whatever you do, don't scare them!" This was just a few months before the fall of the Berlin wall.

Anther example: Eleven years later, in June 2001, at a Defense Zone meeting on the same subject at Marseilles in the south of France, a high-ranking defense official who had come down to the meeting from Paris interrupted me. He announced: "I cannot let this continue. In France things are under control. I am optimistic." Strong words from the defense official. However, during the cocktail party afterwards the same official came to me and confided, "You were right, but I couldn't let that be said to the heads of regions (Préfects)." This was just 2 months before 9/11, and 3 months before the explosion of the AZF chemical plant in France, one of the largest industrial catastrophes in Europe in the last 50 years.

To any suggestion of work or new ideas on the subject, the most favorable response today is, "Let me think about the best way of selling the idea; otherwise we will immediately come up against a wall of resistance." Surely, the time has come for ideas on the issue to be received more creatively.

The problem is not even of resistance to change. The blockage goes far deeper. The stakes are very high and it is these same stakes that we must try to understand.

TESTING THE RESISTANCE

On this issue, a number of fault lines converge. The situation is very worrying and calls for very strong corrective action.

Intellectual Handicap

Anything that is unusual, exceptional and nonlinear is instinctively rejected by our society. It is as if our approach has remained stationary since the natural philosophers of the seventeenth century. The ordinary processes are the only relevant issue (Buffon, 1749).

Rosenthal, one of the pioneers in crisis study, underlines that this tradition has remained central and currently blocks crisis management (Rosenthal, Charles, & 't Hart, 1989). Scientists feel very uncomfortable with anything outside "normal" circumstances and events, which indicates that crises, by definition, are not welcomed.

Perhaps Weinberg (1985) best expresses a division into two separate worlds: *Science,* which deals with regularities on one side, and *Art,* which deals with singularities on the other. It would seem that unconventional problems must remain orphaned. They repel scientists who like phenomena to be regular, reproducible, and measurable. However, leaving the governance of these problems to the artists, although creative, is certainly not going to be enough. Moreover, whoever takes an interest in these phenomena will have great trouble to be taken seriously.

Managerial Handicap

Stacey (1996), a professor of strategic management, has forcefully stated that a vast majority of textbooks on strategic management concentrate on surprise-free issues, when the real priority should be "instability," "irregularity," and "disorder." The fact is that today when flung into these situations, managers are highly likely to react clumsily or simply be confused. To make matters worse, any invitation to prepare for the abnormal is taken as unfounded, illegitimate, or even provocative.

Governance Handicap

Because crises and unconventional events are unplanned, the arguments opposing any real strategic preparation and any personal engagement by people in governance positions are recurrent. The positive results of personal engagement are very clearly illustrated in the way in which the then Mayor Rudolf Giuliani of New York City, totally involved himself in crisis exercises for the city, the last time being in July for an exercise simulating a chemical attack against the city.

Psychological Handicap

This is probably the most determining problem. A crisis event can effectively strip the manager of all his sense of direction, casting him adrift of all his structuring and supporting frameworks, with the loss of everything justifying his social position (power, identity, responsibility, and respectability). Consequently, crisis situations confront the manager with the risk of facing total surprise. Clearly, this is profoundly destabilizing and destructuring for somebody unprepared. It cannot be sufficiently emphasized that a crisis is not a calculable event and no perfect model can be made to fit. Rather it places the manager in front of an incomprehensible precipice, and there are no quick fixes to fill this void.

At this point the analysis of the situation becomes almost psychoanalytical because of the powerful and often irrepressible emotions that surface among both individuals and official groups in critical situations (even a planned exercise regularly evokes the same type of destabilizations). When void and ignorance surface, defensive reactions quickly follow. I have observed with surprise many times the way in which people in charge suddenly physically disappear from the EOC (Emergency Operations Center) when a piece of information comes in that does not fit within their normal frameworks and mindsets. Fabre (2004), a psychoanalyst and specialist of Descartes, is right when commenting on Descartes' refusal to consider the existence of any vacuum (a famous controversy with Pascal) and insisting that he vitally feared considering any system with the slightest chink. We still suffer this very fear in the arena of crisis management: it is so frequent to see people in charge who are focused on their plans and scripts and who refuse open questions and any thinking outside the box. In the same vein, if we want to better understand the why behind modern crises and unstable contexts, a very useful analogy can be found in the early days of psychoanalysis. Freud (1977) warned his audience that their entire cultural background had necessarily made them opponents of the new continent to explore.

Although these references may seem out of context, they are essential. The crisis situation and the loss of references almost automatically make psychology the major issue, both at the group and individual levels. In practice, collective fear repeatedly exacerbates managerial, governance, and intellectual handicaps. Profound destabilization leads to denial, compulsive/extreme rationalization, or avoidance.

These handicaps would not be such a cause for concern if ignorance in the field was diminishing rather than growing and that our technologies and understanding were constantly pushing back the frontiers of uncertainty. However, as highlighted by Bernstein in his seminal book (1998), this is not the case. After a detailed historical study of uncertainty, Bernstein concludes with considerable insight that discontinuities and volatilities seem to be proliferating, not diminishing.

The Straightjacket of Daily Routine

The task of decision makers is exacerbated by the tyranny of daily routine, which complicates the fundamental difficulties described in the preceding text. The complexity is real time and it engenders saturation at all levels. All available time and energy is swallowed up in the tactical management of daily operations. This in itself is the leitmotiv of decision makers who see no time available for temporally projected reflections, open-minded questioning, initiatives, and cross fertilization of ideas.

The avalanche of contributing factors caused by current trends including the acceleration and march of globalization in the business world, the violence of the shocks which seem to call for ever more stringent and weighty administrative operations (whether for control, accompaniment, repair, etc.) and the focus of everyone on stable features among the universal changes constantly taking place, leaves very little room for maneuver. The immediate tactical obstacles can be overcome only if the "wiggle" factor is increased.

The meagerness of the room for maneuver has to be measured and understood before any real progress can be made. If not, failure is inevitable, accompanied by all of the regular ritual. This can be stated as follows: announcement of a new national priority every 2 days depending on the ups and downs of the news; communication instead of governance; compensation for the lack of personal involvement with poorly defined rules to be imposed on others; with the final conclusion every time that the ultimate learning lesson is that children need to be taught these things from primary school onwards.

Clearly, given all the problems, there are no easy solutions. But the pressure of reality is upon us. The risk threshold is repeatedly exceeded and redefined and the handicaps afflicting our capacity for preparation, reaction, implication, and leadership have given rise to very disturbing responses. Three seemingly accelerating factors appear to govern destabilization:

1. The disarray of specialists and managers, confronted with the new interconnected complexity of vulnerability, in a context of exacerbated instability, about which our ignorance appears ever increasing and invasive.
2. The increasing mistrust of the people involved who have experienced the hollow traditional verbal assurances, on the lines of "everything is under control," and observed the U-turn to the new theme "we have no control over events but we guarantee good, transparent communication."
3. The threat of decoupling between decision makers and managers on one side and the wider public on the other. The danger is that, on a rapidly approaching horizon, radical shift occurs in reaction, from the consensual "Never again" to the "Let them all go to hell!" The dynamics of this shift can be characterized as going from explosion to implosion.

These difficulties are being studied and must be addressed.

THE CREATIVE DYNAMICS NEEDED

These issues cannot be solved by any quick and easy recommendations, which come with their own attached checklist. They are real challenges, with real twists and turns, each one characterized by a unique set of surprise, shock, unthinkable, but also positive opportunities.

There are two basic lines of approach and both must be engaged. The first is in-depth groundwork, to provide the basic information to address the new challenges, even if the boundaries are sometimes chaotic. The second is an effort toward adjustment/safeguarding to provide a better basis for dealing with immediate turbulence.

BUILDING FUNDAMENTAL STRENGTHS

We must try to generate a radical turnaround on a number of fronts. There has to be rupture but in a positive and creative sense. The following suggestions are not exhaustive.

A Radical Change in Intellectual Approach

The road map is nearly a clean white page and, as such, it invokes all the paralysis that goes with this information vacuum. The perspective of the issues must be literally up-ended. Issues that had previously existed on the periphery have been brought center stage and must now be treated as core issues and not freak events. The "known world" no longer exists, the comfortable world where we conducted our activities and projects, with recognized measures of excellence with a few discrete little uncertainties at the edges.

In the past these marginal uncertainties were worthy of attention only if they fell into validated theories supported by robust statistical evidence, neatly cleaned free of untidy outliers. The new frontiers of knowledge and the focus of intense and urgent intellectual effort must now concentrate on events and data excluded until now: discontinuity, irreversibility, extremes, volatility, radical change, crystallization, and resonance. This work must be conducted both vertically in all disciplines and horizontally across all disciplines. These subjects must stop being taboo and the work undertaken must not be lip service paid to the wild peripheries, a small concession simply to maintain basic order. The challenge is there and ready to be taken up by the best brains and specialists. If this movement is not tackled with determination and conviction, the intellectual world will disengage. When turbulence and mind numbing events occur, challenging the reference points of our world and disturbing the tranquility of our accepted paradigms, arguments that anything "out of the box" is not science are not acceptable. We need new tools for the new challenges and the closer these tools can be brought to the people at the front line of the management procedure, the less they will refuse the obstacles which confront them.

Intense Involvement at Highest Levels

When confronted with such weighty matters that concern identity, survival, plans and visions for the future, nothing can be done without intense, personal, direct involvement by the key players in the organizations concerned. For example, during the "9/11" crisis, the actions of Mayor Giuliani went far beyond mere circumstantial "media communication" and were a determining factor in the management of the entire situation. But this was not done by "accident." "Prepare relentlessly" had been a personal rule for the Mayor (Giuliani, 2002). Those who occupy the highest offices are expected to be on the front lines, where the stakes are high, mobilizing people capable of taking charge. Those involved must receive a powerful message, that nothing less is expected of them. To date, this type of direct and personal implication by leaders is very much the exception, in all countries.

There is a shrinking ability to think on our feet. Plunged into a world of violent turbulence, organizations must be led, mobilized, and empowered in new terms. The acquisition of a specific, rigid technical arsenal to respond to an unusual situation is no longer adequate. Advance planning and a high level of responsiveness to weak signals at the highest level are essential in order to anticipate sudden change, counter ethically unacceptable reactions, and build the necessary networks of actors. Because of the elements of surprise and complexity and the aberrant nature of the events, organizations must develop new ways of monitoring situations. Leaders must be able to rely on people accustomed to operating in a crisis, people capable of objective stepping back and assessment, whenever a sensitive situation arises. This skill is particularly necessary to counteract the dangerous "bunker mentality" trap where individuals seem unable to think. Perhaps the most seriously pathological reaction to the new forms of crisis is "in a crisis, you don't have time to think," and adopt the easiest approach to problems, usually purely technical, without examining the underlying positions.

Today, more than ever before, great crises will lead to great disaster unless sufficient thought and ability for strategic leadership are developed. The Spanish catastrophic management of the Prestige disaster and the fiasco of March 11, 2003 (the multi-attacks on Madrid trains, and the Aznar's government pointing at ETA) should serve as a final warning here, for many.

During a recent international simulation in Slovakia, we were able to see the degree to which the lack of strategic ability in these areas was determinant. The European political capability was exhausted in only 2 hours. In fact, the expression "Crises as Institution Killers" was coined to express what we observed then.

The Experience of Exchange Clubs

The critical barrier is the profound anxiety, which instantly emerges with any "out of the box" event, where there are no coded and validated responses. We must all, and this applies particularly to those exercising the highest levels of authority, engage the search for best approaches to these difficult territories. Although still at a very embryonic stage, "clubs" for the sharing and exchange of problems, questions and solutions have proved successful. This type of forum has been much appreciated by those who have taken the step to take part. Together, the participants address the destabilization factor of major surprise, of the unmanageable, the unthinkable, and subsequently prove far more able to cope with situations and actually exercise their responsibilities. These clubs cannot provide easy solutions, that is, no checklists, no standard practice, but they do enable participants to take a more objective approach, to understand that each event is unique and that as such management directions must be tailored to the actual challenge being faced. However, these clubs can continue to be effective only if they are provided with some guidelines and direction from time to time. Rigorous professionalism is needed; organizing a meeting is not enough on its own.

Civil Society Back in the Loop

In the same spirit, we must get past the notion that, in delicate situations, everything is immediately put in the hands of some government agency, under a single command, using a sort of military reasoning that believes that civil society will only "panic and give way to looting." The example of the 1988 Quebec ice storms is quite instructive in this regard. The debriefing, largely open and extremely detailed, strongly emphasized the need to determine the response in close cooperation with citizen and nongovernmental organizations (NGOs). For example, it was said that for such complex network failures the citizen had to be prepared to go it alone, cope with the situation at his or her level, and wait as long as it took for service to be restored. The decision here is that the overriding priority was given to the structural restoration of the networks.

Any other strategy can only lead to overall impotence and horrendous mistrust. This is not a militant view advocating some dangerous oversimplification. The shocks that will accompany the new world of risk will require modes of functioning that can no longer rely on our vision of a state that provides solutions to passive groups of people within a "Command and Control" philosophy.

Here, we touch upon our most fundamental concepts of governance. At a large staff meeting of a large ministry in France, held a few years ago after several serious weather-related events, one of the national administrators argued for a new conception of the role of the state by citing: "To profess to solve all problems and to answer all questions would be impudent boasting, and would argue such extravagant self-conceit as at once to forfeit all confidence." The meeting made known how much it agreed with this statement. A high official expressed his indignation; to emphasize the extent to which, on the contrary, the state had all the resources needed to perform its noble tasks. This issue lies at the core of our discussions on risk: is this an opportunity to raise questions and to take responsibility? Or, on the contrary, a danger that requires reaffirmation of the principle that everything is under control, without, however, there being anything reassuring about it.

Here also there is a need to open, share, and invent. However, achieving this supposes that new approaches are available. For example, a few days before a public meeting on risk in Toulouse after the terrible explosion at the AZF factory, I drew to the organizers' attention the need to build in a new framework for sharing experiences and views. The reply was: "The speeches have been approved." The time has come to move on and to engage different practices. The real problem is that the paralyzing nature of these challenges "freezes" action.

In the same way, citizen involvement must be improved. For example, when emergency exercises are conducted, the heads and managers of institutions such as hospitals, schools, retirement homes, and so forth should be consulted in order to get a better idea in advance of their specific needs and constraints, and so target the testing of certain procedures. This would enable the old approach of "Do nothing until you receive orders" to be overturned in favor of "What would be the most useful for you and then we can test it together?" We can only reap the trust that is sown.

Training

The stakes are high. Until these areas have been explored and become part of the basic training in higher education programs, they are unlikely to find their way onto the agendas of our decision makers. The subjects will remain taboo if they do not become part of the identity, the reference training, and the league tables of excellence for new generations of managers/decision makers. Without this preparation from within, the fear associated with major risk will remain too uncontrollable to enable any creative synergy to be generated.

More positively, the big question is to define the necessary basic grounding, which our future managers, among others, need to be able to find the vision, balance, skills and ability to listen in a world constantly shaken by the shockwaves of permanent schisms. It is no longer sufficient to prepare them for a stable world where the rare and freak event requires "management." On the contrary, they must be trained to manage in a world where the dynamics and schisms engendered by crises are structural realities.

IMMEDIATE CREATIVE INITIATIVES

In addition to long-term action, we must adopt more immediate strategies such as rapid reflection forces. Major crisis events engender closure, seizure, the raising of barriers, and engagement in cul-de-sacs. In real terms, each nation with its own diversity of culture groups must designate a range of people who can be mobilized to deal with all aspects of an emerging major crisis. The same should be developed in industry. The lack of such teams was particularly evident during the Toulouse-AZF crisis and again during the tsunami episode of 2004 and Hurricane Katrina in 2005. The task is to identify the people who are both competent and able to remain operational in the face of unconventional crises and to make them work together to develop flexible but efficient strategies for crisis management. These people do exist but they are often dispersed. They must be brought together in teams and trained in order to extend their experience, skills, and ability to ask questions, so that they may assist decision makers to cope with unconventional situations. In building these teams, we must be careful not to fall into the usual rut of assuming that the members should be drawn from the established elitists. To guarantee the essential open-mindedness, the teams must include a whole range of people including females, foreigners and younger persons that is not the case now. This approach is currently under discussion at the European level, in particular within the framework of the European Crisis Management Academy. The next step is to move from idea to action.

Minimum Preparation for Senior Management

From an institutional point of view, there are two current dominating topics in crisis management strategy. First, the preparations of crisis plans often are subcontracted. Second, "crisis communication" media training is too often seen as the priority. This rather rigid compartmentalization must be broken down. This type of "safe waters" response is no longer adequate and crisis management strategy must now make preparations to survive in the challenging "high seas" of risk today. Preparations for unconventional situations should be at the top of all senior management group agendas, from boards of directors to executive committees and ministerial cabinets, without arguing that they already do this on a daily basis!

Preparations and Active Partnerships

Emerging crises give rise to organizational problems, which have no identifiable frontiers. It is now urgent to engage those involved in their management, in joint preparations and training. That should help to encourage them to ask more as well as the right questions. For the last years, the notion of partnership has dominated meetings on the protection of critical infrastructures. "Partnership is a brilliant idea; the practice of partnership is another matter" (see Lagadec & Michel-Kerjan, forthcoming).

The time has come to move into the action phase. For example, this could involve studying scenarios such as the film "The Day Britain Stopped" (BBC, 2003). In this BBC film drama, Britain faces a national crisis in the country's transport infrastructure that has been operating at virtually saturation point. A series of unfortunate events paralyzes all transport systems such as road, air, and rail, resulting in a snowballing chain of events. The interdependence of the decisions adopted by each of the key actors is ignored and the individually managed strategies all become un-operational. A case of so-called "interdependent security" has recently been introduced and formalized by leading scholars in the United States (Heal & Kunreuther, 2005). This program is only a drama and although it lacks rigor on some points (as often criticized in the UK) the real question ought to be why should the monopoly of creating such scenarios be left to journalists? Why are the actual decision makers involved absent from the reflection and work to be accomplished?

Tough, Targeted, and Bold Initiatives

With a battlefield so vast and complex, it is necessary to move forwards in carefully thought out, very specific, but bold stages. In implementing a very specifically defined plan to achieve progress, the lesson can be learned that action is not suicidal; on the contrary, it can be fertile. The field is so vast it is crucial to focus on specific highly targeted initiatives. Indeed, as already highlighted, the time constraints do not permit implementation of cumbersome plans.

For example, In February 2001, a major snowstorm on the Aix-Nice motorway in the south of France trapped 4000 people on the road for nearly 36 hours. Weather conditions were unprecedented. Three feet of snow fell in a few hours. Instead of claiming "force majeure" ("Act of God"), the Chairman of the road operator (Escota) called a public debriefing. Through the press, all interested parties were invited to share their experiences at a public meeting 3 months later. In addition, at this public meeting, the collective effort was supplemented by joint consideration of how each participant could contribute to the safety of such a large network in the future (e.g., if it were necessary to cut off traffic in Provence, then trucks would be held at the Spanish and Italian borders). The result was particularly interesting, providing a better understanding of the incident itself and the problems to be confronted, and planning for the future. Basically, the meeting provided an opportunity to become better aware of the networks at work, especially to create new networks among the various players such as the toll authority, government authorities, local officials, service stations, the weather service, truckers, and motorists.

As another example, after the anthrax attacks in 2001 in the United States, and thousands of false alarms in Europe, I suggested to postal operators that they should organize an international meeting for experience exchange and to define some strong operational initiatives for the future. The President of the French postal service, *La Poste*, immediately agreed to the idea. In 2002, key representatives of about 30 operators attended the meeting in Paris to share their experience, the lessons they had learned and to set up an inter-network alert and information system. One month later, this new capacity was implemented and was used to deal with a new alert, again originating from the American network. A number of key factors made this operation such a success, a willingness to listen, to consult, and to suggest innovative strategies (Lagadec & Michel-Kerjan, 2006, forthcoming).

How often is this type of information exchange engaged today after some major event? Many of the major actors in the Toulouse tragedy regret today the lack of this type of initiative following the AZF explosion. In the SARS episode, it would also have been important to organize a meeting between the public health actors, representatives of the affected cities and governments, and the transport sector in order to try and identify the big issues and centralize good ideas and strategies for progress.

However, experience exchange is not the only solution. Strong initiatives must be instigated on a number of other fronts: questions need to be asked, simulations created, training organized, international public debate engaged, and so forth. The time has come to be creative. We must be as innovative and proactive as the emerging crises are surprising and furtive. There must be one central belief, namely that it is only by taking the risk to try something new that creative opportunities are made. Only by taking risks do we stop being the prisoners of risk. We must be prepared, so that risking some risks is less terrifying and paralyzing than the perspective of a guaranteed fiasco.

RESEARCH NEEDS AND PERSPECTIVES

At least three lines of investigation should be considered by scholars to help those in charge and the public to meet the unknown developing challenges, and to develop their own strategies:

What is new? In the academic world, at least up to now, the trend has been to treat anything "new" with extreme caution. It should be an acceptable and even a desirable objective, to concentrate on the emerging challenges, surprises, and complexities. Priority must be given to the mapping, clarification, and understanding of the real problems and illusions presented by these new challenges.

What are the difficulties? When organizations and people are suddenly confronted to outside the box issues, they tend to try to implement the three Ds: "deny, deflect, defend." It is absolutely necessary to know more about the cultural and educational traps, the managerial blocks and the learning refusals which all combine to exacerbate situations and make them difficult to change.

What are the best initiatives and best cases? When the issue is so severe and so difficult to grasp, it is vital to search for any success, and study it. An official who launched some bold debriefing or simulation to train people to confront the "unthinkable"; any initiative in street empowerment taken by ordinary citizens; any new tools, new organizations or new paradigms that could help academics to get a hold on these events which, because they do not fit into normal statistics nor any common frameworks, take on the character of strange "unidentified flying objects."

CONCLUSION

In the film *The Hunt for Red October*, there is a key moment in which the Commandant of the Soviet submarine announces to his officers that he has informed the Kremlin of his plan to defect, and take his ship to the West. His officers rebel violently against what seems to be a personal whim of their leader: "Suicidal," they cry. The Commandant calmly replies: "But the problem is not the Russians! I know their tactics!" This scene summarizes the crucial challenge of any high-risk situation: traditional approaches are totally submerged by unexpected events, and so we can expect nothing from people in charge because we know that they have neither the culture nor the tools to rise to the occasion. It is a very different game for which most of them have not been trained.

To me, the major risk today may well be the litany that "everything is under control," that "we mustn't be pessimistic" and therefore there is no point "asking too many questions" while simultaneously insisting that citizens must abandon the notion of zero risk and lamenting society's unhealthy preoccupation with legal action.

If we do not have the courage to take strong, determined, and open-minded initiatives, we run the risk of becoming increasingly bogged down in a bunker mentality. The risks will not wait for us to get ready and if we go from fiasco to fiasco, the will, energy, and confidence to tackle the issues will collapse, reinforcing the suspicions of the public, the fears of the authorities and feed into a morbid loop.

Failure is not an option. We must acquire the entire range of skills needed for the new challenges, intellectual, managerial, governance, psychological. Fear is the major assailant to be conquered at all costs, despite all temptations to the contrary and any collateral benefits which it may procure (Krenz, 2001). Quite on the contrary, we must visit the new frontiers with confidence, improve our intelligence about them, and acquire brand new skills and entire new strategy logic. Ultimately, it will be of our responsibility to take and share strong initiatives, with many, in order to remain actors of our particularly turbulent period of history.

AFTERWORD

This chapter was written before the Hurricane Katrina tragedy. It is clear that this event has yet again brutally clarified the need for a new vision and new paradigms. In the hurricane aftermath, in addition to the usual field studies, we must launch specific projects aiming to track and trace any emerging questions that would require new paradigms, new frameworks, and new research practices. As a final word, in reference to the title of this contribution, it was claimed yet again that the fatal combination of hurricane and levee failure was "unthinkable." This was stated in reports prior to the event. The unthinkable is here to stay. We must address it.

CHAPTER 31

New Dimensions: The Growth of a Market in Fear

FRANK FUREDI

Fear is one of the dominant emotions through which we imagine disaster. It also constitutes an important dimension of contemporary social reality. Public fear and anxiety play a crucial role in deliberations surrounding the environment, health, crime, children, new technologies, and recently and quite dramatically in relation to terrorism. Governments and public organizations often take the view that fear is a problem that they need to understand and manage. Today the discussion of public resilience in response to terrorism reflects this concern. Historically the imperative of maintaining public order and morale or concern about the outbreak of mass panic led governments to speculate about this problem with a view to containing it and minimizing its destructive effects. After the devastating experience of Hurricane Katrina, the problem of fear has also been "rediscovered" in relation to natural disasters.

But although fear is widely discussed in the public domain it is seldom studied by social scientists as a problem in its own right. The dimension of fear is rarely explored in contributions on the subject of how individuals and communities cope with acts of misfortune such as disasters. The study of fear has tended to be confined to the field of psychology, which is understandably interested in the emotional response of the individual to threatening circumstances (Lerner & Keltner, 2001). Otherwise fear tends to be treated as self-evident phenomenon that requires little elaboration. However, the experience of fear has both a social and a historical dimension. Fear, like most emotions, is "fundamentally constituted" through social experience (Bourke, 2005, p. 8). So although the psychological perspective on emotion can often provide interesting insights, it also needs to engage with the wider cultural and social influences in order to develop an understanding of how fear is experienced. Scruton (1986, p. 9) introduced the concept of *sociophobics* "the study of human fear as these occur and are experienced in the context of socio-cultural systems" to point toward the territory for future research.

Fear is situational and is to some extent the product of social construction (Altheide, 2006, p. 24). It is constituted through the agency of the self in interaction with others. It also internalized through a cultural script that instructs people as to how to respond to threats to their security. That is why the specific features of the fear experience are most likely to be captured through an assessment of the influence of culture. Fear gains its meaning through the mode of interpretation offered by the narrative of culture. An orientation toward meaning and the rules and customs governing the display of fear can help take the discussion beyond the stage of merely treating it as a self-evident emotion. One of the most perceptive studies of the history of emotions points to the need for distinguishing between the "collective emotional standards of a society" and subjective feeling of the individual (Lewis & Stearns, 1998, p. 7). Although the emotional experience of the individual is an important dimension of the problem, our attempt to conceptualize the current market in fear requires that we analyze the prevailing cultural narrative of fear. Cultural norms that shape the display and management of emotions influence the way that fear is experienced.

Experience shows that fear and the intensity with which it is felt is not directly proportional to the objective character of a specific threat. Adversity, acts of misfortune, threats to personal security do not directly produce fear. The human response to threat is associated with anxiety. But the conversion of anxiety into fear is mediated through cultural norms that inform people about what is expected of them when confronted with a disaster and how they should respond and feel. Hochschild, in her path-breaking study of the sociology of emotions characterizes, describes these informal expectations of what constitutes an appropriate emotional response to situations as **feeling rules** (Hochschild, 1983). These feeling rules influence behaviour in stressful circumstances and instruct us how and what we ought to fear. But the transformation of anxious responses into fears also requires the intervention of social actors, of fear entrepreneurs. The sociologist David Altheide argues that "fear does not just happen; it is socially constructed and then manipulated by those who seek to benefit" (Altheide, 2006, p. 24). While this formulation of the social construction of fear may inflate the role of self-interest, its emphasis on the role of human agency provides a useful counterpoint to the naturalistic and psychological representation of fear.

Fear is not simply a biological response to an event but a construction of the human imagination. My argument is that through a market in fear claim-makers attempt to convert everyday concerns and anxieties into tangible and imminent fears. But while fear entrepreneurs play a central role in the conversion of existential insecurity into fear, their activity cannot account for the impact of this emotion on the public and on society. These concerns are experienced and mediated through taken-for-granted meanings about the nature of social reality and in particular of personhood. C. Wright Mills has argued that people's consciousness of being threatened is mediated through their system of values. Mills claimed that whether or not people feel well or insecure is influenced by their relationship with the prevailing sense of meaning. So "when people cherish some set of values and do not feel any threat to them, they experience *well-being*" (Mills, 1959, p. 11). In contrast, "when they cherish values but *do* feel them to be threatened, they experience a crisis." "And if all their values seem involved they feel the total threat of panic," adds Mills. Mills also projected a scenario that captures an important dimension of contemporary reality. "Suppose, finally they are unaware of any cherished values, but still are very much aware of a threat," he states before concluding, "that is the experience of *uneasiness*, of anxiety, which, if it is total enough, becomes a deadly unspecified malaise" (Mills, 1959, p. 11).

Following Mill's line of approach it becomes evident that it is not simply the threat to our security but our ability to make sense of it that influences the way we fear. Every community that is affected by a disaster is confronted with the task of making sense of the adversity that it has experienced. As Claude Gilbert argues, a disaster upsets the prevailing system of meaning. He notes that "we may speak of a disaster when actors in modern societies increasingly lose their capacity to define a situation that they see as serious or even worrying through traditional understandings and symbolic parameters." And he adds that for a "community, disaster means the loss of key standpoints in common sense, and the difficulty of understanding reality through ordinary mental frameworks" (Gilbert, 1998, p. 17). It is the difficulty in recovering a common meaning in the aftermath of an extraordinary experience that may account for some of the reports of community disorganization found in recent disaster literature. As Pastor notes, such episodes call into question "the ability of a culture to provide safety, meaning and esteem to its individual members" (Pastor, 2004, p. 619). My basic argument is that claims making intensifies and fuels a competitive market in fear when the prevailing system of meaning lacks the authority to make sense of acts of misfortune and disaster.

The growth of litigation and blaming in the aftermath of a disaster can be interpreted as an outcome of a decline in the authority of shared system of meaning. Our study of floods in England indicates that litigation and claims making activities is a product of the eighties. For example, in the aftermath of the floods of 1952 and 1953, claims making activities were conspicuously absent and blame assignation was muted and relatively restrained (Furedi, 2007). Drabek's review of disasters in the United States draws a similar conclusion. Increasingly, "disaster victims engage in a blame assignation process," he writes (Drabek, 1986, p. 201).

Competing claims framed through fear is not a phenomenon unique to current times. Ideological conflicts, for example, fear of nuclear weapons versus fear of communism, have often been conducted through attempting to convert people's sense of disorientation into a clearly focused fear. But as I argue below projecting alternatives through the prism of fear is very different to the situation today. Fear has lost its specific focused quality. Claims making is not confined to competition between a small number of issues. The sense of foreboding toward a large variety of unspecific threats is linked to the absence of a reliable interpretative mechanism through which people can make sense of distressing events.

THE CONTEMPORARY CULTURE OF FEAR

Disasters and catastrophes have occurred throughout history. But the reaction to these events has varied according to the mood that prevails in society. A comparative study of human response to floods in Britain indicates significant differences in the way that disasters are processed. Destructive floods leading to serious loss of life in 1952 and 1953 were perceived through a very different cultural frame than the far less destructive flood of 2000. The cultural script transmitted to society in the 1950s signaled the expectation that communities and individuals would be able to cope with the calamity they encountered. Indeed people were encouraged to interpret disaster as a test or challenge to be overcome. In contrast, in 2000, the flood was represented as a uniquely threatening event that was likely to overwhelm the coping capacity of individuals. This difference in emphasis is highlighted by the following excerpts from the two scripts: A report from *The Times* on the Queen's visit to the afflicted areas clearly transmitted officially sanctioned expectations that people would respond to the flood with "courage and fortitude." It was reported that the Queen was "impressed by the stoic and heroic manner of the people who had obviously been through a bad and trying time, suffering heavy losses" (*Times*, February 4, 1953).

The familiar sounding rhetoric of the Queen was amplified and transmitted through metaphors and powerful symbols that at once affirmed the sense of loss while communicating the belief that Britain's sturdy folk would prevail over the hardships it faced. In contrast, in 2000 newspapers transmitted the conviction that flood victims would suffer serious psychological damage. According to one account in *The Guardian*, "up to 20% of natural disaster victims may suffer from post-traumatic stress disorder." It added that many feel depressed and isolated, losing their sense of place and attachment, or developing obsessive anxieties as a result of the ordeal" (Hirst, 2000).

These two contrasting representation of events were paralleled by a fundamentally different orientation toward claims making. In 1953 the floods were not politicized. Criticism of officials, public agencies, and professional groups was rarely expressed. A handful of politicians criticized the BBC for its inaccurate weather forecast. Claims makers promoting their own distinct agenda were conspicuous by their absence. The response to the flood of 2000 was totally different. From the outset, the project of blaming was vigorously promoted by claims makers. At various times, greedy property developers, the Environmental Agency, public planning officials, and politicians were blamed for the disaster (Furedi, 2007). Not surprisingly arguments about who to blame encouraged suspicion and mistrust in the aftermath of the floods of 2000.

The different evaluations and responses to the floods are in part linked to the significance and meaning attached to the role of informal networks of the community. If the floods of the 1950s were about a disaster inflicted on communities, those of 2000 are about individual distress. It is striking how in comparison to the disasters of the 1950s, the role of the community, with its altruism and resilience, is rarely endowed with significance in 2000. A review of the press indicates that reports of resilient behavior are virtually absent from the discussion. One of the few examples of community altruism was reported in the *Daily Mail*. Its report focused on a group of 22 people who were stranded in a pub in Yalding for 3 days. The owner of the pub was noted that "we were petrified, but it has been like the Dunkirk spirit." According to this account everyone pitched in and provided help to one another. (Irwin, 2000).

It was the populist tabloid *The Sun* that attempted to resurrect the traditional narrative of the "British Bulldog Spirit" to represent the response to the flood. One of its writers noted that "as the nation comes to terms with the worst deluge in living memory, a small band of people leave us feeling proud to be British (Yates, 2000). But it was a "small band" of emergency workers and not the community that constituted the focus of *The Sun's* celebration of British courage. In contrast, a study of the 1953 floods, observed that thousands of volunteers took part in the rescue and salvaging operations. "Many thousands of civilians, belonging to civil defence or voluntary organizations, played their part, and large drafts of officers and men were sent by the army and the R.A.F." noted a report at the time (*The Times*, February 3, 1953).

In contrast to the representation of the flood in 2000, during the 1950s reports continually valorized the response of the community. Individual stories of human suffering were rare. In *The Times* there is only one story of an individual coping with adversity (*The Times*, February 6, 1953). At all levels of society, the informal community networks that emerged in the course of the disaster were seen as the heroes of the hour. For many flood victims, it was the response of neighbors and other community members that gave them the strength to cope with their perilous circumstances. Christopher Manser, a resident of Canvey Island who lost three of his siblings, recalls "the warmth generated by the spontaneous reaction of local people to the need for clothes." He notes that "women had taken their husband's jackets and trousers straight from the wardrobe without emptying pockets" and gave it to victims of the flood. "I found money, cigarettes, diaries, and so on," he added (Pollard, 1978, p. 89). For scores of individuals a sense of community meant something positive. John Peddler, who was 17 when he rescued his father when the Lynmouth flood engulfed the post office, stated that "we are a very close community, and we remember the kindness of ordinary people who sent us things at the time." He added, "that is how we coped" (*The Sunday Times*, August 31, 1997).

Ideas about how people are likely to cope in an emergency or a disaster are shaped by prior experience but also by a cultural narrative that creates a set of expectations and sensitizes people to some problems more than others. It provides a frame through which people understand and make sense of their experience. Twenty-first century Western culture frequently transmits the view that we live in a uniquely dangerous era in which humanity faces hazards and potential disaster. "The modern era is often cast as an age of catastrophe, of global conflicts, genocides and 'ethnic cleansings', disasters of industrial and agrarian change and of technological hubris, and—increasingly—environmental cataclysms," note two British historians (Gray & Oliver, 2001, p. 1).

There is also a manifest tendency toward expanding the range of events that can be characterized as a disaster to be feared. "These days, disasters may result in modest levels of harm, and perhaps relatively straightforward tasks for the emergency services" and yet still they are called 'disasters,'" notes Tom Horlick-Jones (1995, p. 304). In line with contemporary crisis consciousness, often the line between misfortune, accidents, adversity, and disaster have become blurred. According to the philosopher Marcio Seligmann-Silva (2003, p. 143), the definition of catastrophe has altered. Instead of being represented as an "unusual, unique, unexpected event," it is increasingly seen as an everyday event.

The process outlined by Seligmann-Silva has been conceptualized by social construction-ist sociologists as that of *domain expansion*. Domain expansion—the process through which "the contents of previously accepted social problems expand"—is a constituent element in the construction of social problems today (Loseke, 1999, p. 82). Through the process of domain expansion, a heightened sense of anticipation surrounds the discussion of disasters in Britain. "Our recent history is littered with large scale disasters and catastrophes" is the first line of a book on the subject. Its author believes that the 1980s can be appropriately described as a "decade of disasters" in the United Kingdom (Newburn, 1993, p. 9). Another account writes of "the spate of disasters that hit Britain in the mid-late 1980s" (McLean & Johnes, 2000, p. 120). Its inference that we are living through uniquely dangerous times is testimony to a cultural imagination that perceives the world as uniquely risky. Horlick-Jones observed that the association of disasters in the United Kingdom with the 1980s may have served for many as a symbol of a "political and economic system in crisis" (Horlick-Jones, 1995, p. 307).

Ideas about disaster are culturally specific and are linked to wider attitudes about the meaning of misfortune, blame, and social expectations. It is our contention that contemporary disaster consciousness is not the direct product of a qualitative change in intensity of this threat. Rather, what have changed are attitudes to adversity and ideas about its impact on the individual. Whether or not a decade is associated with disasters is determined by a variety of influences. The scale of damage and the number of casualties may produce fear toward disasters in the future or it may not. Historical examples are quite useful in highlighting the influence of cultural norms on perceptions of adversity and hazards. It could be argued that if there was a decade of disaster in the United Kingdom in recent history, it would be the 1950s. In one year alone—1952—there were a larger number of casualties than in all the U.K. 1980s disasters put together. August 15, 1952 saw one of the worst flash floods ever to have occurred in Britain. It swept through the Devon village of Lynmouth, killing 35 people. Between September 4 and 9, the smog in London killed several hundred people. On October 8, three trains crashed in Harrow railway station, leading to 110 fatalities. And then the really big one: in December the Smog hit London, leading to an estimated 4000 deaths.

Yet, despite the mass scale of fatalities, these disasters were not represented as events that signified that the world had become a more dangerous place. Individuals who recall this event often note that back in 1952 the Smog was not interpreted as a disaster. According to one account, "I think it has to be realised that people thought that these disasters of smogs were the result of the industrialization of our country, and that they were a necessary evil which we had to put up with in order to get the benefits of our industry making us more wealthy" (Berridge & Taylor, 2003, p. 21). Jon Ayres recalls that as a youngster during the 1956 Smog, he and his friends regarded it as "rather fun." He noted that although the adults were worried "for us there was a real chance that school might be cancelled." "It was rather exciting, you could play all sorts of games that young boys did with baddies round the next corner," he recalls (Berridge & Taylor, 2003, pp. 17–18). From the standpoint of today's cultural sensibility such a light-hearted reaction to a major episode of pollution would be unthinkable.

Throughout the 1950s, Britain suffered from a large number of air and rail crashes and mining disasters. Compared to reactions to adversity today, the response to them appears as almost casual. A sense of loss and fear was tempered by the conviction that the effects of these tragedies would be contained and soon overcome with little long-term damage. Despite the fact that far more people died in disasters in the 1950s than in the 1980s, the era was not characterized as a decade of disasters. The experience of disasters—major and minor—is a social phenomenon that is mediated through the public's cultural imagination and attitudes toward loss.

SPECIFYING THE EXPERIENCE OF FEAR

The meaning and experience of fear is subject to cultural and historical modifications. The meaning a society attached to the fear of God or the fear of hell is not quite the same as the fear of pollution or of cancer. Matters are also complicated by the fact that the words and expressions used to describe fear are also culturally and historically specific. The language we use today represents fear through idioms that are unspecific, diffuse, and therapeutic. Bourke, in her important study of the cultural history of fear, points to the importance of the "conversion of fear into anxiety through the therapeutic revolution" today (Bourke, 2005, p. 191). Anxieties about being "at risk" or feeling "stressed" or "traumatized" or "vulnerable" indicate that an individualized therapeutic vocabulary influences out sensibility of fear. Conversion of fear into anxiety represents only one dimension of the process. The fear market also works in the opposite direction and converts anxiety into fear.

Our research suggests that the two distinctive features of today's fear culture are:

1. The independent existence of fear as a problem in its own right.
2. The unstable, free-floating and raw character of fear.

Let's look at each of these developments.

Fear as a Problem in Its Own Right

One of the distinguishing features of fear today is that is appears to have an independent existence. It is frequently cited as a problem that exists in its own right disassociated from any specific object. Classically societies associate fear with a clearly formulated threat—the fear of death or the fear of hunger. In such formulations, the threat was defined as the object of such fears. The problem was death, illness, or hunger. Today we frequently represent the act of fearing as a threat itself. A striking illustration of this development is the fear of crime. Today, it is conceptualized as a serious problem that is to some extent distinct from the problem of crime. As Garland (2001) observes; "fear of crime has come to be regarded as a problem in and of itself, quite distinct from actual crime and victimization, and distinctive policies have been developed that aim to reduce fear levels, rather than reduce crime" (Garland 2001, p. 10).

Frequently, public anxiety and concern are represented as a material factor that can have a significant impact on people's health. Contemporary medical culture contends that stress and fear are likely to increase the risk of heart disease, cancer, and chronic lung disease (Siegel, 2005). In the United Kingdom the conclusion of an enquiry held into alleged health effects from cell phones is now regarded as a model for how to respond to contemporary health fears—particularly related to environmental health. The Independent Expert Group on Mobile Phones (IEGMP) set up "to keep ahead of public anxiety" concluded that there was no known health threat posed by mobile telephony. At the same time, the report stated that anxieties created by the simple presence of mobile phone masts need to be taken seriously since public fear by itself could lead to ill health. (Furedi, 2003, p. 4). There is always a potential for people's health anxiety to turn into a major problem. The medical sociologist Phil Strong writes of an "epidemic of suspicion" that can cause serious public health problems (Strong, 1990, p. 253). However it is only recently that risk perception itself has been represented as a "key component to causing fear" (Guzelian, 2004, p. 52).

With the autonomization of fear the issue is not simply its cause but the potential negative consequences of this emotion. This perspective often encourages the strategy of managing feelings of fear rather than the source of the problem. If people feel that their health is at risk, then this fear is often seen as a risk to people's well being (Furedi, 2004, p. 137). The legal system in the United States and the United Kingdom has also internalized this trend and there is a discernible tendency on the part of courts to compensate fear, even in the absence of a perceptible physical threat. As Guzelian noted, in the past "fright" i.e., a reaction to an actual event, was compensated whereas now the fear that something negative would happen is also seen as grounds for making a claim (Guzelian, 2004).

The autonomization of fear is associated with a growing tendency—to conceptualize risk as an independent variable. This approach is clearly formulated through the recently constructed concept of being *at risk*. The emergence of the "at risk" concept ruptures the traditional relationship between individual action and the probability of some hazard. To be at risk is no longer only about what you do or the probability of some hazard impacting on your life—it is also about who you are. It becomes a fixed attribute of the individual, like the size of a person's feet or hands. Being at risk also implies the autonomy of the dangers that people face. Those who are at risk face hazards that are independent of them. If risk is autonomous, it suggests that it exists independently of any act or individual. Like the Greek gods, risk factors exist in a world of their own. But unlike the gods whose acts conveyed a message with a meaning, the risk factors do not talk to us. Living with risk becomes our fate, encouraging a disposition toward a fatalistic perspective toward uncertainty. This sense of fatalism continually counsels us to avoid risks, to take measures that can promote safety. Underpinned by a sense of weak agency—the vulnerable subject—the development of a fatalistic perspective toward risk has fueled the development of a **fear market**. As the sociologist David Altheide (2002, p. 3) suggests, the prerequisite for the ascendancy of a market in fear is the emergence of fear as a "dominant public perspective." Today, the frequently used idiom "politics of fear" expresses this trend" (Furedi, 2005).

The Unstable Free-Floating and Raw Character of Fear

How we react in general and how we fear in particular is subject to historical and cultural variations. Existing research highlights the importance of the historical dimension. Work by Stearns and Haggerty (1991) provides interesting insights into the changing way that fear in relation to children has been conceptualized in the United States. They point out that with the passing of time children's engagement with fear was increasingly interpreted through the prism of terror. One consequence of this perception of childhood has been the tendency toward eliminating terror from children's books (Stearns & Haggerty, 1991, p. 85, 88). The other is to conceptualize children as "vulnerable" and therefore unlikely to be able to cope with adverse circumstances.

Equating fear with terror is one possible orientation toward a particular object of anxiety. However, historically fear does not always have negative connotations. The sixteenth century English philosopher Thomas Hobbes regarded fear as essential for the realization of the individual and of a civilized society (Robin, 2004). For Hobbes and others, fear constituted a dimension of a reasonable response to new events. Nor does fear always signify a negative emotional response. As David Parkin (1986) argues as late as the nineteenth century the sentiment of fear was frequently associated with an expression of "respect" and "reverence" or "veneration." From this standpoint the act of "fearing the Lord" could have connotations that were culturally valued and affirmed. In contrast, today the act of fearing God is far less consistent with cultural norms. One important reason for this shift is that fearing has tended to become disassociated from any positive attributes. This change in attitude is conceptualized by Parkin as a shift from a concept of fear that "encompassed that of respect" to what he calls "raw fear." The former is described as an "institutionally controlled fear" whereas "raw fear" has more of a free-floating and unpredictable character. (Parkin, 1986, pp. 158–159) Bourke claims that this shift toward more "nebulous anxiety states" is due to the decline of the tangible threats to corporeal existence that are occasioned by war (Bourke, 2005, p. 293).

"Respectful" and "raw" fear express very different relations to human experience. Parkin claims that respectful fear assumes "predictable response to behavior." It is a form of "knowable fear." It is knowable because it is embedded in informal taken-for-granted and culturally sanctioned formal relations. In contrast, "raw fear" has as its premise "an unpredictable aspect sustained by the victim" (Parkin, 1986, p. 159). This is a fear that is not rooted in folk culture and not guided by a generally accepted narrative of meaning, hence its unpredictability. The unpredictable character of fear points to its free-floating and dynamic character. Its volatility is enhanced by its unstable and unfocused trajectory. In contemporary times, fear migrates freely from one problem to the next without there being a necessity for causal or logical connection. When the Southern Baptist leader Reverend Jerry Vines declared that Mohammed was a "demon possessed paedophile" and that Allah led Muslims to terrorism in June 2002 he was simply taking advantage of the logical leaps permitted by the free-floating character of our fear narratives (Filler, 2003, p. 345). This arbitrary association of terrorism and pedophilia can have the effect of amplifying the fear of both. In the same way, constant claims that this or that hurricane, flood, and other natural disasters are symptoms of global warming has the effect of altering perceptions and fears.

Fear today has a free-floating dynamic and can attach itself to wide variety phenomena. The fear of terrorism illustrates this trend. Since September 11th, this fear floats into an ever-expanding territory. Deliberations on this subject have acquired a fantasy-like character. "Corporations must re-examine their definition of risk and take seriously the possibility of scenarios that only science fiction writers could have imagined possible one year ago" argues a leading economist (Hale, 2002). Fear floats into new territory because since 9/11 normal hazards can be turned into exceptional threats by associating them with the action of terrorists. As a result, we do not simply worry about the hazard posed by a nuclear power station; we also fear that it may turn into a terrorist target. The fact that an ever-expanding phenomenon can be perceived as a target is less an outcome of an increase in the capabilities of terrorists than in the growth of competitive claims about what to fear.

The free-floating dynamic of fear is promoted by a culture that communicates hesitancy and anxiety toward uncertainty and continually anticipates the worse possible outcome. The culture that has been described as the culture of fear (Furedi, 1997) or as precautionary culture (Pieterman, 2001) encourages society to approach human experience as a potential risk to our safety. Consequently, every conceivable experience has been transformed into a risk to be managed. One leading criminologist, David Garland, writes of the "Rise of Risk"—the explosion in the growth of risk discourse and risk literature. He notes that little connects this literature other than the use of the word risk (Garland, 2003, p. 52). However, the very fact that risk is used to frame a variety of otherwise unconnected experiences reflects a taken-for-granted mood of uncertainty toward human experience. In contemporary society, little can be taken for granted other than an apprehensive response toward uncertainty. The French social theorist Francois Ewald believes that the ascendancy of this precautionary sensibility is underwritten by a cultural mood that assumes the uncertainty of causality between action and effect. This sensibility endows fear with a privileged status. Ewald suggests that the institutionalization of precaution "invites one to consider the worst hypothesis (defined as the "serious and irreversible" consequence) in any business decision." The tendency to engage with uncertainty through the prism of fear and therefore anticipate the worst possible outcome can be understood as a **crisis of causality**.

The question of causation is inextricably bound up with the way communities attempt to make sense of acts of misfortune. The way people interpret such events—an accident or a catastrophe—is processed through the prevailing system of meaning. Questions like "was it God" or "was it nature" or "was it an act of human error" have important implications in how we understand acts of misfortune. Today such questions are complicated by the fact that Western societies possess a weak sense of shared meaning and therefore often lack a consensus about how to attribute blame and responsibility. The absence of consensus means that the link between cause and negative outcome is continually contested. Confusion about causation encourages speculation, rumors, and mistrust. As a result, events often appear as incomprehensible and beyond human control. The appearance of a loss of control is most clearly expressed through the conceptualization of being "at risk." This new and original way of framing the relationship between everyday life and uncertainty endows fear with a distinct quality.

THE PROBLEM OF MEANING

The difficulty that society has in making sense of uncertainty is what gives contemporary fear its raw character. The distinction that Parkin made between the predictability of respectful fear and the uncontrolled character of raw fear can be understood as an expression of the growing tendency to contest the meaning of misfortune. Increasingly the questions of what we should fear and who to blame have become subjects of acrimonious debate. Lack of consensus over the meaning of misfortune bequeaths fearing a private, individuated, and even arbitrary character. Disagreement about the meaning of misfortune is not new. As Russell Dynes points out, the debate surrounding the meaning of the 1755 Lisbon earthquake led to a confrontation between rival views of the world (Dynes, 2000a). But past debates about the causes of disasters involved a clash of competing systems of meaning. Today, the protagonists in such a debate lack such moral and intellectual support and engage in the controversy as isolated individuals. Instead of a consensus forged around a society's fear, the way we respond to threat tends to often isolate us. "Cancer and crime, pain and pollution: these fears isolate us," notes Bourke (2005, p. 293).

As Quarantelli noted, explanations about the cause of a disaster are subject to historical variation (Quarantelli, 1995a). In the absence of a master-narrative that endows misfortune with shared meaning, people's response to disaster has acquired an increasingly subjective and personalized character. The sense of loss of agency bound up with the state of being at risk means that people feel an intense sense of not being in control over their circumstances. Paradoxically, as we feel less in control the more we are likely to reject the idea that misfortune just happened by accident. At a time when apprehensions toward uncertainty intensify a quest for meaning it is difficult to accept that accidents just happen. As the Dutch sociologist Pieterman, argues there has been a shift "from a situation where the role of chance is seen as crucial to one where it is marginal" (Pieterman, 2001, p. 153).

So the crisis of causality does not mean that our culture discourages society from searching for the causes of misfortune. On the contrary, it has unleashed a ceaseless search for discovering meaning in misfortune and for attributing blame. The cultural mood of fatalism coexists with the belief that accidents do not just happen. There is always some one to blame. Ewald notes that "disasters are no longer, as before, attributed to God and providence, but to human agency" (Ewald, 2002, p. 282). The loss of a sense of causality has encouraged perceptions that associate negative and destructive episodes with intentional malevolent behavior. Such episodes are frequently blamed on the self-serving purposeful acts of politicians, public and business figures, doctors, and scientists—indeed all professionals. One of the most important way in which the sense of diminished subjectivity is experienced is the feeling that the individual is manipulated and influenced by hidden powerful forces—not just spin-doctors, subliminal advertising, and the media, but also powers that have no name. That is why we frequently attribute unexplained physical and psychological symptoms to unspecific forces caused by the food we eat, the water we drink, an extending variety of pollutants and substances transmitted by new technologies, and other invisible processes. The American academic Timothy Melley has characterized this response as agency panic. "Agency panic is intense anxiety about an apparent loss of autonomy, the conviction that one's actions are being controlled by someone else or that one has been 'constructed' by powerful, external agents," writes Melley. The perception that one's behavior and actions are controlled by external agents is symptomatic of a heightened sense of fatalism that is associated with the sense of diminished subjectivity. The feeling of being subject to manipulation and external control—the very stuff of conspiracy theory—is a sensibility that is consistent with the perception "at risk." As Melley observed, this reaction "stems largely from a sense of diminished human agency, a feeling that individuals cannot effect meaningful social action and, in extreme cases, may not be able to control their own behaviour" (Melley, 2000).

A diminished capacity to share meaning endows the act of fearing with an atomized character. This may have implications for how disaster-struck communities cope with their loss. As we note elsewhere, the contemporary individuated narrative of fear may discourage the realization of the potential for a resilient response (Furedi, 2007). Fear that is unrestrained by communal norms tends to have a corrosive impact on community life. As one study of this process notes, an "epidemic of fear is also an epidemic of suspicion" (Strong, 1990, p. 253). Such suspicion tends to undermine social capital and solidarity—key requisites of community resilience in the face of disaster.

A MARKET IN FEAR

The absence of consensus about interpreting adversity encourages competitive claims making about the problems facing society. The consequence of such claims making activity is to convert underlying uncertainties and anxieties into more tangible fears. It also provides a medium through which claims for resources can be made. Claims making involves making statements about problems that deserve or ought to deserve the attention of society. A claim constitutes a warrant for recognition or some form of entitlement. Claims demanding that a newly discovered object of fear is taken seriously draw on prevailing assumptions about being at risk. As Joel Best, in his important analysis of claims-making reports, "how advocates describe a new social problem very much depends on how (they and their audiences—the public, the press, and policy-makers) are used to talking about, already familiar problems" (Best, 1999, p. 164). The narrative of fear provides the idiom for claims making activities. Although claimmakers are sometimes accused of scare mongering they are far more likely to gain authority through their demands that something should be done about the object of their fear. And with the steady expansion of campaigns demanding new assurances of safety the fear market has become a busy environment of competing claims.

There is nothing peculiarly novel about claim making activities based on fear. Throughout history, claim-makers have sought to focus people's anxiety toward what they perceived to be the problem. However, the activities of fear entrepreneurs today do not represent simply a quantitative increase over the past. In the absence of a consensus over meaning competitive claims making is both extensive and intrudes into all aspects of life. As I argue elsewhere, fear now constitutes a distinct narrative that is culturally validated and encouraged (Furedi, 2005). As David Altheide remarked, the fear market has "spawned an extensive cottage industry that promotes new fears and an "army of social scientists and other intellectuals—or "issue fans"— serve as claims makers, marketing their target issues and agendas in various forums, such as self-help books, courses, research funds, and expertise" (Altheide, 2002, pp. 3–4). The trend outlined by Altheide constitutes a crucial dimension of claims-making. The promotion of fear represents a claim on moral authority and on resources. So when the British Geological Society demands that the danger of super-eruptions be recognized by officialdom, it also pleads for "investment in research to improve our understanding of regional and global impacts of major volcanic eruptions" (Report, 2005).

In the private sector, numerous industries have become devoted to promoting their business through the fear market. In some cases, entrepreneurs seek to scare the public into purchasing their products. Appeals to personal security constitute the point of departure for the marketing strategy of the insurance, personal security, and health industries. As Haggerty (2003) states, "personal security has become commodified." He notes that fear is "frequently used to sell security products" and ads "help to channel and focus diffuse and amorphous anxieties about crime and other forms of social breakdown into distinct and personalized fears about someone entering *your* bedroom window, stealing *your* car, or attacking you on your evening jog" (Haggerty, 2003, pp. 194, 205). Fear is used by the IT industry and its army of consultants to sell goods and services.

In certain instances, it is difficult to clearly delineate the line that divides the fear economy from the promotion of anxiety and the anticipation of a disaster. It is worth recalling that for a considerable period of time the Y2K problem, also known as the Millennium bug was regarded as the harbinger of a major disaster. The scale of this major internationally coordinated effort and the massive expenditure of billions of dollars to deal with possible technologically induced crisis were unprecedented. Only a very small minority of IT experts were prepared to question those devoted to constructing the "millennium bug problem" (Anderson, 1999). Even social scientists who usually make an effort to interrogate claims about an impending disaster failed to raise any questions about the threat. One IT industry commentator, Larry Seltzer, noted that "looking back on the scale of the exaggeration, I have to think that there was a lot of deception going on." He added that the "motivation—mostly consulting fees—was all too obvious." But nevertheless it was not simply about money. Seltzer believes that there were also a lot of "experienced people with no financial interest who deeply believed it was a real problem" (Seltzer, 2005).

Despite the growth of the Fear Economy and the exploitation of anxieties about potential catastrophes, the promotion of fear is primarily driven cultural concerns rather than financial expediency. One of the unfortunate consequences of the culture of fear is that any problem or new challenge is liable to be transformed into an issue of survival. So, instead of representing the need to overhaul and update our computer systems as a technical problem, contemporary culture preferred to revel in scaring itself about various doomsday scenarios. The millennium bug was the product of human imagination that symbolized society's formidable capacity to scare itself.

Contemporary language reflects the tendency to transform problems and adverse events into questions of human survival. Terms such as "plague," "epidemic," and "syndrome" are used promiscuously to underline the precarious character of human existence. The word plague has acquired everyday usage. The number of times it has been cited in the U.K. press has increased phenomenally from 45 in 1990 to 2298 in 2000 (Furedi, 2002, p. xiii). The adoption of an apocalyptic vocabulary helps turn exceptional events into a normal risk. This process can be seen in the way that the fortunately very rare occurrence of child abduction has been transformed into a routine risk facing all children. In the same way, threats to human survival are increasingly represented as normal. Kumar (1995, p. 205) argues that the apocalyptic imagination has become almost banal and transmits a sense of "millennial belief without a sense of the future."

The fear market thrives in an environment where society has internalized the belief that since people are too powerless to cope with the risks they face, it is continually confronted with the problem of survival. This mood of powerlessness has encouraged a market where different fears compete with one another in order to capture the public imagination. Since September 2001, claim-makers have sought to use the public's fear of terrorism to promote their own interests. Politicians, business, advocacy organizations, and special interest groups have sought to further their own agendas by manipulating public anxiety about terror. All seem to take the view that they are more likely to gain a hearing if they pursue their arguments or claims through the prism of security. Businesses have systematically used concern with homeland security to win public subsidies and handouts. And paradoxically, the critics of big business use similar tactics—many environmentalist activists have started linking their traditional alarmist campaigns to the public's fear of terror attacks.

So after 9/11, the Worldwatch Institute issued a statement entitled "The Bioterror in Your Burger," which argued that although past attempts to clean up America's food chain had "failed to inspire politicians," a patriotic demand for homeland security could "finally lead to meaningful action." The Detroit Project, a campaign started by liberal commentator Arianna Huffington and Americans for Fuel-Efficient Cars, links its campaign against sports utility vehicles (SUVs) with the war on terrorism, arguing that Americans need to "free ourselves from the nations and terrorists holding us hostage through our addiction to oil." Some environmentalists argue that their program offer the most effective counterterrorist strategy of all. In an article for the online journal *OnEarth,* David Corn, the Washington-based editor of America's left-leaning weekly *The Nation*, claimed that "technologies long challenged by environmental advocates are potential sources of immense danger in an era of terrorism." "Environmentalism will have to be an essential component of counter-terrorism," he added. Those who are hostile to environmentalist campaigns are also happy to play the fear card. One critic of the environmentalist movement's hostility to using DDT argues that after the tsunami the "next Asian plague" will be malaria (Johnson, 2005). And supporters of nuclear power claim that the best thing that can be done to minimize the damaging impact of global warming is to expand this industry.

In a similar vein, Hurricane Katrina has also been adopted by claim-makers to serve their preexisting agenda of promoting fear to advance their cause. For some advocacy groups this catastrophe serves as a warning of much more dangerous disasters to come through global warming. Others represent it as an indictment of greedy property developers while others blame the bankruptcy of the politicians who run central government. Some point the finger at "big bureaucracy" while others denounce the human sins that have provoked God to punish New Orleans.

In this chapter, the working of fear has been considered in relation to Western societies. Given the significant role of culture in the construction of fear, we need comparative research to give us insights into the global dimension of this subject. It is also far from clear what impact the operation of the fear market has on human behavior. Research needs to be oriented toward a fear-rich ecology to gain insights into the impact of competitive claims making on people's behavior. While studies have pointed to patterns of risk-avoidance in distinct spheres such as crime and parenting (Furedi, 2002; Garland, 2001) we know very little about how people react and process alarmist claims-making in relation to potentially catastrophic events such as a terrorist dirty bomb, global warming or flu pandemic. This is an issue that must engage the energies of disaster researchers in the twenty-first century.

CHAPTER 32

Disasters Ever More? Reducing U.S. Vulnerabilities[1]

CHARLES PERROW

Natural disasters, unintended disasters (largely industrial and technological), and deliberate disasters have all increased in number and intensity in the United States in the last quarter century[2] (see Figure 32.1) In the United States we may prevent some and mitigate some, but we can't escape them. At present, we focus on protecting the targets and mitigating the consequences, and we should do our best at that. But our organizations are simply not up to the challenge from the increasing number of disasters. What we can more profitably do is reduce the size of the targets, that is, reduce the concentrations of energy found in hazardous materials, the concentration of power in vital organizations, and the concentrations of humans in risky locations. Smaller, dispersed targets of nature's wrath, industrial accidents, or terrorist's aim will kill fewer and cause less economic and social disruption.

Not all of the dangers confronting us can be reduced through downsizing our targets. Some natural hazards we just have to face: we are not likely to stop settling on earthquake faults nor can we avoid tsunamis, volcanoes, and tornadoes. Epidemics and terrorists with biological and radiological weapons can cause such widespread devastation that even small targets are at risk. But all these are rare. The more common sources of devastation, such as wind, water, and fire damage; industrial and technological accidents; and terrorist attacks on large targets, can be greatly reduced.

Why are we doing so poorly? Because the targets are becoming larger, and because our organizations—relief organizations, Congress, and government at all levels—will never

[1] I am grateful for support from a National Science Foundation Small Grant award, SES-0329546.

[2] The evidence for the increase in industrial disasters comes from the Swiss reinsurance firm, the world's largest, Swiss Re. The world-wide figures can be found in their Sigma reports (Re, 2001). Man-made disasters include road and shipping accidents, major fires, and aerospace incidents, and the threshold for qualifying is 20 deaths, or 50 injured or 2000 homeless, or $70 billion in losses, or insurance losses ranging from 143 million for shipping, 28 billion for aerospace to 35 billion for the rest. Similar criteria are applied to natural disasters. For man-made disasters in the United States, the period from 1970 to 1992 averaged 7.7; from 1993 to 2001 it was 12.8, a 60% rise. (Special tabulation provided by Swiss Re.) Natural disasters rose steadily in this period, well below the man-made ones in the 1970s but rising to almost 30 a year for the period 1993 to 2001. Data on terrorist attacks and casualties is harder to come by, but following the end of Algerian, Italian, and Irish terrorist activity in the 1970s and early 1980s, there was a decline. But there has been a rise in the 1990s to the present.

NATURAL: Increased interdependencies of natural and constructed environments.

| Meteorites | Volcanoes | Hurricanes | Floods | Droughts |
| Earthquakes | Tsunamis | Forest fires | Epidemics | |

UNINTENDED: Increased scale and lethal potential of industry and technology.

Fires, explosions   Transportation accidents   Toxic Wastes
Toxic releases   Genetically engineered crops   Software

DELIBERATE: Increased unrest, vulnerability, lethal weapons

Cyber attacks (beginning) Sabotage (minor) Dementia (rare)
Terrorism (mounting: more lethal weapons, consequential targets, radical religious sects, and more international inequality and political disorder)

FIGURE 32.1. Types of disasters.

be up to the task of reasonably protecting us. I will first go through some of the familiar problems with the agencies responsible for prevention, mitigation, and remediation; then turn to some deconcentration possibilities; and finally, outline the general principles that will allow us to build economical, reliable, decentralized networks in our critical infrastructure, with four examples of such systems.

ORGANIZATIONS: PERMANENTLY FAILING

Remediation, or responding to damage, involves "first responders," such as police and fire and voluntary agencies. We have not done well here. For one thing, a repeated criticism of our new Department of Homeland Security (DHS) by the Government Accountability Office (GAO) and public policy organizations is that first responder funds are woefully inadequate. The title of a 2003 Council of Foreign Relations taskforce report summed up the problems: "Emergency Responders: Drastically Underfunded, Dangerously Unprepared" (Rudman, Clarke, & Metzl, 2003). This was apparent in the 2005 Katrina hurricane. Further, we have a "panic" model of behavior, which mistakenly limits information, which in turn breeds skepticism on the part of the public. Years of research on disasters indicate that panic is rare, as is rioting and looting, and the "very first" responders are citizens whose capacity for innovative response is impressive. The panic model unfortunately legitimizes the tendency to centralize responses, thus both curtailing citizen responses and interfering with the responses of the lowest level agencies, such as police, fire, medical teams, and voluntary agencies. Research shows the most effective response comes when such decentralized units are free to act on the basis of first-hand information and familiarity with the setting (Clarke, 2002; Tierney, 2003).

Limiting damage involves building codes that cover structural standards and require protection of hazardous materials, and evacuation plans. There have been improvements here, but it is unlikely they will ever be enough. Organizations do not enforce codes, evacuation plans are unrealistic or not implemented (as Katrina showed), and inventories of hazmats are not made.

Finally, preventing damage is the most developed, perhaps because there are more profits for private industry to be found in expensive prevention devices than in training and funding first responders or in following building codes. Here we have alarms and warning systems for natural and industrial dangers; and for terrorism we have biochemical snifters and suits, border and airport detection, and encryption for electronic transmissions. The economic opportunities here are substantial. As soon as the DHS was established, the corporate lobbying began. Four of Secretary Tom Ridge's senior deputies in his initial position as Assistant for Homeland Security at the White House left for the private sector and began work as homeland security lobbyists, as did his legislative affairs director in the White House. The number of lobbyists who registered and listed "homeland," "security," or "terror" on their forms was already sizable at the beginning of 2002, numbering 157, but jumped to 569 as of April, 2003. One lawyer for a prominent Washington, DC law firm was up-front about corporate interests. He mentions in his online resume that he authored a newsletter article titled "Opportunity and Risk: Securing Your Piece of the Homeland Security Pie" (Shenon, 2003a, 2003b). It is a very large pie indeed.

The DHS is virtually a textbook of organizational failures that impact all three of our disaster sources.[3] For example, the Federal Emergency Management Agency (FEMA), once a model organization, was moved into the DHS and its budget for natural disaster management slashed, its authority to coordinate emergency responses taken from it, and its staffing positions filled with political appointees throughout (Hsu, 2005; Isikoff & Hosenball, 2005; Writers, 2005). It became an extreme case of what sociologists call "permanently failing organizations" (Meyer & Zucker, 1989), those that we cannot do without but that we underfund, use for ends they are not designed for, shackle with bad rules and regulations, and so on. It is what we would expect, regardless of the political party in power. We can always try harder, but we should be prepared for inevitable failures.

A MORE PROMISING RESPONSE: REDUCING VULNERABILITIES

There is little consideration by policymakers of the possibility of reducing our vulnerabilities, rather than just prevention, remediation, and damage limitation. (Steven Flynn's 2004 book, *America the Vulnerable,* is one of the few attempts to explore this.) It would be the most effective in the long run.

The sources of our vulnerabilities are threefold:

- The first are *concentrations of energy*, such as explosive and toxic substances (largely industrial storage and process industries), highly flammable substances (e.g., dry or diseased woods, brush), and dams (one of the concentrations we can do little about).
- The second are *concentrations of populations* (in risky, though desirable areas), especially when high-density populations also have high concentrations of explosive and toxic substances.
- The third are *concentrations of economic/political power*, as with concentrations in the electric power industry, in the Internet (e.g., the "monoculture" Microsoft has created), and in food production such as beef and milk.

The three are interrelated. Concentrations of economic and political power allow the concentrations of energy, generally by means of deregulation, and these tend to be where

---

[3] For details, see C. Perrow, "The second disaster: the department of homeland security and the intelligence reorganization," unpublished manuscript, Department of Sociology, Yale University, 2004, available upon request from charles.perrow@yale.edu.

there are concentrations of populations. To give a minor example, the airline industry, and its catastrophic potential, increased with deregulation. Deregulation started with President Carter, and led initially to more airlines, more competition, and lower fares—all favorable results. But starting in the 1990s the number of airlines declined with reconcentration, made possible because of weakened antitrust concerns of government. They concentrated their routes through the hub and spoke system; and this encouraged ever larger aircraft. Because of the concentrated hub and spoke system, simple industrial accidents or computer breakdowns at major airports now paralyze whole sections of the nation. The attempted terrorist attack on the Los Angeles airport in December, 1999 would have disrupted far more traffic than an attack under the regulated system. And when nature, software failures, or terrorists bring down the new airplanes with more than 500 passengers aboard we will realize our vulnerability has increased. But the concentrated airline industry is only a minor instance of increasing the size of our targets.

Deconcentrating Chemical Production and Storage

More important is the massive concentrations of hazardous materials in our chemical plants. The industry has seen extensive consolidation since the 1960s and increasing plant size (Lieberman, 1987). The industry averages five accidents a day, and kills from 250 to 260 people a year (Purvis & Bauler, 2004). But this is hardly noticed since it is usually only two or three at time, and they are almost always workers. (Think of the outrage if we had comparable fatalities from two 727 crashes each year, killing businessmen and others who are able to afford air travel.) Economies of scale abound in this business. A doubling of plant capacity increases the capital costs by only about 60%, so bigger is cheaper (Ashford, 1993, III-9). Bigger facilities also mean bigger targets and bigger catastrophes, and the losses have been increasing. Writing in 1993, Ashford et al. say "A survey of the largest property losses over the past 30 years indicates an increase of 500 percent in the average size of the loss, holding prices constant." They add that a study by the Organization for Economic Cooperation and Development (OECD) notes that, in the post–World War II period, "The incidence of major industrial accidents was only one every five years or so, until 1980. Since 1980, the incidence has risen to two major accidents per year" (Ashford, 1993, III-9). The industry claims that it is safer than manufacturing industries, but the workers most at risk are "contract workers," hired for short-term jobs from companies that the government classifies in various construction industry categories rather than the chemical industry. Since 30% of the workforce is contract workers, and they are the most likely to have accidents, the claim that the industry has one of the highest safety records is without merit (Perrow, 1999, pp. 361–362).

The potential for catastrophe is immense, and the trigger could be a storm, an industrial accident, or a terrorist attack. Facilities with significant amounts of chemicals had to prepare worst case scenarios for the Environmental Protection Agency (EPA). A remarkable Washington Post story summarizes some of the findings (Grimaldi & Gugliotta, 2001). A single railcar of chlorine, if vaporized near Los Angeles, could poison 4 million people. Four million people could be harmed by the release of 400,000 pounds of hydrogen fluoride that a refinery near Philadelphia keeps on hand. A chlorine railcar release near Detroit would put three million at risk. Union Carbide's Institute, WV plant near Charleston once again has 200,000 pounds of methyl isocyanate, the chemical that did so much damage in Bhopal, which would threaten 60,000 people. (Union Carbide had removed the methyl isocyanate storage from the Institute plant after the Bhopal accident, but the Institute plant was reported to be storing it again in

2001 [Staff Writers, 2001]). And close by New York City, a plant in New Jersey has 180,000 pounds of chlorine and sulfur dioxide that could create a toxic cloud that would put 12 million people at risk (Grimaldi & Gugliotta, 2001). These scenarios assume that there is no collateral damage to nearby processes or storage facilities in the plant, but that damage could make it worse.[4]

Is it possible to reduce these concentrations? There are some significant examples of both substituting safer processes or substances, and reducing storage inventories, indicating that it is quite possible and not economically damaging (Ashford, 1993, II-18; Purvis & Bauler, 2004, p. 10). But considering the thousands of vulnerable sites, a dozen examples are only a drop taken from the chemical bucket. Nor is bigger safer. Both Howard Kleindorfer and Don Grant have studies showing the larger the plant the more unwanted releases, even controlling for size of inventory Grant & Jones, 2003; Grant, Jones, & Bergesen, 2002; Kleindorfer et al., 2003).

One objective that is certainly possible is to reduce these concentrations in concentrated populations. Regulations here are very weak, and the concentrations have only very small economic justifications. Large amounts of diesel fuel were stored in the deepest basement of the World Trade Center, and the fuel almost ignited when the building was destroyed. Its ignition would have wreaked much greater devastation than we already had. The economic savings of such storage were trivial. Railroad cars containing 60 tons of deadly chlorine gas sit idly on side tracks within blocks of the White House in Washington, DC, vulnerable to a railroad accident, a lightening strike, or a suitcase bomb. They either should not be there or should not go through downtown Washington; alternatively, they could be transported in smaller amounts in more rugged containers.

Would more containers increase the likelihood of more disasters? Smaller containers are easier to protect, and easier for workers to handle; they present less surfaces for storms to attack; and their value to terrorists would be much lower. Assume one storage facility is dispersed over 10 widely spaced locations, say a few miles. Terrorist would have to coordinate 10 attacks to realize the damage of a single concentrated one. A disaster at the concentrated facility is more likely to endanger nearby containers or processes with hazmats, and interfere with the ability to man safety systems and recovery efforts. The drawback is that more transportation, and its accident potential, is involved with dispersion, but the quantities are smaller and protection easier. In the face of all three threats, smaller means safer, and this can justify the increased costs.

Deconcentrating Populations

Deconcentrating populations in risky areas is much more difficult. Katrina has done it temporarily in New Orleans, but given the economic importance of the port, it is likely to be rebuilt. It not only drains our Midwest river system of most of the nation's agricultural products, but is the inlet for Latin American raw materials and the distribution node for a quarter of our oil and gas supplies. Given the absence of tough, enforced, building regulations in a state such as Louisiana, a rebuilt New Orleans is not likely to be significantly safer from a direct hit from a future force 4 or 5 hurricane. (Katrina was a softened blow; had it been a few miles west the inrush of water from the storm surge would have meant only 2 to 3 minutes, instead of several

---

[4] For details, see C. Perrow, "Better Vulnerability Thru Chemistry," unpublished manuscript, Department of Sociology, Yale University, 2004, available upon request from charles.perrow@yale.edu.

hours, to get up to the attic and break through to the roof. Katrina is a certified "worst case," but as Lee Clarke says, worst cases can always be even worse (Clarke, 2005). We are not going to abandon the San Andreas, California, earthquake fault with its cities, hazmat storage tanks, and it nuclear plant. (A large earthquake would depopulate it thoroughly.) The ports at and around Los Angeles are marvels of concentrated economic efficiency. An earthquake, tidal wave, domino of explosions, or a dirty bomb in a shipping container would halt much of the economic activity of California (and Hawaii) for months (Flynn, 2004).

Little can be done, beyond what nature, industrial accidents, or terrorists would do, to deconcentrate risky areas. But effective regulation would make a dent and reduce the amount that the nation pays to subsidize the losses of those who enjoy the water views and warm climates. The United States tries and fails each time there is a disaster to withhold funds from those who failed to buy insurance, already heavily subsidized. (This goes for Midwest floods of farm lands, where the water views are not the incentive to settlement.) Gradually, we improve building standards and impose zoning requirements that limit our vulnerability, but the real estate interests' goal of growth and our appetite for lovely settings makes it difficult. As the seas rise and move inland, and populations continue to move to the coast, we should look to the system that the Netherlands has imposed. Most of that lovely country is below sea level, and while it does not have hurricanes, it has significant storm surges that have drowned a good part of it in the past. A strong central government builds and maintains dikes, houses in some areas must be built to float, and zoning disperses the population. The erosion that industry and government has allowed to happen in the alluvial Louisiana delta would be unthinkable in Northern Europe. The ocean and the storm surges are moving closer to New Orleans every year, and experts and government officials have been aware of it for at least since the middle of the last century. Our "permanently failing organizations" could be up to the job of reducing vulnerabilities rather than just increasing our protection and recovery attempts. We make a little progress with each disaster. With increased awareness of our vulnerabilities we could make much more.

Deconcentrating Organizations

The case for deconcentrating large organizations that are at the center of our critical infrastructure will be limited to only two illustrations: the Internet, and even more vital to our connected society, the electric power grid. (Cases can be made for deconcentration in the raising of cattle, bulk milk processing, chemicals, medical care, pharmaceuticals, and others.) Both the Internet and the grid, as we shall see, were exemplary examples of efficient, decentralized, reliable networks, but are in danger of concentration. Regarding the Internet, Microsoft, allegedly through illegal anticompetitive practices, has gained 90 to 95% of the operating systems that computers use. In doing so, it is charged, it paid little attention to reliability, stifled innovations by buying up innovators that threatened it, and, having a near monopoly, did not have to pay attention to security. A report by several experts on computers and security concludes, "The presence of this single, dominant operating system in the hands of nearly all end users is inherently dangerous" (Geer et al., 2003). Microsoft's near monopoly left the Internet open to malicious hackers, who have disrupted parts of the critical infrastructure represented by the Internet from time to time, and to terrorist organizations that have expressed an interest in using the Internet as a terrorist tool, but so far have failed to do successfully do so, as far we know. Had the concentrated power of Microsoft been checked, as a federal lawsuit tried to do, but failed, there would have been more room for competitors who could have competed on the basis of higher reliability and higher security. Now, even the Defense Department has few alternatives to using insecure and "buggy" Microsoft products for its mission-critical systems. (It can get the secure codes from Microsoft and reconfigure Windows, for example, to be safer. Others cannot.)

The increasing concentration in the media industry also poses security problems. Media conglomerates are attempting to reduce the number of independent Internet Service Providers (ISPs) that are available from thousands to a handful. Access to Web pages would be limited to those the cable or DSL company subscribes to (Krugman, 2002; Levy, 2004). A system with a few ISPs is arguably more vulnerable to our three sources of disasters than a highly distributed one with thousands of points of access. (Terrorists should have no trouble breaking into and shutting down a Comcast ISP; hackers break into the more highly protected Defense Department computers almost daily, though they appear not to be disposed to shutting down vital systems. Terrorists could be so disposed.)

The most vital element of our critical infrastructure is electric power, and blackouts the most disastrous event. Deregulation appears to be the "root cause" of the August 14, 2003 blackout in the Northeast, since deregulation led to concentration in the industry. It was supposed to increase competition and drive down prices. Prices did not decline, and it did not produce the competition that would encourage greater innovations and more efficient and reliable transmission. Rather, competition among consolidated utilities was strictly in terms of profits that could be increased by cutting maintenance and requiring "the grid to be operated closer to its reliability limits more of the time than was the case in the past," according to the North American Electric Reliability Council (NAERC). It removed the incentive to add transmission lines to increase reliability, since their costs would not be reimbursed through the regulatory process as they had been in the past. Consequently, investment in transmission has lagged. Competition and consolidation in the industry, after deregulation in the 1990s, replaced the company heads, largely engineers, with lawyers and MBAs without technical experience. Reserve margins of electricity to reduce shortages have been replaced by lower margins; lower margins will drive up prices and increase profits (Wald, 2005). This was apparent in the rigged California market, where the utilities and the larger energy companies such as Enron created artificial shortages to drive up prices (McLean & Elkind, 2003).

Since electric power is the preeminent item in our critical infrastructure, the decline in reliability because of economic concentration is troubling. With decreasing reliability, terrorist attacks are more possible, and storms that disable substations more consequential. Congress deregulated the industry; it could re-regulate it. Its only watchdog, the North American Electric Reliability Council (NAERC), is a voluntary association funded by the utilities, and has no authority to require, as a prime example, the utilities to invest in new transmission lines.

THINKING ABOUT INTERCONNECTEDNESS

How can we reduce our vulnerabilities? This will certainly be difficult since it will impose costs upon business and industry, and local and state governments, and runs counter to our prevailing economic wisdom, which favors large organizations on the grounds that they have economies of scale. It would mean widespread dispersion not only of "hazmats" but of settlements in hurricane zones and flood plains as well, and the breakup of large organizational concentrations of power, or at least their decentralization. It would require a great deal more regulation than these organizations, and our Congress and governmental agencies, are now willing to entertain. But the vulnerabilities are not necessarily inherent in our society; they were less in past decades and could be reversed.

It is my argument that many, though not all, of such vulnerabilities stem from dependencies, and their reduction will be achieved by creating interdependencies. This requires that be clear about interconnectedness.

We speak loosely of a highly interdependent, networked world, but true interdependency is rather rare. Everything is indeed connected, but most of the connections exhibit far more *dependency* than *inter*dependency; more control than cooperation.[5]

True interdependency means reciprocal influence. Behavior by A not only affects B, but B's response changes A in turn. This is the normal interaction of two people with roughly equal power. When power is unequal we can still have some reciprocity, but the reciprocal effect of B on A may be small. Say General Motors asks the Quiet Door Company to bid on making a part of its door, and the Door Company gets the contract and makes the doors. The door company is dependent upon GM. But suppose the door company suggests to GM that there is a better way to design their part of the door and this will save both GM and the door company money. There is a least a small bit of reciprocal influence here. In some industrial networks, especially in Japan and northern Europe, this *inter*dependency is enlarged; for example, the supplier may participate in the initial design of the buyer's product. The supplier changes the buyer. Some industrial networks consist of firms with roughly equal power, and a great deal of interaction or reciprocity.

Reciprocal effects can occur when the interactions are programmed with self-adapting mechanisms. Take some segments of our power grids. Here, A and B are nodes in a network, and component A sends information or commands to component B, and B evaluates the information or command in terms of its view of the system's state—say its links to C, D, and E. If B does not accept the information as complete or valid, or finds the command violates something in the network at that time, it responds in a way that requires A to alter the command or expand the information to clarify it. B is not fully dependent upon A, and an instant later, B may be sending commands to A.

The Interdependency Opportunity

To an increasing degree this automatic reciprocity appears in highly sophisticated electronic systems. Over time, the components, called "intelligent agents," acquire a "memory" that guides their interpretation. Computer speech recognition programs such as Adobe Naturally Speaking are a primitive version of these responses. The program is designed to learn, making subtle decisions as to when to type "knot" instead of "not," expanding and adjusting its initial memory to respond to your tone of voice and phrasing. It must be trained. More important for reciprocity, the interaction is not solely one way. Indeed, I find I speak more clearly when I use it. My behavior is changed.

Sophisticated segments of the electric power grid show learning and collaboration, and the industry aspires to have intelligent agents deployed at critical nodes (Amin, 2001, 2002). It also occurs in the Internet, especially when packets are rerouted because of congestion. No human intervention is involved in either of these operations, and while a few nodes are much more significant than the vast majority—the organizing principle follows a "power law"—there

---

[5] The discussion in this section takes off from some seminal distinctions by three engineers. I have modified their scheme extensively, renamed some key variables, and introduced the notion of the difference between interdependency and dependency (see Rinaldi, Peerenboom, & Kelly, 2001).

is considerable interdependency, largely achieved through redundancies.[6] Let us call this form of interdependency *"reciprocal interdependence."* It is to be highly valued.

A second form of interdependency, also to be valued, I will call *"commonality interdependency,"* though I wish I had a better term. (It involves interoperability, but that term is usually not applied to symbols such as laws.) If two systems have different languages, metrics, or voltages, they cannot communicate. If they are governed by laws or regulations that are not shared and compatible, they cannot coordinate. If their reputations are disparate, dependency will prevail over interdependency. Nations with incompatible laws and legal structures have minimal reciprocal interdependency with each other. Police and fire departments with incompatible communication systems cannot communicate. China, with a policy of secrecy, could not alert the world to the SARS epidemic before it was too late; it did not have an openness policy in common with other nations. The Mars Lander failed because of incompatible metrics within its system. Firms with low reputations for reliability are assigned to a dependent role, if they are not simply forced out of business, as Arthur Anderson was after the Enron scandal. Commonalities may be physical, as in the case of voltages or standardized screws, but the most interesting are these "logical" commonalities.

The Dependency Problem

When we enter the world of nations, firms, and public service departments such as police and fire, or the Central Intelligence Agency and the Federal Bureau of Investigation, we should not assume a high degree interdependency, in the form of logical commonalities. As noted, while the world is getting more interconnected, the connections are increasingly ones of *de*pendency, though we may mistake this for interdependency.

There are two attributes of systems that are often cited as evidence of a society's high degree of interdependency, but should be cited as examples of *de*pendency. The first is called *physical dependency*, and occurs when a system requires a specific kind of input from another system. (The inputs do not have to be physical, but this is the most common example.) The railroad engine needs coal to operate, so it is dependent upon coal suppliers, but it is hardly *interdependent* with any one supplier. Just as the railroad is dependent upon fuel suppliers, the fuel suppliers are dependent upon railroads to buy their fuel, and we like to see this as interdependency, but no reciprocity is required; there are only two examples of dependency, both of which can be exploited.

But this dependency can be reduced if the railroad engine can burn either coal or oil, increasing the range of suppliers it can draw upon, just as the fuel company is less dependent if it has both coal and oil and many railroad customers and other users. Physical dependency is high when the railroad engine can only burn coal, lower if it can shift to oil; or high if the coal company has only one customer, the railroad, but lower if it has several customers, and lower still if the several are not all railroad engine customers. While there may be economies

---

[6] The sender's message is broken up into packets, and these are directed by routers to find the shortest way to the receiver, via servers. If there is congestion at a server or on the route, or a failure in delivery for any reason, the receiving machine checks a packet that has arrived for the address of the missing packet or packets and asks that it be sent again. Each packet contains not only the addresses of all other packets of the message, but a "table of contents" of the message, which provides a further redundancy. There is no cost to these redundancies; indeed, they allow packets to find the shortest uncongested route and thus increase efficiency. It is a bit of a stretch to label all this "interdependency," or "reciprocity," but it is close to that.

associated with an engine built for only one fuel rather than two or three, or a coal supplier with only one customer, there are vulnerabilities associated with single-purpose machines and single source suppliers or customers. There is a high degree of dependency, rather than interdependency. Flexible, multipurpose machines, and multifirm suppliers and customers, reduce these dependencies, and involves more multinode, complex networks, which are partially self-regulating. More important for the argument on vulnerabilities, it also results in smaller concentrations of hazardous materials and lower economic and political power for any one organization.

The flexibility and multipurpose characteristics do not necessarily create *inter* dependencies, but it greatly increases the opportunities for them. While there is some movement toward multiplex networks in a few new industries and research areas, overall we are seeing increased concentration and dependencies.

The second example of *de*pendency will be called "spatial dependency." This is similar to what engineers call "common modes," as in common mode failures. These occur when the failure of an electric power source shuts down not only the nuclear reactor, but also the cooling system in a quite different, but spatially adjacent, system that keeps used fuel rods cool while their radioactivity decays and they await shipment to a permanent storage place. The two systems, power generation and spent fuel rod cooling, need not be linked, but are for minor economic reasons. Or, if a bridge carries not only vehicle traffic but also communication and power lines, its collapse would stop not just traffic but communication and power as well. A vehicle bridge does not require telephone and power lines on it to function.

There are clear economic efficiencies associated with most spatial dependencies. It would be expensive to build two bridges. But it would cost only a little bit more to move the spent storage pool to a distant site that is not dependent upon the nuclear power plant for power. Where catastrophic failures might be experienced, as in the nuclear power case, the risks seem very high compared to the economic benefits.

Spatial vulnerabilities with catastrophic potential abound in our society. We settle on flood plains and hurricane-washed coasts with inadequate building codes and evacuation routes and build cities on known earthquake faults and suburbs on unstable bay fills. We allow unnecessarily large storage of hazardous materials in with dense population concentrations, making them vulnerable to terrorist, industrial, and natural disasters. These vulnerabilities could be eliminated or reduced through better system design that recognizes and reduces this form of dependency. (Fortunately, just-in-time manufacturing and processing practices may lead to a dispersal of some hazardous materials in smaller storage containers.)

Physical dependencies abound because of concentrations of economic and organizational power and can be reduced through reducing these concentrations. But reductions of both forms of dependency run afoul of the economic argument that economies of scale justify these concentrations.

FOUR EXAMPLES OF LARGE, EFFICIENT, RELIABLE AND DECENTRALIZED SYSTEMS

There is ample evidence that very large scales only sometimes produce production economies, but instead produce the social inefficiencies of market power and the political power that can flow from it. It is possible to have very large systems that are highly decentralized, very efficient (they have economies of network scale, rather than economies of organizational scale), innovative, and very reliable, minimizing their vulnerability to the three disasters.

Here are four examples. They are all heavily networked systems, low in physical and spatial dependencies, where the *pathologies* of networks reside, and high in reciprocal and commonality interdependency which represent the *potentials* of networking. Not everything we do in society could be organized in this form, nor is everything that involves our critical infrastructure, but there may be many systems that could be so reconfigured.

They are the Internet, the electric power grid (two essentials for our critical infrastructure); networks of small firms (most prominently in Europe and Japan, but some in the United States); and, alas, the global terrorist network associated with radical, fundamentalist Islamic religion.

We will start with *size*. The Internet is the world's largest system, embracing the globe. Nothing compares to it in terms of size. The U.S. power grid has been called the world's largest machine, reaching from coast to coast and into Mexico and Canada (though made up of three regional systems, they are connected to each other).

Networks of small firms are much smaller of course, but their output can be much larger than that of one or two large companies making the same products. In fact, typically they displace a few large firms. The point is that the small size of most of the firms in the networks is not an economic drawback, but turns out to be a virtue. They are most famously prominent in northern Italy, where an industry making machinery, scientific instruments, furniture, or textiles and clothing will range from a few dozen firms to hundreds, all interacting.[7] Finally, although reliable information is not available, it is estimated that the Al Qaeda terrorist network is made up of thousands of cells.

Our four examples point to two important size considerations: the systems can expand easily in size, and can increase in size without increasing their hierarchies, that is, without encumbering themselves with layers of managers and all the associated costs and complexities. Thousands of new users have joined the Internet every day for years. The power grid can add new lines, territories, and capacities rather easily as can networks of small firms and terrorist groups. This is associated with the "power law" distribution of nodes in these networks. While there are a very tiny number of absolutely essential nodes, the vast majority of nodes have only a few connections to other nodes, so adding them does not affect the vertical structure. But only a few connections are needed to be able to reach the whole vast network of Internet users, power suppliers, small firms or terrorists cells, so efficiency is not decreased with size. Even the criticality of a tiny number of key nodes in the Internet and the power grid is rarely a source of vulnerability because of extensive redundancies designed into these systems. In all these respects, the networks are very different from traditional organizations, such as firms.

Next, consider *reliability*. The Internet is remarkably reliable, considering its size and what it has to do. Computers crash many more times than the Internet, and Internet crashes are generally very brief (excepting deliberate attacks). The reliability of the U.S. power grid has been very high, with major outages occurring only about once a decade. It is true that there have been very serious blackouts in the United States, and "normal accident" theory would say they are to be expected because of interactively complexity and tight coupling (Perrow, 1999). But these kinds of accidents are not just rare, as normal accident theory would expect, but must be considered exceedingly rare given the excessive demands on the system and its size and complexity. Much more likely to cause failures are production pressures, forcing the

---

[7] There is a vast literature on this. For starters, look at the classic Piore and Sabel book that gave the notion, discovered by Italian demographers, its first prominence (Piore & Sable, 1984). It is developed in (Lazerson, 1988). For a synthetic overview, see (Perrow, 1992). For more recent extensions, see Amin (2000) and Lazerson and Lorenzoni (1999).

system beyond design limits, and of course deliberate destabilization to manipulate prices, as in the Enron case in California.

Between 1990 and 2000 the U.S. demand increased 35% but capacity only 18% (Amin, 2001). One does not need a fancy theory such as normal accident theory to explain large failures under those conditions. (Indeed, one does need a fancy theory, such as a network theory that gives a role to interdependencies and redundancies, to explain why there were so few failures under these conditions.) One failure in 1996 affected 11 U.S. states and 2 Canadian provinces, with an estimated cost of $1.5 to $2 billion. Even more serious was the 2003 Northeast blackout. Since the extensive deregulation of the 1990s we can expect more failures as maintenance is cut and production pressures increase. But I am struck more by the high technical reliability of the power grids than by the few serious cascading failures it has had in some 35 years. Without centralized control, despite the production pressures of mounting demand, and despite increased density and scope, it muddles through remarkably well, if it is not manipulated by top management and banks.

The reliability of networks of small firms is more difficult to assess, since there is no convenient metric. But students of small firm networks attest to their robustness, even in the face of attempted consolidations by large organizations. Saxenian effectively contrasts the decline of the non-networked group of high-technology firms around Boston's Route 128 when federal funding declined and Japanese mass production techniques matured, with the networks of small firms in California's Silicon Valley, who charged forward with new innovations for new markets (Saxenian, 1996). Despite predictions of their imminent demise (Harrison, 1994), dating back to the 1980s when they were first discovered and theorized, the small firm networks of northern Italy have survived. In the United States the highly networked biotech firms are prospering, for the time, despite their linkages with the huge pharmaceutical firms (Powell, 1996). Particular firms in small firm networks come and go, but the employees and their skills stay, moving from one firm to another as technologies, products, and markets change.

The reliability of terrorists' networks also seems quite high. Rounding up one cell does not affect the other cells; new cells are easily established; the loosely organized Al Qaeda network has survived at least three decades of dedicated international efforts to eradicate it. There are occasional defections and a few penetrations, but the most serious challenge to it has been the lack of a secure territory for training, once the Taliban was defeated in Afghanistan. (Some argue that Al Qaeda per se is increasingly just one part of a leaderless network of Islamic terrorists.)

Can huge, decentralized networks of small units be *efficient*? It appears so. The Internet is incredibly efficient. Power grids are becoming more so as they add "intelligent agents" (though the concentration of generation and distribution firms reduces maintenance and thwarts needed expansion of the grid). Small firm networks routinely out-produce large, vertically integrated firms. Network economies of scale replace those of firm size, and rely, in part, on trust and cooperation, allowing strong competitive forces only when the overall health of the network is not endangered. Transaction costs are low and handled informally. And finally, terrorist networks live off the land, largely, can remain dormant for years with no maintenance costs and few costs from unused invested capital, and are expendable.

I have tried to establish that decentralized systems can be reliable and efficient, but does it follow that the systems responsible for our basic vulnerabilities could be organized like this? The Internet already is, though that is changing. The security vulnerability of the Internet, making it open to terrorist attacks, could be greatly reduced, for instance, by making providers such as Microsoft liable for having a code that is easily "hacked." The electric power grids will remain reliable if maintenance and improvements are required, which could be done through legislation and liability legislation. Deconcentrating industries that deal in hazardous materials, such as petroleum and chemical industries, could greatly reduce vulnerabilities there (heavy regulation would also be needed), and the power the firms would lose would be market power. Without market power they will be more sensitive to their accident potential. Research and development, which might need large amounts of capital and might have to be centralized, could be detached from production, storage, and delivery, which could be decentralized. Population concentrations in risky areas is not a "system" that could be decentralized along the lines of our four examples, so in this case the reform must depend upon regulations and improvements in the insurance and liabilities area (e.g., stop federal subsidization of disaster insurance; allow federal aid only if federal standards have been met; increased inspection and penalties; etc.). None of this would be easy, but none of it is inconceivable.

In every case of vulnerabilities I have mentioned, we have had laws and regulations that address these issues, but they have been dropped, weakened, or are not enforced. Take a trivial example. The government has tried to withhold disaster relief from those who failed to take out subsidized insurance or failed to conform to regulations, but it has backed off when the flood or hurricane actually came. This could be corrected. More important, we have precedents for deconcentrating organizations; 30 years ago we had effective antitrust legislation; it could be reinstated. We tried to break up Microsoft; we could try again. It doesn't even produce many innovations on its own; it has the market power to buy them up. We could once again regulate the Internet as a common carrier.

Unfortunately, we appear to be moving in the opposite direction. The power of Microsoft to shape computing and the Internet does not seem to have declined, but to be increasing. It is gaining control of the new technologies such as the Internet, browsers, and music that were supposed to check its power. Concentration in the electric power industry is proceeding apace under deregulation. Even networks of small firms may prove to have had only a half-century of efflorescence, as giant retailers control the "commodity chain" that forces producers into mass production in low-wage countries where exploitation is easy and the only alternative to workers is rural starvation.

All of these developments will make us less safe because they will increase our vulnerabilities to natural, industrial, and deliberate disasters.

References

Abrams, C.B., Albright, K., & Panofsky, A. (2004). Contesting the New York community: From liminality to the "new normal" in the wake of September 11. *City & Community, 3*, 189–220.

Acar, F., & Ege, G. (2001). *Women's human rights in disaster contexts: How can CEDAW help?* Paper prepared for the United Nations Division for the Advancement of Women Expert Working Group Meeting. Ankara, Turkey. Retrieved November 6–9, 2001, http://www.un.org/womenwatch/daw/csw/env_manage/documents. html.

Adams, G.B., & Balfour, D.L. (1998). *Unmasking administrative evil*. Thousand Oaks, CA: SAGE.

Adger, W.N., Hughes, T.P., Folke, C., Carpenter, S.R., & Rockström, J. (2005). Social-ecological resilience to coastal disasters. *Science, 309*(5737), 1036–1039.

Adya, A., Bahl, P., & Qiu, L. (2002). *Characterizing alert and browse services for mobile clients*. Monterey, CA: USENIX Annual Technical Conference.

Aguirre, B.E. (2002). Can sustainable development sustain us? *International Journal of Mass Emergencies and Disasters, 20*(2), 111–125.

Aguirre, B. (2004). Homeland security warnings: Lessons learned and unlearned. *International Journal of Mass Emergencies and Disasters, 22*, 103–115.

Aguirre, B.E. (2005). Emergency evacuations, panic, and social psychology. *Psychiatry, 68*(2), 121–129.

Aguirre, B.E., Anderson, W.A., Balandran, S., Peters, B.E., & White, H.M. (1991). *Saragosa, Texas, tornado, May 22, 1987: An evaluation of the warning system*. Washington, DC: National Academy Press.

Aguirre, B.R., Dynes, J.M., Kendra, J., & Connell, R. (2005). Institutional resilience and disaster planning for new hazards: Insights from hospitals. *Journal of Homeland Security and Emergency Management, 2*(2), Article 1. http://www.bepress.com/jhsem/vol2/iss2/1.

Aguirre, B., Wenger, D., Glass, T. A., Diaz-Murillo, M., & Vigo, G. (1995). The social organization of search and rescue: Evidence form the Guadalajara gasoline explosion. *International Journal of Mass Emergencies and Disasters, 13*(1), 67–92.

Aguirre, B.E., Wenger, D., & Vigo, G. (1998). A test of emergency norm theory of collective behavior. *Sociological Forum, 13*, 301–320.

Ahern, M., Kovats, S., Wilkinson, P., Few, R., & Matthies, F. (2005). Global health impacts of floods: A systematic review of epidemiological evidence. *Epidemiologic Reviews, 27*, 36–46.

Ahmed, S. (2004). *The gendered context of vulnerability: Coping/adapting to floods in Eastern India*. Paper prepared for the Gender Equality and Disaster Risk Reduction Workshop. Honolulu, Hawaii, August 11, 2004, http://www.ssri.hawaii.edu/research/GDW website/pages/proceeding.html.

Alba, R.D., & Logan, J.R. (1992). Assimilation and stratification in the homeownership patterns of racial and ethnic groups. *International Migration Review, 26*, 1314–1341.

Albala-Bertrand, J.M. (1993). *The political economy of large natural disasters, with special reference to developing countries*. New York: Clarendon Press.

Albala-Bertrand, J.M. (1999). Industrial interdependence change in Chile 1960–90: A comparison with Taiwan and South Korea. *International Review of Applied Economics, 2*, 161–191.

Albala-Bertrand, J.M. (2000a). Complex emergencies versus natural disasters. An analytical comparison of causes and effects. *Oxford Development Studies, 2*, 187–204.

Albala-Bertrand, J.M. (2000b). Responses to complex humanitarian emergencies and natural disasters: An analytical comparison. *Third World Quarterly, 2*, 215–227.

Albala-Bertrand, J.M. (2004). Natural disaster situations and growth: A macroeconomic model for sudden disaster impact. In H. Kunreuther & A. Rose (Eds.), *The economic of natural hazards* (pp. 453–470). Cheltenham: Elgar.

Albala-Bertrand, J.M., & Mamatzakis, E.C. (2004). The impact of infrastructures on the productivity of the Chilean economy. *Review of Development Economics, 2*, 266–278.

Aldrich, H. (1979). *Organizations and environments.* Englewood Cliffs, NJ: Prentice-Hall.

Alesch, D.J. (2005). *Complex urban systems and extreme events: Toward a theory of disaster recovery.* Paper presented at the 1st International Conference of Urban Disaster Reduction. Kobe, Japan, January 8.

Alesch, D.J., & Holly, J.N. (1997). Small business failure, survival, and recovery: Lessons from the January 1994 Northridge earthquake. In *Proceedings of the NEHRP Conference and Workshop on Research on the Northridge, California Earthquake of January 17, 1994* (pp. 48–55). Richmond, CA: California Universities for Research in Earthquake Engineering.

Alesch, D.J., Holly J.N., Mittler E., & Nagy, R. (2001). *Organizations at risk: What happens when small businesses and not-for-profits encounter natural disasters.* Fairfax, VA: Public Entity Risk Institute, www.riskinstitute.org.

Alesch, D.J., Holly, J.N., Mittler, E., & Nagy, R.A. (n.d). *After the disaster... What should I do now? Information to help small business owners make post–disaster decisions.* Green Bay, WI: University of Wisconsin, Green Bay, Center for Organizational Studies.

Alesch, D.J., & Petak, W.J. (1986). *The politics and economics of earthquake hazard mitigation: Unreinforced masonry buildings in Southern California.* Boulder, CO: University of Colorado, Institute of Behavioral Science, Program on Environment and Behavior, Natural Hazards Research and Applications Information Center.

Alesch, D.J., Taylor, C., Ghanty, A.S., & Nagy, R.A. (1993). Earthquake risk reduction and small business. In K.J. Tierney & J.M. Nigg (Eds.), *National Earthquake Conference Monograph No. 5: Socioeconomic impacts* (pp. 133–160). Memphis: Central U.S. Earthquake Consortium.

Alexander, D. (1980). The Florence floods—What the papers said. *Environmental Magazine*, 27–34.

Alexander, D. (1990). Behavior during earthquakes: A southern Italian example. *International Journal of Mass Emergencies and Disasters, 8*(1), 5–29.

Alexander, D.A. (1993). *Natural disasters.* New York: Chapman and Hall.

Alexander, D. (1997). The study of natural disasters, 1977–1997: Some reflections on a changing field of knowledge. *Disasters, 21*(4), 284–204.

Alexander, D. (2002b). From civil defense to civil protection—and back again. *Disaster Prevention and Management, 11*(3), 209–213.

Alexander, D.A. (2005). An interpretation of disaster in terms of changes in culture, society and international relations. In R.W. Perry, & E.L. Quarantelli (Eds.), *What is a disaster: New answers to old questions* (pp. 25–38). Philadelphia: Xlibris.

Alexander, Y. (2002). Conclusion. In Y. Alexander (Ed.), *Combating terrorism: Strategies of ten countries* (pp. 375–393). Ann Arbor: University of Michigan Press.

All India Disaster Mitigation Institute website. Livelihood Relief Fund, http://www.southasiadisasters.net/lrf.htm

Allison, G.T. (1971). *Essence of decision: Explaining the Cuban missile crisis.* Boston: Little Brown.

Allison, G. (2004). *Nuclear terrorism: The ultimate preventable catastrophe.* New York: Times Books.

Almond, G.A., Flanagan, S., & Mundt, R (Eds.). (1973). *Crisis, choice and change: Historical studies of political development.* Boston: Little Brown.

Alterman, E. (2005). Found in the flood. *The Nation, 281*(9), 33.

Altheide, D.L. (2002). *Creating fear: News and the construction of crisis.* New York: Aldine De Gruyter.

Altheide, D.L. (Forthcoming 2006). *Terrorism and the politics of fear.* Lanham: AltaMira Press.

Alway, J., Belgrave, L.L., & Smith, K. J. (1998). Back to normal: Gender and disaster. *Symbolic Interaction, 21*(2), 175–195.

Amabile, T.M. (1997). Entrepreneurial creativity through motivational synergy. *Journal of Creative Behavior, 31*(1), 18–26.

Ambrosia, V.G., Buechel, S.W., Brass, J.A., Peterson, J.R., Davies, R.H., Kane, R.J., et al. (1998). An integration of remote sensing, GIS, and information distribution for wildfire detection and management. *Photogrammetric Engineering and Remote Sensing, 64*(10), 977–985.

American Red Cross. (2005). Northridge earthquake remembered today: American Red Cross urges Americans to prepare for earthquakes and other disasters. Retrieved July 15, 2005, http://www.redcross.org/pressrelease/ 0,1077,0_489_2172,00.html.

Amin, A. (2000). Industrial districts. In E. Sheppard & T. J. Barnes (Eds.), *A companion to economic geography* (pp. 149–168). Oxford: Blackwell.

Amin, M. (2001). Toward self–healing energy infrastructure systems. *IEEE Computer Applications in Power*, 20–28.

Amin, M. (2002). Restructuring the electric enterprise: Stimulating the evolution of electric power industry with intelligent adaptive agents. In A. Faraqui & K. Eakin (Eds.), *Electricity pricing in transition* (pp. 27–50). Norwell, MA: Kluwer Academic.

Anagnostopoulos, S.A., & Whitman, R.V. (1977). On human loss prediction in buildings during earthquakes. In *Proceedings of the Sixth World Conference on Earthquake Engineering* (vol. 1, pp. 671–676).

Andersen, T.J. (2003). Globalization and natural disasters: An integrative risk management approach. In A. Kreimer, M. Arnold, & A. Carlin (Eds.), *Building safer cities: The future of disaster risk* (pp. 57–74). Washington, DC: World Bank, Disaster Management Facility.

Anderson, M.B. (1991). Vulnerability to disaster and sustainable development: A general framework for assessing vulnerability. http://www.crid.or.cr/crid/CD_ Inversion/pdf/eng/doc6539/doc9539–a.pdf.

Anderson, M.B., & Woodrow, P.J. (1998). *Rising from the ashes: Development strategies in times of disaster*. Boulder, CO: Lynne Reiner.

Anderson, R. (1999). The Millennium Bug: Reasons not to Panic. Retrieved May 23, 2005, http://www.ftp.cl.cam. ac.uk/ftp/users/rja14.y2k.html, accessed 18 April 2006.

Anderson, W.A. (1965). *Some observations on a disaster subculture: The organizational response of Cincinnati, Ohio, to the 1964 flood*. Columbus, OH: Research Note 6, The Ohio State University Disaster Research Center, Department of Sociology.

Anderson, W.A. (1969a). *Disaster and organizational change: A study of the long–term consequences in anchorage of the 1964 Alaska earthquake*. Newark, DE: University of Delaware, Disaster Research Center.

Anderson, W.A. (1969b). Disaster warning and communication processes in two communities. *Journal of Communication, 19*, 92–104.

Anderson, W.A. (1969c). *Local civil defense in natural disaster: From office to organization*. Columbus, OH: Ohio State University, Disaster Research Center.

Angus, L. (2004). *Future challenges in disaster management in New Zealand*. Wellington: Ministry of Civil Defense & Emergency Management: Mimeo.

Annan, K. (1999). *Introduction to secretary-general's annual report on the work of the organization of United Nations, 1999* (document A/54/1).

Aptekar, L. (1994). *Environmental disasters in global perspective*. New York: GO Hall.

Aristotle (1952). *Meteorologica*. Cambridge, MA: Harvard University Press.

Ariyabandu, M.M. (2003). Women: The risk managers in natural disasters, http://online.northumbria.ac.uk/ geography_research/gdn/.

Ariyabandu, M.M., & Wickramasinghe, M. (2004). *Gender dimensions in disaster management: A guide for South Asia*. Colombo, Sri Lanka: ITDG.

Armenian, H.K., Noji, E.K., & Oganessian, A.P. (1992). Case control study of injuries due to the earthquake in Soviet Armenia. *Bulletin World Health Organization, 70*, 251–257.

Armstrong, E., & Rosen, H. (1986). *Effective emergency response: The Salt Lake valley floods of 1983, 1984 and 1985*. Chicago: Public Works Historical Society.

Aroni, S., & Durkin, M.E. (n.d.) *Injuries and occupant behavior in earthquakes*. Los Angeles, CA: UCLA Graduate School of Architecture and Urban Planning. Unpublished manuscript.

Arrowwood, J.C. (2003). *Living with wildfires: Prevention, preparation, and recovery*. Denver, CO: Bradford.

artsACT (2004). *A bushfire memorial for the ACT: Community consultation discussion paper*. Bushfire Consultation Advisory Committee, artsACT: Department of Urban Services.

artsACT. (2005). *ACT bushfire memorial update*. Canberra. Retrieved May, 2005, http://www.arts.act.gov.au.

Arvedlund, E. (2005, May 26). Blackout disrupts Moscow after fire in old power station. *The New York Times*, A12.

Arvidson, E. (1999). Remapping Los Angeles, or taking the risk of class in postmodern urban theory. *Economic Geography, 75*(2), 134–156.

Aschauer, D.A. (1988). *Does public capital crowd out private capital?* Memorandum (pp. 88–10). Chicago: Federal Reserve Bank of Chicago.

Ashford, N.A. (1993). *The encouragement of technological change for preventing chemical accidents: Moving from secondary prevention and mitigation to primary prevention*. Cambridge, MA: MIT, Center for Technology, Policy and Industrial Development.

Ashley, C., & Carney D. (1999). *Sustainable livelihoods: Lessons from early experience*. United Kingdom: Department for International Development.

Asian American Federation of New York. (2002). *Chinatown: One year after September 11th: An economic impact study*. New York: Asian American Federation of New York.

Asian Disaster Reduction Center. (2005). Retrieved October 1, 2005, http://www.adrc.or.jp/.

Assilzadeh, H., & Mansor, S.B. (2004). *Natural disaster data and information management systems: Geo imagery bridging continents, XXth ISPRS Congress*, July 12–23, 2004 Istanbul, Turkey, Commission 7, V11, WG V11/5.

Auf der Heide, E. (1989a). *Disaster response: Principles of preparation and coordination*. St. Louis, MO: Mosby-Year Book.

Auf der Heide, E. (2004). Common misconceptions about disasters: Panic, the disaster syndrome, and looting. In M. O'Leary (Ed.), *The first 72 hours: A community approach to disaster preparedness* (pp. 340–381). Lincoln, NE: Universe.

Averill, J.D., Mileti, D.S., Peacock, R.D., Kuligowski, E.D., Groner, N., Proulx, G., et al. (2005). *Federal building and fire safety inspection of the World Trade Center disaster: Occupant behavior, egress and emergency communications*. Washington, DC: National Institute of Standards and Technology.

Babbie, E. (1995). *The practice of social research*. Belmont, CA: Wadsworth.

Bahk, C.M., & Neuwirth, K. (2000). Impact of movie depictions of volcanic disaster on risk perception and judgments. *International Journal of Mass Emergencies and Disasters, 18,* 63–84.

Baker, E.J. (1979). Predicting response to hurricane warnings: A reanalysis of data from four studies. *Mass Emergencies, 4,* 9–24.

Baker, E.J. (1987). *Evacuation in response to hurricanes Elena and Kate*. Unpublished draft report. Tallahassee, FL: Florida State University.

Baker, R. (2001). *The Journal on the Run*. Columbia Journalism Review November/December, pp. 16–17.

Baker, T., & Simon, J. (Eds.). (2002). *Embracing risk: The changing culture of insurance and responsibility*. Chicago: The University of Chicago Press.

Ballman, J. (2003). The great blackout of 2003. *Disaster Recovery, 10,* 17–18.

Balluz, L., Schieve, L., Holmes, T., Kiezak, S., & Malilay, J. (2000). Predictors for people's response to a tornado warning: Arkansas, 1 March 1997. *Disasters, 24*(1), 71–77.

Balter, M. (2005). The seeds of civilization. *Smithsonian, 36,* 68–74.

Banba, M., Hayashi, H., Maki, N., Kondo, T., Hasegawa, K., & Tamura, K. (2004). Analysis of land use management policies for earthquake disaster reduction through Marikina Case Study. *Proceedings of an International Symposium on City Planning* (pp. 473–482). City Planning Institute of Japan. University of Hokkaido.

Bandy, R., Johnson, A., Peek, L., & Sutton, J. (2004). *Public hazards communication: Annotated bibliography*. Boulder, CO: University of Colorado, Natural Hazards Center. Retrieved October 3, 2005, http://www.colorado.edu/hazards/informer/pubhazbibann.pdf.

Bangladesh Flood Forecasting and Warning Centre, (2005). http://www.ffwc.gov.bd/

Bankoff, G. (2003). *Cultures of disaster: Society and natural hazard in the Philippine*. London: Routledge Curzon.

Bankoff, G., Frerks, G., & Hilhorst, T. (Eds.). (2003). *Vulnerability: Disasters, development and people*. London: Earthscan.

Bankoff, G., & Hilhorst, D. (2004). Differing perceptions of disaster preparedness, management and recovery: The case of the Philippines and its applicability to New Zealand. In S. Norman (Ed.), *Proceedings of the New Zealand recovery symposium* (pp. 220–232). Wellington: Ministry of Civil Defense & Emergency Management.

Barber, J., & Schweithelm, J. (2000). *Trial by fire: Forest fires*. New York: World Resources Institute.

Bardo, J. (1978). Organizational response to disaster: A typology of adaptation and change. *Mass Emergencies, 4,* 145–149.

Bari, F. (1998). Gender, disaster, and empowerment: A case study from Pakistan. In E. Enarson, & B. H. Morrow (Eds.), *The gendered terrain of disaster: Through women's eyes* (pp. 125–131). Westport, CT: Praeger.

Barnecut, C. (1998). Disaster prone: Reflections of a female permanent disaster volunteer. In E. Enarson & B.H. Morrow (Eds.), *The gendered terrain of disaster: Through women's eyes* (pp. 151–159). Westport, CT: Praeger.

Barron, R.A. (2004). International disaster mental health. *Psychiatric Clinics of North America, 27,* 505–519.

Barry, J.M. (1997). *Rising tide: The great Mississippi flood of 1927 and how it changed America*. New York: Simon and Schuster.

Barth, F. (Ed.). (1969). *Ethnic groups and boundaries*. Boston: Little, Brown.

Barton, A.H. (1962). The emergency social system. In G.W. Baker & D.W. Chapman (Eds.), *Man and society in disaster* (pp. 222–267). New York: Basic Books.

Barton, A.H. (1963). *Social organization under stress*. Washington, DC: National Research Council, National Academy of Sciences.

Barton, A.H. (1969). *Communities in disasters: A sociological analysis of collective stress situations*. Garden City, NY: Doubleday.

Barton, A.H. (1970). *Communities in disaster*. New York: Anchor.

Barton, A.H. (1989). Taxonomies of disaster and macrosocial theory. In G.A. Kreps (Ed.), *Social structure and disaster* (pp. 346–350). Newark, DE: University of Delaware Press.

Barton, A.H. (2005). Disaster and collective stress. In R.W. Perry & E.L. Quarantelli (Eds.), *What is a disaster: New answers to old questions* (pp. 125–152). Philadelphia: Xlibris.

Bateman, J., & Edwards, B. (2002). Gender and evacuation: A closer look at why women are more likely to evacuate for hurricanes. *Natural Hazards Review, 3*(3), 107–117.

Bates, F.L. (Ed.) (1982). *Recovery, change and development: A longitudinal study of the Guatemalan Earthquake.* Athens, GA: Department of Sociology.

Bates, F., Fogleman, C., Parenton, V., Pittman, R., & Tracy, G. (1963). *The social and psychological consequences of a natural disaster: A longitudinal study of Hurricane Audrey.* NRC Disaster Study No. 18. Washington, DC: National Academy of Science.

Bates, F., & Harvey, C.C. (1975). *The structure of social systems.* New York: Gardner Press.

Bates, F.L., & Peacock, W.G. (1987). Disasters and social change. In R. R. Dynes, B. Demarchi, & C. Pelanda (Eds.), *The sociology of disasters* (pp. 291–330). Milan, Italy: Franco Angeli Press.

Bates, F., & Peacock, W.G. (1989a). Conceptualizing social structure. *American Sociological Review, 54*, 565–578.

Bates, F.L., & Peacock, W.G. (1989b). Long-term recovery. *International Journal of Mass Emergencies and Disasters (IJMED), 7*, 349–365.

Bates, F.L., & Peacock, W.G. (1992). Measuring disaster impact on household living conditions: The domestic assets approach. *International Journal of Mass Emergencies and Disasters (IJMED), 10*, 133–160.

Bates, F.L., & Peacock, W.G. (1993). *Living conditions, disasters and development.* Athens, GA: University of Georgia Press.

Bates, F.L., & Pelanda, C. (1994). An ecological approach to disasters. In R.R. Dynes & K.J. Tierney (Eds.), *Disasters, collective behavior, and social organization* (pp. 149–159). Newark, DE: University of Delaware Press.

Baum, J.A.C., & Oliver, C. (1991). Institutional linkages and organizational mortality. *Administrative Science Quarterly, 36*, 187–218.

Baumgartner, F.R., & Jones, B.D. (1993). *Agendas and instability in American politics.* Chicago: The University of Chicago Press.

BBC News. (2003). *The day Britain stopped.* BBC Two, Tuesday 13, May 2003.

BBC News. (2004). *Victim rebukes Madrid commission.* London (15 December 2004); http//news.bbc.co.uk.

BBC News. (2004a). *Bombed city centre reopens.* Retrieved November 24, 1999, http://news.bbc.co.uk.

BBC News. (2004b). *Service for Estonia ferry deaths.* Retrieved September 25, 2004, http://www.time.com/time/europe.

BBC News. (2004c).*Victim Rebukes Madrid Commission.* Retrieved December 15, 2004, http://news.bbc.co.uk.

BBC News. (2005a). *Prince marks VJ Day at Cenotaph.* Retrieved August 21, 2005, http://news.bbc.co.uk.

BBC News. (2005b). *Thai tsunami IDs' may take years.* Retrieved August 22, 2005, http://news.bbc.co.uk.

BBC News. (2005c). *Candle vigil for tsunami victims.* Retrieved January 8, 2005, http://news.bbc.co.uk.

BBC News. (2005d). *NI tribute to tsunami victims.* Retrieved January 5, 2005, http://news.bbc.co.uk.

BBC News. (2005e). *Mosques warned of Muslim backlash.* Retrieved July 11, 2005, http://news.bbc.co.uk.

BBC News. (2005f). *Europe's silent tribute.* Retrieved January 5, 2005, http://news.bbc.co.uk.

BBC News. (2005g). *MP condemns three-minute silence.* Retrieved January 5, 2005, http://news.bbc.co.uk.

BBC News. (2005h). *Tsunami memorial event.* Retrieved April 4, 2005, http://news.bbc.co.uk.

BBC News. (2005i). *Pakistan dam burst deaths hit 35.* 2005, http://newsvote.bbc.co.uk/mpapps/pagetools/print/news/bbc.co.uk/2/hi.

Bean, J. (2002). The implementation of the incident control system in NSW: Span of control and management by objectives. *The Australian Journal of Emergency Management, 17*(3), 8–16.

Beatley, T. (1995). *Promoting sustainable land use: Mitigating natural hazards through land use planning.* Hazard Reduction and Recovery Center Publication No. 133A (6 pp.). College Station, TX: Texas A&M University, College of Architecture.

Beatley, T. (1998). The vision of sustainable communities. In R. Burby (Ed.), *Cooperating with nature: Confronting natural hazards with land use planning for sustainable communities* (pp. 233–262). Washington, DC: Joseph Henry Press.

Beck, U. (1992). *Risk society: Towards a new modernity.* London: SAGE.

Beck, U. (1999). *World risk society.* Cambridge: Polity Press.

Becker, H.S. (1967). Whose side are we on? *Social Problems, 14*, 239–247.

Becker, W.S. (1994a). *Rebuilding for the future. . . A guide to sustainable redevelopment for disaster-affected communities.* Washington, DC: U.S. Department of Energy. Retreived September, 2005, www.sustainable.doe.gov/articles.

Becker, W.S. (1994b). The case for sustainable redevelopment. *Environment And Development (American Planning Asociation).* November, 4.

Becker, W.S., & Stauffer, R. (1994). *Rebuilding the future: A guide to sustainable redevelopment for disaster-affected communities* (25 pp.). Golden, CO: U.S. Department of Energy, Office of Energy Efficiency and Renewable Energy, Center of Excellence for Sustainable Development.

Begum, R. (1993). Women in environmental disasters: The 1991 cyclone in Bangladesh. *Focus on Gender, 1*(1), 34–39.

Belardo, S., Karwan, K.R., & Wallace, W.A. (1984). Managing the response to disasters using microcomputers. *Interfaces, 14*, 29–39.

Bell, B.D., Kara, G., & Batterson, C. (1978). Service utilization and adjustment patterns of elderly tornado victims in an American disaster. *Mass Emergencies, 1*, 71–81.

Bell, C., & Newby, H. (1971). *Community studies*. London: Unwin.

Bell, M. (2004). *An invitation to environmental sociology* (2nd ed.). Thousand Oaks, CA: Pine Forge.

Bellah, R. (1975). *The broken covenant: American civil religion in time of trial*. New York: Seabury.

Benini, J.B. (1998). Getting organized pays off for disaster response. *Journal of Contingencies and Crisis Management, 6*, 61–63.

Benson, C., & Clay, E.J. (2004). *Understanding the economic and financial impacts of natural disasters*. Washington, DC: World Bank.

Benson, C. & Twigg, J. (2004a). *Measuring mitigation: Methodologies for assessing natural hazard risks and the net benefits of mitigation—A scoping study*. Decemeber. Geneva: ProVention Consortium.

Benson, C., & Twigg, J. (2004b). *Integrating disaster reduction into development: recommendations for policy-makers*. December. Geneva: ProVention Consortium.

Benson, J.K. (1982). A framework for policy analysis. In D.L. Rogers, D.A. Whetten et al. (Eds.), *Interorganizational coordination: Theory, research and implementation* (pp. 137–176). Ames, IA: Iowa State University Press.

Berg, J. (1988). *Uncovering Soviet disasters*. New York: Random House.

Bergtrom, W. (Ed.). (1995). *Measuring and interpreting business cycles*. Oxford: Oxford University Press.

Berke, P. R. (1995a). Natural hazard reduction and sustainable development: A global assessment. *Journal of Planning Literature, 9*(4), 370–382.

Berke, P.R. (1995b). Natural hazard reduction and sustainable development: A global reassessment. *Working Paper No. S95-02*. University of North Carolina: Center for Urban and Regional Studies.

Berke, P.R., & Beatley, T. (1992). *Planing for earthquakes: Risk, politics and policy*. Baltimore, MD: Johns Hopkins University Press.

Berke, P.R., & Beatley, T. (1997). *After the hurricane: Linking recovery to sustainable development in the Caribbean*. Baltimore, MD: Johns Hopkins University Press.

Berke, P.R., Beatley, T., & Wilhite, S. (1989). Influences on local adoption of planning measures for earthquake hazard mitigation. *International Journal of Mass Emergencies and Disasters, 7*, 33–56.

Berke, P., Kartez, J., & Wenger, D. (1993). Recovery after disaster: Achieving sustainable development, mitigation, and equity. *Disasters, 17*, 93–109.

Berke, P., & Wenger, D. (1991). *Linking hurricane disaster recovery to sustainable development strategies: Montserrat, West Indies*. Hazard Reduction and Recovery Center: Texas A&M University, College Station, TX.

Bernstein, P. (1998). *Against the gods: The remarkable story of risk*. New York: Wiley.

Berridge, V., & Taylor, S. (Eds.). (2003). *The big smoke: Fifty years after the 1952 London Smog: A commemorative conference*. Witness Seminar held at the Brunei Gallery, SOAS, December 9–10, 2002. London: London School of Hygiene & Tropical Medicine.

Best, J. (1999). *Random violence: How we talk about new crimes and new victims*. Berkeley, CA: University of California Press.

Bhatt, E. (1998). Women victims' view of urban and rural vulnerability. In J. Twigg & M. Bhatt (Eds.), *Understanding vulnerability: South Asian perspectives* (pp. 12–26). Colombo, Sri Lanka: ITDG.

Biderman, A.D. (1966). Anticipatory studies and stand-by research capabilities. In R. Bauer (Ed.), *Social indicators* (pp. 68–153). Cambridge, MA: Harvard University Press.

Biel, S. (2001). *American disasters*. New York: New York University Press.

Bigoness, W.J., & Perreault, W.D. Jr. (1981). A conceptual paradigm and approach for the study of innovators. *Academy of Management Journal, 24*, 68–82.

Bimber, B. (2003). *Information and American democracy: Technology in the evolution of political power*. Cambridge, UK: Cambridge University Press.

Birkland, T.A. (1997). *After disaster: Agenda setting, public policy, and focusing events*. Washington, DC: Georgetown University Press.

Blaikie, P., Cannon, T., Davis, I., & Davis, B. (1994). *At risk: Natural hazards, people's vulnerability, and disasters*. New York: Routledge.

Blanchard, B.W. (2004). *Historical overview of U.S. Emergency Management*. Unpublished draft prepared for college courses for emergency managers.

Blanchard-Boehm, D. (1997). *Risk communication in Southern California: Ethnic and gender response to 1995 revised, upgraded earthquake probabilities.* Quick response report 94. Boulder, CO: Natural Hazards Research and Applications Information Center, University of Colorado, http://www.colorado.edu/hazards/qr/qr94.html.

Blanchard-Boehm, R.D. (1998). Understanding public response to increased risk from natural hazards: Application of the hazard risk communication framework. *International Journal of Mass Emergencies and Disasters, 16*(3), 247–278.

Blanshan, S., & Quarantelli, E.L. (1981). From dead body to person: The handling of fatal mass casualties in disasters. *Victimology: An International Journal, 6*(1–4), 275–287.

Bleich, A., Gelkopf, M., & Solomon, Z. (2003). Exposure to terrorism, stress-related mental health symptoms, and coping behaviors among a nationally representative sample in Israel. *Journal of the American Medical Association, 290*, 612–620.

Bloom, S. (1998). By the crowd they have been broken, by the crowd they shall be healed: The social transformation of trauma. In R. Tedeschi, C. Park, & L. Calhoun (Eds.), *Posttraumatic growth: Positive change in the aftermath of crisis* (pp. 179–214). Mahwah, NJ: Erlbaum.

Blumer, H. (1939). Collective behavior. In R. Park (Ed.), *Principles of sociology* (pp. 65–121). New York: Barnes and Noble.

Blumer, H. (1948). Public opinion and public opinion polling. *American Sociological Review, 13*, 542–552.

Blumer, J., & Gurevitch, M. (1995). *The crisis of public communication.* London: Routledge.

Bogard, W.C. (1989). Bringing social theory to hazards research: Conditions and consequences of the mitigation of environmental hazards. *Sociological Perspectives, 31*, 147–168.

Bohle, H.G., Downing, T.E., & Watts, M.J. (1994). Climate change and social vulnerability: the sociology and geography of food insecurity. *Global Environmental Change, 4*, 37–48.

Boin, R.A., & Lagadec, P. (2000). Preparing for the future: Critical challenges in crisis management. *Journal of Contingencies and Crisis Management, 8*, 185–191.

Boin, R.A., Lagadec, P., Michel-Kerjan, E., & Overdijk, W. (2003). Critical infrastructure under threat: Learning from the anthrax scare. *Journal of Contingencies and Crisis Management, 11*(3), 99–106.

Boin, R.A. (2005). From crisis to disaster: Towards an integrative perspective. In R.W. Perry & E.L. Quarantelli (Eds.), *What is a disaster? New answers to old questions* (pp. 153–172). Philadelphia: Xlibris.

Boin, R.A., & 't Hart, P. (2003). Public leadership in times of crisis: Mission impossible? *Public Administration Review, 63*(6), 544–553.

Boin, R.A., 't Hart, P., Stern, E., & Sundelius, B. (2005). *The politics of crisis management: Public leadership under pressure.* Cambridge, UK: Cambridge University Press.

Boin, R.A., Kofman-Bos, C., & Overdijk, W. (2004). Crisis simulations: Exploring tomorrow's vulnerabilities and threats. *Simulation & Gaming, 35*, 378–393.

Boin, R.A., & Rattray, W.A.R. (2004). Understanding prison riots: Towards a threshold theory. *Punishment & Society, 6*, 47–65.

Bolin, R.C. (1976). Family recovery from natural disaster: A preliminary model. *Mass Emergencies, 1*, 267–277.

Bolin, R.C. (1982). *Long-term family recovery from disaster.* Boulder, CO Program on Environment and Behavior, Institute of Behavioral Science, University of Colorado, Monograph No. 36.

Bolin, R.C. (1985). Disasters and long-term recovery policy: A focus on housing and families. *Policy Studies Review, 4*(4), 704–715.

Bolin, R.C. (1986). Disaster impact and recovery: A comparison of black and white victims. *International Journal of Mass Emergenciesy and Disaster (IJMED), 4*, 35–50.

Bolin, R.C. (1993). Post-earthquake shelter and housing: Research findings and policy implications. In K.J. Tierney & J.M. Nigg (Eds.), *Socioeconomic impacts* (pp. 107–131). Memphis, TN: Central United States Earthquake Consortium, Monograph No. 5.

Bolin, R.C. (1994). *Household and community recovery after earthquakes.* Boulder, CO: Program on Environment Behavior, Institute of Behavioral Science, University of Colorado, Monograph No. 56.

Bolin, R.C., & Bolton, P. (1983). Recovery in Nicaragua and the USA. *International Journal of Mass Emergencies and Disasters, 1*(1), 125–152.

Bolin, R.C., & Bolton, P. (1986). Race, religion and ethnicity in disaster recovery. Monograph No. 42. Boulder, CO: University of Colorado.

Bolin, R.C., Grineski, S., & Collins, T. (2005). The geography of despair: Environmental racism and the making of South Phoenix, Arizona, USA. *Human Ecology Review, 12*(2), 156–168.

Bolin, R.C., Jackson, M., & Crist, A. (1998). Gender inequality, vulnerability, and disaster: Issues in theory and research. In E. Enarson & B.H. Morrow (Eds.), *The gendered terrain of disaster: Through women's eyes* (pp. 27–44). Westport, CT: Praeger.

Bolin, R.C., & Stanford, L. (1990). *Shelter and housing issues in Santa Cruz County. The Loma Prieta Earthquake: Studies of short-term impacts.* Program on Environment and Behavior Monograph No. 50. Institute of Behavioral Science, University of Colorado.

Bolin, R.C., & Stanford, L. (1991). Shelter, housing and recovery: A comparison of U.S. disasters. *Disasters, 15*(1), 24–34.

Bolin, R.C., & Stanford, L. (1998a). The Northridge earthquake: Community based approaches to unmet recovery needs. *Disasters, 22*(1), 21–38.

Bolin, R.C., & Stanford, L. (1998b). *The Northridge earthquake: Vulnerability and disaster.* London: Routledge.

Bolin, R.C., & Stanford, L. (1999). Constructing vulnerability in the first world: The Northridge earthquake in Southern California, 1994. In A. Oliver-Smith, & S. Hoffman (Eds.), *The angry earth: Disasters in anthropological perspective* (pp. 89–112). New York: Routledge.

Bolin, R.C., & Trainer, P. (1978). Modes of family recovery following disaster: A cross-national study. In E. Quarantelli (Ed.), *Disasters: Theory and research* (pp. 234–247). Beverly Hills, CA: SAGE.

Bolton, P., Liebow, E., & Olson, J. (1993). Community conflict and uncertainty following a damaging earthquake: Low-income Latinos in Los Angeles, California, *Environmental Professional, 15*, 240–247.

Bommer, J., & Ledbetter, S. (1987). The San Salvador earthquake of 10th October 1986. *Disasters, 11*, 83–95.

Bonnell, V.E., & Hunt, L. (1999). *Beyond the cultural turn.* Berkeley, CA: University of California Press.

Boone, C., & Modarres, A. (1999). Creating a toxic neighborhood in Los Angeles county: A historical examination of environmental inequity. *Urban Affairs Review, 35*(2), 163–187.

Bos, C.K., Ullberg, S., & Hart, P. (2005). The long shadow of disaster: Memory and politics in Holland and Sweden. *International Journal of Mass Emergencies and Disasters, 23*, 5–26.

Bosner, L. (2001). Disaster management in Japan. Mike Mansfield Fellowship study report. Washington, DC: FEMA.

Bosner, L. (2002). Disaster preparedness: How Japan and the United States compare. *Asia Perspectives, 4*(2), 17–20.

Bosworth, S.L., & Kreps, G. A. (1986). Structure as process: Organization and role. *American Sociological Review, 51*, 699–716.

Bourdieu, P. (1984). *Distinction: A social critique of the judgment of taste.* London: Routledge and Kegan Paul.

Bourke, J. (2005). *Fear: A cultural history.* London: Virago Press.

Bourque, L.B., Peek-Asa, C., Mahue, M., Shoaf, K.I., Kraus, J.F., Weiss, B., et al. (1997). Health implications of earthquakes: Physical and emotional injuries during and after the Northridge earthquake. In *Vulnerability reduction, preparedness, and rehabilitation* (pp. 22–31). *Proceedings of the WHO Symposium on Earthquakes and People's Health,* Kobe, Japan.

Bourque, L.B., Shoaf, K.I., & Nguyen, L.H. (1997). Survey research. *International Journal of Mass Emergencies and Disasters, 15*, 71–101.

Bourque, L.B., Siegel, J.M., & Shoaf, K. (2001). Psychological distress and use of health services following urban earthquakes in California. In *Proceedings of the first workshop for comparative study on urban earthquake disaster management* (pp. 77–87), Kobe, Japan.

Bovens, M., & 't Hart, P. (1996). *Understanding policy fiascoes.* New Brunswick, NJ: Transaction.

Brabrooke, D., & Lindblom, C.E. (1970). *A strategy of decision: Policy evaluation as a social process.* New York: Macmillan.

Bradshaw, S. (2001a). *Dangerous liaisons: Women, men, and Hurricane Mitch.* Managua, Nicaragua: Fundacion Puntos de Encuentro.

Bradshaw, S. (2001b). Reconstructing roles and relations: Women's participation in reconstruction in post-Mitch Nicaragua. *Gender and Development, 9*(3), 79–87.

Bradshaw, S. (2002). Exploring the gender dimensions of reconstruction processes post-Hurricane Mitch. *Journal of International Development, 14*, 871–879.

Brändström, A., & Kuipers, S.L. (2003). From "normal incidents" to political crises: Understanding the selective politicization of policy failures. *Government and Opposition, 38*, 279–305.

Bratt, R., Hartman, C., & Meyerson, A. (1986). *Critical perspectives on housing.* Philadelphia: Temple University Press.

Brecher, M. (1993). *Crises in world politics: Theory and reality.* Oxford: Pergamon Press.

Breed, W. (1955). Social control in the newsroom. *Social Forces, 33*, 326–335.

Breznitz, S. (1984). *Cry wolf: The psychology of false alarms.* Hillsdale, NJ: Erlbaum.

Briceño, S. (2002). Gender mainstreaming in disaster reduction. Paper presented at the United Nations Commission on the Status of Women panel discussion on Environmental management and mitigation of natural disasters: A gender perspective. New York, March 4–15, 2002. http://www.un.org/womenwatch/daw/csw/csw46/panel–briceno.pdf.

BRIDGE. (1996). Integrating gender into emergency responses. Briefings on *development and gender, Issue 4*. Sussex: Institute of Development Studies.

Briere, J., & Elliott, D. (2000). Prevalence, characteristics, and long-term sequelae of natural disaster exposure in the general population. *Journal of Traumatic Stress, 13*, 661–679.

Britton, N.R. (1984). Australia's organized response to natural disaster: Background and theoretical analysis. *Disasters, 8*(2), 124–137.

Britton, N.R. (1986a). An appraisal of Australia's disaster management system following the 'Ash Wednesday' bushfires in Victoria, 1983. *Australian Journal of Public Administration, 45*, 112–127.

Britton, N.R. (1986b). Developing an understanding of disaster. *Australian and New Zealand Journal of Sociology, 22*, 254–272.

Britton, N.R. (1991). Constraints or effectiveness in disaster management: The bureaucratic imperative versus organizational mission. *Canberra Bulletin of Public Administration, 64*, 54–64.

Britton, N.R. (1999a). Political commitment. In J. Ingleton (Ed.), *Natural disaster management* (pp. 214–216). Leicester: Tudor Rose.

Britton, N.R. (1999b). Whither the emergency manager? *International Journal of Mass Emergencies and Disasters, 17*(2), 223–235.

Britton, N.R. (2002). Institutional arrangements for total risk management in New Zealand: Issues and solutions. In *Proceedings of regional workshop on best practices in disaster mitigation* (pp. 47–58). Bangkok: Asian Disaster Preparedness Center.

Britton, N.R. (2004). Management of multi-lateral, multi-disciplinary projects. In *Proceedings of the safety engineering symposium* (pp. 135–138). July 1–2, 2004, Tokyo, Japan.

Britton, N.R. (2005). What's a word—opening up the debate. In R.W. Perry & E.L. Quarantelli (Eds.), *What is a disaster: New answers to old questions* (pp. 60–78). Philadelphia: Xlibris.

Britton, N.R., & Clark, G. J. (2000). From response to resilience: Emergency management reform in New Zealand. *Natural Hazards Review, 1*(3), 145–150.

Britton, N.R., & Wettenhall, R.L. (1990). Evolution of a disaster focal point: Australia's Natural Disasters Organization. *International Journal of Mass Emergencies and Disasters, 8*(3), 237–274.

Bromet, E., & Dew, M.A. (1995). Review of psychiatric epidemiologic research on disasters. *Epidemiologic Reviews, 17*, 113–119.

Brooks, B., Kennedy G., Moon, D.R., & Ranly, D. [The Missouri Group]. (1992). *News reporting & writing* (228 pp.). New York: St. Martin's Press.

Brouillettee, J.R., & Quarantelli, E.L. (1971). Types of patterned variation in bureaucratic adaptations to organizational stress. *Sociological Inquiry, 41*, 39–46.

Browne, R.B., & Neal, A.G. (2001). *Ordinary reactions to extraordinary events*. Bowling Green, OH: Bowling Green State University Popular Press.

Bruneau, M., Chang, S.E., Eguchi, R.T., Lee, G.C., O'Rourke, T.D., Reinhorn, A.M., Shinozuka, M., Tierney, K., Wallace, W.A., & Von Winterfeldt, D. (2003). *Earthquake Spectra, 19*(4), 733–752.

Brunhuber, K. (1998). The real story at Peggy's Cove. *The Sunday Herald*, September 13.

Bryson, B. (2003). *A short history of nearly everything*. New York: Broadway Books.

Buchanan, M. (2000). *Ubiquity: Why catastrophes happen*. New York: Three Rivers Press.

Bucher, R. (1957). Blame and hostility in disaster. *American Journal of Sociology, 62*, 467–475.

Buck, W.B. (1987) Environmental pollution, including toxic wastes. *Journal of the American Veterinary Medical Association, 190*, 793–796.

Buckle, P. (2005). Mandated definitions, local knowledge and complexity. In R.W. Perry & E.L. Quarantelli (Eds.), *What is a disaster: New answers to old questions* (pp. 173–200). Philadelphia: Xlibris.

Buckle, P., Mars, G., & Smale, S. (2000). New approaches to assessing vulnerability and resilience. *Australian Journal of Emergency Management, 15*(2), 8–14.

Buffoon. (1749). Théorie de la Terre. In J. Delumeau, & Y. Lequin, *Les Malheurs des temps—Histoire des fléaux et des calamités en France, Mentalités: vécu et representations* (397 pp.). Paris: Larousse.

Bullard, R. (1990). *Dumping in dixie*. Boulder, CO: Westview Press.

Bullard, R. (1993). *Confronting environmental racism: Voices from the crossroads*. Boston: South End Press.

Bullard, R. (1994). *Unequal protection: Environmental justice and communities of color*, San Francisco: Sierra Club Books.

Bullard, R., Johnson, G., & Torres, A. (2000). Environmental costs and consequences of sprawl. In R. Bullard, G. Johnson, & A. Torres (Eds.), *Sprawl city: Race, politics and planning in Atlanta* (pp. 21–38). Covelo, CA: Island Press.

Bullock, J.A., Haddow, G.D., & Bell, R. (2004). Communicating during emergencies in the United States. *The Australian Journal of Emergency Management, 19*(2), 7.

Bullock, J.A., Haddow, G.D., Coppola, D., Ergin, E., Westerman, L., & Yeletaysi, S. (2005). *Introduction to homeland security*. New York: Elsevier.

Bunge, M. (1998). *Social science under debate*. Toronto: University of Toronto Press.

Burawoy, M. (2005). 2004 Presidential Address: For public sociology. *American Sociological Review, 70*, 4–28.

Burby, R.J. (Ed). (1998). *Cooperating with nature: Confronting natural hazards with land-use planning for substainable*. Washington, DC: Joseph Henry Press.

Burby, R.J. (2000). Land-use planning for flood hazard reduction. In D.J. Parker (Ed.), *Floods* (pp. 6–18). New York: Routledge.

Burby, R.J. (2001b). Building disaster resilient and sustainable communities. Federal Emergency Management Agency; Emergency Management Institute, higher education project. The course is available online at: http://training.fema.gov/emiweb/edu/completeCourses.asp.

Burby, R.J., & French, Steven. (1981). Gaping with floods: The land use management paradox. *Journal of the American Planning Association, 47*, 289–300.

Burby, R.J. (2005). Have state comprehensive planning mandates insured losses from natural disasters? *Natural Hazards Review, 6*(2), 67–81.

Burby, R., Beatley, T., Berke, P.R., Deyle, R.E., French, S.P., Godschalk, D.R., et al. (1999). Unleashing the power of planning to create disaster-resistant communities. *Journal of the American Planning Association, 65*, 247–258.

Burby, R., & Dalton, L. (1994). Plans can matter: The role of land use and state planning mandates on limiting development of hazardous areas. *Public Administration Review, 54*(3), 229–238.

Burkle, F.M. (1996). Acute-phase mental health consequences of disasters: Implications for triage and emergency medical services. *Annals of Emergency Medicine, 28*, 119–128

Burt, C. (2004). *Extreme weather, A guide & record book*. New York: Norton.

Burton, I. (1981) *The Mississauga evacuation, Final report*. Toronto: Institute for Environmental Studies, University of Toronto.

Burton, I. (2005). The social construction of natural disasters: An evolutionary process. In United Nations, *Know risk* (pp. 35–36). Leicester: Tudor Rose Publications.

Burton, I., & Kates, R. (1964). The perception of natural hazards in resource management. *Natural Resources Journal, 3*, 412–441.

Burton, I., Kates, R., & White, G. (1978). *The environment as hazard*. New York: Oxford University Press.

Burton, I., Kates R.W., & White, B.F. (1993). *The environment as hazard* (2nd ed.). New York: Guilford Press.

Bush, G.W. (2002). *State of the Union Address*. Washington, DC: www.whitehouse.gov.

Buss, S., Stern, E.K., & Newlove, L. (2005). *Value complexity in crisis management: The Lithuanian transition*. CRISMART Series. Stockholm: Elanders Gotab.

Buvinić, M. (1999). Hurricane Mitch: Women's needs and contributions. Washington, DC: Inter–American Development Bank. Retrieved, http://www.iadb.org/sds/doc/ SOC%2D115E.pdf.

Bynander, F., & Chemilievski, P. (Eds.). (Forthcoming). *The politics of crisis management in transitional Poland*. Stockholm: Elanders Gotab.

Cabinet Office. (2003). *Dealing with disaster* (3rd ed.). London: Crown Copyright.

Cabinet Office. (2005). *Disaster management in Japan*. Tokyo: Government of Japan. Retrieved, http://www.bousai.go.jp.

Çabuk, A. (2001). A proposal for a method to establish natural-hazard-based land-use planning: The Adapazarı case study. *Turkish Journal of Earth Sciences, 10*, 143–152.

Campbell, J.R. (1990). Disasters and development in historical context: Tropical cyclone response in the Banks Islands, Northern Vanuatu. *International Journal of Mass Emergencies and Disasters, 8*(3), 401–424.

Camus, A. (1947). *La peste*. Paris: Gallimard.

Canadian International Development Agency [CIDA]. (2003). Gender equality and humanitarian assistance: A guide to the issues. Gatineau, Quebec. Retrieved May 3, 2005, http://www.acdi–cida.gc.ca/INET/IMAGES.NSF/ vLUImages/Africa/$file/Guide–Gender.pdf.

Cann, M. (1990) Hagersville! *Emergency Preparedness Digest, 17*, 2–7.

Cannon, T. (1993). A hazard need not a disaster make: Vulnerability and the causes of natural disasters. In P.A. Merriman & C.W.A. Browitt (Eds.), *Natural disasters: Protecting vulnerability communities*. London: Thomas Telford.

Cannon, T. (1994). Vulnerability analysis and the explanation of 'natural' disasters. In A. Varley (Ed.), *Disasters, development and environment*. London: Wiley.

Cannon, T. (2000). Vulnerability analysis and disasters. In D. Parker (Ed.), *Flood hazards and disasters*. London: Routledge.

Caplow, T., Bahr, H.M., & Chadwick, B.A. (1984). *Readiness of local communities for integrated emergency management planning*. Final Report. Charlottesville, VA: United Research Services Incorporated.

CARE International. (2002). Flood impact on women and girls: Prey Veng Province, Cambodia. Australia. Retrieved June 2002, http://www.adpc.net/pdrsea/publications /FLdWG %20 Flood.pdf.

Carley, K.M., & Harrald, J. R. (1997). Organizational learning under fire: Theory and practice. *American Behavioral Scientist, 40*, 310–332.

Carlin, G. (2001). *Napalm and silly putty.* New York: Hyperion.

Carlos, C. (2001). *The Philippine disaster management story: Issues and challenges.* Quezon City: National Defense College of the Philippines, Camp Aguinaldo.

Carr, L.J. (1932). Disaster and the sequence-pattern concept of social change. *American Journal of Sociology, 38*, 207–218.

Carter, A.O., Millson, M.E., & Allen, D.E. (1989). Epidemiologic study of deaths and injuries due to tornadoes. *American Journal of Epidemiology, 130*, 1209–1218.

Castenfors, K., & Svedin, L. (2001). Crisis communication: Learning from the 1998 LPG near miss in Stockholm. *Journal of Hazardous Materials, 88*, 235–254.

Castillo, F. (2005). *Verbal report provided to the workshop on development of disaster risk management master plan for metro Manila.* Manila: Metro Manila Development Authority.

Cavallin A., Floris, B., & Cerutti, P. (1995). GIS potential for regional and local scale groundwater hazard assessment. In A. Carrara, & F. Guzzetti (Eds.), *Geographical information systems in assessing natural hazards* (pp. 259–272). Dordrecht: Kluwer Academic.

Cavanaugh, M. (2000). *The Loma Prieta earthquake and hurricane Andrew: A comparative study in disaster preparedness activities.* Newark DE: M. A. thesis, Department of Sociology and Criminal Justice, University of Delaware.

Ceciliano, N., Pretto, E., Watoh, Y., Angus, D.C., & Abrams, J.I. (1993). The earthquake in Turkey in 1992: A mortality study. *Prehospital and Disaster Medicine, 8*, S139.

Center for Advanced Engineering. (1991). *Lifelines in earthquakes.* Wellington case study project report. Christchurch: Centre for Advanced Engineering, University of Canterbury.

Center for Advanced Engineering. (1995). *Wellington after the 'quake: The challenge of rebuilding cities.* Earthquake Commission. Christchurch: Centre for Advanced Engineering, University of Canterbury.

Centers for Disease Control (CDC). (1982). Public health impact of a snow disaster. *Morbidity and Mortality Weekly Report, 31*, 695–696.

Centers for Disease Control (CDC). (1983). Flood disasters and immunization—California. *Morbidity and Mortality Weekly Report, 32*, 171–172,178.

Centers for Disease Control (CDC). (1984a). Heat-associated mortality—New York City. *Morbidity and Mortality Weekly Report, 33*, 518–521.

Centers for Disease Control (CDC). (1984b). Illness and death due to environmental heat—Georgia and St. Louis, Missouri, 1983. *Morbidity and Mortality Weekly Report, 33*, 325–326.

Centers for Disease Control (CDC). (1984c). Tornado disaster—North Carolina, South Carolina, March 28, 1984. *Morbidity and Mortality Weekly Report, 34*, 211–213.

Centers for Disease Control (CDC). (1986a). Cytotoxicity of volcanic ash: Assessing the risk for Pneumonoconiosis. *Morbidity and Mortality Weekly Report, 35*, 265–267.

Centers for Disease Control (CDC). (1986b). Hurricanes and hospital emergency-room visits—Mississippi, Rhode Island, Connecticut. *Morbidity and Mortality Weekly Report, 34*(51), 765.

Centers for Disease Control (CDC). (1986c). Tornado Disaster—Pennsylvania. *Morbidity and Mortality Weekly Report, 34*, 233–235.

Centers for Disease Control (CDC). (1988). Tornado disaster—Texas. *Morbidity and Mortality Weekly Report, 37*, 454–456, 461.

Centers for Disease Control (CDC). (1989a). Current trends in heat-related deaths—Missouri, 1979–1988. *Morbidity and Mortality Weekly Report, 38*, 437–439.

Centers for Disease Control (CDC). (1989b). Deaths associated with Hurricane Hugo—Puerto Rico. *Morbidity and Mortality Weekly Report, 38*, 680–682.

Centers for Disease Control (CDC). (1989c). Earthquake-associated deaths—California. *Morbidity and Mortality Weekly Report, 38*, 767–770.

Centers for Disease Control (CDC). (1989d). Medical examiner/coroner reports of deaths associated with Hurricane Hugo—South Carolina. *Morbidity and Mortality Weekly Report, 38*, 759–762.

Centers for Disease Control (CDC). (1989e). Update: Work-related electrocutions associated with hurricane Hugo—Puerto Rico. *Morbidity and Mortality Weekly Report, 38*, 718–725.

Centers for Disease Control (CDC). (1991). Tornado disaster—Illinois. *Morbidity and Mortality Weekly Report, 40*, 33–36.

Centers for Disease Control (CDC). (1992a). Emergency mosquito control associated with Hurricane Andrew—Florida and Louisiana, 1992. *Morbidity and Mortality Weekly Report, 42,* 240–242.

Centers for Disease Control (CDC). (1992b). Preliminary report: Medical examiner reports of deaths associated with Hurricane Andrew—Florida, August 1992. *Morbidity and Mortality Weekly Report, 41,* 641–644.

Centers for Disease Control (CDC). (1992c). Rapid health needs assessment following Hurricane Andrew—Florida and Louisiana, 1992. *Morbidity and Mortality Weekly Report, 41,* 685–688.

Centers for Disease Control (CDC). (1992d). Tornado disaster—Kansas, 1991. *Morbidity and Mortality Weekly Report, 41,* 181–183.

Centers for Disease Control (CDC). (1993a). Comprehensive assessment of health needs 2 months after Hurricane Andrew—Dade County, Florida, 1992. *Morbidity and Mortality Weekly Report, 42,* 434–437.

Centers for Disease Control (CDC). (1993b). Flood-related mortality—Missouri, 1993. *Morbidity and Mortality Weekly Report, 42,* 941–943.

Centers for Disease Control (CDC). (1993c). Injuries and illnesses related to Hurricane Andrew—Louisiana, 1992. *Morbidity and Mortality Weekly Report, 42,* 242–243,250–251.

Centers for Disease Control (CDC). (1993d). Morbidity surveillance following the Midwest flood—Missouri, 1993. *Morbidity and Mortality Weekly Report, 42,* 797–798.

Centers for Disease Control (CDC). (1993e). Public health consequences of a flood disaster—Iowa, 1993. *Morbidity and Mortality Weekly Report, 42,* 653–656.

Centers for Disease Control (CDC). (1994a). Flood-related mortality—Georgia, July 4–14, 1994. *Morbidity and Mortality Weekly Report, 43,* 526–530.

Centers for Disease Control (CDC). (1994b). Heat-related deaths—Philadelphia and United States, 1993–1994. *Morbidity and Mortality Weekly Report, 43,* 453–455.

Centers for Disease Control (CDC). (1994c). Tornado disaster—Alabama, March 27, 1994. *Morbidity and Mortality Weekly Report, 43,* 356–359.

Centers for Disease Control (CDC). (1995a). Heat-related illnesses and deaths—United States, 1994–1995. *Morbidity and Mortality Weekly Report, 44,* 465–468.

Centers for Disease Control (CDC). (1995b). Heat-related mortality—Chicago, July 1995. *Morbidity and Mortality Weekly Report, 44,* 577–579.

Centers for Disease Control (CDC). (1995c). Work-related injuries associated with falls during ice storms—National Institutes of Health, January 1994. *Morbidity and Mortality Weekly Report, 44,* 920–922.

Centers for Disease Control (CDC). (1996a). Deaths associated with Hurricanes Marilyn and Opal—United States, September–October 1995. *Morbidity and Mortality Weekly Report, 45,* 32–38.

Centers for Disease Control (CDC). (1996b). Heat-wave-related mortality—Milwaukee, WI, July 1995. *Morbidity and Mortality Weekly Report, 45,* 505–507.

Centers for Disease Control (CDC). (1996c). Surveillance for injuries and illnesses and rapid-health-needs assessment following Hurricanes Marilyn and Opal, September–October 1995. *Morbidity and Mortality Weekly Report, 45,* 81–85.

Centers for Disease Control (CDC). (1997a). Heat-related deaths—Dallas, Wichita and Cooke Counties, Texas, and United States, 1996. *Morbidity and Mortality Weekly Report, 46,* 528–531.

Centers for Disease Control (CDC). (1997b). Tornado disaster—Texas, May 1997. *Morbidity and Mortality Weekly Report, 46,* 1069–1073.

Centers for Disease Control (CDC). (1997c). Tornado-associated fatalities—Arkansas, 1997. *Morbidity and Mortality Weekly Report, 46,* 412–416.

Centers for Disease Control (CDC). (1998a). Community needs assessment and morbidity surveillance following an ice storm—Maine, January 1998. *Morbidity and Mortality Weekly Report, 47,* 351–354.

Centers for Disease Control (CDC). (1998b). Deaths associated with Hurricane Georges—Puerto Rico, September, 1998. *Morbidity and Mortality Weekly Report, 47,* 897–898.

Centers for Disease Control (CDC). (1999). Needs assessment following Hurricane Georges—Dominican Republic, 1998. *Morbidity and Mortality Weekly Report, 48,* 93–95.

Centers for Disease Control (CDC). (2000a). Heat-related illnesses, deaths, and risk factors—Cincinnati and Dayton, Ohio, 1999, and United States, 1979–1997. *Morbidity and Mortality Weekly Report, 49,* 470–473.

Centers for Disease Control (CDC). (2000b). Storm-related mortality—Central Texas, October 17–31, 1998. *Morbidity and Mortality Weekly Report, 49,* 133–135.

Centers for Disease Control (CDC). (2001). Heat-related deaths—Los Angeles County, California, 1999–2000, and United States, 1979, 1997–1998. *Morbidity and Mortality Weekly Report, 50,* 623–626.

Centers for Disease Control (CDC). (2002a). Deaths in World Trade Center terrorist attacks—New York City, 2001. *Morbidity and Mortality Weekly Report, 51* (Special issue), 16–18.

Centers for Disease Control (CDC). (2002b). Impact of September 11 attacks on workers in the vicinity of the World Trade Center—New York City. *Morbidity and Mortality Weekly Report, 51* (Special issue), 8–10.

Centers for Disease Control (CDC). (2002c). Injuries and illnesses among New York City Fire Department rescue workers after responding to the World Trade Center attacks. *Morbidity and Mortality Weekly Report, 51* (Special issue), 1–5.

Centers for Disease Control (CDC). (2002d). Injuries and illnesses among New York City Fire Department rescue workers after responding to the World Trade Center attacks. *Journal of the American Medical Association, 288,* 1581–1584.

Centers for Disease Control (CDC). (2002e). Occupational exposures to air contaminants at the World Trade Center disaster site New York, September–October, 2001. *Morbidity and Mortality Weekly Report, 51,* 453–456.

Centers for Disease Control (CDC). (2002f). Rapid assessment of injuries among survivors of the terrorist attack on the World Trade Center. *Morbidity and Mortality Weekly Report, 51,* 1–5.

Centers for Disease Control (CDC). (2002g). Self–reported increase in asthma severity after the September 11 attacks on the World Trade Center—Manhattan, New York, 2001. *Morbidity and Mortality Weekly Report, 51,* 782–784.

Centers for Disease Control (CDC). (2003a). Heat-related deaths—Chicago, Illinois, 1996–2001, and United States, 1979–1999. *Morbidity and Mortality Weekly Report, 52,* 610–613.

Centers for Disease Control (CDC). (2003b). Potential exposures to airborne and settled surface dust in residential areas of lower Manhattan following the collapse of the World Trade Center—New York City, November 4–December 11, 2001. *Morbidity and Mortality Weekly Report, 52,* 131–136.

Centers for Disease Control (CDC). (2004a). Mental health status of World Trade Center rescue and recovery workers and volunteers—New York City, July 2002–August 2004. *Morbidity and Mortality Weekly Report, 53,* 812–815.

Centers for Disease Control (CDC). (2004b). Physical health status of World Trade Center rescue and recovery workers and volunteers—New York City, July 2002–August 2004. *Morbidity and Mortality Weekly Report, 53,* 807–812.

Centers for Disease Control (CDC). (2004c). Preliminary medical examiner reports of mortality associated with Hurricane Charley—Florida, 2004. *Morbidity and Mortality Weekly Report, 53,* 835–842.

Centers for Disease Control (CDC). (2004d). Rapid community health and needs assessments after Hurricanes Isabel and Charley—North Carolina, 2003–2004. *Morbidity and Mortality Weekly Report, 53,* 840–842.

Centers for Disease Control (CDC). (2005). Epidemiologic assessment of the impact of four hurricanes—Florida, 2004. *Morbidity and Mortality Weekly Report, 54,* 693–697.

Center for Research on the Epidemiology of Disasters (CRED). (2005). Retrieved October 1, 2005, http://www.cred.be/.

Chakrabarty, S.K. (1978). *The evolution of politics in Bangladesh 1947–1980.* New Delhi: Association Publishing House.

Chalmers, J. (1995). *Japan— who governs? The rise of the developmental state.* New York: W. W. Norton.

Chambers, R. (1997). *Whose reality counts? Putting the first last.* London: Intermediate Technology Publications.

Chambers, R., & Conway, G. (1992). *Sustainable rural livelihoods: Practical concepts for the 21st century.* IDS Discussion Paper 296. Brighton: Institute for Development Studies.

Chang, H.J. (1996). *The political economy of industrial policy.* London: Macmillan.

Chang, H.J., & Grabel, I. (2004). *Reclaiming development.* London: Zed Books.

Chang, S.E. (2001). Structural change in urban economies: Recovery and long–term impacts in the 1995 Kobe Earthquake." *The Kokumin Keizai Zasshi Journal of Economics and Business Administration, 183,* 47–66.

Chang, S.E. (2005). *Modeling how cities recover from disasters.* Paper presented at the 1st international conference on urban disaster reduction, Kobe, Japan. January (p. 6).

Chang, S.E., & Falit–Baiamonte, A. (2003). Disaster vulnerability of businesses in the 2001 Nisqually earthquake. *Environmental Hazards, 4,* 59–71.

Chang, S.E., & Miles, S. B. (2004). The dynamics of recovery: A framework. In Y. Okuyama & S. E. Chang (Eds.), *Modeling spatial and economic impacts of disasters* (pp. 181–204). Berlin: Springer-Verlag.

Charing cross bottleneck was big killer. (1991, November 2). *San Francisco Chronicle,* A14, 2.

Charles, C.Z. (2003). The dynamics of racial residential segregation. *Annual Review of Sociology, 29,* 167–207.

Charveriat, C. (2000). Natural disasters in Latin America and the Caribbean: An overview of risk. *Inter-American Development Bank Working Paper Series,* 434.

Cherkasin, N. (2001). *Unesenniye Bezdnoi. Gibel 'Kurska': Khronika, Versii, Sud'bi.* (Gone to Abyss. The Death of 'Kursk': Chronicles, Versions, Fates). Moscow: Sovershenno Secretno.

Childers, C. (1999). Elderly female-headed households in the disaster loan process. *International Journal of Mass Emergencies and Disasters, 17*(1), 99–110.

Chiles, J.R. (2001). *Inviting disaster: Lessons from the edge of technology.* New York: Harper Business.

Chiyers, C. (2005). *New sight in Chernobyl's dead zones: Tourists*. Retrieved January 16, 2005, www.nytimes.com/2005/06/15/international/europe/15schernobyl.

Chong, D. (1991). *Collective action and the Civil Rights Movement*. Chicago: The University of Chicago Press.

Chowdhury, M. (2001). *Women's technological innovations and adaptations for disaster mitigation: A case study of charlands in Bangladesh*. Paper prepared for the United Nations Division for the Advancement of Women Expert Working Group Meeting. Ankara, Turkey (November 6–9, 2001); Retrieved December 5, 2005, http://www.un.org/womenwatch/daw/csw/env_manage/documents.html.

Cisin, I.H., & Clark, W.B. (1962). The methodological challenge of disaster research. In G. Baker & D. Chapman (Eds.), *Man and society in disaster* (pp. 23–54). New York: Basic Books.

City of Oklahoma City. (1996) *Alfred P. Murrah federal building bombing, April 19, 1995: Final report*. Stillwater, OK: Fire Protection Publications, Oklahoma State University.

Civil Defense Review Panel. (1992). *Report on the Emergency Services Review Task Force*. Wellington: Department of Internal Affairs.

Clancy, T. (2000). *The bear and the dragon*. London: Michael Joseph.

Clarke, L.B. (1999). Mission improbable: Using fantasy documents to tame disaster. Chicago: The University of Chicago Press.

Clarke, L. (2002). Panic: Myth or reality? *Contexts, 1*(3), 21–27.

Clarke, L. (2005). *Worst cases: Terror and catastrophe in the popular imagination*. Chicago: The University of Chicago Press.

Clausen, L. (1992). Das Konkrete und das abstrakte. Frankfurt: Suhrkamp.

Clay, E. (2005). *Learning from the Indian Ocean disaster: ODI opinions*. Retrieved January 31, 2005, http://www.odi.org.uk/publications/opinions/31_tsunami_jan05R.pdf

Clifford, R.A. (1956). The Rio Grande flood: A comparative study of border communities. *National Research Disaster Study No. 7*. Washington, DC: National Academy Press.

Coburn, A.W., & Hughes, R.E. (1987). Fatalities, injury and rescue in earthquakes. In *Proceedings of the 2nd Conference of the Development Studies Association*. Manchester, England: University of Manchester.

Coburn, A.W., Spence, R.J.S., & Pomonis, A. (1992). Factors determining human casualty levels in earthquakes: Mortality prediction in building collapse. In *Proceedings of the First International Forum on Earthquake-Related Casualties*. Madrid Spain, July 1992. Reston, VA: US Geological Survey.

Cochrane, H.C. (1975). *Natural hazards and their distributive effects*. Boulder, CO: Institute of Behavioral Science.

Cochrane, H.C. (1991). Hazards research is not affecting practice. *Natural Hazards Observer, 15*(6), 1–2.

Cohen, B.P. (1980). *Developing sociological knowledge*. Englewood Cliffs, NJ: Prentice-Hall.

Cohn, A. (2005). FEMA's new challenges. *Washington Times*. May 20, 2005.

Cole, E.E. (Ed.) (1991). *Reflections on the Loma Prieta Earthquake October 17, 1989*. Sacramento, CA: Structural Engineers Association of California.

Cole, E., & Buckle, P. (2004). Developing community resilience as a foundation for effective disaster recovery. *Australian Journal of Emergency Management, 19*(4), 6–15.

Cole, P.M.S. (2003). *An empirical examination of the housing recovery process following disaster*. Doctoral dissertation, College Station, TX: Texas A&M University.

Collins, L. (2002). Collapse rescue operations at the Pentagon 9–11 attack: A case study on urban search and rescue disaster response. Retrieved September, 2005,: http://www.ukfssart.org.uk/files/pentagon%20report.PDF.

Columbia Accident Investigation Board (CAIB). (2003). *Columbia accident investigation report 1*. Burlington: Apogee Books.

Combs, D.L., Quenemoen, L.E., Parrish, R.G., & Davis, J.H. (1999). Assessing disaster-attributed mortality: Development and application of a definition and classification matrix. *International Journal of Epidemiology, 28*, 1124–1129.

Comeau, E. (1996). *Oklahoma City Rescue Operations Report*. Fire Investigation Report. National Fire Protection Association (NFPA).

Comerio, M.C. (1995). *Northridge housing losses: A study of the California governor's office of emergency services*. Berkeley, CA: University of California, Berkeley, Center for Environmental Design Research.

Comerio, M.C. (1998). Disaster hits home: New policy for urban housing recovery. Berkely, CA: University of California Press.

Comerio, M.C. (2005). *Key elements in a comprehensive theory of disaster recovery*. Paper presented at the 1st International Conference on Urban Disaster Reduction. Kobe, Japan. January.

Comerio, M.C., Landis, J.D., & Rofe, Y. (1994). *Post-disaster residential rebuilding*. Working Paper 608. Berkeley, CA: University of California, Institute of Urban and Regional Development.

Comfort, L.K., (1996). Self organization in disaster response: The Great Hanshin, Japan earthquake of January 17, 1995. *Quick Response Report No. 78*. Boulder, CO: Natural Hazards Research and Applications Information Center: University of Colorado.

Comfort, L.K. (1999b). *Shared risk: Complex systems in seismic response*. Pittsburgh, PA: Pergamon.

Comfort, L.K., Wisner B., Cutter, S., Pulwarty, R., Hewitt, K., Oliver-Smith, A., et al. (1999). Reframing disaster policy: The global evolution of vulnerable communities. *Environmental Hazards, 1*, 39–44.

Commission Report. (2004). What do we do with the SARS reports? *Health Quarterly, 7*, 28–34.

Committee of Concerned Journalists. (1999). Framing the news: The triggers, frames and messages in newspaper coverage. Retrieved January 13, 2005, www.journalism.org/ publ_research/framing.html.

Committee of Concerned Journalists. (2001). Before and after: How the war on terrorism has changed the news agenda. Retrieved July 17, 2005, http://www.journalistm.org/publ_ research/befandaftl.html.

Congressional Budget Office. (2005) Federal funding for homeland security: An update. *CBO Economic and Budget Issue Brief*, July 20.

Cooper, S, & Coxe, D. (2005). An investor's guide to Avian Flu, BMO Nesbitt Burns research, special report August 2005. Retrieved December 5, 2005, http://www.sherrycooper. com/article.php3

Cooperman, A. (2005). Some see wrath of God in storm's disaster. *Wilmington News Journal*. September 4, 2004.

Coppock, J.T. (1995). GIS and natural hazards: An overview from a GIS perspective. In A. Carrara, & F. Guzzetti (Eds.), *Geographical information systems in assessing natural hazards* (pp. 21–34). Dordrect: Kluwer Academic.

Corbridge, S. (1986). *Capitalist world development: A critique of radical development geography*. London: Macmillan.

Corbridge, S. (1990). Post-Marxism and development studies: Beyond the impasse. *World Development, 18*(5), 623–639.

Couch, S.R., & Kroll–Smith, J.S. (1985). The chronic technical disaster: Toward a social scientific perspective. *Social Science Quarterly, 66*, 564–575.

Couch, S.R., & Wade, B.A. (2003). I want to barbecue bin Laden: Humor after 9/11. *International Journal of Mass Emergencies and Disasters, 21*, 67–86.

Cova, T.J. (1997). Modeling community evacuation vulnerability using GIS. *International Journal of Geographic Information Science, 11*, 763–784.

Cox, H. (1998). Women in bushfire territory. In E. Enarson & B.H. Morrow (Eds.), *The gendered terrain of disaster: Through women's eyes* (pp. 133–142). Westport, CT: Praeger.

Culver, C.G., Lew, H.S., Hart, G.C., & Pinkham, C.W. (1975). *Natural hazards evaluation of existing buildings*. NBS Building Science Series Report No. 61. Washington, DC: National Bureau of Standards, Institute for Applied Technology, Center for Building Technology.

Cunningham, S. (2005). Incident, accident, catastrophe: Cyanide on the Danube. *Disasters, 29*, 99–128.

Cuny, F.C. (1983). *Disaster and development*. Oxford: Oxford University Press.

Cuny, F.C., & Hill, R.B. (1999). *Famine, conflict and response: A basic guide*. New West Hartford, CT: Kumarian Press.

Curry, M.R. (1997). The digital individual and the private realm. *Annals of the Association of American Geographers, 87*(4), 681–699.

Curson, P. (1989). Introduction. In J.I. Clarke, P. Curson, S.L. Kayastha, & P. Nag (Eds.), *Population and disaster* (pp. 1–23). Oxford: Blackwell and Institute of British Geographers.

Curtice, J. (1985). Government. In A. Kuper & J. Kuper (Eds.), *The social science ncyclopedia* (pp. 340–341). London: Routledge and Kegan Paul.

Cushman, J.G., Pachter, H.L., & Beaton, H.L. (2003). Two New York City hospitals' surgical response to the September 11, 2001, terrorist attack in New York City. *The Journal of Trauma, 54*, 147–155.

Cuthbertson, B.H., & Nigg, J.M. (1987). Technological disaster and the nontherapeutic community: A question of true victimization. *Environment and Behavior, 19*, 462–488.

Cutter, S. (1991). Fleeing from harm: International trends in evacuation from chemical accident. *International Journal from Mass Emergencies and Disasters, 9*, 267–285.

Cutter, S. (1994). *Environmental risks and hazards*. Englewood Cliffs, NJ: Prentice-Hall.

Cutter, S. (1995a). The forgotten casualties: Women, children, and environmental change. *Global Environmental Change, 5*(3), 181–194.

Cutter, S. (1995b). Race, class, and environmental justice. *Progress in Human Geography, 19*, 107–118.

Cutter, S. (1996). Vulnerability to environmental hazards. *Progress in Human Geography, 20*(4), 529–539.

Cutter, S. (Ed.). (2002). *American hazardscapes: The regionalization of hazards and disasters*. Washington, DC: Joseph Henry Press.

Cutter, S. (2003a). The vulnerability of science and the science of vulnerability. *Annals of the Association of American Geographers, 93*(1), 1–12.

Cutter, S. (2003b). GI Science, disasters, and emergency management. *Transactions in GIS, 7*(4), 439–445.

Cutter, S. (2005a). Pragmatism and relevance. In R.W. Perry & E.L. Quarantelli (Eds.), *What is a disaster: New answers to old questions* (pp. 104–106). Philadelphia: Xlibris.

Cutter, S. (2005b). Are we asking the right question?. In R.W. Perry & E.L. Quarantelli (Eds.), *What is a disaster: New answers to old questions* (pp. 39–48). Philadelphia: Xlibris.

Cutter, S., & Barnes, K. (1982). Evacuation behavior at Three Mile Island. *Disasters, 6*, 116–124.

Cutter, S., Boruff, B., & Shirley, W. (2003). Social vulnerability to environmental hazards. *Social Science Quarterly, 84*, 242–261.

Cutter, S., Hodgson, M., & Dow, K. (2001). Subsidized inequities: The spatial patterning of environmental risks and federally assisted housing. *Urban Geography, 22*(1), 29–53.

Cutter, S., Mitchell J.T., & Scott, M.S. (2000). Revealing the vulnerability of people and places: A case study of Georgetown County, South Carolina. *Annals of the Association of American Geographers, 90*(4), 713–737.

Cutter, S., Richardson, D.B., & Wilbanks, T.J. (Eds.). (2003). *The geographical dimensions of terrorism.* New York: Routledge.

Cutter. S., Tiefenbacher, J., & Soleci, W. (1992). Engendered fears: Femininity and technological risk perception. *Industrial Crisis Quarterly, 6*, 5–22.

Cyert, R., & March, J. (1963) *A behavioral theory of the Firm.* Englewood Cliffs, NJ: Prentice-Hall.

Dacy, D.C., & Kunreuther, H. (1969). *The economics of natural disasters.* New York: Free Press.

Daft, R.L. (2004). *Organization theory and design* (8th ed.). Mason, OH: Southwestern.

Dahlburg, J.-T. (2005, May 30). Towns in big storms' path still winded. *Los Angeles Times*, A16.

Dahlhamer, J.M. (1998). *Rebounding from environmental holts: Organizational and ecological factors affecting business disaster recovery.* Doctoral dissertation. Newark, DE: Department of Sociology and Criminal Justice, University of Delaware.

Dahlhamer, J.M., & D'Souza, M.J. (1997). Determinants of business disaster preparedness in two U.S. metropolitan areas. *International Journal of Mass Emergencies and Disasters, 15*, 265–281.

Dahlhamer, J.M., & Tierney, K.J. (1998). Rebounding from disruptive events: Business recovery following the Northridge Earthquake. *Sociological Spectrum, 18*, 121–141.

Daines, G.E. (1991). Planning, training and exercising. In G.J. Hoetmer & T.E. Drabek (Eds.), *Emergency management: Principles and practice for local government.* (pp. 161–200). Washington, DC: ICMA.

Daley, W.R., Brown, S., Archer, P., Kruger, E., Jordan, F., Batts, D., et al. (2005). Risk of tornado-related death and injury in Oklahoma, May 3, 1999. *American Journal of Epidemiology, 161*, 1144–1150.

Damanpour, F., & Gopalakrishnan, S. (1998). Theories of organizational structure and innovation adoption: The role of environmental change. *Journal of Engineering and Technology Management, 15*, 1–24.

Damill, M., Frenkel, R., & Maurizio, R. (2003). Políticas macroeconómicas y vulnerabilidad social: La Argentina en la década de los noventa. *Serie Financiamiento del Desarrollo, 135.* Santiago de Chile: CEPAL.

Dann, S., & Wilson, P. (1993). *Women and emergency services.* Paper presented at the Symposium on Women in Emergencies and Disasters. Brisbane, Queensland.

Dash, N. (1997). The use of geographic information systems in disaster research. *International Journal of Mass Emergencies and Disasters, 15*(1), 135–146.

Dash, N. (2002). The use of geographic information systems in disaster research. In R. A. Stallings (Ed.), *Methods of disaster research* (pp. 320–333). Philadelphia, Pennsylvania: Xlibris.

Dash, N., & Morrow, B.H. (2001). Return delays and evacuation order compliance: The case of Hurricane Georges and the Florida Keys. *Environmental Hazards, 2*, 119–128.

Dash, N., Peacock, W., & Morrow, B. (1997). And the poor get poorer: A neglected black community. In W. Peacock, B. Morrow, & H. Gladwin (Eds.), *Hurricane Andrew: Ethnicity, gender, and the sociology of disaster* (pp. 206–225). New York: Routledge.

Davis, I. (1978). *Shelter after disaster.* Oxford: Oxford Polytechnic Press.

Davis, I. (Ed.). (1981). *Disaster and small dwelling.* Oxford: Pergamon Press.

Davis, I., & Quarantelli, E. (Forthcoming). A selective research agenda for the future: Some major topics worthwhile exploring. In G. Webb & E. Quarantelli (Eds.), *The Popular culture of disasters: Views from the social sciences and from the humanities and history.* Philadelphia: Xlibris.

Davis, M. (1992). *City of quartz: Excavating the future in Los Angeles.* London: Verso.

Davis, M. (2005). *Planet of slums.* London: Verso.

Dawson, G. (1993). A comparison of research and practice: A practitioner's view. *International Journal of Mass Emergencies and Disasters, 11*, 55–62.

Dearing, J.W., & Kazmierczak, J. (1993). Making iconoclasts credible: The Iben Browning earthquake prediction. *International Journal of Mass Emergencies and Disasters, 11*, 391–403.

De Brucycker, M., Greco, D., & Lechat, M.F. (1985). The 1980 earthquake in Southern Italy—Morbidity and mortality. *International Journal of Epidemiology, 14*(1), 113–117.

Delaney, P., & Shrader, E. (2000). *Gender and post-disaster reconstruction: The case of Hurricane Mitch in Honduras and Nicaragua.* Preliminary report commissioned by the World Bank. Retrieved August 26, 2005, http://online.northumbria.ac.uk/geography _ research/gdn/resources/reviewdraft.doc.

Demuth, J. (2002) *Countering terrorism: Lessons learned from natural and technological disasters.* Natural Disaster Roundtable. Washington, DC: National Academy Press.

Dengler, L., & Preuss, J. (n.d.). *EERI reconnaissance study of the July 17, 1998 Papua New Guinea tsunami.* Humboldt State University. Retrieved November 11, 2004, http://sorrel.humboldt.edu/~geodept/Faculty/Dengler/final_PNG_report.html.

Denis, H. (1995). Coordination in a government disaster mega-organization. *International Journal of Mass Emergencies and Disasters, 13*, 25–43.

Denis, H. (1997). Technology, structure, and culture in disaster management. *International Journal of Mass Emergencies and Disasters, 15*, 293–308.

Densham, P. (1991). Spatial decision support systems. In D.J. Maguire, M.F. Goodchild, & D.W. Rhind (Eds.), *Geographical information systems: Principles and applications* (vol. 1, 403–412). New York: Wiley.

Department of Homeland Security. (2003). The Office for Domestic Preparedness Guidelines for Homeland Security. Washington, DC, U.S. Department of Homeland Security.

Department of Internal Affairs. (1995). *Report of the emergency services review task force.* Wellington: Department of Internal Affairs, New Zealand Government.

Deppa, J., Russell, M., Hayes, D., & Flocke, E.L. (1994). *The media and disasters Pam Am 103* (29 pp.). New York: New York University Press.

De Silva, F.N. (2001). Providing spatial decision support for evacuation planning: A challenge in integrating technologies. *Disaster Prevention and Management: An International Journal, 10*, 11–20.

De Silva, F., Pidd, M., & Eglese, R. (1993). Spatial decision support systems for emergency planning: An operational research/geographic information systems approach to evacuation planning. In J. Sullivan (Ed.), *International Emergency Management and Engineering Conference, Society for Computer Simulation* (pp. 130–133).

de Tocqueville, A. (1947). *Democracy in America.* New York: Oxford University Press.

de Ville de Goyet, C. (2004). Epidemics caused by dead bodies: A disaster myth that does not wish to die [Editorial]. *Pan American Journal of Public Health, 15*, 297–299.

Dewey, J. (1938). *Logic, the nature of inquiry.* New York: Holt, Rinehart, & Winston.

Deyle, R.E., & Smith, R.A. (1996). *State planning mandates: State implementation and local government response.* Tallahassee, FL: The Florida Planning Laboratory, Department of Urban and Regional Planning, Florida State University.

DFID. (2005). *Disaster Risk Reduction: A Development Concern.* Department For International Development (DFID) ODG.

Dietz, V.J., Rigau-Perez, J.G., Sanderson, L., Diaz, L., & Gunn, R.A. (1990). Health assessment of the 1985 flood disaster in Puerto Rico. *Disasters, 14*, 164–170.

Difede, J., Apfeldorf, W.J., Cloitre, M., Spielman, L.A., & Perry, S. W. (1979). Acute psychiatric responses to the explosion at the World Trade Center: A case series. *Journal of Nervous and Mental Disease, 185*, 519–522.

Di Justo, P. (2005). Asteroids are coming. *Wired.* August 8, 42.

Dillman, D., Schwalbe, M., & Short, J. (1983). Communication behavior and social impacts following the May, 18, 1980, eruption of Mt. St. Helens. In S.A.C. Keller (Ed.), *Mt. St. Helens one year later* (pp. 191–198). Cheny, WA: Eastern University Press.

Disaster Research Center, University of Delaware. http://www.udel.edu/DRC/.

Disaster Watch. (2005). Retrieved November 3, 2005, http://www.disasterwatch.net/.

Dobson, N. (1994). From under the mud-pack: Women and the Charleville floods. *Australian Journal of Emergency Management, 9*(2), 11–13.

Doherty, N.A. (2000). *Integrated risk management: Techniques and strategies for reducing risk.* New York: McGraw-Hill.

Dombrowsky, W.R. (1981). *Another step toward a social theory of disaster.* Newark, DE: Disaster Research Center Preliminary Paper Number 70.

Dombrowsky, W.R. (1998). Again and again: Is a disaster what we call a disaster? In Quarantelli, E.L. (Ed.), *What is a disaster: Perspectives on the question* (pp. 19–30). London: Routledge.

Dombrowsky, W.R. (2005). Not every move is a step forward. In R.W. Perry & E.L. Quarantelli (Eds.), *What is a disaster: New answers to old questions* (pp. 79–98). Philadelphia: Xlibris.

Dominici, F., Levy, J.I., & Louis, T.A. (2005). Methodological challenges and contributions in disaster epidemiology. *Epidemiologic Reviews, 27*, 9–12.

Donahue, A. (2003). *Incident management teams: All-risk operations and management study.* Storrs, CT: Center for Policy Analysis and Management, University of Connecticut.

Doocy, S., Rofi, A., Robinson, C., Burnham, G., & Shanker, A. (2005). *Assessing tsunami related mortality in Aceh Province, Panel 2.1: Assessing needs and measuring impact.* Paper presented at the World Health Organization Conference on the Health Impacts of the Tsunami Disaster in Asia, Phuket, Thailand.

Dory, A.J. (2003). *Civil security: Americans and the challenge of homeland security.* Washington, DC: The CSIS Press.

Douglas, M. (1992). *Risk and blame: Essays in cultural theory.* London: Routledge.

Dove, M.R., & Khan, M.H. (1995). Competing constructions of calamity: The April 1991 Bangladesh cyclone. *Population and Environment, 16*, 445–471.

Dow, K. (1992). Exploring differences in our common future(s): The meaning to global environmental change, *Geoforum, 23*, 417–436.

Dow, K., & Cutter, S. (1998). Crying wolf: Repeat responses to hurricane evacuation orders. *Coastal Management, 26*, 237–252.

Dow, K., & Cutter, S. (2000). Public orders and personal opinions: Household strategies for hurricane risk assessment. *Environmental Hazards, 2*, 143–155.

Dow, K., & Downing, T.E. (1995). Vulnerability research: Where things stand. *Human Dimensions Quarterly, 1*, 3–5.

Downey, L. (1998). Environmental injustice: Is race or income a better predictor? *Social Science Quarterly, 79*(4), 766–778.

Downey, R. (1995). Task force operations: An overview. *Fire Engineering, 11*, 25–36.

Drabek, T.E. (1968). *Disaster in aisle 13.* Columbus, OH: Ohio State University.

Drabek, T.E. (1969). Social processes in disaster: Family evacuation. *Social Problems, 16*, 336–349.

Drabek, T.E. (1970). Methodology of studying disasters. *American Behavioral Scientist, 13*, 331–343.

Drabek, T.E. (1983). Shall we leave? A study of family reactions when disaster strikes. *Emergency Management Review, 1*, 25–29.

Drabek, T.E. (1985). Managing the emergency response. *Public Administration Review, 45*, 85–92.

Drabek, T.E. (1986). *Human system responses to disaster: An inventory of sociological findings.* New York: Springer-Verlag.

Drabek, T.E. (1987a). Emergent structures. In R.R. Dynes, B. DeMarchi, & C. Pelanda (Eds.), *Sociology of disasters: Contribution of sociology in disaster research.* (pp. 190–259, 259–290). Milano, Italy: International Sociological Association Research Committee on Disasters: Franco Angeli.

Drabek, T.E. (1987b). *The professional emergency manager: Structures and strategies for success.* Boulder, CO: University of Colorado.

Drabek, T.E. (1989). Taxonomy and disaster: Theoretical and applied issues. In G.A. Kreps (Ed.), *Social structure and disaster* (pp. 317–345). Newark, DE: University of Delaware Press.

Drabek, T.E. (1990). *Emergency management: Strategies for maintaining organizational integrity.* New York: Springer-Verlag.

Drabek, T.E. (1991a). The *Evolution of emergency management.* In T.E. Drabek, & G.J. Hoetmer (Eds.), *Emergency management: Principles and practice for local government* (pp. 3–29). Washington, DC: International City Management Association.

Drabek, T.E. (1991b). *Microcomputers in emergency management: Implementation of computer technology.* Boulder, CO: University of Colorado.

Drabek, T.E. (1994). *Disaster evacuation and the tourist industry.* Boulder, CO: Institute of Behavioral Science, Program on Environment and Behavior, Natural Hazards Center.

Drabek, T.E. (1996). *Disaster evacuation behavior—Tourists and other transients.* Boulder, CO: Institute of Behavioral Science, University of Colorado.

Drabek, T.E. (1999). *Disaster-induced employee evacuation.* Boulder, CO: Institute of Behavioral Science, University of Colorado.

Drabek, T.E. (2003a). *Strategies for coordinating disaster responses.* Boulder, CO: University of Colorado.

Drabek, T.E. (2003b). Presentation at the Natural Disasters Roundtable, National Academies, Retrieved August 30, 2005, http://dels.nas.edu/dr/f8.shtml.

Drabek, T.E. (2004). *Social dimensions of disaster* (2nd ed.). Emmitsburg, MD: Emergency Management Institute, Federal Emergency Management Agency.

Drabek, T., & Boggs, K. (1968). Families in disaster: Reactions and relatives. *Journal of Marriage and Family, 30*, 443–451.

Drabek, T.E., & Haas, J.E. (1969). Laboratory simulation of organizational stress. *American Sociological Review, 34*, 223–238.

Drabek, T.E., & Haas, J.E. (1974). *Understanding complex organizations.* Dubuque, IA: William C. Brown.

Drabek, T.E., & Hoetmer, G.J. (1991). Introduction. In T.E. Drabek & G.J. Hoetmer (Eds.), *Emergency management: Principles and practice for local government* (pp. xvii– xxxiv). Washington, DC: International City Management Association.

Drabek, T.E., & Key, W.H. (1984). *Conquering disaster: Family recovery and long-term consequences.* New York: Irvington.

Drabek, T.E., & McEntire, D.A. (2002). Emergent phenomena and multiorganizational coordination in disasters: Lessons from the research literature. *International Journal of Mass Emergencies and Disasters, 20,* 197–224.

Drabek, T.E., & McEntire, D. A. (2003). Emergent phenomena and the sociology of disaster: Lessons, trends and opportunities from the research literature. *Disaster Prevention and Management, 12,* 97–112.

Drabek, T.E., Mushkatel, A., & Kilijanek, T.S. (1983). *Earthquake mitigation policy: The experience of two states.* Boulder, CO: Institute of Behavioral Science, University of Colorado.

Drabek, T.E., & Quarantelli, E.L. (1967). Scapegoats, villains, and disasters. *Transaction, 4,* 12–17.

Drabek, T., & Quarantelli, E. (1969). Blame in disaster: Another look, another viewpoint. In D. Dean (Ed.), *Dynamic social psychology* (pp. 604–615). Chicago: Rand McNally.

Drabek, T.E., & Stephenson, J.S. (1971). When disaster strikes. *Journal of Applied Social Psychology, 1,* 187–203.

Drabek, T.E., Tamminga, H.L., Kilijanek, T.S., & Adams, C.R. (1981). *Managing multiorganizational emergency responses: Emergent search and rescue networks in natural disasters and remote area settings.* Boulder, CO: Institute of Behavioral Science, University of Colorado.

Drew, C. (2005) Efforts to hide sensitive data pit 9/11 concerns against safety. *New York Times.* Retrieved March 5, 2005, www.newyorktimes.com.

Dreze, J., & Sen, A. (1990/91). *The political economy of hunger.* Oxford: Clarendon Press.

Dror, Y., Lagadec, P., Porfiriev, B., & Quarantelli, E. (2001). Crises to come: Comments and findings. In U. Rosenthal, A. Boin, & L. Comfort (Eds.), *Managing crises, threats, dilemmas, opportunities* (pp 342–349). Springfield, IL: Charles C Thomas.

Dubin, R. (1978). *Theory building.* New York: Free Press.

Duclos, P., Binder, S., & Riester, R. (1989) Community evacuation following the Spencer metal processing plant fire, Nanticoke, Pennsylvania. *Journal of Hazardous Materials, 22,* 1–11.

Duffield, M. (1996). The symphony of the damned: Racial discourse, complex political emergencies, and humanitarian aid. *Disasters, 20*(3), 173–193.

Dufka, C. (1988). The Mexico City earthquake disaster. *Social Casework: The Journal of Contemporary Social Work, 69,* 162–170.

Durkheim, E. (1915). *Elementary forms of religious life.* New York: Tr. J. W. Swain Free Press.

Durkheim, E. (1984). *The division of labor in society.* New York: Free Press.

Durkin, M.E. (1985). Behavior of building occupants in earthquakes. *Earthquake Spectra, 1*(2), 271–283.

Durkin, M.E. (1989). The role of the physical setting in earthquake injuries: The Mexico experience. *Proceedings from the Third U.S.–Mexico Workshop on 1985 Mexico earthquake Research,* March 16–18.

Durkin, M.E. (1995). Fatalities, nonfatal injuries, and medical aspects of the Northridge earthquake. In W.R. Seiple (Ed.), *The Northridge, California earthquake of 17 January 1994 (Special Publication 116)* (pp. 187–213). Sacramento, CA: California Department of Conservation, Division of Mines and Geology.

Durkin, M.E., Coulson, A.H., Hijar, M., Kraus, J., & Ohashi, H. (1987). *The survival of people in collapsed buildings.* Report. Michael E. Durkin and Associates.

Durkin, M.E., & Murakami, H.O. (1988). Casualties, survival and entrapment in heavily damaged buildings. *Proceedings of the Ninth World Conference on Earthquake Engineering* (pp. 2–8). Tokyo-Kyoto, Japan, August 2–9.

Dymon, U.J. (1993). *Map use during and after Hurricane Andrew.* University of Colorado, Institute of Behavioral Science, Natural Hazards Research and Applications Information Center, The University of Colorado.

Dynes, R.R. (1970). *Organized behavior in disaster.* Lexington, MA: Heath Lexington Books.

Dynes, R.R. (1972). Cross cultural studies of disaster. *Proceedings of the Japan–United States Disaster Research Seminar: Organizational and community responses to disaster* (pp. 235–256). Columbus, OH: Disaster Research Center.

Dynes, R.R. (1978a). Interorganizational relations in communities under stress. In E.L. Quarantelli (Ed.), *Disaster: Theory and research* (pp. 49–64). Beverly Hills, CA: SAGE.

Dynes, R.R. (1978b). Review of *"Everything in its path: Destruction of community in the Buffalo Creek flood,"* by K. T. Erikson. *Social Forces, 57,* 721–722.

Dynes, R.R. (1983). Problems in emergency planning. *Energy, 8,* 653–660.

Dynes, R.R. (1987). The concept of role in disaster research. In R.R. Dynes, B. De Marche, & C. Pelanda (Eds.), *Sociology of disasters: Contributions of sociology to disaster research* (pp. 71–103). Milano, Italy: Franco Angelo.

Dynes, R.R. (1988). Cross–cultural international research: Sociology and disaster. *International Journal of Mass Emergencies and Disasters, 6*(2), 101–129.

Dynes, R.R. (1993). Disaster reduction: The importance of adequate assumptions about social organization. *Sociological Spectrum, 13,* 175–192.

Dynes, R.R. (1994). Community emergency planning: False assumptions and inappropriate analogies. *International Journal of Mass Emergencies and Disasters, 12*(2), 141–158.

Dynes, R.R. (1998). Coming to terms with community disaster. In E.L. Quarantelli (Ed.), *What is a disaster: Perspectives on the question* (pp. 109–126). London: Routledge.

Dynes, R.R. (2000a). The Dialogue between Voltaire and Roussseau on the Lisbon earthquake: The emergence of a social science view. *International Journal of Mass Emergencies and Disasters, 18,* 97–115.

Dynes, R.R. (2000b). The Lisbon earthquake in 1755: Contested meanings in the first modern disaster. *TsuInfo Alert, 2,* 10–18.

Dynes, R.R. (2002). Disaster and development: Again. Newark, DE: University of Delaware, Disaster Research Center.

Dynes, R.R. (2003). Finding order in disorder: Continuities in the 9–11 response. *International Journal of Mass Emergencies and Disasters, 21,* 9–23.

Dynes, R.R. (2004). Expanding the horizons of disaster research. *Natural Hazards Observer, 28,* 4.

Dynes, R.R. (2005). Community social capital as the primary basis for resilience. Preliminary paper no. 344. Newark, DE: Univeristy of Delaware, Disaster Research Center.

Dynes, R.R., & Aguirre, B.E. (1979). Organizational adaptation to crises: Mechanisms of coordination and structural change. *Disasters, 3,* 71–74.

Dynes, R.R., DeMarchi, B., & Pelanda, C. (Eds.). (1987). *Sociology of disasters: Contributions of sociology to disaster research.* Milan, Italy: Franco Angeli.

Dynes, R.R., & Drabek, T.E. (1994). The structure of disaster research: Its policy and disciplinary implications. *International Journal of Mass Emergencies and Disasters, 12*(1), 5–23.

Dynes, R.R., Haas, J.E., & Quarantelli, E.L. (1967). Administrative, methodological, and theoretical problems of disaster research. *Indian Sociological Bulletin, 4,* 215–227.

Dynes, R.R., & Quarantelli, E.L. (1968). What looting in civil disturbances really means. *Trans-Action, 5,* 9–4.

Dynes, R.R., & Quarantelli, E.L. (1977). *Organizational communications and decision making in crises.* (Report Series no. 17). Columbus, OH: Disaster Research Center, Ohio State University.

Dynes, R.R., & Quarantelli, E.L. (1980). *Helping behavior in large scale disasters.* Newark, DE: University of Delaware, Disaster Research Center, article no. 132.

Dynes, R.R, Quarantelli, E.L., & Kreps, G.A. (1972). *A perspective on disaster planning.* Columbus, OH: Disaster Research Center, The Ohio State University.

Dynes, R.R., Quarantelli, E.L., & Wenger, D. (1990). *Individual and organizational response to the 1985 earthquake in Mexico City, Mexico.* Newark, DE: University of Delaware, Disaster Research Center, Book and Monograph Series No. 24.

Dynes, R.R., & Rodriguez, H. (2005). Finding and framing Katrina: The social construction of disaster. In *Understanding Katrina: Perspectives from the social sciences.* Social Science Research Council, http://understandingkatrina.ssrc.org/Dynes_Rodriguez/.

Dynes, R.R., & Tierney K. (Eds.). (1994). *Disasters, collective behavior and social organization.* Newark, DE: University of Delaware Press.

Eadie, C., Emmer, R.E., Esnard, A.M., Michaels, S., Monday, J., Philipsborn, C., et al. (2001). *Holistic disaster recovery: Ideas for building local sustainability after a natural disaster.* Boulder, CO: Natural Hazards Research and Applications Information Center, University of Colorado.

Eads, M. (2002). Marginalized groups in times of crisis: Identity, needs, and response. Quick Response Report No. 152. Boulder, CO: Natural Hazards Research and Applications Information Center, University of Colorado. Retrieved March 25, 2005, http://www.colorado.edu/hazards/qr/qr152/qr152.html.

Earthquake Engineering Research Institute (EERI). (2004, December 26). *Sumatra-Andaman Islands earthquake virtual clearinghouse.* Retrieved July 15, 2005, World Wide Web: http://www.eeri.org/lfe/clearinghouse/sumatra_tsunami/overview.html.

Earthquake Engineering Research Institute (EERI). (2005a). *Earthquake rebuilding in Gujarat, India: EERI recovery reconnaissance report.* Oakland, CA.

Earthquake Engineering Research Institute (EERI). (2005b). *Preliminary observations: San Simeon, California, earthquake December 22, 2003.* Report no. 2005–01. Oakland, CA.

East Bay Hills Fire Operations Review Group. (1992). *The East Bay Hills Fire—A multi-agency review of the October 1991 fire in the Oakland/Berkeley Hills.* Sacramento, CA: Governor's Office of Emergency Services.

Eberhart-Phillips, J.E., Saunders, T.M., Robinson, A.L., Hatch, D.L., & Parrish, R. G. (1994). Profile of mortality from the 1989 Loma Prieta earthquake using coroner and medical examiner reports. *Disasters, 18*, 160–170.

ECLAC (1999). *Manual for estimating the socio-economic effects of natural disasters*. Santiago of Chile: ECLAC.

Economic principles, issues, and research priorities in natural hazard loss estimation. In U. Okuyama, & S.E. Chang (Eds.), *Modeling Spatial Economic Impacts of Natural Disasters* (pp. 13–36). New York: Springer-Verlag.

Economist (2004). Pocket world in figures, 2005 edition. London: *The Economist*.

Edelman, M.J. (1977). *Political language: Words that succeed and policies that fail*. New York: Academic Press.

Edelman, M.J. (1988). *Constructing the political spectacle*. Chicago: The University of Chicago Press.

Eichengreen, B. (2001). Capital account liberalization: What do cross–country studies tell us. *World Bank Economic Review, 3*, 341–365.

Eichengreen, B. (2002). *Financial crises: And what to do about them*. New York: Oxford University Press.

Eisentadt, S. (1996). *Japanese civilization: A comparative view*. Chicago: The University of Chicago Press.

Eisner, R. (2000). Initial response: The Great Hanshin-Awaji Earthquake. *Assessment reports of the global assessment pf earthquake countermeasures, 1, Set–up for disaster countermeasures*. Kobe: Hyogo Prefectural Government.

Elias, N. (1987). *Involvement and detachment*. Oxford: Blackwell.

Elias, T., Sutton, A.J., Stokes, J.B., & Casadevall, T.J. (1998). *Sulfur dioxide emission rates of Kilauea Volcano, Hawaii, 1979–1997*. (Open file report 98–462). Menlo Park, CA: United States Geological Survey, Hawaiian Volcano Observatory.

Elwood, S., & Leitner, H. (1998). GIS and community–based planning: Exploring the diversity of neighborhood perspectives and needs. *Cartography & Geographic Information Systems, 25*(2), 77.

Emani, S., & Kasperson, J.X. (1996). Disaster communication via the information superhighway: Data and observations on the 1995 hurricane season. *International Journal of Mass Emergencies and Disasters, 14*, 321–342.

Emergency Management Institute (EMI). (1998). *Basic incident command system (ICS): Independent study*. Emmitsburg, MD: Emergency Management Institute, Federal Emergency Management Agency.

Enarson, E. (1998). *Surviving domestic violence and disasters*. Vancouver, BC: The FREIDA Centre for Research on Violence Against Women and Children.

Enarson, E. (1999a). Women and housing issues in two U.S. disasters. *International Journal of Mass Emergencies and Disasters, 17*(1), 39–63.

Enarson, E. (1999b). Violence against women in disasters: A study of domestic violence programs in the U.S. and Canada. *Violence Against Women, 5*(7), 742–768.

Enarson, E. (2000a). *A gender analysis of work and employment issues in natural disasters*. Final report prepared for the International Labour Organization's In Focus Programme on Crisis and Reconstruction, http://www.ilo.org/public/english/ employment/ recon/crisis/ gender.htm.

Enarson, E. (2000b). We will make meaning out of this: Women's cultural responses to the Red River Valley flood. *International Journal of Mass Emergencies and Disasters, 18*, 39–62.

Enarson, E. (2001a). We want work: Rural women in the Gujarat drought and earthquake. Quick Response Report No. 135. Boulder, CO: Natural Hazards Research and Applications Information Center, University of Colorado, www.colorado.edu/hazards/ qr/qr135/ qr135.html.

Enarson, E. (2001b). What women do: Gendered labor in the Red River Valley Flood. *Environmental Hazards, 3*, 1–18.

Enarson, E., Childers, C., Morrow, B.H., Thomas, D., & Wisner, B. (2003). *A social vulnerability approach to disasters*. Emmitsburg, MD: Emergency Management Institute, Federal Emergency Management Agency.

Enarson, E., & Fordham, M. (2001). From women's needs to women's rights in disasters. *Environmental Hazards, 3*, 133–136.

Enarson, E., & Fordham, M. (2004). Lines that divide, ties that bind: Race, class, and gender in women's flood recovery in the U.S. and U.K. *Australian Journal of Emergency Management, 15*(4), 43–52.

Enarson, E., & Meyreles, L. (2004). International perspectives on gender and disaster: Differences and possibilities. *International Journal of Sociology and Social Policy, 24*(10/11), 49–93.

Enarson, E., Meyreles, L., Gonzáles, M., Morrow, B.H., Mullings, A., & Soares, J. (2003). Working with women at risk: Practical guidelines for assessing local disaster risk. Retrieved June 30, 2003, http://online.northumbria.ac.uk/geography_research/gdn/resources/Working%20w%20Women%20English%20.pdf.

Enarson, E., & Morrow, B. (1997). A gendered perspective: The voices of women. In W. Peacock, B. Morrow, & H. Gladwin (Eds.), *Hurricane Andrew: Ethnicity, gender and the sociology of disasters* (pp. 116–140). New York: Routledge.

Enarson, E., & Morrow B.H. (Eds.). (1998). The gendered terrain of disaster: Through women's eyes. Wesport, CT: Greenwood Publications.

Enarson, E., & Phillips, B. (Forthcoming). Invitation to a new feminist disaster sociology: Integrating feminist theory and methods. In B. Phillips & B.H. Morrow (Eds.), *Women and disasters*. Philadelphia: Xlibris.

Enarson, E., & Scanlon, J. (1999). Gender patterns in a flood evacuation: A case study of couples in Canada's Red River Valley. *Applied Behavioral Science Review, 7*(2), 103–125.

Engineering Field Investigation Team (EEFIT). Retrieced July 15, 2005; http://www.istructe.org.uk/eefit/index.asp?bhcp=1.

EQE International Inc. (1997). *The Northridge Earthquake of January 17, 1994: Report of data collection and trends; Part B: Analysis and trends.* Warrington, UK.

Erharuyi, N., & Fairbain, D. (2003). Mobile geographic information handling technologies to support disaster management. *Geography, 88*(4), 312–319.

Erickson, P.E., Drabek, T.E., Key, W.H., & Crowe, J.L. (1976). Families in disaster: Patterns of recovery. *Mass Emergencies, 1,* 203–216.

Ericson, R.V., & Doyle, A. (Ed.). (2003). *Risk and morality.* Toronto: University of Toronto Press.

Eriksen, T. (1991). The cultural contexts of ethnic differences. In W.H. Form & S. Nosow (Eds.), *Community in disaster* (pp. 127–144). New York: Harper.

Erikson, K.T. (1966). *Wayward puritans: A study in the sociology of deviance.* New York: Wiley.

Erikson, K.T. (1976). *Everything in its path: Destruction of community in the Buffalo Creek flood.* New York: Simon and Schuster.

Erikson, K. (1994). *A new species of trouble: Explorations in disaster, trauma, and community.* New York: W. W. Norton.

Escobar, A. (1995). *Encountering development.* Princeton, NJ: Princeton University Press.

Etzioni, A. (1964). *Modern organizations.* Englewood Cliffs, NJ: Prentice-Hall.

EU-MEDIN. (2005). Retrieved October 1, 2005, http://www.eu–medin.org/.

Ewald, F. (2002). The return of Descartes's malicious demon: An outline of a philosophy of precaution. In T. Baker & J. Simon (Eds.), *Embracing risk: The changing culture of insurance and responsibility* (pp. 273–301). Chicago, IL: The University of Chicago Press.

Eyre, A. (1989). *After Hillsborough: An ethnographic account of life in Liverpool in the first few weeks.* Unpublished.

Eyre, A., Wachtendorf, T., & Webb, G.R. (Eds.). (2000). The popular culture of disaster. *International Journal of Disasters and Mass Emergencies, 18,* 5–115.

Fabbri, K.P. (1998). A methodology for supporting decision making in integrated coastal zone management: An application to agricultural land use in The Netherlands. *Journal of Ocean & Coastal Management, 39*(1), 51–62.

Fabre, N. (2004). *L'inconscient de Descartes.* Paris: Bayard.

Fahy, R.F. (1995). Study of occupant behavior during the World Trade Center evacuation: Preliminary report of results. In D.P. Lund & E.A. Angell (Eds.), *International Conference on Fire Research and Engineering (ICFRE). Proceedings,* September 10–15, 1995, Orlando, FL, pp. 197–202.

Falkenrath, R.A., Newman, R.D., & Thayer, B.A. (1998). *America's Achilles' heel: Nuclear, biological and chemical terrorism and covert attack.* Cambridge, MA: MIT Press.

Falkiner, L. (2005). Availability of Canadian social science disaster management education. *International Journal of Mass Emergencies and Disasters, 23*(1), 85–110.

Farazmand, A. (2001). *Handbook of crisis and emergency management.* New York: Marcel Dekker.

Faris, R.E.L. (1970 [1967]). *Chicago sociology 1920–1932.* Chicago and London: The University of Chicago Press.

Farley, J.E. (1998). Down but not out: Earthquake awareness and preparedness trends in the St. Louis metropolitan area, 1990–1997. *International Journal of Mass Emergencies and Disasters, 16,* 303–319.

Faure, M., Gupta, Y., & Nentjes, A. (2003). *Climate change and the Kyoto Protocol.* Cheltenham: Elgar.

Feagin, J.R., & Sikes, M. P. (1994). *Living with racism: The black middle class experience.* Boston: Beacon.

Fearn-Banks, K. (1996). *Crisis communications: A casebook approach.* Mahwah, NJ: Erlbaum.

Federal Bureau of Investigations (FBI). (n.d.). *Terrorism 2000/2001 (FBI Publication no. 0308).* U.S. Department of Justice. Retrieved September 1, 2005, http://www.fbi.gov/publications /terror/terror2000_2001.pdf

Federal Emergency Management Agency (FEMA). (1980). *An assessment of the consequences and preparations for a catastrophic California earthquake: Findings and actions taken.* Washington, DC: Federal Emergency Management Agency.

Federal Emergency Management Agency (FEMA). (1994). Hurricane Andrew Tent Cities: After Action Special Report.

Federal Emergency Management Agency (FEMA). (1997). *Multi-hazard identification and risk assessment: A cornerstone of the national mitigation strategy.* Washington, DC: Federal Emergency Management Agency.

Federal Emergency Management Agency (FEMA). (1998). Protecting business operations: Second report on costs and benefits of natural hazard mitigation. (FEMA Report 331).Washington, DC: Federal Emergency Management Agency.

Federal Emergency Management Agency (FEMA). (2000a). Planning for a sustainable future: The link between hazard mitigation and livability. (FEMA Report 364). Washington, DC: Federal Emergency Management Agency.

Federal Emergency Management Agency (FEMA). (2000b). Rebuilding for a more sustainable future: An operational framework. (FEMA Report 365). Washington, DC: Federal Emergency Management Agency.

Federal Emergency Management Agency (FEMA). (2004a). *The National Response Plan*. Washington, DC: Federal Emergency Management Agency.

Federal Emergency Management Agency (FEMA). (2004b). Responding to incident of national consequences: Recommendations for America's fire and emergency services based on the events of September 11, 2001 and other similar incidents. (FA-282-May 2004). Retrieved September, 2005, http://www.usfa.fema.gov/downloads/pdf/publications/fa-282.pdf.

Federal Emergency Management Agency, National Earthquake Hazards Reduction Program. (2005). *The earthquake hazard*. Retrieved July 15, 2005, http://www.fema.gov/hazards /earthquakes/nehrp/about.shtm.

Federal Emergency Management Agency (FEMA). (2005a). Retrieved October 1, 2005, http://www.hazardmaps.gov/atlas.php.

Federal Emergency Management Agency (FEMA). (2005b). Retrieved October 1, 2005, http://www. fema.gov/hazus/.

Fennell, G. (2002). An alternative to the incident cgommand system. *Contingency Planning & Management, 7*(1), 35–38.

Fernandez, A.L. (2005). *A comparative study of disaster-related science and technology policies in five countries: A discussion paper*. EDM Technical Report 20. Kobe: Earthquake Disaster Mitigation Research Centre.

Fernandez, A.L., & Britton, N.R. (2004). *Dealing with disasters from the risk perspective: Practices from India, Japan and New Zealand*. Paper delivered at the International Joint Conference on Risk Assessment and Management, November 4–6, 2004, Seoul, Korea.

Fernando, P., & Fernando, V. (1997). *South Asian women facing disasters, securing life*. Colombo, Sri Lanka: ITDG.

Filler, D.M. (2003). Terrorism, panic and pedophilia. *Virginia Journal of Social Policy & the Law*, Spring 2003.

Fink, S. (1986). *Crisis management: Planning for the inevitable*. Saranac Lake: AMACOM.

Finlay, C. (1998). Floods, they're a damned nuisance: Women's flood experiences in rural Australia. In E. Enarson & B. H. Morrow (Eds.), *The gendered terrain of disaster: Through women's eyes* (pp. 143–150). Westport, CT: Praeger.

Fire & Emergency Management Agency. (2005). Actual conditions and prospects of fire and emergency management administration. Ministry of Internal Affairs and Communications. Retrieved September 22, 2005, http://www.fdma.go.jp/disaster.

Fiscal Policy Institute. (2001). *World Trade Center job impacts take a heavy toll on low-wage workers: Occupational and wage implications of job losses related to the September 11 World Trade Center attack*. New York: Fiscal Policy Institute.

Fischer, H.W. III. (1994). *Response to disaster: Fact versus fiction and its perpetuation: The sociology of disaster*. New York: University Presses of America.

Fischer, H. (1998a). *Response to disaster: Fact versus fiction & its perpetuation: The sociology of disaster*. Lanham, MD: University Presses of America.

Fischer, H.W. III. (1998b). The role of the new information technologies in emergency mitigation, planning, response and recovery. *Disaster Prevention and Management, 7*(1), 28–37.

Fischer, H.W. III. (1999). Dimensions of biological terrorism: To what must we mitigate and respond. *Disaster Prevention and Management, 8*(1), 27–32.

Fischer, H. (2003). The sociology of disaster: Definitions, research questions and measurements. *International Journal of Mass Emergencies and Disasters, 21*, 91–108.

Fischer, S. (2003). Globalization and its challenges. *American Economic Review*, May, 1–30.

Fisher, S. (2005). Gender based violence in Sri Lanka in the aftermath of the 2004 Tsunami crisis: The role of international organizations and international NGOs in prevention and response to gender based violence. Unpublished paper. Retrieved October 11, 2005, http://online.northumbria.ac.uk/geography_research/gdn/.

Flin, R. (1996). *Sitting in the hot seat: Leaders and teams for critical incidents*. Chichester: Wiley.

Flippen, C. (2004). Unequal returns to housing investments? A study of real housing appreciation among black, white, and Hispanic households. *Social Forces, 82*, 1523–1551.

Flynn, C. (1979) *Three Mile Island telephone survey –NUREG/CR–1093*. Washington, DC: U.S. Nuclear Regulatory Commission.

Flynn, S. (2004). *America the vulnerable : How our government is failing to protect us from terrorism*. New York: HarperCollins.

Foley, D.L. (1980). The Sociology of Housing. *Annual Review of Sociology, 6*, 457–478.

Fordham, M. (1999). The intersection of gender and social class in disaster: Balancing resilience and vulnerability. *International Journal of Mass Emergencies and Disasters, 17*(1), 15–36.

Fordham, M. (2003). Gender, disaster and development: The necessity for integration. In Pelling Mark (Ed.), *Natural disasters and development in a globalizing world*. London: Routledge.

Fordham, M. (2004). Gendering vulnerability analysis: Towards a more nuanced approach. In G. Bankoff, G. Frerks, & D. Hillhorst (Eds.), *Mapping vulnerability: Disasters, development, and people* (pp. 174–182). London: Earthscan.

Fordham, M., & Ketteridge, A. (1998). Men must work and women must weep: Examining gender stereotypes in disasters. In E. Enarson, & B.H. Morrow (Eds.), *The gendered terrain of disaster: Through women's eyes* (pp. 81–94). Westport, CT: Praeger.

Forester, J. (1987). Planning in the face of conflict. *Journal of the American Planning Association, 53*(3), 303–314.

Forester, J. (1989). *Planning in the face of power*. Berkeley, CA: University of California Press.

Form, W.H., & Nosow, S. (1958). *Community in disaster*. New York: Harper & Brothers.

Forrest, T.R. (1973). Needs and group emergence: Developing a welfare response. *American Behavioral Scientist, 16*, 313–325.

Forrest, T.R. (1978). Group emergence in disasters. In E.L. Quarantelli (Ed.), *Disasters: Theory and research* (pp. 106–125). Beverly Hills, CA: SAGE.

Forrest, T. (1993). Disaster anniversary: A social reconstruction of time. *Sociological Inquiry, 63*(4), 444–456.

Fothergill, A. (1996). Gender, risk, and disaster. *International Journal of Mass Emergencies and Disasters, 14*(1), 33–56.

Fothergill, A. (1999). Women's roles in a disaster. *Applied Behavioral Science Review, 7*(2), 125–143.

Fothergill, A. (2000). Knowledge transfer between researchers and practitioners. *Natural Hazards Review, 1*(2), 91–98.

Fothergill, A. (2003). The stigma of charity: Gender, class, and disaster assistance. *The Sociological Quarterly, 44*(4), 659–680.

Fothergill, A. (2004). *Heads above water: Gender, class, and family in the Grand Forks flood*. Albany, NY: State University of New York Press.

Fothergill, A., Maestas, E.G.M., & Darlington, J. D. (1999). Race, ethnicity, and disasters in the United States: A review of the literature. *Disasters, 23*(2), 156–173.

Fothergill, A., & Peek, L.A. (2004). Poverty and disasters in the United States: A review of recent sociological findings. *Natural Hazards, 32*, 89–110.

Foundation for Research, Science and Technology. (2003). *Requests for proposals for research in natural physical hazards*. New Zealand: Wellington.

Francaviglia, R.V. (1978). Xenia rebuilds: Effects of predisaster conditioning on post-disaster redevelopment. *Journal of the American Institute of Planners, 44*(1), 13–24.

Franke, M.E., & Simpson, D.M. (2004). *Understanding community response to Hurricane Isabel: An Examination of the Role and Function of Community Emergency Response Team (CERT) Organizations in Virginia*. Quick Response Report #170, Boulder, CO: Natural Hazards Center at the University of Colorado, Boulder.

Franks, J. (2005). BP Texas plant had fire day before blast. *The New York Times*, March 25.

Freeman, P.K., Martin, L.A., Mechler, R., & Warner K. (2002). Catastrophe and development: Integrating natural catastrophes into developing planning. *Disaster Risk Management Working Papers Series 4*. Washington, DC: World Bank.

French, J.G., & Holt, K.W. (1989). Floods. In M.B. Gregg (Ed.), *The public health consequences of disaster* (pp. 69–78). Atlanta: U.S. Department of Health and Human Services, Public Health Service, Centers for Disease Control.

Frenkel, R. (2003). Globalization and financial crises in Latin America. *CEPAL Review, 80*, 39–52.

Freud, S. (1977). *Introductory lectures on psychoanalysis*, New York: Liveright.

Freud, S. (1984). *On metapsychology: The theory of psychoanalysis: 'Beyond the Pleasure Principle', 'The Ego and the Id' and other works*, Harmondsworth.

Freudenburg, W.R. (1997). Contamination, corrosion, and the social order: An overview. *Current Sociology, 45*, 19–39.

Friedman, J. (1981). *Retracking America.*. Emmaus, PA: Rodale Press.

Friesema, H.P., Caporaso J., Goldstein G., Lineberry, R., & McCleary, R. (1979). Aftermath: Communities after natural disasters. Beverly Hills, CA: SAGE.

Fritz, C.E. (1952). The social psychology of disaster: Some theoretical notes and suggested problems for research. Unpublished paper.

Fritz, C.E. (1961a). Disasters. In R.K. Merton & R.A. Nisbet (Eds.), *Contemporary social problems. An introduction to the sociology of deviant behavior and social disorganization* (pp. 651–694). Riverside, CA: University of California Press.

Fritz, C.E. (1961b). *Disaster and community therapy*. Washington, DC: National Research Council, National Academy of Sciences.

Fritz, C.E. (1968). Disasters. In D.L. Sills (Ed.), *Encyclopedia of the social sciences.* (pp. 202–207). New York: Collier-Macmillan.

Fritz, C., & Marks, E. (1954). The NORC studies of human behavior in disaster. *Journal of Social Issues, 10*(3), 26–41.

Fritz, C.E., & Mathewson, J.H. (1957). *Convergence behavior in disasters: A problem in social control.* Washington, DC: National Academy of Sciences, National Research Council.

Fujita, T.T. (1987). *U.S. tornadoes part 1: 70-year statistics, satellite and mesom research project (SMRP.)* (Research Paper Number 218). Chicago: The University of Chicago Press.

Furedi, F. (1997). *The culture of fear; Risk taking and the morality of low expectations* (2nd ed.). London: Cassel.

Furedi, F. (2002). *The Culture of Fear; Risk Taking and the Morality of Low Expectations* (2nd ed.). London: Continuum Press.

Furedi, F. (2003). Proof of evidence on health effects and risk. Local public Inquiry—1 July 2003. www.bexley.gov.uk.

Furedi, F. (2004). *Therapy culture; Cultivating vulnerability in an uncertain age.* London: Routledge.

Furedi, F. (2005). *The politics of fear; Beyond left and right.* London: Continuum Press.

Furedi, F. (2007). *The fear market; Explorations in the sociology of fear.* London: Continuum Press.

Galea, S., Ahern, J., Resnick, H., Kilpatrick, D., Bucuvalas, M., Gold, J., & Vlahov, D. (2002). Psychological sequelae of the September 11 terrorist attacks in New York City. *New England Journal of Medicine, 346,* 982–987.

Galea, S., Vlahov, D., Resnick, H., Ahern, J., Susser, E., Gold, J., et al. (2003). Trends of probable post-traumatic stress disorder in New York City after the September 11 terrorist attacks. *American Journal of Epidemiology, 158,* 514–524.

Gans, H. (1980). *Deciding what's news.* New York: Vintage Press.

Garland, D. (2001). *The culture of control: Crime and social order in contemporary society.* Oxford: Oxford University Press.

Garland, D. (2003). The rise of risk. In R.V. Ericson, & A. Doyle (Ed.), *Risk and morality* (pp. 48–86). Toronto: University of Toronto Press.

Garrison, C.Z., Bryant, E.S., Addy, C.L., Spurrier, D.G., Freedy, J.R., & Kilpatrick, D.G. (1995). Posttraumatic stress disorder in adolescents after Hurricane Andrew. *Journal of the American Academy of Child and Adolescent Psychiatry, 34,* 1193–1201.

Geer, D., Bace, R., Gutmann, P., Metzger, P., Pfleeger, C., Quarterman, J., et al. (2003). *CyberInsecurity: The cost of monopoly: How the dominance of Microsoft's products poses a risk to security.* Computer & Communications Industry Association.

Geipel, R. (1982). *Disaster and reconstruction. The Fruili (Italy) earthquake of 1976.* London: Allen & Unwin.

Geis, D.E. (2000). By design: The disaster resilient and quality of life community. *Natural Hazards Review, 1*(3), 151–160.

Gender and Disaster Network. (2005). Retrieved December 5, 2005, http://online.northumbria.ac.uk/geography_research/gdn/.

George, A.L. (Ed.). (1991). *Avoiding war: Problems of crisis management.* Boulder, CO: Westview Press.

Giacalone, R.A., & Rosenfeld, P. (1989). *Impression management in the organization.* Hillsdale, NJ: Erlbaum.

Giarini, O. (Ed.). (1984). *The Geneva papers on risk and insurance.* Geneve: The Geneva Association.

Gibbs, S. (1990). *Women's role in the Red Cross/Red Crescent.* Geneva: Henry Dunant Institute.

Gibson-Graham, J.K., Resnick, S., & Wolff, R. (Eds.). (2001). *Re/Presenting class: Essays in postmodern marxism.* London: Duke University Press.

Gilbert, C. (1998). Studying disaster: Changes in the main conceptual tools. In E.L. Quarantelli (Ed.), *What is a disaster: Perspectives on the question* (pp. 11–18). London: Routledge.

Gillespie, D.F. (1991). Coordinating community resources. In T.E. Drabek & G.J. Hoetmer (Eds.), *Emergency management: Principles and practice for local government* (pp. 55–78). Washington, DC: International City Management Association.

Gillespie, D.F., & Colignon, R.A. (1993). Structural change in disaster preparedness networks. *International Journal of Mass Emergencies and Disasters, 11,* 143–162.

Gillespie, D.F., Colignon, R.A., Banerjee, M.M., Murty, S.A., & Rogge, M. (1993). *Partnerships for community preparedness.* Boulder, CO: Institute of Behavioral Science, University of Colorado.

Gillespie, D., & Perry, R.W. (1974). An integrated systems and emergent norm approach to mass emergencies. *Mass Emergencies, 1,* 303–312.

Gillespie, D.F., & Streeter, C.L. (1987). Conceptualizing and measuring disaster preparedness. *International Journal of Mass Emergencies and Disasters, 5,* 155–176.

Gioia, D.A., & Chittipeddi, K. (1991). Sensemaking and sensegiving in strategic change initiation. *Strategic Management Journal, 12*, 433–448.

Girard, C., & Peacock, W. (1997). Ethnicity and segregation: Post-hurricane relocation. In W. Peacock, B. Morrow, & H. Gladwin (Eds.), *Hurricane Andrew: Ethnicity, gender, and the sociology of disaster* (pp. 191–205). New York: Routledge.

Gitlin, T. (1980). *The whole world is watching*. Berkeley, CA: University of California Press.

Giuliani, R. (2002). *Leadership*. New York: Miramax Books.

Gladwin, H., & Peacock, H. (1997). Warning and evaluation: A night for hard houses. In W. Peacock, B. Morrow, & H. Gladwin (Eds.), *Hurricane Andrew—Ethnicity, gender and the sociology of disaster* (pp. 52–74). London: Routledge.

Glass, R.I., Craven, R.B., Bregman, D.J., Stoll, B.J., Horowitz, N., Kerndt, P., et al. (1980). Injuries from the Wichita Falls tornado: Implications for prevention. *Science, 207*, 734–738.

Glass, R.I., O'Hare, P., & Conrad, J. L. (1979). Health Consequences of the Snow Disaster in Massachusetts, February 6, 1978. *American Journal of Public Health, 69*, 1047–1049.

Glass, R.I., Urrutia, J.J., Sibony, S., Smith, H., Garcia, B., & Rizzo, L. (1977). Earthquake injures related to housing in a Guatemalan village. *Science, 197*, 638–643.

Glassman, J. (2003). Rethinking overdetermination, structural power and social change: A critique of Gibson-Graham, Resnick, and Wolff. *Antipode, 35*(4), 678–698.

Glickman, T., Golding, D. & Silverman, E. (1992). *Acts of God and acts of man: Recent trends in natural disasters and major industrial accidents*. Washington, DC: Resources for the Future.

Global Disaster Information Network. (1997). Harnessing Information and Technology for Disaster Management. Disaster Information Task Force Report. Washington, DC: Global Disaster Information Network.

Godschalk, D.R. (1991). Disaster mitigation and hazard management. In G.J. Hoetmer & T.E. Drabek (Eds.), *Emergency management: Principles and practice for local government* (pp. 131–160). Washington, DC: International City Management Association.

Godschalk, D.R. (1992). Negotiating intergovernmental development policy conflicts: Practice-based guidelines. *Journal of the American Planning Association, 58*(2), 368–378.

Godschalk, D.R., Beatley, T., Berke, P., Brower, D., & Kaiser, E. (1998). *Making mitigation work: Recasting natural hazard planning and implementation*. Washington, DC: Island Press.

Godschalk, D., Beately T., Berke, P., Brower, D., Kaiser, E., Bohl, C.C., et al. (1999). *Natural hazard mitigation: Recasting disaster policy and planning*. Washington, DC: Island Press.

Godschalk, D.R., Brower, D., & Beatley, T. (1989). *Catastrophic coastal storms: Hazard mitigation and development management*. Durham, NC: Duke University Press.

Goenjian, A.K., Najarian, L.M., Pynoos, R.S., Steinberg, A.M., Manoukian, G., Tavosian, A., et al. (1994). Posttraumatic stress disorder in elderly and younger adults after the 1988 earthquake in Armenia. *American Journal of Psychiatry, 151*, 895–901.

Goldstone, J.A., & Useem, B. (1999). Prison riots as microrevolutions: An extension of state-centered theories of revolution. *American Journal of Sociology, 104*, 985–1029.

Goltz, J.D. (2006). *Initial behavioral response to a rapid onset disaster: A social psychological study of three California earthquakes* (draft). Unpublished dissertation. Los Angeles: University of California.

Gopalan, P. (2001). *Responding to earthquakes: People's participation in reconstruction and rehabilitation*. Paper prepared for the United Nations Division for the Advancement of Women Expert Working Group Meeting. Ankara, Turkey (November 6–9, 2001). Retrieved December 5, 2005, http://www.un.org/womenwatch/daw/csw/env_manage /documents.html.

Gordon, J.A. (2002). *Comprehensive emergency management for local governments: Demystifying emergency planning*. Brookfield, CT: Rothstein Associates Inc.

Gordon, P., Richardson H.W., & Davis, B. (1997). Transport-related impacts of the Northridge earthquake. *Journal of Transportation and Statistics, 1*, 21–36.

Gordon, R. (2004). The social system as site of disaster impact and resource for recovery. In S. Norman (Ed.), *Proceedings of the New Zealand Recovery Symposium*, July 12–13, 2004. New Zealand: Ministry of Civil Defense & Emergency Management.

Gorer, G. (1965). *Death, grief & mourning in contemporary Britain*. London: Cresset.

Gori, P.L. (1991). Communication between scientists and practice: The important link in knowledge utilization. *Earthquake Spectra, 7*(1), 89–95.

Gorman, C. (2005). Design unveiled for bushfire memorial. *ABC Canberra*. Retrieved January 18, 2005, http://www.abc.net.au.

Government Accountability Office. (2005). Homeland security: Federal and industry efforts are addressing security issues at chemical facilities, but additional action is needed. GAO-05-631T. Washington, DC: Government Accountability Office.

Government of Japan. (2005). *National report of Japan on disaster reduction for the World Conference on Disaster Reduction*. Geneva: International Strategy for Disaster Reduction. Retrieved December 5, 2005, http://www.unisdr.org/wcdr/nationalreports.

Grabel, I. (2002). Neoliberal finance and crisis in the developing world. *Monthly Review 11*, 34–46.

Graff, J. (2005). The Voices of the Victims: Why survivors of the attack think Spain's leaders are playing politics with 3/11 Time Europe (March 13, 2005); http://www.time.com/time/europe.

Graham, B. (2005). War plans prafted to counter terror attacks in U.S. *Washington Post*, August 8, A1.

Gramsci, A. (1971). *Selections from the prison notebooks*. London: Lawrence and Wishart.

Granot, H. (1997). Emergency inter-organizational relationships. *Disaster Prevention and Management: An International Journal, 6*, 305–310.

Grant, D., & Jones, A.W. (2003). Are subsidiaries more prone to pollute? New evidence from the EPA's Toxics Release Inventory. *Social Science Quarterly, 84* (March), 162–171.

Grant, D., Jones, A.W., &. Bergesen, A.J. (2002). Organizational size and pollution: The case of the U.S. chemical industry. *American Sociological Review, 67* (June), 389–407.

Gray, P., & Oliver, K. (2001). The memory of catastrophe. *History Today*, February 2001.

Gray, P., & Oliver, K. (2004). *The memory of catastrophe*. Manchester: Manchester University Press.

Green, S. (1977). *International disaster relief: towards a responsive system*. New York: McGraw-Hill.

Greenberg, J. (November 2, 2003). Saturday's Developments. *Los Angeles Times*, p. A28.

Grenier, G., & Morrow, B. (1997). Before the storm: The socio-political ecology of miami. In W. Peacock, B. Morrow, & H. Gladwin (Eds.), *Hurricane Andrew: Ethnicity, gender, and the sociology of disaster* (pp. 36–51). NY: Routledge.

Grimaldi, J.V., & Gugliotta, G. (2001). Chemical plants feared as targets. *Washington Post*, December 16, 2001.

Gruntfest, E. (1977). *What people did during the Big Thompson Flood*. Working paper No. 32. Boulder, CO: Institute of Behavioral Science, University of Colorado.

Gruntfest, E., & Huber, C. (1989). Status report on flood warning systems in the United States. *Environmental Management, 13*, 279–286.

Gruntfest, E., & Weber, M. (1998). Internet and emergency management: Prospects for the future. *International Journal of Mass Emergencies and Disasters, 16*, 55–72.

Guadagni, A.A., & Kaufmann, J. (2004). Comercio internacional y pobreza mundial. *CEPAL Review, 84*, 83–97.

Guarnizo, C.C. (1993). Integrating disaster and development assistance after natural disasters: NGO response in the Third World. In D. Neal (Guest Ed.), Special issue: Disaster research and practice: Bridging the gap. *International Journal of Mass Emergencies and Disasters, 11*(1), 111–122.

Guehenno, J. (1995). *The end of the nation state*. Minneapolis: University of Minnesota Press.

Gupta, A., & Ferguson, J. (Eds.). *Culture, power, place: Explorations in critical anthropology*. Durham, NC: Duke.

Gusfield, J.R. (1984). On the side: Practical action and social constructivism in social problems theory. In J. W. Schneider, & J.I. Kitsuse (Eds.), *Studies in the Sociology of Social Problems* (pp. 31–51). Norwood, NJ: Ablex.

Guss, C.D., & Pangan, O.I. (2004). Cultural influences on disaster management: A case study of the Mt. Pinatubo eruption. *International Journal of Mass Emergencies and Disasters, 22*(2), 31–58.

Gustin, J.F. (2004). *Disaster and recovery planning: A guide for facility managers* (3rd ed.). New York: Marcel Dekker.

Guy, R.F., Pol, L.G., & Ryker, R. (1982). Discrimination in mortgage lending: The Mortgage Disclosure Act. *Population Research and Policy Review, 1*, 283–296.

Guzelian, C.P. (2004). *Liability and fear*. Stanford Public Law and Legal Theory Working Paper Series. Stanford, CA: Stanford Law School.

Haas, P. (Ed.) (2003). *Environment in the new global economy*. Cheltenham: Elgar.

Haas, J.E., & Drabek, T.E. (1973). *Complex organizations: A sociological perspective*. New York: Macmillan.

Haas, J.E., Kates, R., & Bowden, M. (1977). *Reconstruction following disaster*. Cambridge, MA: MIT Press.

Habermas, J. (1975). *Legitimation crisis*. Boston: Beacon Press.

Habermas, J. (1994). *The structural transformation of the public sphere*. Cambridge, MA: MIT Press.

Haddow, G.D., & Bullock, J.A. (2003). *Introduction to emergency management*. Amsterdam: Butterworth-Heinemann.

Hage, J., & Aiken, M. (1970). *Social change in complex organizations*. New York: Random House.

Hagen, C.A., Ender, M.G., Tiemann, K.A., & Hagen, C.O. (1999). Graffiti on the great plains: A social reaction to the Red River Valley flood of 1997. *Applied Behavioral Science Review, 7*, 145–158.

Haggerty, K.D. (2003). From risk to precaution: The rationalities of personal crime prevention. In R.V. Ericson & A. Doyle (Eds.), *Risk and morality* (pp. 193–214). Toronto: University of Toronto Press.

Haines, V.A., Hurlbert, J.S., & Beggs, J.J. (1999). The disaster framing of the stress process: A test of an expanded model. *International Journal of Mass Emergencies and Disasters, 17*, 367–397.

Hale, D. (2002). Insuring a nightmare. *Worldlink, March 19, 2002*.

Hall, K. (2005). Japan paper runs censored A-bomb stories. *News.yahoo.com/s/at/20050619/ap_on_re_as/ japan_nagasaki*

Hall, R.H. (1962). Intraorganizational structural variation: Application of the bureaucratic model. *Administrative Science Quarterly, 7*, 295–308.

Hall, R.H. (1987). *Organizations: Structures, processes, and outcomes*. Englewood Cliffs, NJ: Prentice-Hall.

Halvorson, S.J. (2004). Women's management of the household health environment: Responding to childhood diarrheal disease in the northern areas, Pakistan. *Health and Place, 10*, 43–58.

Handmer, J. (2000). Are emergency services becoming private? *Australian Journal of Emergency Management, 15*(3), 42–45.

Hanley, N., & Owen, A.D. (2004). *The economics of climate change*. London: Routledge.

Hansén, D., & Stern, E. (2000). *Crisis management in a transitional society: The Latvian experience. CRISMART Series*. Stockholm: Elanders Gotab.

Hansen, J. (1998). Handling the media in times of crisis: Lessons from the Oklahoma City Bombing. In P. Patterson & L. Wilkins, (Ed.), *Media ethics issues cases* (pp. 56–57). New York: McGraw-Hill.

Hanson, C. (2001). Over here we're all war correspondents now. *Columbia Journalism Review*, Nov/Dec, 25–28.

Harrel-Bond, E. (1986). *Imposing aid*. Oxford: Oxford University Press.

Harrison, B. (1994). *Lean and mean: The changing landscape of corporate power in the age of flexibility*. New York: Basic Books.

Hart, G.C. (1976). *Natural hazards: Tornado, hurricane, and severe wind loss models*. Redondo Beach, CA: J. H. Wiggins.

't Hart, P. (1993). Symbols, rituals and power: The lost dimension in crisis. *Journal of Contingencies and Crisis Management, 1*, 36–50.

't Hart, P. (1994). *Groupthink in government: A study of small groups and policy failure*. Baltimore: Johns Hopkins University Press.

't Hart, P., Rosenthal, U., & Kouzmin, A. (1993). Crisis decision making: The centralization thesis revisited. *Administration and Society, 25*, 12–45.

't Hart, P., Stern, E.K., & Sundelius, B. (Eds.). (1997). *Beyond groupthink: Political group dynamics and foreign policymaking*. Ann Arbor: University of Michigan Press.

Harvey, D. (1990). *The condition of postmodernity*. Cambridge, MA: Blackwell.

Harvey, D. (1996a). *Justice, nature, and the geography of difference*. Oxford: Blackwell.

Harvey, D. (1996b). The environment of injustice. In A. Merrifield & E. Swyngedouw (Eds.), *The urbanization of injustice* (pp. 65–99). New York: New York University Press.

Harvey, D. (2001). *Spaces of capital: Toward a critical geography*. Routledge: London.

Harvey, L. (1990). *Critical social research*. London: Unwin Hyman.

Hasselman, T., Equchi, R., & Wiggins, J. (1980). *Assessment of damageability for existing buildings in a natural hazards environment* (Technical Report No. 80-1332-1, September). Redondo Beach, CA.

Hauer, J. (2004). Emergency unpreparedness. *The New York Times*, March 15, 2004. On line at http://www.nytimes.com.

Hayashi, H. (2004). A comparison of the emergency management system between Japan and the United States. In K. Meguro (Ed.), *Assessment of post-event management processes using multi-media disaster simulation* (pp. 2-25–2-30). Kyoto: US–Japan Cooperative Research on Urban Earthquake Disaster Mitigation Project.

Haydon, G. (2004). Educational aims and the question of priorities. In J.P. Stoltman, et al. (Eds.), *International perspectives on natural disasters: Occurrence, mitigation and consequence* (pp. 359–367). Dordrecht: Kluwer.

Hays, W. (1999). The IDNDR in perspective. In J. Ingleton (Ed.), *Natural disaster management* (pp. 276–279). Leicester: Tudor Rose.

Hazards Management Group (HMG). (n.d.) *Southeast states hurricane evacuation traffic study: Floyd behavioral reports*, www.fhwaetis.com/etis

Heal, G., & Kunreuther, H. (2005). IDS models for airline security. *Journal of Conflict Resolution, 49*, 201–217.

Healy, G. (2003). Deployed in the USA: The creeping militarization of the home front. Policy Analysis No. 303, December 17. Washington, DC: The Cato Institute.

Heath, R. (1998). *Crisis management for managers and executives*. London: Financial Times–Pitman Publishing.

Heath, S., Kass, P., Beck, A., & Glickman, L. (2001a). Risk factors for pet evacuation failure after a slow-onset disaster. *Journal of the American Veterinary Association, 218*, 1905–1910.

Heath, S., Kass, P., Beck, A., & Glickman, L. (2001b). Human and pet-related risk factors for household evacuation failure during a natural disaster. *American Journal of Epidemiology 53*, 659–665.

Heinz Center, (2002). *Human links to coastal disasters*. Washington, DC: Heinz Center.

Hempel, C.G. (1952). *Fundamentals of concept formation in empirical science*. Chicago: The University of Chicago Press.

Hengjian, L., Kohiyama, M., Horie, K., Maki, N., Hayashi, H., & Tanaka, S. (2000). Building damage and casualty after earthquakes. Relationship between building damage pattern and casualty determined using housing damage photos in the 1995 Hanshin-Awaji Earthquake Disaster. *Eighth International Symposium on Natural and Technological Hazards*, May 2000.

Herman, J. (1997). *Trauma and recovery: The aftermath of violence—from domestic abuse to political terror.* Basic Books, New York.

Hermann, C.F. (1972). *International crises: Insights from behavioral research*. New York: Free Press.

Hewitt, K. (1983a). *Interpretations of calamity from the viewpoint of human ecology*. London: Allen and Unwin.

Hewitt, K. (1983b). The idea of calamity in a technocratic age. In K. Hewitt (Ed.), *Interpretations of calamity from the perspective of human ecology* (pp. 3–32). London: Allen and Unwin.

Hewitt, K. (1997). *Regions of risk: A geographical introduction to disasters*. Reading, MA: Addison Wesley Longman.

Hewitt, K. (1998). Excluded perspectives in the social construction of disaster. In E.L. Quarantelli (Ed.), *What is a disaster?* (pp. 75–91). London: Routledge.

Hewitt, K., & Burton, I. (1971). *The hazardousness of a place*. Toronto: University of Toronto Press.

Heymann, P.B. (1998). *Terrorism and America*. Cambridge, MA: MIT Press.

Hickey, R., & Jankowski, P. (1997). GIS and environmental decision making to aid smelter reclamation planning. *Environment and Planning, A 29*(1), 5–19.

Higashida, M. (2005). *Tonankai and Nankai earthquake preparedness measures: Lessons learned from the Great Hanshin-Awaji earthquake*. Paper presented at *1st* international conference on urban disaster reduction, Kobe, Japan.

Hiles, A. (2000). *Business continuity: Best practices, world-class business continuity management*. Brookfield, CT: Rothstein Associates Inc.

Hilhorst, D. (2003). Responding to disasters: Diversity of bureaucrats, technocrats and local people. *International Journal of Mass Emergencies and Disasters, 21*(1), 37–55.

Hiroi, O., Mikami, S., & Miyata, K. (1985). A study of mass media reporting in emergencies. *International Journal of Mass Emergencies and Disasters, 3*, 21–49.

Hirscleifer, J. (1975). Disaster behavior: altruism or alliance. *American Economic Review, 1*, 45–57.

Hirst, J. (2000). In deep trouble. *The Guardian,* December 6, 2000.

Hochschild, A.R. (1983). *Managed heart: Commercialization of human feeling*. Los Angeles: University of California Press.

Hochschild, A.R. (1989). *The second shift: Working parents and the revolution at home*. New York: Viking.

Hocker, C. (2005). Enterprises owned by African Americans have the lowest survival rates among ethnic businesses. *Black Enterprise, 35*, 38.

Hodder, R. (2000). *Development geography*. London: Routledge.

Hodgson, M., & Cutter, S. (2001). Mapping and the spatial analysis of hazardscapes In S.L. Cutter (Ed.), *American hazardscapes: The regionalization of environmental risks and hazards* (pp. 37–60). Washington, DC: Joseph Henry Press.

Hoelscher, S. (2003). Making place, making race: Performances of whiteness in the Jim Crow south. *Annals of the Association of American Geographers, 93*(3), 657–686.

Hoetmer, G.J. (1982). *Assessing local government emergency management needs and priorities*. Technical Report. Washington, DC: International City Management Association.

Hoetmer, G.J. (1991). *Introduction*. In G.J. Hoetmer & T.E. Drabek (Eds.), *Emergency management: principles and practice for local government* (pp. xvii–xxxiv). Washington, DC: International City Management Association.

Hoffman, B. (1999). Terrorism trends and prospects. In I.O. Lesser, B. Hoffman, J. Arquilla, D. Ronfeldt, & M. Zanini (Eds.), *Countering the new terrorism* (pp. 7–38). With a Foreword by Brian Michael Jenkins. Santa Monica, CA: RAND.

Hoffman, S.H., & Oliver-Smith, A. (2002). *Catastrophe and culture*. Santa Fe, NM: School of American Research Press.

Hoffman, S.M. (1998). Eve and Adam among the embers: Gender patterns after the Oakland Berkeley firestorm. In E. Enarson & B.H. Morrow (Eds.), *The gendered terrain of disaster: Through women's eyes* (pp. 55–61). Westport, CT: Praeger.

Hogg, S. (1980). Reconstruction following seismic disaster in Venzone, Friuli. *Disasters, 2*, 173–185.

Holifield, R. (2001). Defining environmental justice and environmental racism. *Urban Geography, 22*(1), 78–90.

Holsti, O.R. (1979). Theories of crisis decision making. In P. G. Lauren (Ed.), *Diplomacy: New approaches in history, theory, and policy* (pp. 99–136). New York: Free Press.

Homans, G.C. (1967). *The nature of social science.* New York: Harcourt, Brace & World.

Home quake measures still lax. (2005, January 15). *The Daily Yomiuri.*

Honeycombe, B. (1994). Special needs of women in emergency situations. *Australian Journal of Emergency Management, 8*(4), 28–31.

Hooper, M. (1999). Disaster preparedness: An analysis of public safety agency and community preparedness during the Northridge earthquake. *International Journal of Public Administration, 22,* 679–710.

Hopkins, A. (1999). Counteracting the cultural causes of disaster. *Journal of Contingencies and Crisis Management, 7,* 141–149.

Horkheimer, M., & Adorno, T. (1996). *Dialectic of enlightenment.* New York: Continuum.

Horlick-Jones, T. (1995). Modern disasters as outrage and betrayal. *International Journal of Mass Emergencies and Disasters, 13*(3), 305–316.

Horlick-Jones, T. (2001). Urban disasters and megacities in a risk society. In A. Giddens (Ed.) *Sociology: Introductory readings* (pp. 339–345). Cambridge: Polity.

Horton, H.D. (1992). Race and wealth: A demographic analysis of black homeownership. *Sociological Inquiry, 62,* 480–489.

Hossain, H., Dodge, C., & Abel, H. (Eds.). (1992). *From crisis to development: Coping with disasters in Bangladesh.* Dhaka: University Press Limited.

House of Representatives. (2002). *Learning from 9/11—Understanding the collapse of the World Trade Center.* (Hearing before the Committee on Science. 107th Congress, Second Session. March 6, 2002. Serial No. 107–46). Retrieved September 2005, http://www.house.gov/science.

Howell, S.E. (1998). *Evacuation behavior in Orleans and Jefferson parishes, Hurricane Georges.* New Orleans: Survey Research Center, University of New Orleans.

Howell, S., & Bonner, D.E. (2005). *Citizen hurricane and evacuation behavior in southeastern Louisiana: A twelve parish study.* New Orleans: Survey Research Center, University of New Orleans.

Hsu, S.S. (2005). Leaders lacking disaster experience *Washington Post,* September 9, A01.

Hughes, E.C. (1946). Institutions in process. In A. McClung Lee (Ed.), *New outline of the principles of sociology* (pp. 236–247). New York: Barnes & Noble.

Human Development Report (2004). *Human development report 2004.* New York: UNDP.

Humboldt State University, Geology Department. (n.d.). *Tsunamis that have affected North Coast California in historic times.* Retrieved November 11, 2004, http://www.humboldt.edu/~geodept/earthquakes/tsunami!/n_coast_tsunamis.html

Humphrey, C. (2003). Rethinking infrastructure: Siberian cities and the great freeze of January 2001. In J. Schneider & I. Susser (Eds.), *Wounded cities: Destruction and reconstruction in a globalized world.* (pp. 91–107). New York: Berg.

Hurley, A. (1995). *Environmental inequalities: Class, race, and industrial pollution in Gary, Indiana, 1945–1980.* Chapel Hill, NC: University of North Carolina Press.

Hushon, J., Kelly, R.B., & Rubin, C. (1989). *Identification and analysis of factors affecting emergency evacuations.* Report prepared for the Nuclear Management and Resources Council, Inc. (NUMARC), Washington, DC.

Ibrahim, M.A. (2005). Unfortunate, but timely (editorial). *Epidemiologic Reviews, 27,* 1–2.

Iceland, J., Weinberg D.H., & Steinmetz, E. (2002). *Racial and Ethnic Residential Segregation in the United States: 1980–2000.* Washington, DC: U.S. Census.

Ikeda, K. (1995). Gender differences in human loss and vulnerability in natural disasters: A case study from Bangladesh. *Indian Journal of Gender Studies, 2*(2), 171–193.

Ikle, F. (1951). The effects of war destruction upon the ecology of cities. *Social Forces, 29,* 383–391.

Imai, N. (2002). Sociological research on the "memory" of the Great Hanshin earthquake: A consideration of monuments erected in the stricken area. *Soshioroji, 47,* 89–127.

Independent Expert Group on Mobile Phones (2000). *Mobile Phones and Health.* Chilton, Didcot, UK: IEGMP.

Ingleton, J., Ed. (1999). *Natural disaster management.* A presentation to commemorate the international decade for natural disaster reduction (IDNDR), Leicester, England: Tudor Rose.

Institute for Business and Home Safety. (2005). *Open for business: A disaster planning toolkit for the small to mid-sized business owner.* Tampa, FL: Institute for Business and Home Safety and Public Entity Risk Institute.

Institute for Community Innovation. Global Entrepreneurship Center. Florida International University, Miami. Retrieved October 11, 2005, http://www.entrepreneurship. fiu.edu/community_innovation.htm.

Institute for Crisis, Disaster, and Risk Management (2002). *Observing and documenting the inter-organizational response to the September 11th attack on the Pentagon.* The George Washington University. Retrieved September 2005, http://www.gwu.edu/~ icdrm/publications/nsf9/11.

Integrated Regional Information Networks (2004). *The eight plagues: West Africa's locust invasion.* Retrieved October 1, 2004; http://www.IRINnews.org.

Inter-Agency Standing Committee (2005). Retrieved October 1, 2005, http://www.hewsweb.org/home_page/default.asp

Intermediate Technology Development Group (2005). *Earthquake resistant housing.* Retrieved November 2005, http://www.itdg.org/?id=earthquake_housing

International Federation of Red Cross (2002). *World Disasters Report: Focus on reducing risk.* Geneva: International Federation of Red Cross and Red Crescent Societies.

International Journal of Mass Emergencies & Disasters (1993). Special Issue: Disaster research and practice: Bridging the gap. D. Neal (Guest Ed.), *International Journal of Mass Emergencies and Disasters, 11*(1).

International Strategy for Disaster Reduction (2005). *Platform for the promotion of early warning.* Retrieved October 3, 2005, www.unisdr.org/ppew/ew-actors/main-participants.htm.

Irvine, L. (2004). *Providing for pets during disaster: An exploratory study.* (Quick Response Report No. 171). Boulder, CO: Natural Hazards Research and Applications Information Center, University of Colorado.

Irvine, R.B. (1987). *When you are the headline—Managing a major news story.* Homewood, IL: Dow Jones-Irwin.

Irwin, A. (1995). *Citizen science: A study of people, expertise and sustainable development.* London and New York: Routledge.

Irwin, J. (2000). Anguish as flood Victims return to find their homes looted. *The Daily Mail*, October 16, 2000.

Isikoff, M., & Hosenball, M., (2005). *Wrong priorities? Newsweek* Edition. Retrieved September 7, 2005, msnbc.msn.com/id/9246373/site/newsweek.

Jain, S.K., Murty, C.V.R., Rai, D.C., Malik, J.N., Sheth, A.R., Jaiswal, A., et al. (2006). *The great Sumatra earthquake and Indian Ocean tsunami of December 26, 2004: The effects in Mainland Indian and in the Andaman-Nicobar Islands* (EERI Special Report, Learning from Earthquakes, Report No. 3). Oakland, CA: Earthquake Engineering Research Institute.

Janis, I.L. (1982). *Groupthink: Psychological studies of policy decisions and fiascos.* Boston: Houghton Mifflin.

Janis, I.L. (1989). *Crucial decisions: Leadership in policymaking and crisis management.* New York: Free Press.

Janis, I., Herek, G., & Huth, P. (1987). Decision-making during international crises: Is quality of process related to outcome? *Journal of Conflict Resolution, 31*(3), 542.

Janis, I.L., & Mann, L. (1977). *Decision-making: A psychological analysis of conflict, choice and commitment.* New York: Free Press.

Japanese Standards Association (2001). *Guidelines for development and implementation of risk management system.* Japanese Industrial Standard JIS Q 2001. Tokyo: Japanese Standards Association.

Jeggle, T. (2005). Governance and institutional policy: Introduction. In United Nations. *Know risk* (pp. 38–39). Leicester: Tudor Rose.

Jemphrey, A., & Eileen, B. (2000). Surviving the media: Hillsborough, Dunblane and the press. *Journalism Studies, 1*(3), 469–484.

Jenkins, P. (2002). *Images of terror.* New York: Aldine de Gruyter.

Jervis, R. (1976). *Perception and misperception in international politics.* Princeton: Princeton University Press.

Jigyasu, R. (2005a). Disaster: A reality or construct? In R.W. Perry & E.L. Quarantelli (Eds.), *What is a disaster: New answers to old questions* (pp. 49–59). Philadelphia: Xlibris.

Jigyasu, R. (2005b). Cultural heritage concerns in WCDR. *International Journal of Mass Emergencies and Disasters, 23*(1), 141–160.

Joh, H. (1997). Disaster stress of the 1995 Kobe earthquake. *Psychologia, 40*, 192–200.

Johnson, B. (2005). The next Asian plague. *FrontPage Magazine*, 14 January 2005.

Johnson, L.A. (2005). *Toward a comprehensive theory of disaster recovery: Comparing post-disaster financing in Los Angeles and Kobe and the long-term effects on land use and local finance.* Paper presented at the 1st International Conference on Urban Disaster Reduction January, Kobe, Japan.

Johnson, N.R. (1988). Fire in a crowded theater: A descriptive investigation of the emergence of panic. *International Journal of Mass Emergencies and Disasters, 6*(1), 7–26.

Johnston, B. (1994). *Who pays the price? The sociocultural context of the environmental crisis.* Washington, DC: Island Press.

Johnston, H., & Klandermans, B. (1995). *Social movements and culture.* Minneapolis: University of Minnesota Press.

Jones, B.D. (1994). *Reconceiving decision-making in democratic politics: Attention, choice, and public policy.* Chicago: The University of Chicago Press.

Jones, B., & Chang, S.E. (1995). Economic aspects of urban vulnerability and disaster mitigation. In F.Y. Chang & M.S. Sheu (Eds.), *Urban disaster mitigation: The role of engineering and technology* (pp. 311–320). Oxford: Elsevier.

Jones, B., & Malik, A.M. (1996). The building stock in Memphis: Relating structural type and use. In *Proceedings of the Eleventh World Conference on Earthquake Engineering.* Oxford: Elsevier.

Jones, N.P., Noji, E.K., Smith, G.S., & Krimgold, F. (1990). Preliminary earthquake injury epidemiology report. In R. Bolin (Ed.), *The Loma Prieta earthquake: Studies of short–term impacts* (pp. 33–42). Boulder, CO: Institute of Behavioral Science, University of Colorado.

Jones, N., Noji, E., Smith, G., & Wagner, R. (1993). Casualty in earthquakes. In K. Tierney & J. Nigg (Eds.), *Socioeconomic Impacts. 1993 National Earthquake Conference* (pp. 19–68). Memphis: Central United States Earthquake Consortium.

Jones, S. (1999). Religious "memorial" tiles rejected at Columbine. *Cybercast News Service,* October 5, http://www.cnsnews.com/ViewReligion.asp?Page=%5 Creligion%5 Carchive%5CREL19991005a.html.

Jonnes, J. (2004). New York unplugged 1889. *The New York Times,* August 13, 2004.

Jordan, M.H., Hollowed, K.A., Turner, D.G., Wang, D.S., & Jeng, J.C. (2005). The Pentagon attack of September 11, 2001: A burn center's experience. *Journal of Burn Care and Rehabilitation, 26,* 109–116.

Joy, B. (2000). Why the future doesn't need us. *Wired, 8,* 238–262.

Kafi, S.A. (1992). *Disaster and destitute women: Twelve case studies.* Dhaka: Disaster Resource Unit, Bangladesh Development Partnership Centre.

Kahn, J. (2005). China to shed secrecy over its natural disasters. *The New York Times,* September 12, 2005, http://www.nytimes.com/2005/09/12/international/asia/12cnd–china.

Kaiser, R., Spiegel, P.B., Henderson, A.K., & Gerber, M.L. (2003). The application of geographic information systems and global positioning systems in humanitarian emergencies: Lessons learned, programme implications and future research. *Disasters 27*(2), 127–140.

Kamrava, A. (1996). *Understanding comparative politics. A framework for analysis.* London: Routledge.

Kaniasty, K., & Norris, F.H. (1993). A test of the social support deterioration model in the context of natural disaster. *Journal of Personality and Social Psychology, 64,* 395–408.

Kaniasty, K., & Norris, F.H. (1994). *Social support from family and friends following catastrophic events: The role of cultural factors.* Paper presented at the 7th International Conference on Personal Relationships, Groningen, Netherlands.

Kaniasty, K., & Norris, F.H. (1995). In search of altruistic community: Patterns of social support mobilization following Hurricane Hugo. *American Journal of Community Psychology, 23,* 447–477.

Kanihan, S.F., & Gae, K.L. (2003). Within 3 hours, 97 percent learn about 9/11 attacks. *Newspaper Research Journal, 24*(1), 89.

Kano, M. (2005). Characteristics of earthquake-related injuries treated in emergency departments following the 2001 Nisqually earthquake in Washington. *Journal of Emergency Management, 3,* 33–45.

Kano, M., Siegel, J.M., & Bourque, L.B. (2005). First-aid training and capabilities of the lay public: A potential alternative source of emergency medical assistance following a natural disaster. *Disasters, 29,* 58–74.

Kaplan, A. (1964). *The conduct of inquiry.* San Francisco: Chandler Press.

Kario, K., & Ohashi, T. (1997). Increased coronary heart disease mortality after the Hanshin-Awaji earthquake among the older community on Awaji Island. *Journal of the American Geriatrics Society, 45,* 610–613.

Kartez, J. (1991). Problems and alternatives in the disaster assistance system. In *A study on improving earthquake mitigation (draft).* Washington, DC: Federal Emergency Management Agency.

Kartez, J., & Faupel, C. (1994). Comprehensive hazard management and the role of cooperation between local planning departments and emergency management offices. Unpublished paper.

Kasperson, J., & Kasperson, R. (Eds.). (2005). *The social contours of risk: Risk communication and the social amplification of risk.* New York: Earthscan.

Kasperson, R., Kasperson, J., & Dow, K. (2001). Vulnerability, equity, and global environmental change. In J. Kasperson & R. Kasperson (Eds.), *Global environmental risk* (pp. 247–272). New York: United Nations University Press.

Kasperson, R., Renn, O., Slovic, P., Brown, H., Eemel, J., Goble, A., et al. (1988). The social amplification of risk: A conceptual framework. *Risk Analysis, 8,* 177–187.

Kates, R.W. (1970). Human adjustment to earthquake. In Committee on the Alaska Earthquake of the National Research Council (Eds.), *The great Alaska earthquake of 1964: Human ecology* (pp. 7–31). Washington, DC: National Academy Press.

Kates, R.W. (1977). Major insights: A summary and recommendations. In E.J. Haas, R.W. Kates, & M.J. Bowden (Eds.), *Reconstruction following disaster* (pp. 261–293). Cambridge, MA: MIT Press.

Kates, R.W. (1985). The interaction of climate and society, In R.W. Kates, J.H. Ausubel, & M. Berberian (Eds.), *Climate impact assessment.* New York: Wiley.

Kates, R., & Pijawka, D. (1977). From rubble to monument: The pace of reconstruction. In J.E. Haas, E. Kates, & M. Bowden (Eds.), *Reconstruction following disaster* (pp. 1–23). Cambridge, MA: MIT Press.

Keenan, P.B. (1998). Spatial decision support systems for vehicle routing. *Decision Support Systems, 22*(1), 64–71.

Keipel, K., & Tyson, J. (2002). Planificacion y proteccion financiera para sobrevivir desastres, Washington, DC: Banco Inter-Americano de Desarrollo, ENV-139.

Kelly, C., & Chowdhury, M.H.K. (2005). *Poverty, disasters and the environment in Bangladesh: A quantitative and qualitative assessment of causal linkages.* DFID Bangladesh Issues Paper.

Kendra, J., & Wachtendorf, T. (2003a). Reconsidering convergence and converger legitimacy in response to the World Trade Center disaster. *Research in Social Problems and Public Policy, 11*, 97–122.

Kendra, J., & Wachtendorf, T. (2003b). Elements of community resilience in the World Trade Center attack: Reconstituting New York City's emergency operations center *Disasters, 27*(1), 37–53.

Kendra, J., & Wachtendorf, T. (2003c). Creativity in emergency response to the World Trade Center disaster. In Natural Hazards Research and Applications Information Center, Public Entity Risk Institute, and Institute for Civil Infrastructure Systems (Eds.), *Beyond September 11th: An account of post-disaster research, No. 39* (pp. 121–146). Special Publication. Boulder, CO: Natural Hazards Research and Applications Information Center, University of Colorado.

Kendra, J., & Wachtendorf, T. (2004). Creativity and coordination in disaster response. In *Proceedings of the 4th Workshop for Comparative Study on Urban Earthquake Disaster Management,* Kobe, Japan. January 29–30, 2004, pp. 73–86.

Kendra, J., & Wachtendorf, T. (In preparation). *The waterborne evacuation of lower Manhattan on September 11: A case of distributed sensemaking.*

Kendra, J., Wachtendorf, T., & Quarantelli, E. (2002). Who was in charge of the massive evacuation of lower Manhattan by water transport on September 11? No one was, yet it was an extremely successful operation. Implications? *Securitas, 1*, 3–5.

Kendra, J., Wachtendorf, T., & Quarantelli, E. (2003). The evacuation of lower Manhattan by water transport on September 11: An unplanned success. *Joint Commission of Quality and Safety, 29*, 316–318.

Kent, R.C. (1987). *Anatomy of disaster relief: The international network in action.* London: Pinter Publishers.

Khondker, H.H. (1996). Women and floods in Bangladesh. *International Journal of Mass Emergencies and Disasters, 14*(3), 281–292.

Khondker, H.H. (2002). Problems and prospects of disaster research in the developing world: A case study of Bangladesh. In R.A. Stallings (Ed.), *Methods of disaster research* (pp. 334–348). Philadelphia: Xlibris.

Khong, Y.F. (1992). *Analogies at war: Korea, Munich, Dien Bien Phu, and the Vietnam decisions of 1965.* Princeton: Princeton University Press.

Kilijanek, T.S., & Drabek, T.E. (1979). Assessing long-term impacts of a natural disaster: A focus on the elderly. *The Gerontologist, 19*, 555–566.

Killian, L.M. (1954). Some accomplishments and some needs in disaster study. *Journal of Social Issues, 10*, 66–72.

Killian, L.M. (1994). Are social movements irrational or are they collective behavior? In R. Dynes, & K. Tierney (Eds.), *Disasters, collective behavior and social organization* (pp. 273–280). Newark, DE: University of Delaware Press.

Killian, L.M. (2002). An introduction to the methodological problems of field studies in disasters. In R. A. Stallings (Ed.), *Methods of disaster research* (pp. 49–93). Philadelphia: Xlibris.

King, D. (2004). Understanding the message: Social and cultural constraints to interpreting weather generated natural hazards. *International Journal of Mass Emergencies and Disasters, 22*(1), 57–74.

King, L., & McCarthy, D. (2005). (Eds.), *Environmental sociology: From analysis to action.* New York: Rowman-Littlefield.

Kingdon, J.W. (1984). *Agendas, alternatives and public policies.* Boston: Little, Brown.

Kirby, A. (Ed.) (1990). *Nothing to fear: Risks and hazards in American society.* Tucson, AZ: The University of Arizona Press.

Kirschenbaum, L., Keene, A., O'Neill, P., & Astiz, M.E. (2005). The experience at St. Vincent's Hospital, Manhattan, on September 11, 2001: Preparedness, response, and lessons learned. *Critical Care Medicine, 33* (Suppl.), S48–S52.

Kitch, C. (2003). Mourning in America: Ritual, redemption and recovery in news narrative after September 11. *Journalism Studies, 4*(2), 213–224.

Kitz, J. (1989). *Shattered city: The Halifax explosion and the road to recovery.* Halifax: Nimbus Press.

Klein, G. (2001). *Sources of power: How people make decisions* (7th ed.). London: MIT Press.

Klein, N. (2005). The rise of disaster capitalism. *The Nation, 280*(17), 9–11.

Kleindorfer, P.R., Belke, J.C., Elliott, M.R., Lee, K., Lowe R.A., & Feldman, H.I. (2003). Accident epidemiology and the U.S. chemical industry: Accident history and worst-case data from risk management program info. *Risk Analysis, 23*, 865–881.

Klinenberg, E. (2002). *Heat wave: A social autopsy of disaster in Chicago.* Chicago: The University of Chicago Press.

Kloner, R.A., Leor, J.U., Poole, W.K., & Perritt, R. (1997). Population-based analysis of the effect of the Northridge earthquake on cardiac death in Los Angeles County. *California Journal of the American College of Cardiology, 30,* 1174–1180.

Klonglan, G.E., Beal, G.M., Bohlen, J.M., & Shaffer, T.G. (1964). *Local civil defence directors attitudes, opinions, knowledge, and activities, 1962. Rural Sociology Report No. 29.* Ames, IA: Iowa State University.

Koerner, B. (2003). In computer security, a bigger reason to squirm. *The New York Times,* September 5, 2003.

Kohiyama, M., Kroehl, H.W., Elvidge, C.D., Hobson, V.R., Hayashi, H., Maki, et al. (2004). Early damaged area estimation system using DMSP-OLS night-time imagery. *International Journal of Remote Sensing, 25*(11), 2015–2036.

Kopala, M., & Keitel, M.A. (1998). Groups for traumatic stress disorders. In K.C. Stoiber & T.R. Kratochwill (Eds.), *Handbook of group intervention for children and families.* Boston: Allyn and Bacon.

Koppe, C., Kovats, S., Jendritzky, G., & Menne, B. (2004). *Heat waves: Risks and responses.* Denmark: World Health Organization.

Kory, D.N. (1998). Coordinating intergovernmental policies on emergency management in a multi-centered metropolis. *International Journal of Mass Emergencies and Disasters, 16,* 45–54.

Kouznetsov, B. (2005). *"Ona utonula … ": Pravda o "Kurske", Kotoruyu Skril Genprokuror Ustinov. (Zapiski advokata). ("It sank … ": The Truth About Kursk Hidden by the General Prosecutor Ustinov. (The Lawyer's Notes).* Moscow: De Facto.

Kouzmin, A., Jarman, A.M.G., & Rosenthal, U. (1995). Interorganizational policy processes in disaster management. *Disaster Prevention and Management: An International Journal, 4,* 20–37.

Kratzer, R.M., & Kratzer, B. (2003). How newspapers decided to Run disturbing 9/11 photos. *Newspaper Research Journal, 21*(1), Winter 2003, AEJMC.

Krenz, G. (2001). Failure is not an option: Mission control from mercury to Apollo 13 and beyond, Thorndike paperback bestsellers.

Kreps, G.A. (1978). The organization of disaster response: Some fundamental theoretical issues. In E.L. Quarantelli (Ed.), *Disasters: Theory and research* (pp. 65–87). London: SAGE.

Kreps, G.A. (1981). The worth of the NAS-NRC and DRC studies of individual and social responses to disasters. In J.D. Wright & P. Rossi (Eds.), *Social science and natural hazards* (pp. 91–122). Cambridge, MA: Abt Books.

Kreps, G.A. (1984). Sociological inquiry and disaster research. *Annual Review of Sociology, 10,* 309–330.

Kreps, G.A. (1985). Disaster and the social order. *Sociological Theory, 3,* 49–65.

Kreps, G.A. (1989a). Description, taxonomy, and explanation in disaster research. *International Journal of Mass Emergencies and Disasters, 7,* 277–280.

Kreps, G.A. (1989b). Disaster and the social order. In G.A. Kreps (Ed.), *Social structure and disaster* (pp. 31–51). Newark, DE: University of Delaware Press.

Kreps, G.A., Ed. (1989c). *Social structure and disaster.* Newark, London, and Toronto: University of Delaware and Associated University Presses.

Kreps, G.A. (1990). The federal emergency management system in the United States: A research assessment. *International Journal of Mass Emergencies and Disasters, 8,* 275–300.

Kreps, G.A. (1991a). Answering organizational questions: A brief for structural codes. In G. Miller (Ed.), *Studies in organizational sociology* (pp. 143–177). Greenwich, CT: JAI Press.

Kreps, G.A. (1991b). Organizing for emergency management. In T.E. Drabek & G.J. Hoetmer (Eds.), *Emergency management: Principles and practice for local government* (pp. 30–54). Washington, DC: International City Management Association.

Kreps, G.A. (1994). Disaster archives and structural analysis: Uses and limitations. In R.R. Dynes & K.J. Tierney (Eds.), *Disaster, collective behavior, and social organization* (pp. 45–71). Newark, Toronto, and London: University of Delaware and Associated University Presses.

Kreps, G. (1995). Disaster as systemic event and social catalyst: A clarification of the subject matter. *International Journal of Mass Emergencies and Disasters, 13*(3), 255–284.

Kreps, G.A. (1998). Disaster as systemic event and social catalyst: A clarification of subject matter. In E.L. Quarantelli, (Ed.), *What is a disaster: Perspectives on the question* (pp. 31–55). New York and London: Routledge.

Kreps, G.A. (2001). Disasters, sociology of. In N. Smelser & P. Bates (Eds.), *International encyclopedia of the social and behavioral sciences* (vol. 6, pp. 3719–2721). Oxford, UK: Elsevier.

Kreps, G.A., & Bosworth, S.L. (1993). Disaster, organizing, and role enactment: A structural approach. *American Journal of Sociology, 99,* 428–63.

Kreps, G.A., & Bosworth, S.L. (1994). *Organizing, role enactment and disaster: A structural theory.* Newark, Toronto, and London: University of Delaware and Associated University Presses.

Kreps, G.A., & Drabek, T.E. (1996). Disasters are non-routine social problems. *International Journal of Mass Emergencies and Disasters, 14*, 129–153.

Kroll-Smith, S., & Couch, S. (1991). *The real disaster is above ground: A mine fire and social conflict.* Lexington: University of Kentucky Press.

Kroll-Smith, S. & Gunter, V. (1998). Legislators, interpreters and disasters. In E.L. Quarantelli (Ed.), *What is a disaster: Perspectives on the question* (pp. 160–176). London: Routledge.

Krugman, P. (2002). Digital robber barons? *The New York Times,* December 6, 2002.

Kueneman, R.M., & J.E. Wright (1975). New policies of broadcast stations for civil disturbances and disasters. *Journalism Quarterly, 52*(4), 670–677.

Kuhn, T. (1970). Reflections on my critics. In I. Lakatos & A. Musgrave (Eds.), *Criticism and the growth of knowledge* (pp. 231–278). Cambridge, UK: Cambridge University Press.

Kumar, K. (1995). Apocalypse, millenium and utopia today. In M. Bull, (Ed.), *Apocalypse theory and the ends of the world.* Oxford: Blackwell.

Kunii, O., Akagi, M., & Kita, E. (1995). The medical and public health response to the great Hanshin-Awaji earthquake in Japan: A case study in disaster planning. *Medicine and Global Survival, 2*(4), 214–226.

Kunkle, R.F. (1989). Medical care of entrapped patients in confined spaces. *Proceedings of the workshop on earthquake epidemiology* (pp. 338–344), Baltimore: Johns Hopkins University Press.

Kunreuther, H. (1973). *Recovery from natural disasters: Insurance or federal Aid?* Washington, DC: American Enterprise Institute for Public Policy.

Kunreuther, H. (1996). Mitigating disaster losses through insurance. *Journal of Risk and Uncertainty, 12*, 171–187.

Kunreuther, H. (1997). Rethinking society's management of catastrophic risks. *Geneva Papers on Risk and Insurance 83*, 151–176.

Kunreuther, H. (1998). Insurability conditions and the supply of coverage. In H. Kunreuther & R.J. Roth (Eds.), *Paying the price: The status and role of insurance against natural disasters in the United States* (pp. 17–50). Washington, DC: Joseph Henry Press.

Kunreuther, H., & Heal, G. (2003). Interdependent security. *Journal of Risk and Uncertainty, 26*, 231–249.

Kunreuther, H., & Michel-Kerjan, E. (2004). Policy watch: New challenges for terrorism risk coverage in the US. *Journal of Economic Perspectives, 18*, 201–214.

Kunreuther, H. & Rose, A. (Eds.). (2004). *The economics of natural hazards.* Cheltenham: Elgar.

Kunreuther, H., & Roth, A. (Eds.). (1998). *Paying the price: The status and role of insurance against natural disasters in the United States.* Washington, DC: National Academy Press.

Kurtz, R.S., & Browne, W.P. (2004). Crisis management, crisis response: An introduction to the symposium. *Review of Policy Research, 21*, 141–143.

Kuwata, Y., & Takada, S. (2002). Instantaneous instrumental seismic intensity and evacuation. *Journal of Natural Disaster Science, 24*, 24–35.

Lachman, R., Tatsuoka, M., & Bonk, W. (1961). Human behavior during the tsunami of May, 1960. *Science, 133*, 1405–1409.

LaCorte, R. (2005). Barren ground at Mount St. Helens reawakens. *Wilmington News Journal*, May 15, 2005.

Lagadec, P. (1993). *Preventing chaos in a crisis: Strategies for prevention, control and damage limitation* (J.M. Phelps, Trans.). New York: McGraw-Hill.

Lagadec, P. (1997). Learning processes for crisis management in complex organizations. *Journal of Contingencies and Crisis Management, 5*, 24–31.

Lagadec, P. (2000). *Ruptures creatrics.* Paris: Editions d'Organisation.

Lagadec, P. (2004). Understanding the French 2003 heat wave experience: Beyond the heat, a multi-layered challenge. *Journal of Contingencies and Crisis Management, 12, 160–169.*

Lagadec, P. (2005). Crossing the Rubicon. *Crisis Response, 1*, 38–41.

Lagadec, P., & Guilhou, X. (2002). *La fin du risque zero.* Paris: Eyrolles.

Lagadec, P., & Michel-Kerjan, E. (2006, Forthcoming). A framework for senior executives to meet the challenge of interdependent critical networks under threats: In Auerswald, Branscomb, LaPorte, & Michel-Kerjan (Eds.), *Protecting critical infrastructure. Private efficiency, public Vulnerability.* Cambridge, UK: Cambridge University Press.

Lagadec, P., & Rosenthal, U. (Eds.). (2003). Anthrax and beyond: New challenges, new responsibilities. *Journal of Contingencies and Crisis Management, Special Issue, 11*, 97–98.

Laird, R. (1991). *Ethnography of a disaster.* Unpublished MA Thesis. San Francisco: San Francisco State University.

Lake, R.W. (1980). Racial transition and Black homeownership in American suburbs. In G. Sternlieb & J.W. Hughes (Eds.), *America's housing* (pp. 419–438). New Brunswick, NJ: Center for Urban Policy Research.

Lang, B. (1985). Non-semitic deluge stories and the Book of Genesis. A bibliographic and critical survey. *Anthropos, 80*, 605–616.

Lang, G.E., & Lang, K. (1980). Newspaper and TV archives: Some thoughts about research on disaster news. In *Disasters and the mass media* (pp. 269–280). Washington, DC: The National Research Council.

Lanza, L., & Siccardi, F. (1995). The role of GIS as a tool for the assessment of flood hazard at the regional scale. In A. Carrara & F. Guzzetti (Eds.), *Geographical information systems in assessing natural hazards* (pp. 199–217). Dordrecht: Kluwer Academic.

LaPlante, J.M., & Kroll-Smith, J.S. (1989). Coordinated emergency management: The challenge of the chronic technological disaster. *International Journal of Mass Emergencies and Disasters, 7*, 134–150.

Larabee, A. (2003). Empire of fear: Imagined community and the September 11 attacks. *Research in Social Problems and Public Policy, 11*, 19–31.

Lasora, D. (2003). News media Perpetuate Few Rumors About 9/11 Crisis. *Newspaper Research Journal, 24*(1), 10–21.

Lateef, N.V. (1982). *Crisis in the Sahel: A case study in development cooperation*. Boulder, CO: Westview Press.

La Trobe, S. (2005). Tearfund. *International Journal of Mass Emergencies and Disasters, 23*(1), 141–160.

Lavell, A. (1999). *The impact of disasters on development gains: Clarity or controversy*. Paper presented at the International Decade for Natural Disasters Reduction Programme Forum, Geneva, July 5–9, 1999.

Lavell, A. (2002). *Local level risk management. Concepts and experience in Central America*. Paper presented at the Disaster Preparedness and Mitigation Summit, November 21–23, 2002. New Delhi, India.

Lavell, A. (2003). The Lower Lempa River Valley, El Salvador: From risk to Sustainability. Experience with a risk reduction project. In G. Bankoff, G. Frerks, & T. Hilhorst (Eds.), *Mapping vulnerability: Disasters, development and people*. London: Earthscan.

Law Commission. (1991). *Final report on emergencies*. Report No. 22. Wellington: New Zealand Law Commission.

Laye, J. (2002). *Avoiding disaster: How to keep your business going when catastrophe strikes*. Hoboken, NJ: Wiley.

Lazerson, M. (1988). Organizational growth of small firms: An outcome of markets and hierarchies? *American Sociological Review 53*, 330–342.

Lazerson, M., & Lorenzoni, G. (1999). The networks that feed industrial districts: A return to the Italian source. *Industrial and Corporate Change, 8*, 235–266.

Lebow, R.N. (1981). *Between peace and war: The nature of international crisis*. Baltimore: Johns Hopkins University Press.

Lechat, M.F. (1976). The epidemiology of disasters. Section of epidemiology and community medicine. *Proceedings of the Royal Society of Medicine, 69*, 421–426.

Lechat, M.F. (1989). *Corporal damage as related to building structure and design. The need for an international survey*. Unpublished manuscript.

Ledingham, J.A., & Masel Walters, L. (1989). The sound and fury: Mass media and hurricanes. In L. Masel Walters, L. Wilkins, & T. Walters (Eds.), *Bad tidings communications and catastrophe* (pp. 43). Hillsdale: Lawrence Erlbaum and Associates.

Leik, R.K., Carter, T.M., & Clark J.P., et al. (1981). *Community response to natural hazard warnings: Final report*. Minneapolis, Minnesota: University of Minnesota.

Lenski, G., Lenski, J., & Nolan, P. (1991). *Human societies: An introduction to macrosociology*. New York: McGraw-Hill.

Leor, J., Poole, W.K., & Kloner, R.A. (1996). Sudden cardiac death triggered by an earthquake. *The New England Journal of Medicine, 334*, 413–419.

Lerner, J.S., & Keltner, D. (2001). Fear, anger, and risk. *Journal of Personality and Social Psychology, 81*(1), 146–159.

Levi, D., & Lawn, M. (1993). The driving and restraining forces which affect technological innovations in organizations. *The Journal of High Technology Management Research, 4*, 225–240.

Levinthal, D., & March, J. (1981). A model of adaptive organizational search. *Journal of Economic Behavior and Organization, 2*, 307–333.

Levy, S. (2004). Net of control. *Newsweek*. Retrieved March 3, 2004, http://www.msnbc.msn. com/id/4439682/site/newsweek/.

Lewis, J. (1999). *Development in disaster-prone places*. IT Press.

Lewis, J., & Stearns, P.N. (Eds.). (1998). *An emotional history of the United States*. New York: New York University Press.

Lieberman, M.B. (1987). Market growth, economies of scale, and plant size in the chemical processing industries. *The Journal of Industrial Economics, 36*, 175–191.

Light, I., & Gold, S.J. (2000). *Ethnic economies*. San Diego: Academic Press.

Lindblom, C.E. (1959). The science of muddling through. *Public Administration Review, 19*, 79–88.

Lindell, M.K. (1994). Are local emergency planning committees effective in developing community disaster preparedness? *International Journal of Mass Emergencies and Disasters, 12*, 159–182.

Lindell, M.K. (1997). Adoption and implementation of hazards adjustments. *International Journal of Mass Emergencies and Disasters, 15*, 325–437.

Lindell, M., Bolton, P., Perry. R., Stoetzel, G., Martin, J., et al. (1985). *Planning concepts and decision criteria for sheltering and evacuation in a nuclear power plant emergency*. Bethesda, MD: Atomic Industrial Forum, Inc.

Lindell, M.K., & Perry, R.W. (1992). *Behavioral foundations of community emergency planning*. Washington, DC: Hemisphere.

Lindell, M.K., & Perry, R.W. (2000). Household adjustment to earthquake hazard, a review of research. *Environment and Behavior, 32*, 590–630.

Lindell, M.K., & Perry, R.W. (2001). Community innovation in hazardous materials management: Profess in implementing SARA Title III in the United States. *Journal of Hazardous Materials, 88*, 169–194.

Lindell, M.K., & Perry, R.W. (2004). *Communicating environmental risk in multiethnic communities*. Thousand Oaks, CA: SAGE.

Lindell, M.K., Perry, R., & Prater, C.S. (Forthcoming). *Emergency management: Principles and practices*. Hoboken, NJ: Wiley.

Lindell, M.K., & Prater, C.S. (2003). Assessing community impacts of natural disasters. *Natural Hazards Review, 4*, 176–185.

Lindell, M.K., Whitney, D.J., Futch, C.J., & Clause, C.S. (1996a). Multi-method assessment of organizational effectiveness in a local emergency planning committee. *International Journal of Mass Emergencies and Disasters, 14*, 195–220.

Lindell, M.K., Whitney, D.J., Futch, C.J., & Clause, C.S. (1996b). The local emergency planning committee: A better way to coordinate disaster planning. In R.T. Sylves & W.L. Waugh, Jr. (Eds.), *Disaster management in the U.S. and Canada: The politics, policymaking, administration and analysis of emergency management* (pp. 274–295). Springfield, IL: Charles C Thomas.

Linn, J.R., & Kreps, G.A. (1989). Disaster and the restructuring of organization. In G.A. Kreps (Ed.), *Social structure and disaster* (pp. 108–135). Newark, Toronto, and London: University of Delaware and Associated University Presses.

Linz, J.J., & Stepan, A.C. (1978). (Eds.). *The breakdown of democratic regimes*. Baltimore: Johns Hopkins University Press.

Logan, J. & Molotch, H. (1987). *Urban fortunes: The political economy of place*. Berkeley, CA: University of California Press.

Lombardi, M. (2002). Media studies. In R.A., Stallings (Ed.), *Methods of disaster research* (pp. 251–265). International Research Committee on Disasters.

Lorber, J. (1998). *Gender inequality: Feminist theories and politics*. Los Angeles: Roxbury.

Loseke, D.R. (1999). *Thinking about social problems: An introduction to constructionists perspectives*. Hawthorne, NY: Aldine De Gruyter.

Lovekamp, W. (Forthcoming). Gender and disaster: A synthesis of flood research in Bangladesh. In B. Phillips & B.H. Morrow (Eds.), *Women and disasters*. Philadelphia: Xlibris.

Lowe, S., & Fothergill, A. (2003). A need to help: Emergent volunteer behavior after September 11th. In J.L. Monday (Ed.), *Beyond September 11th: An account of post-disaster research* (pp. 293–314). Boulder, CO: University of Colorado, Institute of Behavioral Science, Natural Hazards Research and Applications Information Center, Special Publication No. 39.

Lowenstein, R. (2004). *When genius fails*. New York: Random House.

Luna, E.M. (2000). *NGO natural disaster mitigation and preparedness: The Philippine case study*. Report prepared for NGO natural disaster mitigation and preparedness projects: An assessment and way forward. ESCOR Award R7231, http://www.benfieldhrc.org/disaster_studies/ngo_intiatives/ngo_ini_risk_red_index.htm.

MacDougall, C. (1982). *Interpretative reporting*. New York: Macmillan.

Macrae, J. (1998). Purity or political engagement?: Issues in food and health security interventions in complex political emergencies. *The Journal of Humanitarian Assistance*. Retrieved June 3, 2000, http://www.jha.ac/articles/a037.htm.

Macrae, J. & Zwi, A. (Eds.). (1994). *War and hunger: Rethinking international approaches to complex emergencies*. London and New Jersey: Zed Books.

Mader, G.G., Spangle, W.E. , & Blair, M.L. (1980). *Land use planning after earthquakes*. Portola Valley, CA: William Spangle and Associates, Inc.

Mahue-Giangreco, M., Mack, W., Seligson, H., & Bourque, L.B. (2001). Risk factors associated with moderate and serious injuries attributable to the 1994 Northridge earthquake, Los Angeles, California. *Annals of Epidemiology, 2001*, 347–357.

Major, A.M. (1999). Gender differences in risk and communication behavior: Responses to the New Madrid earthquake prediction. *International Journal of Mass Emergencies and Disasters, 17*(3), 313–338.

Mallonee, S., Shariat, S., Stennies, G., Waxweiler, R., Hogan, D., & Jordan, F. (1996). Physical injuries and fatalities resulting from the Oklahoma City bombing. *Journal of the American Medical Association, 276*, 382–387.

Mann, M. (1997). Has globalization ended the rise of the nation-state? *Review of International Political Economy, 4*, 472–496.

Mansoob, M. (Ed.). (2002). *Globalization, marginalization and development.* London: Routledge.

Marshall, B., Picou, J., & Gill, D. A. (2003). Terrorism as disaster: Selected commonalities and long–term recovery for 9/11 survivors. *Research in Social problems and Public Policy, 11*, 73–96.

Martindale, D. (1979). Ideologies, paradigms and theories. In W. Snizek, E. Fuhrman, & M. Miller (Eds.), *Contemporary issues in theory and research* (pp. 7–24). Westport, CT: Greenwood Press.

Maskrey, A. (1989). *Disaster mitigation: A community based approach.* Oxford: Oxfam Disaster and Development.

Maskrey, A. (1993). *Los Desastros No Son Naturales.* Bogota: La Red/ITDG.

Maskrey, A. (1994). Disaster mitigation as a crisis of paradigms: Reconstruction after the Alto Mayo earthquake, Peru. In A. Varley (Ed.), *Disaster, development and environment.* Chichester, UK: Wiley.

Massard-Guilbaud, G., Platt, H., & Schott, D. (Eds.). (2002). *Cities and catastrophes: Coping with emergency in European history.* Frankfurt: Peter Lang.

Massey, D.D., & Denton, N.A. (1993). *American apartheid: Segregation and the making of the underclass.* Cambridge, MA: Harvard University Press.

Masterman, M. (1970). The nature of a paradigm. In I. Lakatos & A. Musgrave (Eds.), *Criticism and the growth of knowledge* (pp. 58–89). Cambridge, UK: Cambridge University Press.

May, P.J. (1985). *Recovering from catastrophes: Federal disaster relief policy and politics.* Westport, CT: Greenwood Press.

May, P.J. (1994). Analyzing mandate design: State mandates governing hazard prone areas. *The Journal of Federalism, 24*, 1–16.

May, P.J., & Deyle, R.E. (1998). Governing land use in hazardous areas with a patchwork system. In R. Burby (Ed.), *Cooperating with nature: Confronting natural hazards with land-use planning for sustainable communities* (pp. 57–82). Washington, DC: Joseph Henry Press.

May, P.J., Burby, R.J., Ericksen, N.J., Handmer, J.W., Dixon, J.E., Michaels, S. et al. (1996). *Environmental management and governance: Intergovernmental approaches to hazards and sustainability.* London: Routledge.

May, P.J., & Williams, W. (1986). *Disaster policy implementation: Managing programs under shared governance.* New York and London: Plenum Press.

Mayhorn, C. (2004). Emerging issues in risk communication: Older adults and information processing of hazard warnings, Research abstract R04–21. Boulder Hazards Workshop. Boulder, CO: Natural Hazard Center, University of Colorado. http://www.colorado.edu/hazards/workshop/.

McAdam, D., McCarthy, J.D., & Zald, M.N. (1996). *Comparative perspectives on social movements.* Melbourne: Cambridge University Press.

McAneney, J. (2005). December 26, 2004 Sumatra earthquake and tsunami. *Risk Frontiers Newsletter, 1*, 3.

McConnell, A. (2003). Overview: Crisis management, influences, responses and evaluation. *Parliamentary Affairs, 56*, 363–409.

McDonnell, S., Troiano, R.P., Barker, N., Noji, E., Hlady, W.G., & Hopkins, R. (1995). Long-term effects of Hurricane Andrew: Revisiting mental health indicators. *Disasters, 19*, 235–246.

McEntire, D.A. (1997). Reflecting on the weaknesses of the international community during the IDNDR: Some implications for research and its application. *Disaster Prevention and Management, 6*(4), 221–233.

McEntire, D.A. (1998a). Pendulum policies and the need for relief and invulnerable development. *International Journal of Mass Emergencies and Disasters, 16*(2), 213–216.

McEntire, D.A. (1998b). *Towards a theory of coordination: Umbrella organization and disaster relief in the 1997–98 Peruvian el niño disaster.* Quick Response Report No. 105. Boulder, CO: University of Colorado.

McEntire, D.A. (1999). Correspondence. In N. Middleton & P.O'Keefe (Eds.), *Disaster and development: The politics of humanitarian aid* (pp.78–79). London: Pluto Press.

McEntire, D.A. (2000). *Sustainability or invulnerable development? Justifications for a modified disaster reduction concept and policy guide.* Ph.D. dissertation. Denver, CO: University of Denver.

McEntire, D.A. (2001a). The Internationalization of emergency management: Challenges and opportunities facing an expanding profession. *International Association of Emergency Managers Bulletin*, October, 3–4.

McEntire, D.A. (2001b). Multi-organizational coordination during the response to the March 28, 2000, Fort Worth tornado: An assessment of constraining and contributing factors. Quick Response Report No. 143. Boulder, CO: Natural Hazards Research and Applications Information Center.

McEntire, D.A. (2003). Causation of catastrophe: lessons from hurricane Georges. *Journal of Emergency Management,* *1*(2), 22–29.

McEntire, D.A. (2004a). *The status of emergency management theory.* Paper presented at the FEMA Higher Education Conference, Emmitsburg, MD.

McEntire, D.A. (2004b). Tenets of vulnerability: an assessment of a fundamental disaster concept. *Journal of Emergency Management,* *2*(2), 23–29.

McEntire, D.A., Fuller, C., Johnson, C.W., & Weber, R. (2002). A comparison of disaster paradigms: The search for a holistic policy guide. *Public Administration Review, 62*(3), 267–281.

McEntire, D.A., & Myers, A. (2004). Preparing communities for disasters: issues and processes for government readiness. *Disaster Prevention and Management, 13*(2), 140–152.

McEntire, D., Robinson, R.J., & Weber, R.T. (2003). Business responses to the world trade center disaster: A study of corporate roles, functions, and interaction with the public sector. In J.L. Monday (Ed.), *Beyond September 11th: An account of post-disaster research* (pp. 431–457). Boulder, CO: University of Colorado, Institute of Behavioral Science, Natural Hazards Research and Applications Information Center, Special Publication No. 39.

McGuigan, J. (1992). *Cultural populism.* London: Routledge.

McGuire, W. (2000). *Apocalypse.* London: Blanford.

McIntosh, N. (1989). *Lockerbie: A local authority responds to disaster.* Dumfries: Dumfries and Galloway Regional Council.

McIntyre, M. (2002). The coproduction of race and class in Brazil and the United States. *Antipode, 34*(2), 168–175.

McKean, J., Buechel S., & Gaydos L. (1991). Remote sensing and landslide hazard assessment. *Photogrammetric Engineering and Remote Sensing, 57*(9), 1185–1193.

McKenna, M.A.J. (2005). Deadly 1918 flu reborn for study. *Atlanta Journal-Constitution* (October 6), pp. A1, A12.

McLean, B., & Elkind P. (2003). *The smartest guys in the room; The amazing rise and scandalous fall of Enron.* New York: Penguin Group.

McLean, I., & Johnes, M. (2000). *Aberfan; Government & disasters.* Cardiff: Welsh Academic Press.

McLuckie, B.F. (1970). *The study of three functional responses to stress in three cities.* Ph.D. dissertation. Ohio: Ohio State University.

McMillen, J.C., North, C.S., & Smith, E.M. (2000). What parts of PTSD are normal: Intrusion, avoidance, or arousal? Data from the Northridge, CA earthquake. *Journal of Traumatic Stress, 13,* 57–75.

Mechler, R. (2003). Natural disaster risk and cost–benefit analysis. In A. Kreimer, M. Arnold & A. Carlin. *Building safer cities: The future of disaster risk* (pp. 45–56). Washington, DC: World Bank, Disaster Management Facility.

Medvedev, G. (1991). *The truth about Chernobyl.* New York: Basic Books.

Meli, R. (1989). Modes of failure of buildings under seismic actions. In *Proceedings of the Workshop on Earthquake Injury Epidemiology* (pp. 366–377). Baltimore: John Hopkins University Press.

Melley, T. (2000). *Empire of conspiracy; The culture of paranoia in postwar America.* Ithaca, NY: Cornell University Press.

Mendonca, D. (2001). *Improvisation in emergency response organizations: A cognitive approach.* Ph.D. dissertation. Rensselaer Polytechnic Institute. Ann Arbor MI: UMI Dissertation Services.

Mendonca, D. (Forthcoming). Decision support for improvisation in response to extreme events: Learning from the response to the 2001 World Trade Center attack. *Decision Support Systems.*

Mendonca, D., Lee, E.E. II, & Wallace, W.A. (2004). Impact of the 2001 World Trade Center attack on critical interdependent infrastructures. In *Proceedings of the IEEE International Conference on Systems, Man, and Cybernetics* (vol. 5, 4053–4058).

Mendonca, D., & Wallace, W.A. (2002). Development of a decision logic to support improvisation: An application to emergency response. *Hawaii International Conference on System Sciences,* HICSS-35, 220b-221.

Mendonca, D., & Wallace, W.A. (2004). Studying organizationally situated improvisations in response to extreme events. *International Journal of Mass Emergencies and Disasters, 22,* 5–31.

Menker, R.E., & Floren, T.M. (1986). White phosphorus ignites in the Miamisburg derailment. *Fire Command,* October, 30–34, 41.

Merchant, J.A., Baxter, P.L., Bernstein, R., McCawley, M., Falk, H., Stein, G., et al. (1982). Health implications of the Mount St. Helens' eruption: Epidemiological considerations. *Annals of Occupational Hygiene, 26,* 911–919.

Merrifield, A. (2000). General law of US capitalist accumulation: Contingent work and the working class. *Antipode, 32,* 176–198.

Merton, R.K. (1957). *Social theory and social structure.* New York: Free Press.

Meyer, A. (1982). Adapting to environmental jolts. *Administrative Science Quarterly, 27,* 515–537.

Meyer, M.W., & Zucker, L.G. (1989). *Permanently failing organizations.* Newbury Park, CA: SAGE.

Meyers, G.C., & Holusha, J. (1986). Managing crisis: A positive approach. London: Unwin.

Michaels, S. (2003). Perishable information, enduring insights? Understanding quick response research. In J.L. Monday (Ed.), *Beyond September 11th: An account of post-disaster research* (pp. 15–48). Boulder, CO: Natural Hazards Research and Applications Information Center.

Michel-Kerjan, E. (2003): New challenges in critical infrastructures: A U.S. perspective. *Journal of Contingencies and Crisis Management, 11*, 132–141.

Mikheev, V. (Ed.). (2005). *Kitai: Ugrozi, Riski, Vizovi Razvitiyu. (China: Threats, Risks and challenges to development).* Moscow: Carnegie Center.

Miles, S.B., & Chang, S.E. (2003). *Urban disaster recovery: A framework and simulation model* (Multidisciplinary Center for Earthquake Engineering Research. Technical Report no. MCEER-03-0005). Buffalo, NY.

Miles, S.B., & Chang, S.E. (2004). Foundations for modeling community recovery from earthquake disasters. In *Proceedings of the 13th World Conference on Earthquake Engineering*, Vancouver, Canada.

Mileti, D. (1975). *Natural hazard warnings systems in the United States*. Boulder, CO: Institute of Behavioral Science, University of Colorado.

Mileti, D. (1987). Sociological methods and disaster research. In R.R. Dynes, B. de Marchi, & C. Pelanda (Eds.), *Sociology of disasters: Contributions of sociology to disaster research* (pp. 57–69). Milan, Italy: Franco Angeli.

Mileti, D. (1999). *Disasters by design: A reassessment of natural hazards in the United States*. Washington, DC: Joseph Henry Press.

Mileti, D., & Beck, E.M. (1975). Communication in crisis: Explaining evacuation symbolically. *Communication Research, 2*, 24–49.

Mileti, D.S., Cress, D., & Darlington, J.D. (2002). Earthquake culture and corporate action. *Sociological Forum, 17*, 161–180.

Mileti, D., Drabek, T., & Haas, J. (1975). *Human systems in extreme environments, Monograph 21*. Boulder, CO: University of Colorado Institute of Behavioral Science.

Mileti, D., Nathe, S., Gori, P., Greene, M., & Lemersal, E. (2004). Public hazards communication and education: The state of the art. *The Hazards Center, University of Colorado–Boulder*. Retrieved October 3, 2005, http://www.colorado.edu/hazards/informer/informerupdate.pdf.

Mileti, D., & Sorensen, J. (1987). Determinants of organizational effectiveness in crisis. *Columbia University Journal of World Business, 12*, 13–21.

Mileti, D., & Sorensen, J. (1988). Planning and implementing warning systems. In M. Lystad (Ed.), *Mental health and care in mass emergencies: Theory and practice* (pp. 321–345). New York: Brunner/Mazel.

Mileti, D., & Sorenson, J. (1990). *Communication of emergency public warnings: A social science perspective and the state-of-the-art assessment, ORNL–6609*. Oak Ridge, TN: Oak Ridge National Laboratory, Department of Energy.

Mileti, D., Sorensen, J., & O'Brien, P. (1992). Towards an explanation of mass care shelter use in evacuations. *International Journal of Mass Emergencies and Disasters, 10*, 25–42.

Mileti, D.S., Cress, D.M., & Darlington, J.D. (1992). Earthquake culture and corporate action. *Sociological Forum, 17*(1), 161–180.

Mill, J.S. (1872 [1843]). *System of logic: Ratiocinative and inductive. Being a connected view of the principles of evidence and the methods of scientific investigation* (vol. 1, 8th ed.). London: Longmans, Green, Reader, & Dyer.

Miller, J. (1974). *Aberfan: A disaster and its aftermath*. London: Constable.

Millican, P. (1993). *Women in disaster*. Paper presented at the Symposium on Women in Emergencies and Disasters, Brisbane, Queensland.

Mills, C.W. (1959). *The sociological imagination*. New York: Oxford University Press.

Mills, C.W. (1963). The cultural apparatus. In I.L. Horowitz, (Ed.), *C. Wright Mills: Power, politics, and people* (pp. 405–422). New York: Ballantine Books.

Minear, L. (2002). *The humanitarian enterprise: Dilemmas and discoveries*. Bloomfield, CT.: Kumarian Press.

Minear, L. & Weiss, T.G. (1995). *Mercy under fire: War and the global humanitarian community*. Boulder, CO: Westview Press.

Mines, M., Thach, A., Mallonee, S., Hildebrand, L., & Shariat, S. (2000). Ocular injuries sustained by survivors of the Oklahoma City bombing. *Ophthalmology, 107*, 837–843.

Ministry of Civil Defense & Emergency Management (2002a). *Working together: Developing a CEM group plan: Director's guidelines for CDEM groups*. Wellington, New Zealand: Ministry of Civil Defense & Emergency Management.

Ministry of Civil Defense & Emergency Management (2002b). *Working together: The formation of CDEM groups: Director's guidelines for local authorities and emergency services*. Wellington, New Zealand: Ministry of Civil Defense & Emergency Management.

Ministry of Civil Defense & Emergency Management (2004). Resilient New Zealand (A Aotearoa manahau). *National civil defence emergency management strategy (2003–2006)*. Wellington, New Zealand: MCDEM.

Ministry of Civil Defence and Emergency Management. (2005a). *Recovery Management*. Wellington New Zealand: Ministry of Civil Defence and Emergency Management.

Ministry of Civil Defense and Emergency Management. (2005b). *Focus on Recovery: a holistic framework for recovery in New Zealand*. Wellington, New Zealand: Ministry of Civil Defence and Emergency Management.

Mitchell, J.K. (1990). Human dimensions of environmental hazards: Complexity, disparity, and the search for guidance. In A. Kirby (Ed.), *Nothing to fear: Risk and hazards in American society* (pp. 131–175). Tucson, AZ: University of Arizona Press.

Mitchell, J.K. (1999). *Crucibles of hazard: Mega-cities and disasters in transition*. New York: United Nations University Press.

Mitchell, J.K. (2003). The fox and the hedgehog: Myopia about homeland security in U.S. policies on terrorism. *Research in Social Problems and Public Policy, 11*, 53–72.

Mitchell, J.K. (2004). *Re-conceiving recovery*. Keynote address to the Recovery Symposium, Napier, New Zealand, July 12–13, 2004.

Mitchell, J.T., Thomas, D.S.K., Hill, A.A., & Cutter, S.L. (2000). Catastrophe in reel life versus real life: Perpetuating disaster myth through Hollywood films. *International Journal of Mass Emergencies and Disasters, 18*, 383–402.

Mitroff, I.I., & Pauchant, T.C. (1990). We're so big and powerful nothing bad can happen to us: An investigation of America's crisis prone corporations. Secaucus, NJ: Carol Publishing Group.

Mitroff, I.I., Pauchant T.C., Finney, M., & Pearson, C. (1989). Do (some) organizations cause their own crises? Cultural profiles of crisis prone versus crisis prepared organizations. *Industrial Crisis Quarterly, 3*, 269–283.

Miyano, M., Jian, L.H., & Mochizuki, T. (1991). Human casualty due to the Nankai earthquake tsunami, 1946. IUGG/IOC International Tsunami Symposium.

Monmonier, M. (1997). *Cartographies of danger: Mapping hazards in America*. Chicago, IL: The University of Chicago Press.

Moore, H.E. (1958). *Tornadoes over texas*. Austin: University of Texas Press.

Moore, H.E., Bates, F.L., Alston, J.P., Fuller, M.M., Layman, M.V., Mischer, D.L., et al. (1964). ... *and the Winds Blew*. Austin TX: The Hogg Foundation for Mental Health.

Moore, H.E., Bates, F.L., Layman, M.V., & Parenton, V.J. (1963). *Before the wind: A study of response to Hurricane Carla*. National Academy of Sciences/National Research Council Disaster Study No. 19. Washington, DC: National Academy Press.

Moran, C.C. (1990). Does the use of humor as a coping strategy affect stresses associated with emergency work? *International Journal of Mass Emergencies and Disasters, 8*, 361–377.

Morgan Stanley, Deutsche Bank. *Tokyo offices on quake unease*. Retrieved March 14, 2005, http://bloomberg.com.

Morris, P. (1998). *Weaving gender in disaster and refugee assistance*. Washington, DC: Interaction: American Council for Voluntary International Action.

Morrissey, M. (2004). Curriculum innovation for natural disaster reduction: Lessons from the commonwealth Caribbean. In J.P. Stoltman, J. Lidstone, & L.M. Dechano (Eds.), *International perspectives on natural disasters: Occurrence, mitigation and consequence* (pp. 385–396). Dordrecht: Kluwer.

Morrow, B.H. (1992). *The aftermath of Hugo: Social effects on St. Croix*. St. George's, Grenada: Caribbean Studies Association.

Morrow, B.H. (1997). Stretching the bonds: The families of Hurricane Andrew. In W.G. Peacock, B.H. Morrow, & H. Gladwin (Eds.), *Hurricane Andrew: Ethnicity, gender, and the sociology of disasters* (pp. 141–170). New York: Routledge.

Morrow, B. (1999). Identifying and mapping community vulnerability. *Disasters, 23*(1), 1–18.

Morrow, B.H., & Enarson, E. (1996). Hurricane Andrew through women's eyes: Issues and recommendations. *International Journal of Mass Emergencies and Disasters, 14*(1), 1–22.

Morrow, B.H., & Peacock, W.G. (1997). Disasters and social change: Hurricane Andrew and the reshaping of Miami? In W.G. Peacock, B.H. Morrow, & H. Gladwin (Eds.), *Hurricane Andrew: Ethnicity, gender and the sociology of Disasters* (pp. 226–242). New York: Routledge.

Morrow, B.H., & Phillips, B.D. (Guest Eds.). (1999). Special Issue: Women and disasters, *International Journal of Mass Emergencies and Disasters, 17*(1).

Morton, O. (2005). Biology's new forbidden fruit. *The New York Times*. February 11, 2005.

Mozgovaya, A. (2002). Crisis management of the ecological disaster in the town of Karabash. In: B. Porfiriev, B. & L. Svedin (Eds.), *Crisis management in Russia: Overcoming institutional rigidity and resource constraints. CRISMART* (pp. 205–222). Stockholm, Elanders Gotab.

Mueller. J. (2004). A false sense of insecurity? *Regulation, 22*, 42–46.

Mukerji, C., & Schudson, M. (1991). *Rethinking popular culture*. Berkeley, CA: University of California Press.

Mulcahy, M. (2002). Urban catastrophes and imperial relief in the eighteenth-century British Atlantic world: Three case studies. In G., Massard-Guilbaud, H. Platt, & D. Schott (Eds.). *Cities and catastrophes: Coping with emergency in European history* (pp. 105–122). Frankfurt: Peter Lang.

Mulford, C.L., & Klonglan, G. E. (1981). *Creating coordination among organizations: An orientation and planning guide*. Ames, IA: Iowa State University.

Mulford, C.L., Klonglan, G.E., & Kopachevsky, J.P. (1973). *Securing community resources for social action*. Ames, IA: Iowa State University.

Mulford, C.L., Klonglan, G.E., & Tweed, D.L. (1973). *Profiles on effectiveness: A systems analysis*. Sociology Report No. 110. Ames, IA: Iowa State University.

Mulford, C.L., & Mulford, M.A. (1977). Community and interorganizational perspectives on cooperation and conflict. *Rural Sociology, 42*, 569–590.

Muller, J.C. (1993). Latest developments in GIS/LIS. *International Journal of Geographical Information Systems, 7*(4), 293–303.

Murakami, H. (2000). Translated by A. Birnbaum & P. Gabriel, *Underground: The Tokyo gas attack and the Japanese psyche*. New York: Vintage International.

Murnane, L., Fortney, J., & Connell, T. (Eds.). (2003). *Technical rescue for structural collapse*. Stillwater, OK: Fire Protection Publications.

Murria, J. (2004). A disaster by any other name. *International Journal of Mass Emergencies and Disasters, 22*, 117–129.

Mustafa, D. (2005). The terrible geographicalness of terrorism: Reflections of a hazards geographer. *Antipode, 37*(1), 72–92.

Myers, M.F. (1993). Bridging the gap between research and practice: The natural hazards research and information applications center, Special Issue: Disaster research and practice: Bridging the gap. D. Neal (Guest Ed.), *International Journal of Mass Emergencies and Disasters, 11*(1), 41–54.

Nafziger, W., & Vayrynen, R. (Eds.). (2002). *The prevention of humanitarian emergencies*. London: Palgrave MacMillan.

Nakagawa, Y., & Shaw, R. (2004). Social capital: A missing link to disaster recovery. *International Journal of Mass Emergencies and Disasters, 22*(1), 5–34.

Nakamura, A. (2000). The need and development of crisis management in Japan's Public Administration: Lessons from the Kobe Earthquake. *Journal of Contingencies and Crisis Management, 8*(1), 23–29.

Nakamura, A. (2001). Preparing for the inevitable: Japan's ongoing search for best crisis management practices. In U. Rosenthal, R.A. Boin, & L.A. Comfort (Eds.), *Managing crises: Threats, dilemmas, opportunities* (pp. 307–315). Springfield, IL: Charles C Thomas.

Nakane, C. (1997). *Japanese society*. Tokyo: Charles Tuttle.

National Academy of Sciences, Advisory Committee on the International Decade of Natural Hazard Reduction (1987). *Confronting natural disasters*. Washington, DC: National Academy Press.

National Aeronautics and Space Administration. (2005). Retrieved October 1, 2005, http://earthobservatory.nasa.gov/NaturalHazards/.

National Association of Broadcasters. (1980). *Natural disasters: A broadcasters' guide* Washington, DC: National Association of Broadcasters.

National Commission on Terrorist Attacks Upon the United States. (2004). *The 9/11 commission report*. New York: W. W. Norton.

National Disaster Coordinating Council. (2004). Philippine Report on Disaster Reduction. Report to the World Conference on Disaster Reduction, Kobe. Hyogo. Japan January 2005.

National Economic and Development Agency. (2004). Medium-Term Philippine Development Plan 2004-1010. Government of the Philippines. Manila.

National Fire Protection Association. (2004). *NFPA 1600: Standard on disaster/emergency management and business continuity programs, 2004 Ed.* Quincy, MA: National Fire Protection Association.

National Governors' Association. (1979). *Comprehensive emergency management: A governor's guide*. Washington, DC: U.S. Government Printing Office.

Natural Hazards Research and Applications Center, Public Risk Institute, & Institute for Civil Infrastructure Systems. (2003). *Beyond September 11th: An account of post disaster research*. No. 39. Boulder, CO: University of Colorado, Natural Hazards and Applications Information Center.

National Information Service for Earthquake Engineering (n.d.). Northridge California earthquake January 17, 1994. University of California, Berkeley. Retrieved July 15, 2005, http://nisee.berkeley.edu/northridge.html

National Oceanic and Atmospheric Administration: Coastal Services Center. (2005). Retrieved September 23, 2005, http://www.csc.noaa.gov/bins/mapping.html.

National Oceanic and Atmospheric Administration: National Weather Service. (2005). Retrieved October 1, 2005, http://weather.gov/.

National Oceanic and Atmospheric Administration: Satellite Services Division, Fire Products. (2005). Retrieved October 1, 2005, http://www.firedetect.noaa.gov/viewer.htm.

National Research Council. (1989). *Growing vulnerability of the public switched networks: Implications for national security emergency preparedness*. Washington, DC: National Academy Press.

National Research Council, Board on Natural Disasters, Commission on Geosciences, Environment, & Resources. (1999). *Reducing natural disasters through better information*. Washington, DC: National Academy Press.

National Science and Technology Council. (1996). *Natural disaster reduction: A plan for the nation*. Washington, DC: National Science and Technology Council.

National Science Foundation. (2002). *Workshop report: Integrated research in risk analysis and decision making in a democratic society*. Workshop held in Arlington, Virginia, July 17–18, 2002. NSF03209. Posted May 22, 2003. Retrieved December 5, 2005, http://www.nsf.gov/pubs/2003/nsf03209/nsf03209.pdf.

National Task Force on Interoperability (2003). *Why can't we talk? Working together to bridge the communications gap to save lives: A guide for public officials*. Denver, CO: University of Denver, National Law Enforcement and Corrections Technology Center, Rocky Mountain.

Naum, C.J. (1993). Trends in integrated collapse rescue operations. *Fire Engineering, 146*, 61–68.

Nayyar, D. (Ed.). (2002). *Governing globalization: Issues and institutions*. Oxford: Oxford University Press.

Neal, D.M. (1993). Integrating disaster research and practice: An overview of issues. *International Journal of Mass Emergencies and Disasters, 11*, 5–13.

Neal, D.M. (1994). The consequences of excessive unrequested donations: The case of Hurricane Andrew. *Disaster Management, 6*, 23–28.

Neal, D.M. (1997). Reconsidering the phases of disaster. *International Journal of Mass Emergencies and Disasters, 15*(2), 239–264.

Neal, D.M. (2000). Developing degree programs in disaster management. *International Journal of Mass Emergencies and Disasters, 18*(3), 417–437.

Neal, D.M. (2004). Teaching introduction to disaster management: A comparison of classroom and virtual environments. *International Journal of Mass Emergencies and Disasters, 22*(1), 103–116.

Neal, D.M. (2005). Higher education and the profession of disaster management: A brief commentary on the past, current and future directions. *International Journal of Mass Emergencies and Disasters, 23*, 73–76.

Neal, D., & Phillips, B. (1990). Female-dominated local social movement organizations in disaster-threat situations. In G. West, & R. Blumberg (Eds.), *Women and social protest* (pp. 243–255). New York: Oxford University Press.

Neal, D.M., & Phillips, B.D. (1995). Effective emergency management: Reconsidering the bureaucratic approach. *Disasters: The Journal of Disaster Studies, Policy and Management, 19*, 327–337.

Neiman, S. (2005). The moral cataclysm: Why we struggle to think and feel differently about natural and man-made disasters. *New York Times Magazine*, January 16, 15–16.

Nelson, C.E., Crumley, C., Fritzsche, B., & Adcock, B. (1989). *Lower Southwest Florida hurricane study*. Tampa, FL: University of South Florida.

Newburn, T. (1993). *Disaster and after: Social work in the aftermath of disaster*. London: Jessica Kingsley.

Newlove, L., Stern, E.K., & Svedin, L. (2003). *Auckland unplugged*. Stockholm: OCB: The Swedish Agency for Civil Emergency Planning: Lexington Books.

Newsom, D.E., & Mitrani, J.E. (1993). Geographic information system applications in emergency management. *Journal of Contingencies and Crisis Management, 1*, 198–202.

Newtown, J. (1999). Converging approaches to disaster management. In J. Ingleton, (Ed.), *Natural disaster management* (pp. 264–265). Leicester: Tudor Rose.

Nguyen, L.H., Shen, K.I., Rottman, S.J., & Bourque, L.B. (1997). Examining self-perceived first-aid abilities after the Northridge Earthquake. *Prehospital and Disaster Medicine, 12*, 293–299.

Nguyen, L.H., Shen, H., Ershoff, D., Afifi, A.A., & Bourque, L.B. (in press). Exploring the causal relationship between exposure to the 1994 Northridge earthquake and pre- and post-earthquake preparedness activities. *Earthquake Spectra*.

Nicholls, R.J.N., Mimura, N., & Topping, J.C. (1995). Climate change in south and southeast Asia: Some implications for coastal areas. *Journal of Global Environment Engineering, 1*, 137–154.

Nigg, J.M. (1987). Communication and behavior: Organizational and individual response to warnings. In R. Dynes, Bruna de Marchi, & C. Pelanda (Eds.), *Sociology of disasters: Contributions of sociology to disaster research* (pp. 103–118). Milan, Italy: Franco Angeli.

Nigg, J.M. (1994). Influences of symbolic interaction on disaster research. In G. Platt & C. Gordon (Eds.), *Self, collective behavior, and society: Essays honoring the contributions of Ralph H. Turner* (pp. 33–50). Greenwich, CT: JAI Press.

Nigg, J.M. (1995a). Disaster recovery as a social process. *Wellington after the quake: The challenge of rebuilding* (pp. 81–92). Wellington, New Zealand: The Earthquake Commission.

Nigg, J.M. (1995b). Risk communication and warning systems. In T. Horlick-Jones, A. Amendola, & R. Casale (Eds.), *Natural risk and civil protection* (pp. 369–382). London: E & FN Spon.

Nigg, J., & Tierney, K. (1990). *Explaining differential outcomes in the small business disaster loan application process*. Preliminary Paper 156. Newark, DE: Disaster Research Center, University of Delaware.

Nimmo, D. (1984). TV network news coverage of Three Mile Island: Reporting disasters as technological tables. *International Journal of Mass Emergencies and Disasters, 2*, 115–145.

Noel, G.E. (1998). The role of women in health-related aspects of emergency management: A Caribbean perspective. In E. Enarson & B.H. Morrow (Eds.), *The gendered terrain of disaster: Through women's eyes* (pp. 213–223). Westport, CT: Praeger.

Noji, E.K. (1991). Medical consequences of earthquakes: Coordinating medical and rescue response. *Disaster Management, 4*, 32–40.

Noji, E. (2000). Public health consequences of disasters. *Prehospital and Disaster Medicine, 15*, 21–31.

Noji, E.K. (2003). *Public health consequences of earthquakes*. Web Lecture: Retrieved September, 2005, http://www.pitt.edu/~super1/lecture/lec13021/index.htm.

Noji, E.K. (2005). Disasters: Introduction and state of the art. *Epidemiologic Reviews, 27*, 3–8.

Noji, E.K., Kelen, G.D., Armenian, H.K., Oganessian, A., Jones, N.P., & Sivertson, K.T. (1990). The 1988 earthquake of Soviet Armenia: A case study. *Annals of Emergency Medicine, 19*(8), 891–897.

Noon, J.M. (2001). Revisiting key issues about collective behavior, organizing, and role enactment. *Sociological Spectrum, 21*, 479–506.

Norman, S. (2004). *New Zealand recovery symposium proceedings*. Wellington, New Zealand: Ministry of Civil Defence and Emergency Management.

Norris, D.H. (1998). *Disaster recovery: Salvaging photograph collections*. Philadelphia: Conservation Center for Art and Historic Artifacts.

Norris, F.H., Friedman, M.J., & Watson, P.J. (2002). 60,000 disaster victims speak: Part II. Summary and implications of the disaster mental health literature. *Psychiatry, 65*, 240–260.

Norris, F.H., Friedman, M.J., Watson, P.J., Byrne, C.M., Diaz, E., & Kaniasty, K. (2002). 60,000 disaster victims speak: Part I. An empirical review of the empirical literature, 1981–2001. *Psychiatry, 65*, 207–239.

North, C.S., Nixon, S.J., Shariat, S., McMillen, J.C., Spitnagel, E.L., & Smith, E.M. (1999). Psychiatric disorders among survivors of the Oklahoma City bombing. *Journal of the American Medical Association, 282*, 755–762.

Norton, J. (2004). Setting the scene. In S. Norman (Ed.), *Proceedings of the New Zealand recovery symposium* (pp. 25–26). Wellington: Ministry of Civil Defence & Emergency Management.

Nuclear Regulatory Commission. (1986). 23 Nuclear Regulatory Commision 294. *Atomic safety and licensing board in the matter of Carolina Power and Light Company* (Nuclear Regulatory Comission Docket No. 50-400-0L).

Nuclear Regulatory Commission. (2005). NRC Incident Response Plan, NUREG-0728, Rev. 4. Washington, DC: U.S. Nuclear Regulatory Commission, Division of Preparedness and Response, Office of Nuclear Security and Incident Response.

Nuzzo, J. (2004). The next pandemic? *Biosecurity Bulletin, 6*, 1–8.

O'Brien, G.O., & Read, P. (2005). Future UK emergency management: New wine, old skin? *Disaster Prevention and Management, 14*(3), 353–361.

O'Brien P., & Atchison, P. (1998). Gender differentiation and aftershock warning response. In E. Enarson & B.H. Morrow (Eds.), *The gendered terrain of disaster: Through women's eyes* (pp. 173–180). Greenwood, CT: Praeger.

Office for the Coordination of Humanitarian Affairs. (1998, August 7). *Papua New Guinea: Tsunami*. Retrieved November 11, 2004, http://www.cidi.org/disaster/98b/0032.html.

Ofman, P.S., Mastria, M.A., & Steinberg, J. (1995). Mental health response to terrorism: The World Trade Center bombing. *Journal of Mental Health Counseling, 17*, 312–320.

Ohlsen, C. & Rubin, C. (1993). *Planning for disaster recovery*. MIS report 25(7), 23. Washington, DC: International City Management Association.

O'Keefe, P., Westgate, K., & Wisner, B. (1976). Taking the naturalness out of natural disasters. *Nature, 260*, 566–567.

Okuyama, U., & Chang, S.E. (Eds.). (2004). *Modeling spatial economic impacts of natural disasters*. New York: Springer-Verlag.

Oliver, J. (1980). The disaster potential. In J. Oliver (Ed.), *Response to disaster* (pp. 3–28). North Queensland: Center for Disaster Studies, James Cook University.

Oliver, M.L., & Shapiro, T.M. (1995). *Black wealth/white wealth: A new perspective on racial inequality.* New York: Routledge.

Oliver-Smith, A. (1986). *The martyred city: Death and rebirth in the Peruvian Andes.* Albuquerque: University of New Mexico Press.

Oliver-Smith, A. (1990). Post-disaster housing reconstruction and social inequality: A challenge to policy and practice. *Disasters, 14,* 7–19.

Oliver-Smith, A. (1991). Success and failures in post-disaster resettlement. *Disasters, 15.1,* 12–23.

Oliver-Smith, A. (1994). Peru's five hundred year earthquake: Vulnerability in historical context. In A. Varley (Ed.). *Disasters, development and environment.* London: Wiley.

Oliver-Smith, A. (1996). Anthropological research on hazards and disasters. *Annual Review of Anthropology, 25,* 303–328.

Oliver-Smith, A. (1998). Global challenges and the definition of disaster. In E.L. Quarantelli (Ed.), *What is a disaster: Perspectives on the question* (pp. 177–194). London: Routledge.

Oliver-Smith, A. (1999a). Anthropological research on hazards and disasters. *Annual Review of Anthropology, 25,* 303–328.

Oliver-Smith, A. (1999b). *What is a disaster?* In A. Oliver-Smith & S. Hoffman (Eds.), *The angry earth: Disasters in anthropological perspective* (pp. 18–34). New York: Routledge.

Oliver-Smith, A. (1999c). Peru's five-hundred year earthquake: Vulnerability. In A. Oliver-Smith & S. Hoffman (Eds.), *The angry earth: Disasters in anthropological perspective* (pp. 74–88). New York: Routledge.

Oliver-Smith, A., & Hoffman, S. (Eds.). (1999). *The angry earth: Disasters in anthropological perspective.* New York: Routledge.

Ollenburger, J.C., & Tobin, G.A. (1998). Women and postdisaster stress. In E. Enarson & B.H. Morrow (Eds.), *The gendered terrain of disaster: Through women's eyes* (pp. 95–108). Greenwood, CT: Praeger.

Ollenburger, J.C., & Tobin, G.A. (1999). Women, aging, and post disaster stress: Risk factors for psychological morbidity. *International Journal of Mass Emergencies and Disasters, 17,* 65–78.

Olshansky, R.B. (2005). *Toward a theory of community recovery from disaster: A review of existing literature* (8 pp.). Paper presented at the 1st International Conference on Urban Disaster Reduction, Kobe, Japan.

Olshansky, R.B., & Kartez, J.D. (1998). Managing land use to build resilience. In R. Burby (Ed.), *Cooperating with nature: Confronting natural hazards with land-use planning for sustainable communities* (pp. 167–201). Washington, DC: Joseph Henry Press.

Olson, R.S. (2000). Toward a politics of disaster: Losses, values, agendas, and blame. *International Journal of Mass Emergencies and Disasters, 18*(2), 265–287.

Olson, R.S., & Drury, A.C. (1997). Un-therapeutic communities: A cross–national analysis of post–disaster political unrest. *International Journal of Mass Emergencies and Disasters, 15*(2), 221–238.

Olson, R.S., & Olson, R.A. (1987). Urban heavy rescue. *Earthquake Spectra, 3*(4), 645–658.

Olson, R.S., & Olson, R.A. (1993). The rubble's standing up in Oroville, California: The politics of building safety. *International Journal of Mass Emergencies and Disasters, 11*(2), 163–188.

Olson, R.S., Olson, R.A., & Gawronski, V.T. (1998). Night and day: Mitigation policy making in Oakland, California, before and after the Loma Prieta earthquake. *International Journal of Mass Emergencies and Disasters, 16,* 145–179.

Olson, R.S., Olson, R.A., & Gawronski, V.T. (1999). *Some buildings just can't dance: Politics, life safety, and disaster.* Stanford, CT: JAI Press.

Omi, M., & Winant, H. (1994). *Racial formation in the United States.* New York: Routledge.

Osborne, D., & Plastrik, P. (1998). *Banishing bureaucracy: The five strategies for reinventing government.* New York: Plume.

Oxfam International. (2005). *The tsunami's impact on women.* Oxfam Briefing Note, http://www.oxfam.org.uk/what_we_do/issues/conflict_disasters/downloads/bn_tsunami_women.pdf.

Oyola-Yemaiel, A., & Wilson, J. (2005). Three essential strategies for emergency management professionalization in the U.S. *International Journal of Mass Emergencies and Disasters, 23*(1), 77–84.

Palinkas, L., Downs, M., Petterson, J., & Russel, J. (1993). Social, cultural, and psychological impacts of the Exxon Valdez oil spill. *Human Organization, 52*(1), 1–13.

Palm, R. (1995). *Earthquake insurance: A longitudinal study of California homeowners.* Boulder, CO: Westview Press.

Palm, R. (1998). Urban earthquake hazards: The impacts of culture on perceived risk and response in the USA and Japan. *Applied Geography, 18*(1), 35–46.

Palm, R., & Carroll, J. (1998). *Illusions of safety: Culture and earthquake hazard response in California and Japan.* Boulder, CO: Westview Press.

Palm, R., Hodgson, M., Blanchard, D., & Lyons, D. (1990). *Earthquake insurance in California: Environmental policy and individual decision making*. Boulder, CO: Westview Press.

Pan American Health Organization (2004). *Management of dead bodies in disaster situations*. Washington, DC: Pan American Health Organization.

Pan American Health Organization (n.d.). *Natural disasters: Myths & realities*. Retrieved July 15, 2005, http://www.paho.org/English/PED/myths.htm.

Pangi, R.L. (2003). After the attack: The psychological consequences of terrorism. In J.N. Kayyem & R.L. Pangi (Eds.), *First to arrive: State and local responses to terrorism* (pp. 135–162). Cambridge, MA: MIT Press.

Pangi, R.L. (2003). Consequence management in the 1995 Sarin attacks on the Japanese subway system. In A.M. Howitt & R.L. Pangi (Eds.), *Countering terrorism: Dimensions of preparedness* (pp. 371–410). Cambridge, MA: MIT Press.

Paolisso, M., Ritchie, A., & Ramirez, A. (2002). The significance of the gender division of labor in assessing disaster impacts: A case study of Hurricane Mitch and hillside farmers in Honduras. *International Journal of Mass Emergencies and Disasters, 20*(2), 171–195.

Parachini, J.V. (2000). The World Trade Center bombers (1993). In J.B. Tucker (Ed.), *Toxic terror: Assessing terrorist use of chemical and biological weapons* (pp. 185–206). Cambridge, MA: MIT Press.

Parker, D., & Mitchell, J.K. (1995). Disaster vulnerability of megacities: An expanding problem that requires rethinking and innovative responses. *GeoJournal, 37*(3), 295–301.

Parker, E.C. (1980). What is right and wrong with media coverage of disaster? *Disasters and the mass media* (pp. 237–240). Washington, DC: The National Research Council.

Parkes, C.M. (1972). *Bereavement: Studies of grief in adult life*. London: Tavistock.

Parkin, D. (1986). Toward an apprehension of fear. In D.L. Scruton (Ed.), *Sociophobics: The anthropology of fear*. Boulder: Westview Press.

Parsons, T. (1971). Belief, unbelief and disbeleif. In R. Caporale & A. Grumelli (Eds.), *The culture of unbelief*. Berkeley, CA: University of California Press.

Partnership for Public Warning (2003). *A national strategy for integrated public warning policy and capability*, http://www.unisdr.org/ppew/info-resources/docs/EWCII–conclusions.pdf, (October 2, 2005).

Partnership for Public Warning (2005). Public *alert & warning: A national duty, a national challenge*. Retrieved October 2, 2005, http://www.partnershipforpublicwarning.org/ppw/natlstratsumm.html.

Pastor, L.H. (2004). Culture as casualty. *Psychiatric Annals, 34*(8), 616–625.

Pastrick, E.T. (1998). The national flood insurance program. In H. Kunreuther & R.J. Roth (Eds.), *Paying the price: The status and role of insurance against natural disasters in the United States* (pp. 125–154). Washington, DC: Joseph Henry Press.

Patel, T. & Nanavaty, R. (2005). Case Study 4: The experience of SEWA. *UNISDR 2005 Invest to prevent disaster*. Geneva: UNISDR.

Paton, D., & Johnson, D. (2001). Disasters and communities: Vulnerability, resilience and preparedness. *Disaster Prevention and Management: An International Journal, 10*, 270–277.

Paton, D., Smith, L., & Violanti, J. (2000). Disaster response: Risk, vulnerability and resilience. *Disaster Prevention and Management, 9*(3), 173–179.

Patterson, M. (2002). *Community schools in community development: Democracy, education, and social change*. PhD dissertation. New Brunswick, NJ: Rutgers University.

Pauchant, T.C., & Mitroff, I.I. (1992). *Transforming the crisis-prone organization: Preventing individual, organizational and environmental tragedies*. San Francisco: Jossey-Bass.

Paul, B.K., Brock, V.T., Csiki, S., & Emerson, L. (2003). Public response to tornado warnings: A comparative study of the May 4, 2003 tornadoes in Kansas, Missouri, and Tennessee. *Quick Response Research Report No. 165*. Boulder, CO: Natural Hazards Center, University of Colorado.

Peacock, W.G. (1997). Cross-national and comparative disaster research. *International Journal of Mass Emergencies and Disasters, 15*(1), 117–133.

Peacock, WG. (2002). Cross–national and comparative disaster research. In R.A. Stallings (Ed.), *Methods of disaster research* (pp. 235–250). Philadelphia: Xlibris.

Peacock, W.G., & Girard, C. (1997). Ethnic and racial inequalities in hurricane damage and insurance settlements. In W. Peacock, B. Morrow, & H. Gladwin (Eds.), *Hurricane Andrew: Ethnicity, gender, and the sociology of disaster* (pp. 171–190). New York: Routledge.

Peacock, Walter Gillis with A. Kathleen Ragsdale. (1997). Social systems, ecological networks, and disasters: Toward a socio-political ecology of disasters. In Peacock, Walter Gillis, Betty Hearn Morrow, & Hugh Galdwin (Eds.), *Hurricane Andrew: Ethnicity, gender, and the sociology of disasters* (pp. 20–35). London and New York: Routledge.

Peacock, W.G., Killian, C.D., & Bates, F.L. (1987). The effects of disaster damage and housing aid on household recovery following the 1976 Guatemalan earthquake. *International Journal of Mass Emergencies and Disasters, 5*, 63–88.

Peacock, W.G., Morrow, B.H., & Gladwin, H. (Eds.). (1997). *Hurricane Andrew: Ethnicity, gender and the sociology of disaster.* London: Routledge.

Peacock, W.G., Morrow, B., & Gladwin H. (Eds.). (2000). *Hurricane Andrew: Ethnicity, gender, and the sociology of disasters.* Miami, FL: International University, International Hurricane Center.

Peacock, W.G., Morrow, B., & Gladwin, H. (2001). (Eds.), *Hurricane Andrew and the reshaping of Miami.* Miami, FL: International Hurricane Center.

Peacock, W.G., & Ragsdale, A.K. (1997). Social systems, ecological networks, and disasters: Toward a socio-political ecology of disasters. In W.G. Peacock, B.H. Morrow, & H. Gladwin (Eds.), *Hurricane Andrew: Ethnicity, gender, and the sociology of disasters* (pp. 20–35). New York: Routledge.

Peacock, W.G., Zhang, Y., & Dash, N. (2005). *Single family housing recovery after Hurricane Andrew in Miami–Dade county.* College Station, TX: Hazard Reduction & Recovery Center, Texas A&M University.

Peek-Asa, C., Kraus, J.F., Bourque, L.B., Vimalachandra, D., Yu, J., & Abrams, J. (1998). Fatal and hospitalized injuries resulting from the 1994 Northridge earthquake. *International Journal of Epidemiology, 27*, 459–465.

Peek-Asa, C., Ramirez, M., Seligson, H., & Shoaf, K. (2003). Seismic, structural, and individual factors associated with earthquake related injury. *Injury Prevention, 9*, 62–66.

Peek-Asa, C., Ramirez, M., Shoaf, K., Seligson, H., & Kraus, J.F. (2000). GIS mapping of earthquake-related deaths and hospital admissions from the 1994 Northridge California, earthquake. *Annals of Epidemiology, 10*, 5–13.

Peek, L., & Sutton, J. (2003). An exploratory comparison of disasters, riots and terrorist acts. *Disasters, 27*, 319–335.

Peet, R. (1998). *Modern geographical thought.* London: Blackwell.

Peet, R., & Watts, M. (Eds.). (2004). *Liberation ecologies: Environment, development, social movements* (2nd ed.). London: Routledge.

Pelling, M. (2005). *Comments on the world conference on disaster reduction* (WCDR). Kobe, Hyogo, Japan. January 18–22.

Pellow, D. (2000). Environmental inequality formation: Toward a theory of environmental injustice. *American Behavioral Scientist, 43*(4), 581–601.

Pellow, D., Weinberg, A., & Schnaiberg, A. (2005). The environmental justice movement: Equitable allocation of the costs and benefits of environmental management outcomes. In L. King & D. McCarthy (Eds.), *Environmental sociology: From analysis to action* (pp. 240–252). Lanham, MD: Rowman Littlefield.

Peluso, N., & Watts, M. (2001). *Violent environments.* Ithaca, NY: Cornell University Press.

Pennings, J.M. (1981). Strategically interdependent organizations. In P.C. Nystrom & W.H. Starbuck (Eds.), *Handbook of organizational design: Adapting organizations to their environments* (pp. 433–455). New York: Oxford University Press.

Pereau, M.J. (1991). *First-world/third world: Disasters in context: A study of the Saragosa and Wichita Falls, Texas tornadoes.* Paper presented at the UCLA International Conference on the Impact of International Disasters. Los Angeles.

Pérez-Lugo, M. (2001). The mass media and disaster awareness in Puerto Rico: A case study of the floods in Barrio Tortugo. *Organization and Environment, 14*(1), 55–73.

Perrow, C. (1992). *Small firm networks: Networks and organizations.* Boston: Harvard Business School Press.

Perrow, C. (1999). *Normal accidents: Living with high-risk technologies* (2nd ed.). Princeton, NJ: Princeton University Press.

Perry, R.W. (1979). Evacuation decision-making in natural disasters. *Mass Emergencies, 4*, 25–38.

Perry, R.W. (1982). *The social psychology of civil defense.* Lexington, MA: Lexington Books.

Perry, R.W. (1985). *Comprehensive emergency management.* Greenwich, CT: JAI Press.

Perry, R.W. (1987). Disaster preparedness and response among minority citizens. In R. Dynes, B. DeMarchi, & C. Pelanda (Eds.), *Sociology of disasters.* Milan: Agnelli.

Perry, R.W. (1989). Taxonomy, classification and theories of disaster phenomena. In G.A. Kreps (Ed.), *Social structure and disaster* (pp. 351–359). Newark, DE: University of Delaware Press.

Perry, R.W. (1991). Managing disaster response operations. In T.E. Drabek & G. Hoetmer (Eds.), *Emergency management: Principles and practice for local government* (pp. 201–223). Washington, DC: International City Management Association.

Perry, R.W. (1991). Managing response operations. In T. E. Drabek & G. J. Hoetmer (Eds.), *Emergency management: Principles and practice for local government* (pp. 201–223). Washington, DC: International City Management Association.

Perry, R.W. (2003). Municipal terrorism management in the United States. *Disaster Prevention and Management, 12*(3), 190–202.

Perry, R.W. (2004). Disaster exercise outcomes for professional emergency personnel and citizen volunteers. *Journal of Contingencies and Crisis Management, 12*, 63–75.

Perry, R.W. (2005). Disasters, definitions and theory construction. In R.W. Perry & E.L. Quarantelli (Eds.), *What is a disaster? New answers to old questions.* (pp. 311–324). Philadelphia: Xlibris.

Perry, R.W., & Greene, M.R. (1982). The role of ethnicity in the emergency decision-making process. *Sociological Inquiry, 52*, 309–334.

Perry, R.W., & Greene, M. (1983). *Citizen response to volcanic eruptions: The case of Mount St. Helens.* New York: Irvington Publishers.

Perry, R.W., & Lindell, M.K. (1989). Communicating threat information for volcano hazards. In L.M. Walters, L. Wilkins, & T. Walters (Eds.), *Bad tidings communications and catastrophe* (62 pp.). Hillsdale, NJ: Erlbaum.

Perry, R.W., & Lindell, M.K. (2003). Understanding citizen response to disasters with implications for terrorism. *Journal of Contingencies and Crisis Management, 11*, 49–60.

Perry, R.W., & Lindell, M.K. (2004). Disaster exercise outcomes for professional emergency personnel and citizen volunteers. *Journal of Contingencies and Crisis Management, 12*, 64–75.

Perry, R.W., Lindell, M.K., & Greene, M.R. (1981). *Evacuation planning in emergency management.* Lexington, MA: Lexington Books.

Perry, R.W., Lindell, M.K., & Greene, M.R. (1982). Threat perception and public response to volcano hazard. *The Journal of Social Psychology, 116*, 199–204.

Perry, R.W., Lindell, M., & Prater, C. (2005). *Introduction to emergency management in the United States.* Washington, DC: Federal Emergency Management Agency.

Perry, R.W., & Mankin, L. (2004). Terrorism challenges for human resource management. *Review of Public Personnel Administration, 24*, 3–17.

Perry, R.W., & Mushkatel, A. (1984). *Disaster management: Warning response and community relocation.* Westport, CT: Quorum Books.

Perry, R.W., & Mushkatel, A. (1986). *Minority citizens in disaster.* Athens, GA: University of Georgia Press.

Perry, R.W., & Quarantelli, E.L. (2005). *What is a disaster? New answers to old questions.* Philadelphia: Xlibris.

Petak, W.J. (1984). Natural hazard mitigation: Professionalization of the policy making process. *International Journal of Mass Emergencies and Disasters, 2*, 285–302.

Petak, W.J. (1985). Emergency management: A challenge for public administration. *Public Administration Review, 54*, 3–7.

Peterson, J. (2005). Enron tapes show blackout scheme. *The New York Times,* February 6.

Petrescu-Prahova, M. & Butts, B.T. (2005). *Emergent coordination in the World Trade Center Disaster.* Paper No. 36. Institute for Mathematical Behavioral Sciences. University of California, Irvine. Retrieved September, 2005, http://repositories.cdlib.org/imbs/36.

Petroff, C., Bourgeois, J., & Yeh, H. (1996). *The February 21, 1996 Chimbote tsunamis in Peru: EERI Special earthquaker Report, Learning from earthquakes.* Oakland, CA: Earthquake Engineering Research Institute.

Pettersson, P. (1996). Implicit service relations turned explicit: A case study of the Church of Sweden as service provider in the context of the Estonia disaster. In B. Edvardson & S. Modell (Eds.), *Servicem management: Interdisciplinary perspectives* (pp. 225–247). Stockholm: Nerenius and Santerus.

Pew Research Center for the People and the Press. (2002). Internet sapping broadcast news audience. *Survey reports.* Retrieved September 28, 2002, http://people-press.org/reports/display.php3?ReportID=36,.

Phillippi, N. (1994). Plugging the gaps in flood control policy. *Issues in Science and Technology: Winter,* 71–78.

Phillips, B. (1990). Gender as a variable in emergency response. In R. Bolin (Ed.), *The Loma Prieta earthquake: Studies of short-term impacts* (pp. 84–90). Boulder, CO: Natural Hazards Research and Applications Information Center, University of Colorado.

Phillips, B. (1993). Cultural diversity in disaster: Shelter, housing, and long-term recovery. *International Journal of Mass Emergencies and Disasters, 11*(1), 99–110.

Phillips, B. (2002). Qualitative methods and disaster research. In R. A. Stallings (Ed.), *Methods of disaster research* (pp. 194–211). Philadelphia: Xlibris.

Phillips, B. (2003). Disasters by discipline: Necessary dialogue for emergency management education. Paper presented at the Workshop, Creating Educational Opportunities for the Hazards Manager of the 21st Century. Denver, CO, October 22.

Phillips, B. (2004). Grasping the big picture: Using classic research to generate insight for emergency management education. *Contemporary Disaster Review, 2*(1), 12–17.

Phillips, B. (2005). Disaster as a discipline: The status of emergency management education in the U.S. *International Journal of Mass Emergencies and Disasters, 23*(1), 111–140.

Phillips, B., & Ephraim, M. (1992). *Living in the aftermath: Blaming processes in the Loma Prieta Earthquake*. University of Colorado-Boulder Natural Hazards Research and Applications Information Center, Working Paper 80.

Phillips, B., & Morrow, B.H. (Eds.). (Forthcoming). *Women and Disasters*. Philadelphia: Xlibris.

Phillips L., Bridgeman, J., &. Ferguson-Smith, M. (2001). *The BSE inquiry: Findings and conclusions*. London: Stationary Office.

Pickett, J.H., & Block, B.A. (1991). Day-today management. In G.J. Hoetmer & T.E. Drabek (Eds.), *Emergency management: Principles and practice for local government*. Washington, DC: ICMA.

Picou, J., & Gill, D. (1996). The Exxon Valdez oil spill and chronic psychological stress. In E. Rice, R. Spies, D. Wolfe, & B. Wright (Eds.), *Proceedings of the Evon Symposium* (pp. 100–110). Alaska: American Fisheries Symposium.

Picou, J.S., Marshall, B.K., & Gill, D.A. (2004). Disaster, litigation, and the corrosive community. *Social Forces, 82*, 1497–1526.

Pidgeon, N., Kasperson, R.E., & Slovic, P. (Eds.). (2003). *The social amplification of risk*. Cambridge, UK: Cambridge University Press.

Pielke, R.A., Jr., & Klein, R. (2005). Distinguishing tropical cyclone-related flooding in U.S. presidential disaster declarations. *Natural Hazards Review, 6*, 55–66.

Pieterman, R. (2001). Culture in the risk society. An essay on the rise of a precautionary culture. *Zeitschrift fur Rechtsoziologie, 22*(2), 145–168.

Pieterse, J.N. (2001). *Development theory: Deconstructions/reconstructions*. London: SAGE.

Pijawka, K.D., & Radwan, A.E. (1985). The transportation of hazardous materials: Risk assessment and hazard management. *Dangerous Properties of Industrial Materials Report*, 2–11.

Pilkey, O.H., & Dixon, K.L. (1996). *The corps and the shore*. Washington, DC: Island Press.

Piore, M., & Sable, C. (1984). *The second industrial divide*. New York: Basic Books.

Pizarro, C. (Ed.). (1996). *Social and economic policies in Chile's transition to democracy*, Santiago: CIEPLAN.

Platt, R.H. (1996). *Land use and society: Geography, law, and public policy*. Washington, DC: Island Press.

Platt, R.H. (1998). Planning & land use adjustments in historical perspective. In R. Burby (Ed.), *Cooperating with nature: Confronting natural hazards with land-use planning for sustainable communities* (pp. 29–56). Washington, DC: Joseph Henry Press.

Platt, R.H. (1999). *Disasters and democracy: The politics of extreme natural events*. Washington, DC: Island Press.

Pollack, A. (2004). Can biotech crops be good neighbors? *The New York Times*. Retrieved September 26, www.nytimes.com.

Pollack, A. (2005). *Open-source practices for biotechnology*, http://www.nytimes.com/2005/02/10/technology/10gene.html.

Pollard, M. (1978). *North Sea surge: The story of the east coast floods of 1953*. Lavenham, Suffolk: Terence Dalton Limited.

Pomonis, A. (2005). *Concluding remarks, Indian Ocean Tsunami preliminary field mission report*. Presented to the Institution of Structural Engineers. Earthquake Engineering Field Investigation Team. Retrieved July 15, 2005, http://www.istructe.org.uk/eefit/index. asp?bhcp=1.

Pomonis, A., Sakai, S., Coburn, A.W., & Spence, R.J.S. (1991). *Assessing human casualties caused by building collapse in earthquakes*. Proceedings of the International Conference on the Impact of Natural Disasters. Los Angeles: University of California Los Angeles.

Poncelet, J.L. (2000). *Disaster myths*. Virtual Online Library Presentation. Emergency Information Infrastructure Partnership. Retrieved July 15, 2005, http://www.emforum.org/vlibrary/000405.htm.

Porfiriev, B. (1996). Social aftermath and organizational response to a major disaster: The case of the 1995 Sakhalin earthquake in Russia. *Journal of Contingencies and Crisis Management, 4*, 218–227.

Porfiriev, B. (1998a). Disaster policy and emergency management in Russia. New York: Nova Science Publishers.

Porfiriev, B. (1998b). Issues in the definition and delineation of disasters and disaster areas. In E.L. Quarantelli (Ed.), *What is a disaster: Perspectives on the question*. (pp. 56–72). London: Routledge.

Porfiriev, B. (1999a). Development policy: a driving force of environmental hazard in Russia. *Environmental Hazards 1*, 45–50.

Porfiriev, B. (1999b). Emergency and disaster legislation in Russia: The key development trends and features. *Australian Journal of Emergency Management, 14*(1), 59–64.

Porfiriev, B. (2001a). Institutional and legislative issues of emergency management policy in Russia. *Journal of Hazardous Materials, 88*, 145–168.

Porfiriev, B. (2001b). Managing security and safety risks in the Baltic Sea Region: A comparative study of crisis policy institutional models. *Risk Management, 3*, 51–62.

Porfiriev, B. (2003). Economicheskoye Razvitiye i Chrezvichainiye Situatsii: Mir i Sovremennaia Rossiya. (Economic Development and Disasters: The World and Contemporary Russia). Rossiiskii Ekomicheskii Zhournal (Russian Economic Journal), 5–6, 44–55.

Porfiriev, B., & Quarantelli, E.L. (Eds.). (1996). *Social science research on mitigation of and recovery from disasters and large scale hazards in Russia.* Newark, DE: Disaster Research Center, University of Delaware.

Porfiriev, B., & Svedin, L. (Eds.) (2002). *Crisis management in Russia: Overcoming institutional rigidity and resource constraints.* CRISMART Series. Stockholm, Elanders Gotab.

Post, J. (1977). *The last great subsistence crisis in the Western world.* Baltimore: John Hopkins University Press.

Poteyeva, R. (2005). Urban search and rescue: A multidisciplinary annotated bibliography. *Disaster research center preliminary paper.* Newark, DE: University of Delaware, Disaster Research Center.

Poulin, T.E. (2005). National threat—local response: Building local disaster capacity with mutual aid agreements. *PA Times, 28*(3).

Pourvakhshouri, S.Z., & Mansor, S. (2003). Decision support system in oil spill cases. Literature review. *Disaster Prevention and Management: An International Journal, 12*(3), 217–221.

Powell, W.W. (1996). Inter-organizational collaboration in the biotechnology industry. *Journal of Institutional and Theoretical Economics, 152*, 197–215.

Prater, C.S., & Lindell, M.K. (2000). Politics of hazard mitigation. *Natural Hazard Review, 1*, 73–82.

Prater, C., Vigo, G., Hall, M., & Edmiston, J. (1991). *Search and rescue: A multidisciplinary annotated bibliography.* College Station, TX: Texas A&M University, Hazard Reduction Recovery Center.

Prater, C., Wenger, D., & Grady, K. (2000). *Hurricane Bret post storm assessment: A review of the utilization of hurricane evacuation studies and information dissemination.* College Station, TX: Texas A&M University Hazard Reduction & Recovery Center.

President's Commission on Critical Infrastructure Protection (1998). *Critical foundations, protecting America's infrastructures.* Washington, DC: President's Commission on Critical Infrastructure Protection.

Prezant, D.J., Weiden, M., Banauch, G.I., McGuinness, G., Rom, W.N., Aldrich, T.K., et al. (2002). Cough and bronchial responsiveness in firefighters at the World Trade Center site. *New England Journal of Medicine, 347*, 806–815.

Prince, S.H. (1920). *Catastrophe and social change: Based upon a sociological study of the Halifax disaster.* Doctoral dissertation. New York: Columbia University, Department of Political Science.

Public Safety Wireless Network Program. (2002). *Answering the call: Communications lessons learnt from the Pentagon Attack,* http://knxas1.hsdl.org/homesec/docs/justice/Answering_the_Call_Pentagon_Attack.pdf

Pulido, L. (1996). A critical review of the methodology of environmental racism research. *Antipode, 28*(2), 142–159.

Pulido, L. (2000). Rethinking environmental racism: White privilege and urban development in Southern California. *Annals of the Association of American Geographers, 90*(1), 12–40.

Pulido, L., Sidawi, S., & Vos, R. (1996). An archaeology of environmental racism in Los Angeles. *Urban Geography, 17*(5), 419–439.

Purvis, M., & Bauler, J. (2004). *Irresponsible care: The failure of the chemical industry to protect the public from chemical accidents.* New York: United States Public Interest Research Group Education Fund.

Quarantelli, E.L. (1954). The nature and conditions of panic. *American Journal of Sociology, 60*, 267–275.

Quarantelli, E.L. (1960). Images of withdrawal behavior in disasters: Some basic misconceptions. *Social Problems, 8*, 68–79.

Quarantelli, E.L. (1966). Organization under stress. In R. Brictson (Ed.), *Symposium on emergency operations* (pp. 3–19). Santa Monica, CA: The Rand Corporation.

Quarantelli, E.L. (1978). *Disaster theory and research.* London: SAGE.

Quarantelli, E.L. (1979). *Studies in disaster response and planning.* Newark, DE: University of Delaware, Disaster Research Center.

Quarantelli, E.L. (1980a). *Evacuation behavior and problems: Findings and implications from the research literature.* Columbus, OH: Disaster Research Center, Ohio State University.

Quarantelli, E.L. (1980b). *The study of disaster movies: Research problems, findings, and implications.* Disaster Research Center Preliminary Paper No. 64. Newark, DE: Disaster Research Center, University of Delaware.

Quarantelli, E.L. (1981). The command post view point of view in local mass communication systems. *International Journal of Communication Research, 7*, 57–73.

Quaratelli, E.L. (1982a). What is a disaster?: An agent specific or an all disaster spectrum approach to socio-behavioral aspects of earthquakes. In B. Jones & M. Tomazevic (Eds.), *Social and economic aspects of earthquakes* (pp. 453–478). Ithaca, NY: Cornell University, Program in Urban and Regional Studies.

Quarantelli, E.L. (1982b). General and particular observations on sheltering and housing in American disasters. *Disasters, 6*, 277–281.

Quarantelli, E.L. (1983a). *Delivery of emergency medical services in disasters: Assumptions and realities.* New York: Irvington Publishers.

Quarantelli, E.L. (1983b). *Perceptions and reactions to emergency warnings of sudden hazards.* Disaster Research Center article no. 173, reprinted from Ekistics, 309 (Nov.–Dec.), 511–515.

Quarantelli, E.L. (1984a). *Emergent behavior at the emergency time periods of disaster. Final report.* Columbus, OH: Disaster Research Center, Ohio State University.

Quarantelli, E.L. (1984b). *Organizational behavior in disasters and implications for disaster planning.* Emmitsburg, MD: National Emergency Training Center, Federal Emergency Management Agency.

Quarantelli, E.L. (1984c). Perceptions and reactions to emergency warnings of sudden hazards. *Ekestics, 309*, 511–515.

Quarantelli, E.L. (1985). Realities and mythologies in disaster films. *Communications, 11*, 31–44.

Quarantelli, E.L. (1987a). Disaster studies: an analysis of the social historical factors affecting the development of research in the area. *International Journal of Mass Emergencies and Disasters, 5*(3), 285–310.

Quarantelli, E.L. (1987b). Presidential address: What should we study? *International Journal of Mass Emergencies and Disasters, 5*, 7–32.

Quarantelli, E.L. (1988a). Disaster crisis management: A summary of research findings. *Journal of Management Studies, 25*, 373–385.

Quarantelli, E.L. (1988b). *Disaster crisis management: A summary of research findings.* Newark, DE: University of Delaware, Disaster Research Center.

Quarantelli, E.L. (1988c). Disaster studies: An analysis of the social historical factors affecting the development of research in the area. *International Journal of Mass Emergencies and Disasters, 5*, 285–310.

Quarantelli, E.L. (1988d). The NORC research on the Arkansas Tornado: A Fountainhead study. *International Journal of Mass Emergencies and Disasters, 6*(3), 283–310.

Quarantelli, E.L. (1989a). *Disaster recovery: Comments on the literature and a mostly annotated bibliography.* Miscellaneous Report #44, Newark, DE: University of Delaware, Disaster Research Center.

Quarantelli, E.L. (1989b). Conceptualizing disaster from a sociological perspective. *International Journal of Mass Emergencies and Disasters, 7*, 243–251.

Quarantelli, E.L. (1989c). *Human behavior in the Mexico City earthquake: Some implications from basic themes in survey findings.* Preliminary Paper No. 37. Newark, Delaware: Disaster Research Center, University of Delaware.

Quarantelli, E.L. (1990). Disaster prevention and mitigation in Lada. Paper presented at Colloquium on the Environment and Natural Disaster Management. Washington, DC: World Bank.

Quarantelli, E.L. (1991a). *Converting disaster scholarship into effective disaster planning and managing: Possibilities and limitations.* Disaster Research Center preliminary paper No. 162. Newark, DE: University of Delaware, Disaster Research Center.

Quarantelli, E.L. (1991b). Disaster response: Generic or agent-specific? In A. Kreimer, & M. Mujnasinghe (Eds.) *Managing natural disasters and the environment* (pp. 97–105). Washington, DC: The World Bank.

Quarantelli, E.L. (1991c). *Lessons from research: Findings on mass communications system behavior in the pre, trans and postimpact periods.* Newark, DE: University of Delware, Disaster Research Center.

Quarantelli, E.L. (1992a). The case for a generic rather than agent specific agent approach to disasters. *Disaster Management, 2*, 191–196.

Quarantelli, E.L. (1992b). The environmental disasters of the future will be more and worse but the prospect is not hopeless. *Disaster Prevention and Management, 2*(1), 11–25.

Quarantelli, E. (1993a). Community crises: An exploratory comparison of the characteristics and consequences of disasters and riots. *Journal of Contingencies and Crisis Management, 1*, 67–78.

Quarantelli, E.L. (1993b). Converting disaster scholarship into effective disaster planning and managing: Possibilities and limitations. *International Journal of Mass Emergencies and Disasters, 11*(1), 15–39.

Quarantelli, E.L. (1994). Disaster studies: The consequences of the historical use of a sociological approach in the development of research. *International Journal of Mass Emergencies and Disasters, 12*(1), 25–50.

Quarantelli, E.L. (1995a). *Disaster planning, emergency management and civil protection: The historical development of organized efforts to plan for and to respond to disasters.* Disaster Research Center preliminary paper #227. Newark, DE: University of Delaware, Disaster Research Center.

Quarantelli, E.L. (1995b). Patterns of shelter and housing in US disasters. *Disaster Prevention and Management, 4*, 43–53.

Quarantelli, E.L. (1995c). What is a disaster? *International Journal of Mass Emergencies and Disasters, 13*(3), 221–230.

Quarantelli, E.L. (1996a). Emergent behaviors and groups in the crisis times of disasters. In M.K. Kwan (Ed.), *Individuality and social control: Essays in honor of Tamotsu Shibutani* (pp. 47–68). Greenwich, CT: JAI Press.

Quarantelli, E.L. (1996b). Just as a disaster is not simply a big accident, so a catastrophe is not just a bigger disaster. *The Journal of the American Society of Professional Emergency Planners, 3,* 68–71.

Quarantelli, E.L. (1996c). *Ten criteria for evaluating the management of community disasters.* Preliminary paper no. 241. Newark, DE: University of Delaware, Disaster Research Center.

Quarantelli, E.L. (1996d). The future is not the past repeated: Projecting disasters in the 21st century from current trends. *Journal of Contingencies and Crisis Management, 4,* 228–240.

Quarantelli, E.L. (1997a). Problematical aspects of the information/communication revolution for disaster planning and research: Ten non-technical issues and questions. *Disaster Prevention and Management, 5,* 94–106.

Quarantelli, E.L. (1997b). Ten criteria for evaluating the management of community disasters. *Disasters, 21,* 39–56.

Quarantelli, E.L. (Ed.). (1998). *What is a disaster? Perspectives on the question.* New York: Routledge.

Quarantelli, E.L. (1998a). *What is a disaster: Perspectives on the question.* London: Routledge.

Quarantelli, E.L. (1998b). Epilogue: Where we have been and where we might go. In E.L. Quarantelli (Ed.), *What is a disaster: Perspective on the question* (pp. 234–273). London: Routledge.

Quarantelli, E.L. (1999a). *Disaster related social behavior: Summary of 50 years of research findings.* Preliminary Paper No. 280. Newark, DE: University of Delaware, Disaster Research Center.

Quarantelli, E.L. (1999b). *The disaster recovery process: What we know and do not know from research.* Preliminary paper #286. Newark, DE: University of Delaware, Disaster Research Center.

Quarantelli, E.L. (2000). Disaster research. In E. Borgatta, & R. Montgomery (Eds.), *Encyclopedia of sociology.* (pp 682–688). New York: Macmillan.

Quarantelli, E.L. (2001a). *Disaster planning, emergency management and civil protection: The historical development of organized efforts to plan and to respond to disasters.* Preliminary paper #301. Newark, DE: University of Delaware, Disaster Research Center.

Quarantelli, E.(2001b). Statistical and conceptual problems in the study of disasters. *Disaster Prevention and Management 10,* 325–338.

Quarantelli, E.L. (2002a). The Disaster Research Center field studies of organized behavior in the crisis time period of disasters. In R. A. Stallings (Ed.), *Methods of disaster research* (pp. 94–126). Philadelphia: Xlibris.

Quarantelli, E.L. (2002b). *The protection of cultural properties: The neglected social science perspective and other questions and issues that ought to be considered.* Newark, DE: University of Delaware, Disaster Research Center. Preliminary paper no. 325.

Quarantelli, E.L. (2002c). The role of the mass communication system in natural and technological disasters and possible extrapolation to terrorism situations. *Risk Management: An International Journal, 4,* 7–22.

Quarentelli E.L. (2003). *A half century of social science disaster research: Selected major findings and their applicability.* University of Delaware Preliminary Paper No. 336.

Quarantelli, E.L. (2005a). A social science research agenda for the disasters of the 21st century. In R.W. Perry & E.L. Quarantelli (Eds.), *What is a disaster? New answers to old questions* (pp. 325–396). Philadelphia: Xlibris.

Quarantelli, E.L. (2005b). *Catastrophes are different from disasters.* Social Science Research Council, www.ssrc.org.

Quarantelli, E.L., & Dynes, R.R. (1970). Property norms and looting: Their patterns in community crises. *Phylon, 31,* 168–182.

Quarantelli, E.L., & Dynes, R.R. (1970). Special issue: Organizational and groups behavior in disasters. *American Behavioral Scientist, 13,* 323–480.

Quarantelli, E.L., & Dynes, R.R. (1972). When disaster strikes: It isn't much like what you've heard and read about. *Psychology Today, 5*(9), 66–70.

Quarantelli, E., & Dynes, R.R. (1976). Community conflict: Its absence and its presence in natural disasters. *Mass Emergencies, 1,* 139–152.

Quarantelli, E.L., & Dynes, R.R. (1977). Response to social crisis and disaster. *Annual Review of Sociology, 3,* 23–49.

Quarantelli, E.L., & Dynes, R. (1989). Reconstruction in the context of recovery: thoughts on the Alaskan earthquake. Paper presented at the Conference on Reconstruction after Urban Earthquakes, National Center for Earthquake Engineering Research. Buffalo, NY.

Quarantelli, E.L., & Mozgovaya, A. (Eds.). (1994). *An annotated inventory of the social science research literature on disasters in the former Soviet Union and Contemporary Russia.* Newark, DE: University of Delaware, Disaster Research Center.

Quarantelli, E.L., & Perry, R.W. (Eds.). (2005). *What is a disaster? New answers to old questions.* Philadelphia: Xlibris.

Quarantelli, E. L. 1982. Sheltering and Housing After Major Community Disaster: Case studies and General Conclusions. Newark, Delaware: Disaster Research Center, University of Delaware.

The queen sees the floods. (1953, February 20). *The Times.*

Quon, T.K., & Laube, A. (1991). Do faster rescues save more lives? *Risk Analysis, 11*(2), 291–301.

Radke, J., Cova, T., Sheridan, M.F., Troy, A., Lan, M., & Johnson, R. (2000). Application challenges for GIScience: Implications for research, education, and policy for risk assessment, emergency preparedness and response. *Journal of the Urban and Regional Information Systems Association, 12*, 15–30.

Ragozin, A. (1999). Obschiye polozheniya otsenki I upravleniya prorodnim riskom. (Fundamentals of natural risk assessment and management). *Geoecologia, Ingenernaia Geologia, Gidrogeologia, Geocriologia (Geoecology, Engineering Geology, Hydrogeology, Geocriology), 5*, 417–429.

Ramirez, M., & Peek-Asa, C. (2005). Epidemiology of traumatic injuries from earthquakes. *Epidemiologic Reviews, 27*, 47–55.

Randall, D. (2004). Into the mainstream. *Homeland Protection Professional, 3*(3), 22–24, 26, 28–29.

Raphael, B. (1986). *When disaster strikes: How individuals and communities cope with catastrophe.* New York: Basic Books.

Rapley, J. (2004). Development studies and the post-development critique. *Progress in Development Studies, 4*(4), 350–354.

Rappaport, E.N., & Fernandez-Partagas, J.J. (1997). History of the deadliest Atlantic tropical cyclones since the discovery of the New World. In H. F. Diaz & R. S. Pulwarry (Eds.), *Hurricanes, climate, and socioeconomic impacts* (pp. 93–108). New York: Springer-Verlag.

Rashed, T., & Weeks, J. (2003). Assessing vulnerability to earthquake hazards through spatial multicriteria analysis of urban areas. *International Journal of Geographical Information Science, 17*(6), 547–576.

Re Swiss. (2001). Natural Catastrophes and Man-made Disasters in 2001. Swiss Re, Zurich, January, 2002.

Reason, J. (1990). *Human error.* New York: Cambridge University Press.

Rees, M. (2004). *Our final hour: A scientist's warning: How terror, error and environmental disaster threaten humankind's future in this century–on Earth and beyond.* New York: Basic Books.

Reese, S. (2005). *Risk-based funding in Homeland Security grant legislation: Analysis of issues for the 109th congress.* August 29. (Order Code RL33050). Congressional Research Service and Library of Congress.

Rees, W.E. (1992). Ecological footprints and appropriated carrying capacity: What urban economics leaves out. *Environment and Urbanization, 4*(2), 121–130.

Regester, M. (1989). *Crisis management: What to do when the unthinkable happens.* London: Hutchinson Business.

Report of a geological society working group (2005). *Super-eruptions: Global effects and future threats.* Retrieved June 16, 2005, http://www.geolsoc.org.uk/template.cfm?name=Super2.

Reynolds, A., & Barnett, B. This just in ...How national TV news handled the breaking 'live' coverage of September 11. *Journalism & Mass Communication Quarterly, 80*(3), 698.

Richardson, W. (1993). Identifying the cultural causes of disasters: An analysis of the Hillsborough football stadium disaster. *Journal of Contingencies and Crisis Management, 1*, 27–35.

Richman, J.A., Wislar, J.S., Flaherty, J.A., Fendrich, E., & Rospenda, K. M. (2004). Effect on alcohol use and anxiety of the September 11, 2001, attacks and chronic work stressors: A longitudinal cohort study. *American Journal of Public Health, 94*, 2010–2015.

Richmond, N. (1993). After the flood. *American Journal of Public Health, 83*, 1522–1524.

Rinaldi, S.M., Peerenboom, J.P., & Kelly, T.K. (2001). Critical infrastructure interdependencies. *IEEE Control Systems Magazine*, December, 2001.

Ritzer, G. (1975). *Sociology: A multiple paradigm science.* Boston: Allyn & Bacon.

Ritzer, G. (1979). Toward an integrated sociological paradigm. In W. Snizek, E. Fuhrman, & M. Miller (Eds.), *Contemporary issues in theory and research* (pp. 25–46). Westport, CT: Greenwood Press.

Rivers, J.W. (1982). Women and children last: An essay on sex discrimination in disasters. *Disasters, 6*(4), 256–267.

Robbins, P. (2004). *Political Ecology.* Oxford, UK: Blackwell.

Roberts, K.H. (1989). New challenges in organizational research: High-reliability organizations. *Industrial Crisis Quarterly, 3*, 111–125.

Roberts, K.H., Rousseau, D.M., & LaPorte, T.R. (1993). The culture of high reliability: Quantative and qualitative assessment about nuclear powered aircraft carriers. *High Technology Management Research, 5*, 141–161.

Robin, C. (2004). *Fear: The history of a political idea.* New York: Oxford University Press.

Roces, M.C., White, M.E., Dayrit, M.M., & Durkin, M.E. (1992). Risk factors for injuries due to the 1990 earthquake in Luzon, Philippines. *Bulletin World Health Organization, 70*, 509–514.

Rocheleau, D., Thomas-Slayter, B., & Wangarai, E. (Eds.). (1996). *Feminist political ecology: Global issues and local experiences.* New York: Routledge.

Rodrick, D. (2004). Rethinking growth strategies. WIDER Annual Lectures 8.

Rodríguez, H. (2005). Reflections on the United Nations world conference on disaster reduction: How can we develop disaster resilient communities? *International Journal of Mass Emergencies and Disasters, 23*(1), 141–160.

Rodríguez, H., Díaz, W., & Donner, W. (2005, in progress). *Technology, weather forecasts, and warnings: A perspective from the Oklahoma Emergency Management Organizations*. Newark, DE: University of Delaware, Disaster Research Center.

Rodriguez, H., Wachtendorf, T., Kendra, J., & Trainor, J. (2005). The great Sumatra Earthquake and the Indian Ocean Tsunami of December 26, 2004: A preliminary assessment of societal impacts and consequences. *Earthquake Engineering Research Institute (EERI) Newsletter*, (4), May 2005, *39*(5), 1–7.

Rogers, D.A., Whetten, D.A. and Associates. (1982). *Interorganizational coordination: Theory, research and implementation*. Ames, IA: Iowa State University Press.

Rogers, E.M., & Sood, R. (1981). *Mass media operations in a quick-onset natural disaster: Hurricane David in Dominica Boulder*. Natural Hazards Research and Applications Information Center.

Rogers, G.O. (1994). The timing of emergency decisions: Modeling decisions by community officials during chemical accidents. *Journal of Hazardous Materials, 37*, 353–373.

Rogers, G.O., & Sorensen, J. (1988). Diffusion of emergency warnings. *Environmental Professional, 10*, 281–294.

Rogers, G.O., & Sorensen, J. (1989). Public warning and response to hazardous materials accidents. *Journal of Hazardous Materials, 22*, 57–74.

Rogers, G.O., Sorensen, J.H., Long, J.F., Jr., & Fisher, D. (1989). Emergency planning for chemical agent releases. *The Environmental Professional, 11*, 396–408.

Rogers, G.O., Sorensen, J.H., & Morell, J.A. (1991). Using information systems in emergency management. *Advances in the Implementation and Impact of Computer Systems, 1*, 161–181.

Rose, A., & Guha, G.-S. (2004). Computable general equilibrium modeling of electric utility lifeline losses from earthquakes. In U. Okuyama & S.E. Chang (Eds.), *Modeling spatial economics impacts of natural disasters* (pp. 119–141). New York: Springer-Verlag.

Rose, R. (1993). *Lesson drawaing in public policy: A guide to learning across time and space*. Chatham, NJ: Chatham House.

Rosenblatt, P. (1997). Grief in small-scale societies. In P.C. Murray, L. Pittu, & B. Young (Eds.), *Death and bereavement across culture*. London: Routledge.

Rosengren, K.E., Arvidson P., & Struesson D. (1974). *The barseback panic*. Lund: University of Lund.

Rosenthal, U. (1998). Future disasters, future definitions. In E. L. Quarantelli (Ed.), *What is a disaster: Perspectives on the question* (pp. 146–159). London: Routledge.

Rosenthal, U., Boin, R.A., & Comfort, L.K. (Eds.). (2001). *Managing crises: Threats, dilemmas, opportunities*. Springfield, IL: Charles C Thomas.

Rosenthal, U., Charles, M.T., & Hart, P. (Eds.). (1989). *Coping with crisis: The management of disasters, riots and terrorism*. Springfield, IL: Charles C Thomas.

Rossi, P.H., Wright, J.D., & Weber-Burdin, E. (1982). *Natural hazards and public choice: The state and loc al politics of hazard mitigation*. New York: Academic Press.

Rossman, E.J. (1993). Public involvement in environmental restoration: Disaster research and sociological practice in Superfund community relations plans. *International Journal of Mass Emergencies and Disasters, 11*(1), 123–133.

Rotbart, D. (1999). An intimate look at covering Littleton. *Columbia Journalism Review* May–June, 24–35.

Roth, R.J. (1998). Earthquake insurance protection in California. In H. Kunreuther & R. J. Roth (Eds.), *Paying the price: The status and role of insurance against natural disasters in the United States* (pp. 67–95). Washington, DC: Joseph Henry Press.

Rozario, S. (1997). 'Disasters' and Bangladeshi women. In R. Lentin (Ed.), *Gender and catastrophe* (pp. 255–268). New York: Zed Books.

Rozdilsky, Jack L. (1995). Flood-related relocation, sustainable redevelopment, and alternative energy: Planning recommendations for the use of wind energy in Valmeyer, Illinois. *Thesis, environmental studies*. Springfield, IL: University of Illinois.

Rubin, C.B. (1982). Case studies of communities recovering from natural disasters, Year II, Final report. November 1982. Available from the principle investigator at George Washington University, Washington, DC.

Rubin, C.B. (1985). The community recovery process in the United States after a major natural disaster. *International Journal of Mass Emergencies and Disasters, 3*(2), 9–28.

Rubin, C.B. (1991). Recovery from disaster. In T. E. Drabek & G. J. Hoetmer (Eds.), *Emergency management: Principles and practice for local governments* (pp. 224–259). Washington, DC: International City Management Association.

Rubin, C., & Barbee, D. (1985). Disaster recovery and hazard mitigation: Bridging the intergovernmental gap. In Emergency management: A challenge for public administration. (pp. 57–63). *Public Administration Review*. January, 45.

Rubin, C., Saperstein M., & Barbee, D. (1985). *Community recovery from a major natural disaster. Monograph No. 41* (295 pp.). Boulder, CO: University of Colorado, Institute of Behavioral Science.

Rubin, C.B., & Renda-Tanali, I.R. (2001). *Disaster timeline: Selected events and outcomes (1965–2000).* Arlington, VA: Claire Rubin and Associates. http//www.disastertimeline.com.

Rubonis, A.V., & Bickman, L. (1991). Psychological impairment in the wake of disaster: The disaster–psychopathology relationship. *Psychological Bulletin, 109,* 384–399.

Rudman, W.B., & Clarke, R.A. (2003). *Emergency responders: drastically underfunded, dangerously unprepared.* Washington, DC: Council on Foreign Relations.

Rudra, N. (2002). Globalization and the decline of the welfare state in less-developed countries. *International Organization, 2,* 411–445.

Rules to Survive By. (2005, March 31). *The Japan Times,* 18.

Russell, L.A., Goltz, J.D., & Bourque, L.B. (1995). Preparedness and hazard mitigation actions before and after two earthquakes. *Environment and Behavior, 27,* 744–770.

Ruzicka, G. (2002). *Disaster recovery: Salvaging books.* Philadelphia: Conservation Center for Art and Historic Artifacts.

Sabatier, P., & Jenkins-Smith, H.C. (1993). *Policy change and learning: An advocacy coalition approach.* Boulder, CO: Westview Press.

Sadohara, S., Shigekawa, K,. Hayashi, H., & Chinoi, T. (2005). *A study on the creation of a human resources development system for risk management in Japan.* 1st International conference on urban disaster reduction. Kobe: Kobe Bay Sheraton Hotel. January 18–20, 2005.

Safire, W. (2005). Tsunami: The vocabulary of disaster. *New York Times Magazine.* January 16.

Sagalyn, L.B. (1983). Mortgage lending in older urban neighborhoods: Lessons from past experiences. *Annals of American Academy, 465,* 98–108.

Sagan, S.D. (1993). *The limits of safety: Organizations, accidents and nuclear weapons.* Princeton, NJ: Princeton University Press.

Salter, J. (1997, 1998). Risk management in the emergency management context. *Australian Journal of Emergency Management, 12*(4), 22–28.

Sanderson, D. (2000). Cities, disasters and livelihoods. *Environment and Urbanization, 12*(2), 93–102.

Sandman, P.M., & Paden, M. (1979). At Three Mile Island. *Columbia Journalism Review.* 18, July–August, 48.

Sanford, T. (1967). *Storm over the states.* New York: McGraw-Hill.

Santos, G., & Aguirre, B. (2004). *A critical review of emergency evacuation simulation models.* Proceedings of Conference on building occupant movement during fire emergencies, June 10–11, 2004. Gaithersburg, MD: National Institute of Standards and Technology.

Saunders, S.L., & Kreps, G.A. (1987). The life history of the emergent organization in times of disaster. *The Journal of Applied Behavioral Science, 23,* 443–462.

Saxenian, A. (1996). *Regional advantage culture and competition in Silicon Valley and Route 128* (pp. xi, 226 pp). Cambridge, MA: Harvard University Press.

Scanlon, T.J. (1976). The not so mass media: The role of individuals in mass communication. In G. Stuart Adam (Ed.), *Journalism, communication and the law* (pp.104–111). Scarborough: Prentice-Hall Canada.

Scanlon, T.J. (1977). Post-disaster rumor chains: A case study. *International Journal of Mass Emergencies and Disasters, 2,* 121–126.

Scanlon, T.J. (1988). Disaster's little known pioneer: Canada's Samuel Henry Prince. *International Journal of Mass Emergencies and Disasters, 6,* 213–232.

Scanlon, T.J. (1991). Reaching out: Getting the community involved in preparedness. In G.J. Hoetmer & T.E. Drabek (Eds.), *Emergency management: Principles and practice for local government.* Washington, DC: ICMA.

Scanlon, T.J. (1992). *Disaster preparedness some myths and misconceptions easingwold.* Easingwood, UK: The Emergency Planning College.

Scanlon, T.J. (1994). The role of EOCs in emergency management: A comparison of American and Canadian experience. *International Journal of Mass Emergencies and Disasters, 12,* 51–75.

Scanlon, T.J. (1995). Federalism and Canadian emergency response: Control, co–operation and conflict. *The Australian Journal of Emergency Management, 10*(1), 18–24.

Scanlon, T.J. (1996). Not on the record: Disasters, records and disaster research. *International Journal of Mass Emergencies and Disasters, 14*(3), November, 265–280.

Scanlon, T.J. (1997). Rewriting a living legend: Researching the 1917 Halifax explosion. *International Journal of Mass Emergencies and Disasters, 15,* 147–178.

Scanlon, T.J. (1998a). *ICE STORM 1998: Sharing the lessons learned.* Ottawa: Regional Municipality of Ottawa Carleton.

Scanlon, T.J. (1998b), Military support to civil authorities: The Eastern Ontario ice storm. *Military Review, 4*, 41–51.

Scanlon, T.J. (1998c). The perspective of gender: A missing element in disaster response. In E. Enarson, & B.H. Morrow (Eds.), The *gendered terrain of disaster: Through women's eyes* (pp. 45–52). Greenwood, CT: Praeger.

Scanlon, T.J. (1998d). The search for non-existent facts in the reporting of disaster. *Journalism and Mass Communication Educator, 53*(2), 45.

Scanlon, T.J. (1999a). Emergent groups in established frameworks: Ottawa Carleton's response to the 1998 ice disaster. *Journal of Contingencies and Crisis Management, 7*, 30–37.

Scanlon, T.J. (1999b). Myths of male and military superiority: Fictional accounts of the 1917 Halifax explosion. *English Studies in Canada, 24*, 1001–1025.

Scanlon T.J. (2001). Increasingly intolerable boundaries: Future control of environmental pollution. *Journal of Hazardous Materials, 86*(1–3), 121–133.

Scanlon, T.J. (2002a). Helping the other victims of September 11: Gander uses multiple EOCs to handle 38 diverted flights. *International Journal of Mass Emergencies and Disasters, 20*(3), 369–398.

Scanlon, T.J. (2002b). Rewriting a living legend: Researching the 1917 Halifax explosion. In R.A. Stallings (Ed.), *Methods of disaster research* (pp. 266–301). Philadelphia: Xlibris.

Scanlon, T.J. (2004a). A perspective on North American natural disasters. In J.P. Stoltman, J. Lidstone, & L.M. Dechano (Eds.), *International perspectives on natural disasters: Occurrence, mitigation, and consequences, 157*(53), 4.3.

Scanlon, T.J. (2004b). High alert chemical terrorism and the safety of first responders. *Royal Canadian Mounted Police Gazette, 66*(2), 33.

Scanlon, T.J. (2005a). Foreword. In R. W. Perry & E. L. Quarantelli (Eds.), *What is a disaster? New answers to old questions* (pp. 13–18). Philadelphia: Xilbris.

Scanlon, T.J. (2005b). Strange bed partners: Thoughts on the London Bombings of July 2005 and the link with the Indian Ocean Tsunami of december 26th 2004. *International Journal of Mass Emergencies and Disasters, 23*(2), 149–158.

Scanlon, T.J., & Alldred, S. (1982). Media coverage of disasters: The same old story. In B. G. Jones & M. Tomazevic (Eds.), *Social and economic aspects of earthquakes.* (pp. 363–375) Ithaca, NY: Cornell University and Ljubljana: Institute for Testing and Research in Materials and Structures.

Scanlon, T.J., Conlin, D., Duffy, A., Osborne, G., & Whitten, J. (1984). *The Pemberton Valley floods: BC's Tiniest village responds to a major emergency.* Ottawa: Emergency Communications Research Unit.

Scanlon, T.J., Luukko, R., & Morton, G. (1978). Media coverage of crises: Better than reported, worse than necessary. *Journalism Quarterly, 55*(1), 68–72.

Scanlon, T.J., Osborne, G., & McClellan, S. (1996). *The Peace River ice jam and evacuation: An Alberta Town adapts to a sudden emergency.* Ottawa: Emergency Communications Research Unit.

Scanlon, T.J., & Padgham, M. (1980). *The Peel Regional Police Force & the Mississauga evacuation.* Ottawa: Canadian Police College.

Scanlon, T.J., & Prawzick A. (1991). Not just a big fire: Emergency response to an environmental disaster. *Canadian Police College Journal, 13*(4), 225–229.

Scanlon, T.J., Prawzick, A., Osborne, G., Medcalf, L., & Cote, S. (1985). *The Petawawa train derailment.* Ottawa, Canada: Emergency Preparedness.

Scanlon, T.J., & Taylor, B. (1975). *The warning smell of gas.* Ottawa, Canada: Emergency Preparedness.

Scanlon, T.J., & Taylor, B. (1977). A stand-by research capacity. *Mass Emergencies, 2*, 35–41.

Scawthorn, C., & Wenger, D. (1990). *Emergency response, planning and search and rescue.* HHRC Publication 11P College Station, TX: A&M University, Hazard Reduction and Recovery Center.

Scawthorn, C.R., Porter, K.A., & Blackburn, F.T. (1992). Performance of emergency-response services after the earthquake. In T.D. O'Rourke (Ed.), *The Loma Prieta, California, Earthquake of October 17, 1989—Marina District* (pp. 195–215). Washington, DC: U.S. Department of the Interior, U.S. Geological Survey. USGS Professional Paper. 1551-F.

Schlenger, W.E., Caddell, J.M., Ebert, L., Jordan, B.K., Rourke, K.M., Thalji, L., et al. (2002). Psychological reactions to terrorist attacks: Findings from the national study of Americans' reactions to September 11. *Journal of the American Medical Association, 288*, 581–588.

Schmuck, H. (2000). "An Act of Allah": Religions explanations for floods in Bangladesh as survival strategy. *International Journal of Mass Emergencies and Disasters, 18*, 85–95.

Schneider, J. & Susser, I. (Eds.), (2003). *Wounded cities: Destruction and reconstruction in a globalized world.* New York: Berg Publishers.

Schneider, S.K. (1992).Governmental response to disasters: The conflict between bureaucratic procedures and emergent norms. *Public Administration Review, 52*, 135–145.

Schneider, S.K. (1998). Reinventing public administration: A case study of the Federal Emergency Management Agency. *Public Administration Quarterly, 22*, 35–37.

Schnitter, N. (1994). *A history of dams.* Brookfield: Balkema.

Schoenberger, E. 1998. Discourse and practice in human geography. *Progress in Human Geography, 22*(1), 1–14.

Schoff, J.L. (2004) (Ed.). *Crisis management in Japan & the United States: Creating opportunities for cooperation amid dramatic change.* The Institute for Foreign Policy Analysis, Inc. Dulles, VA: Brassey's.

Schorr, J. (1987). Some contributions German Katastrophensoziologie can make to the sociology of disaster. *International Journal of Mass Emergencies and Disasters, 5*, 115–135.

Schulte, P. (1991). *The politics of disaster: An examination of class and ethnicity in the struggle for power following the 1989 Loma Prieta earthquake in Watsonville, California.* Unpublished MA Thesis. Sacramento, CA: California State University.

Schuster, M.A., Stein, B.D., Jaycox, L.H., Collins, R.L., Marshall, G. N., Elliott, M.N., et al. (2001). A national survey of stress reactions after the September 11, 2001, terrorist attacks. *New England Journal of Medicine, 345*, 1507–1512.

Schwab, J. (2005). Fixing the future. *Planning*, August–September, 14–19.

Schwab, J., Topping, K.C., Eadie, C., Deyle, R., & Smith, R. (1998). Planning for postdisaster recovery and reconstruction. *PAS Report 483/484.* Chicago, IL: American Planning Association.

Schwartz, J. (2003). *Old virus has a new trick: Mailing itself in quantity*, http://www. nytimes.com/2003/08/20/technology/20VIRU.html.

Schwartz, R., & Sulitzneanu-Kenan, R. (2004). Managerial values and accountability pressures: Challenges of crisis and disaster. *Journal of Public Administration Research and Theory, 14*, 79–102.

Scott, W.R. (1981). *Organizations: Rational, natural, and open systems.* Englewood Cliffs, NJ: Prentice-Hall, Inc.

Scott, W.R. (1991). The evolution of organizational theory. In Miller, G. (Ed.), *Studies in organizational sociology* (pp. 53–69). Greenwich, CT: JAI Press.

Scruton, D.L. (1986). (Ed.), *Sociophobics: The anthropology of fear.* Boulder, CO: Westview Press.

Seeger, M.W., Sellnow, T.L., & Ulmer, R.R. (2003). *Communication and organizational crisis.* Westport, CT: Praeger.

Seligmann-Silva, M. (2003). Catastrophe and representation: History as trauma. *Semiotica, 143*, 1–4.

Seligson, H.A., & Shoaf, K. I. (2003). Human impacts of earthquake. In W. F. Chen & C. Scawthorn (Eds.), *Earthquake engineering handbook.* (pp. 28:21–28:29). Boca Raton, FL: CRC Press.

Seltzer, L. (2005). Some Perspective 5 Years After Y2K, *eweek*, January 3, 2005, www.eweek.com/article2/10.1895.1747163.00.asp, accessed 18 April 2006.

Semenza, J.C., McCullough, J.E., Flanders, W.D., McGeehin, M.A., & Lumpkin, J.R. (1999). Excess hospital admissions during the July 1995 heat wave in Chicago. *American Journal of Preventive Medicine, 16*, 269–277.

Serrat Viñas, C. (1998). Women's disaster vulnerability and response to the Colima earthquake. In E. Enarson & B. H. Morrow (Eds.), *The gendered terrain of disaster: Through women's eyes* (pp. 161–172). Greenwood, CT: Praeger.

Seydlitz, R.J., Spencer, W., Laska, S., & Triche, E. (1991). The effects of newspaper reports on the public's response to a natural hazard event. *International Journal of Mass Emergencies and Disasters, 9*, 5–29.

Shaluf, I., Ahmadun, F., & Mustapha, S. (2003). Technological disaster's criteria and models. *Disaster Prevention and Management, 12*, 305–311.

Sharan, P., Chaudhary, G., Kavathekar, S.A., & Saxena, S. (1996). Preliminary report of psychiatric disorders in survivors of a severe earthquake. *American Journal of Psychiatry, 153*, 556–558.

Shaw, G. (1999). *Business and industry crisis management, disaster recovery, and organizational continuity.* Emmitsburg, MD: Emergency Management Institute, National Emergency Training Center, Federal Emergency Management Agency.

Shaw, R., Gupta, M., & Sarma, A. (2003). Community recovery and its sustainability: Lessons from the Gujarat Earthquake of India. *The Australian Journal of Emergency Management, 18*(2), 28–34.

Shearer, A.W. (1991). *Survivors and the media.* London: John Libbey & Company Limited.

Shearer, A.W. (2005). Whether the weather: Comments on: An abrupt climate change scenario and its implications for United States national security. *Futures, 37*(6), 445–463.

Sheehan, L., & Hewitt, K. (1969). *A pilot survey of global natural disasters of the past twenty years.* Working Paper No. 11. Boulder, CO: University of Colorado, Natural Hazards Center.

Shenon, P. (2003a). Antiterror money stalls in congress. *The New York Times, 1*, A21.

Shenon, P. (2003b). Former domestic security aides make a quick switch to lobbying. *The New York Times, 1*, A20.

Shlikova, E. (2002). Social welfare and benefits for the Chernobyl liquidators: Clean-up and rescue workers. In: B. Porfiriev, & L. Svedin (Eds.), *Crisis management in Russia: Overcoming institutional rigidity and resource constraints. CRISMART Series* (pp. 173–204). Stockholm, Elanders Gotab.

Shoaf, K.I., & Bourque, L.B. (1999). Correlates of damage to residences following the Northridge earthquake, as reported in a population-based survey of Los Angeles County residents. *Earthquake Spectra, 15*, 145–172.

Shoaf, K.I., Nguyen, L.H., Sareen, H.R., & Bourque, L.B. (1998). Injuries as a result of California earthquakes in the past decade. *Disasters, 22*, 218–235.

Shrivastava, P. (1987). *Bhopal: Anatomy of a crisis*. Cambridge, MA: Ballinger Publishing Company.

Shrivastava, P. (1992). Bhopal: Anatomy of a crisis (2nd ed.). In *Before Disaster Strikes: Why thousands are dying needlessly each year in preventable disasters*. London: Paul Chapman Tearfund, 2004.

Shroeder, R.A. (1987). *Gender vulnerability to drought: A case study of the Hausa social environment*. Working Paper No. 58. Boulder, CO: University of Colorado, Natural Hazards Research and Applications Information Center.

Shultz, J.M., Russell, J., & Espinel, Z. (2005). Epidemiology of tropical cyclones: The dynamics of disaster, disease and development. *Epidemiologic Reviews, 27*, 21–35.

Siegel, J.M. (2000). Emotional injury and the Northridge California earthquake. *Natural Hazards Review, 1*, 204–211.

Siegler, M. (2005). Stressed to excess: Fear's links to disease. *The Washington Post*, 5.

Simon, H.A. (1977). *Models of discovery*. Boston: D. Reidel.

Simpson, D.M. (2001). Community emergency response training (CERTs): A recent history and review. *Natural Hazards Review, 2*(2), 54–63.

Simpson, D.M., & Howard, G. A. (2001). Issues in the profession: The evolving role of the emergency manager. *The Journal of the American Society of Professional Emergency Planners, 8*, 63–70.

Simpson, R.L. (1959). Vertical and horizontal communication in formal organizations. *Administrative Science Quarterly, 4*, 188–196.

Sims, J., & Bauman, D. (1972). The tornado threat: Coping style of the north and south. *Science, 176*, 1186–1192.

Singer, B.D., & Green, L. (1972). *The social functions of radio in a community emergency*. Toronto: Copp Clark.

Singer, B.D., Osborn, R.W., & Geschwender, J.A. (1970). *Black rioters*. Lexington: D. C. Heath.

Singh, R.B. (2004). Current curriculum initiatives and perspectives in education for natural disaster reduction in India (pp. 409–416). In J.P. Stoltman, J. Lidstone, & L.M. Dechano, (Eds.), *International perspectives on natural disasters: Occurrence, mitigation and consequence*. Dordrecht: Kluwer

Sjoberg, G. (1962). Disasters and social change. In G. Baker & D. Chapman (Eds.), *Man and society in disaster* (pp. 356–384). New York: Basic Books.

Skinner, N., & Becker, B. (1995). *Pattonsburg, Missouri: On higher ground*. Washington, DC: President's Council on Sustainable Development.

Slovic, P. (1993). Perceived risk, trust, and democracy: A systems perspective. *Risk Analysis, 13*, 675–682.

Slovic, P. (2000). Trust, emotion, sex, politics and sciences: Surveying the risk-assessment battlefield. In P. Slovic. (Ed.), *The perception of risk: Risk, society and policy series* (pp. 390–412). London: Earthscan.

Slovic, P., Flynn, J. & Layman, M. (1991). Perceived risk, trust, and the politics of nuclear waste. *Science, 254*, 1603–1607.

Smelser, N.J. (1963). *Theory of collective behavior*. New York: Free Press.

Smelser, N.J. (2004). September 11, 2001, as cultural trauma. In J. Alexander, R. Eyerman, B. Giesen, N. Smelser & P. Sztompka. *Cultural trauma and collective Identity*. (pp. 263–278). Berkeley, CA: University of California Press.

Smith, C. (1992). *Media and apocalypse: News coverage of the Yellowstone forest fires, Exxon Valdez oil spill, and Loma Prieta earthquake*. Westport, CT: Greenwood Press.

Smith, D. (2005). Through a glass darkly. In R.W. Perry & E.L. Quarantelli (Eds.), *What is a disaster: New answers to old questions* (pp. 292–307). Philadelphia: Xlibris.

Smith, G. (2002). *The 21st century emergency manager*. Paper presented at the Federal Emergency Management Higher Education Conference: Florida International University.

Smith, G. (2004). Holistic disaster recovery: Creating a sustainable future. Federal Emergency Management Agency. Emergency Management Institute, Higher Education Project. The course is available online at: http://training.fema.gov/emiweb/edu/completeCourses.asp

Smith, G. (Forthcoming). *Inter-organizational relationships and policymaking: Key factors shaping sustainable disaster recovery in the United States*.

Smith, K. (1992). *Environmental hazards: assessing risk and reducing disaster*. New York: Routledge.

Smith, M., & Feagin, J. (Eds), (1995). *The bubbling cauldron: Race, ethnicity and the urban crisis*. Minneapolis: University of Minnesota Press.

Smithson, A. & Levy, A.L. (2000). *Ataxia: The chemical and biological terrorism threat and the US response*. Report No. 35. Washington, DC: Henry L. Stimson Center.

Soja, E. (1989). *Postmodern geographies*. London: Verso.

Soja, E. (1996a). Los Angeles 1965–1992: From crisis-generated restructuring to restructuring-generated crisis. In A. Scott & E. Soja (Eds.), *The city: Los Angeles and urban theory at the end of the twentieth century*. Berkeley, CA: University of California Press.

Soja, E. (1996b). Margin/Alia: Social justice and the new cultural politics. In A. Merrifield & E. Swyngedouw (Eds.), *The urbanization of injustice* (pp. 180–199). New York: New York University Press.

Soja, E. (2000). *Postmetropolis: Critical studies of cities and regions*. Malden, MA: Blackwell.

Solway, L. (1994). Urban development and megacities: Vulnerability to natural disasters. *Disaster Management, 6*(3), 160–169.

Sood, R., Stockdale, G., Rogers, E. M. (1987). How the news media operate in natural disasters. *Journal of Communication, 37*, 27–41.

Sorensen, A. (2002). *The making of urban Japan: Cities and planning from Edo to the twenty-first century*. London: Routledge.

Sorensen, J.H. (1991). When shall we leave? Factors affecting the timing of evacuation departures. *International Journal of Mass Emergencies and Disasters, 9*, 153–165.

Sorensen, J.H. (1992). *Assessment of the need for dual indoor/outdoor warning systems and enhanced tone alert technologies in the CSEPP, ORNL/TM–12095*. Oak Ridge, TN: Oak Ridge National Laboratory.

Sorensen, J.H. (2000). Hazard warning systems: A review of 20 years of progress. *Natural Hazards Review, 1*, 119–125.

Sorensen, J.H., & Mileti, D. (1987). Decision making uncertainties in emergency warning system organizations. *International Journal of Mass Emergencies and Disasters, 5*, 33–61.

Sorensen, J.H., & Mileti, D. (1989). Warning and evacuation: Answering some basic questions. *Industrial Crisis Quarterly, 2*, 195–210.

Sorensen, J.H., & Mileti, D. (1991). Risk communication for emergencies. In R. Kasperson & P. Stallen (Eds.), *Communicating risks to the public: International perspectives* (pp. 369–394). Boston, MA: Kluwer Academic.

Sorensen, J.H., Mileti, D.S., & Copenhaver, E. (1985). Inter and intraorganizational cohesion in emergencies. *International Journal of Mass Emergencies and Disasters, 3*, 27–52.

Sorensen, J.H., & Rogers, G. (1988). Community preparedness for chemical emergencies: A survey of U.S. communities. *Industrial Crisis Quarterly, 2*, 89–108.

Soresen, J.H., Vogt, B., & Mileti, D. (1987). Evacuation: An Assessment of Planning and Research, ORNL-6376. Oak Ridge, TN: Oak Ridge National Laboratory.

Sorensen, J.H., Vogt, B., & Shumpert, B. (2004). Planning protective action decision making: Evacuate or shelter-in-place. *Journal of Hazardous Materials, 109*, 1–11.

Sorokin, P.A. (1942). *Man and society in calamity*. New York: Dutton.

South, S.J., & Crowder, K.D. (1997). Escaping distressed neighborhoods: Individual, community and metropolitan tnfluences. *American Journal of Sociology, 102*, 1040–1084.

Southern Association of Colleges and Schools. (2003), http://www.sacs.org. Retrieved September 22, 2003.

Southern Region Sustainable Agriculture and Education and Southern Rural Development Center. (2005). *Request for proposals 2005: Sustainable Community Innovation Grants*. Southern SARE Program and Southern Rural Development Center. Retrieved October 16, 2005, www.griffin.uga.edu/sare/currentcalls/sci.doc.

Sowina, U. (2002). Les eaux qui Charrient la mort et les desastres: inondation et pollution des eaux dans les villes polonaises aux Xve et XVIe siecles. In G. Massard-Guilbaud, H. Platt, & D. Schott (Eds.), *Cities and catastrophes: Coping with emergency in European history* (pp. 43–62). Frankfurt: Peter Lang.

Spangle, W. (1987). *Pre-earthquake planning for post-earthquake rebuilding*. Southern California Earthquake Preparedness Project. California Governor's Office of Emergency Services.

Spangle and Associates. (1991). *Rebuilding after earthquakes: Lessons from planners*. Portola, CA: William Spangle and Associates.

Sparks, P.R. (1985). *Building damage in South Carolina caused by the tornadoes of March, 28, 1984*. Washington, DC: National Academy Press.

Sprang, G. (1999). Post-disaster stress following the Oklahoma City bombing: An examination of three community groups. *Journal of Interpersonal Violence, 14*, 169–183.

Spread of 'SobigF' is fastest ever. *The New York Times*, August 21, 2003.

Squires, G.D. (1998). Why an insurance regulation for prohibit redlining? *John Marshall Law Review, 31*, 489–511.

Squires, G.D., & Velez, W. (1987). Insurance redlining and the transformation of an urban metropolis. *Urban Affairs Quarterly, 23*, 63–83.

Squires, G.D., O'Connor, S., & Silver, J. (2001). The unavailability of information on insurance unavailability: Insurance redlining and the absence of geocoded disclosure data. *Housing Policy Debate, 12*, 347–372.

Stacey, R. (1996). *Strategic management & organizational dynamics*. London: Paitman.

Staff Writers. (2001). Chemical plants feared as targets. *Washington Post*, December 16, 2001, A01.

Stallings, R.A. (1978). The structural patterns of four types of organizations in disaster. In E.L. Quarantelli (Ed.), *Disasters: Theory and research* (pp. 87–103). Beverly Hills, CA: SAGE.

Stallings, R.A. (1979). *Preliminary analysis of gubernatorial emergency declarations in California, 1950–1974.* Los Angeles: Working Paper No. 30. University of Southern California: Center for Public Affairs.

Stallings, R.A. (1984). Evacuation behavior at Three Mile Island. *International Journal of Mass Emergencies and Disasters, 2*, 11–26.

Stallings, R.A. (1986). *National Science Foundation field report: The Miamisburg (Ohio) train derailment and toxic fire of July 8, 1986.* Los Angeles: School of Public Administration, University of Southern California.

Stallings, R.A. (1988). Conflict in natural disasters: A codification of consensus and conflict theories. *Social Science Quarterly, 69*, 569–586.

Stallings, R.A. (1991). Disasters as social problems? A dissenting view. *International Journal of Mass Emergencies and Disasters, 9*, 90–95.

Stallings, R.A. (1995). *Promoting risk: Constructing the earthquake threat.* Hawthorne, NY: Aldine de Gruyter.

Stallings, R.A. (1998). Disaster and the theory of social order. In E.L. Quarantelli (Ed.), *What is a disaster: Perspectives on the question* (pp. 127–145). New York: Routledge.

Stallings, R.A. (Ed.). (2002a). *Methods of disaster research.* Philadelphia: Xlibris.

Stallings, R.A. (2002b). Methods of disaster research: Unique or not? In R. A. Stallings (Ed.), *Methods of disaster research.*(pp. 21–44). Philadelphia: Xlibris.

Stallings, R.A.(2002c). Weberian political sociology and sociological disaster studies. *Sociological Forum, 17*, 281–305.

Stallings, R.A. (Ed.). (2003). *Methods of disaster research.* International Research Committee on Disasters, http://www.xlibris.com. Selected articles are available from http://www.ijmed.org through International Journal of Mass Emergencies and Disasters,15,1. Philadelphia: Xlibris.

Stallings, R.A. (2005). Disaster, crisis, collective stress and mass deprivation. In R.W. Perry & E. L. Quarantelli (Eds.), *What is a disaster: New answers to old questions* (pp. 237–274). Philadelphia: Xlibris.

Stallings, R.A., & Quarantelli, E.L. (1985). Emergent citizen groups and emergency management. *Public Administration Review, 45*, 93–100.

Standards Australia. (1999). Risk management standard AS/NZS4360 (2nd ed.). *Standards Australia and Standards New Zealand.* Sydney and Wellington.

Standards New Zealand (2000). *Risk management handbook for local government.* SNZ HB 4360:2000. Wellington: Standards New Zealand.

Staples, C., & Stubbings, K. (1998). *Business impacts in the 1997 Red River Valley Flood.* Paper presented at the Annual Meeting of the Midwest Sociological Society. Kansas City, MO.

Starbuck, W.H. (1983). Organizations as action generators. *American Sociological Review, 48*, 91–103.

State College, Pennsylvania. (2005). Accuweather. Retreived August 29, 2005, http://wwwa.accuweather.com/company.asp?page=about.

Steady, F.C. (Ed.). (1993). *Women and children first: Environment, poverty, and sustainable development.* Rochester, VT: Schenkman Books.

Stearns, P.N., & Haggerty, T. (1991). The role of fear: Transitions in American emotional standards for children, 1850–1950. *American Historical Review, 96*.

Stein, H.F. (1999). A bombing in April: Culture and disaster in the Oklahoma City bombing. *Illness, Crisis & Loss, 7*, 17–36.

Steinberg, T. (2000). *Acts of God: The unnatural history of natural disaster in America.* New York: Oxford University Press.

Steinglass, P., & Gerrity, E. (1990). Natural disasters and post-traumatic stress disorder: Short-term versus long-term recovery in two disaster-affected communities. *Journal of Applied Social Psychology, 20*, 1746–1765.

Stephens, M., & Edison, N. (1982). News coverage of the incident at Three Mile Island. *Journalism Quarterly, 59*, 199.

Stephenson, R., & Anderson, P.S. (1997). Disasters and the information technology revolution. *Disasters: The Journal of Disaster Studies, Policy and Management, 21*, 305–334.

Stern, E.K. (1997). Crisis and learning: A balance sheet. *Journal of Contingencies and Crisis Management, 5*, 69–86.

Stern, E.K., & Nohrstedt, D. (Eds.) (1999) *Crisis management in Estonia: Case studies and comparative perspectives.* CRISMART Series. Stockholm, Elanders Gotab.

Stern, E.K., & Sundelius, B. (2002). Crisis management Europe: An integrated regional research and training program. *International Studies Perspectives, 3*, 771–788.

Stern, P.C., & Easterling, W.E. (Eds.). (1999). *Making climate forecasts matter.* Washington, DC: National Academy Press.

Stewart, F., Humphreys, F.P., & Lea, N. (1997). Civil conflict in developing countries over the last quarter of a century: An empirical overview of economic and social consequences. *Oxford Development Studies, 1*, 11–41.

Stiglitz, J. (1998). More instruments and broader goals: Moving toward the post-Washington consensus. *WIDER Annual Lectures 2.*

Stiglitz, J. (2002). *Globalization and its discontents.* London: Allen Lane.

Stinchcomb, A.L. (1965). Social structure and organizations. In J. G. March (Ed.), *Handbook of organizations* (pp. 142–193). Chicago: Rand McNally.

Stoker, R.P. (1991). *Reluctant partners: Implementing federal policy.* Pittsburg: Pittsburg University Press.

Storey, J. (1998). *An introduction to cultural theory and popular culture* (2nd ed.). Athens, GA: The University of Georgia Press.

Stretton, A. (1976). *The furious days: The relief of Darwin.* Sydney: William Collins.

Strong, P. (1990). Epidemic psychology: A model. *Sociology of Health & Illness, 12*(3), 249–259.

Stubbs, N., & Sikorsky, C. (1987). The structural feasibility of vertical evacuation: Final report. *National Science Foundation Technical Report*, TR–87–106.

Stubbs, N., Sikorsky, C., Lipnick, P., & Lombard, P. (1989). Simulation of fatalities in structures subjected to hurricane loading. In *Simulation in emergency management and technology* (pp. 88–93). San Diego: Simulation Councils, Inc.

Sturken, M. (1997). *Tangled memories: The Vietnam War, the AIDS epidemic, and the politics of remembering.* Berkeley, CA: University of California Press.

Suddards, R.W., Price, L., & Picarda, H. (1987). *Bradford disaster appeal: The administration of an appeal fund.* Sweet and Maxwell.

Sudo, K., Kameda, H., & Ogawa, Y. (2000). Recent history of Japan's disaster mitigation and the impact of IDNDR. *Natural Hazards Review, 1*(1), 10–17.

Sullivan, M. (2003). Integrated recovery management: A new way of looking at a delicate process. *The Australian Journal of Emergency Management, 18*(2), 4–27.

Sultana, F. (Forthcoming). Dying for water, dying from water: Gendered geographies of the drinking water crisis from arsenic contamination in Bangladesh. In S. Raju (Ed.), *Gendered geographies: Interrogating place and space in South Asia.* Oxford: Oxford University Press.

Sun-Tzu. (2005). *The principles of Warfare: The art of war.* http://www.sonshi.com/sun3.html.

Survey: Worm infects 30% of China e-mail users. (2003). www.nyties.com/reuters/technologoy/tech–tech–worm–chian,html

Susman, P., O'Keefe, P., & Wisner, B. (1983). Global disasters, a radical interpretation. In K. Hewitt (Ed.), *Interpretations of calamity* (pp. 263–283). Boston: Allen and Unwin.

Susskind, L., & Cruikshank, J. (1987). *Breaking the impasse: Consensual approaches to resolving public disputes.* New York: Basic Books.

Sutphen, S., & Waugh, W.L. Jr. (1998). Organizational reform and technological innovation in emergency management. *International Journal of Mass Emergencies and Disasters, 16*(1), 7–12.

Sutton, A.J., Elias, T., Hendley, J.W., II, & Stauffer, P. H. (2000). United States geological survey fact sheet 169–97, Online version 1.1. United States Geological Survey. Retrieved November 11, 2004, http://pubs.usgs.gov/fs/fs169–97/.

Sutton, J. (2003). A complex organizational adaptation to the World Trade Center disaster: An analysis of faith-based organizations. In J. L. Monday (Ed.), *Beyond September 11th: An Account of Post-Disaster Research* (pp. 405–428). Boulder, CO: University of Colorado, Institute of Behavioral Science, Natural Hazards Research and Applications Information Center, Special Publication No. 39.

Suzuki, S., Sakamoto, S., Miki, T., & Matsuo, T. (1995). Hanshin-Awaji earthquake and acute myocardial infarction. *Lancet, 345*, 981.

Sweet, S. (1998). The effect of a natural disaster on social cohesion: A longitudinal study. *International Journal of Mass Emergencies and Disasters, 16*, 321–331.

Sylves, R.T. (1991). Adopting integrated emergency management in the United States: Political and organizational challenges. *International Journal of Mass Emergencies and Disasters, 9*, 413–424.

Sylves, R., & Cumming, W.R. (2004). FEMA's path to homeland security. *Journal of Homeland Security and Emergency Management: 1979–2003, 1*(11), 1–21.

Szasz, A., & Meuser, M. (1997). Environmental inequalities: Literature review and proposals for new directions in research and theory. *Current Sociology, 45*(3), 99–120.

Szasz, A., & Meuser, M. (2000). Unintended, inexorable: The production of environmental inequalities in Santa Clara County, California. *American Behavioral Scientist, 43*(4), 602–632.

Talen, E. (1999). Constructing neighborhoods from the bottom up: The case for resident-generated GIS. *Environment and Planning B, 26,* 533–554.

Tarrow, S. (1998). *Power in movement* (2nd ed.). Cambridge, UK: Cambridge University Press.

Taylor, L. (1983). *Structuralist macroeconomics.* New York: Basic Books.

Taylor, L. (1994). Gap models. *Journal of Development Economics, 45,* 17–34.

Taylor, L. (2000). *External liberalization, economic performance, and distribution in Latin America and elsewhere.* WIDER Working Paper No. 215.

Taylor, L. (2004). *Reconstructing macroeconomics. Structuralist proposals and critiques of the mainstream.* Cambridge, MA: Harvard University Press.

Taylor, V.A. (1977). Good news about disasters. *Psychology Today, 11,* 93–96.

Taylor, V.A. (1978). Future directions for study. In E. L. Quarantelli (Ed.), *Disasters: Theory and methods* (pp. 251–280). London and Beverly Hills, CA: SAGE.

Tearfund. (2004). Before disaster strikes: Why thousands are dying needlessly each year in preventable disasters. http://www.tearfund.org/webdocs/Website/Campaiging/Policy%20and%20research/BDS%20Kobe%20Jan%202005.pdf.

Ten Berge, D. (1990). *The first 24 hours: A comprehensive guide to successful crisis communications.* Oxford: Basil Blackwell.

Tenner, E. (1996). *Why things bite back.* New York: Knopf.

Tewari, P. (2005). *Recognition of traditional knowledge.* Retrieved 10 October 2005, www.netaddress.com/tplMessage/623MCWVJP/Read.

Thieler, E., & Bush, D. (1991). Hurricanes Gilbert and Hugo send powerful messages forcoastal development. *Journal of Geological Education, 39,* 291–299.

Thirwall, A.P. (2003). *Growth and development* (7th ed.). London: Macmillan.

Thomas, D.S.K, Cutter, S.L., Hodgson, M.E., Gutekunst, M., & Jones, S. (2003). Use of spatial data and geographic technologies in response to the September 11 terrorist attack on the World Trade Center. In *Beyond September 11th: An account of post-disaster research* (pp.147–164), Special Publication No. 39. Boulder, CO: University of Colorado, Natural Hazards Research and Applications Information Center.

Thomas, D., & Mileti, D.S. (2003). *Designing educational opportunities for the hazards manager of the 21st century.* Working paper no. 109. Boulder, CO: University of Colorado, Natural Hazards Research and Applications Information Center.

Thomas, J.D. (1992). *Informal economic activity.* New York: Harvester.

Thomas, W. & Thomas, D. (1928). *The child in America: Behavior problems and programs.* New York: Knopf.

Thompson, C. (2004). Virus underground. *The New York Times,* March 7, Section 6, p. 10.

Thompson, J.D. (1967). *Organizations in action.* New York: McGraw-Hill.

Thompson, J.D., & Hawkes, R.W. (1962). Disaster organization and administrative process. In G.W. Baker & D.W. Chapman (Eds.), *Man and society in disaster* (pp. 268–300). New York: Basic Books.

Thompson, W.C., Jr. (2002). *One year later: The effects of 9/11 on commercial insurance rates and availability in New York City.* New York: New York City Government, Office of the Comptroller of the City of New York.

Thorson, A., & Ekdahl, K. (2005). Avian influenza—Is the world on the verge of a pandemic and can it be stopped? *Journal of Contingencies and Crisis Management, 13,* 21–28.

Tiedemann, H. (1989). *Casualties as a function of building quality and earthquake intensity.* In *Proceedings of the workshop on earthquake injury epidemiology.* Baltimore: Johns Hopkins University Press, 420–434.

Tiefenbacher, J., & Hagelman, R. (1999). Environmental equity in urban Texas: Race, income, and patterns of acute and chronic toxic air releases in metropolitan counties. *Urban Geography, 20,* 516–533.

Tierney, K.J. (1985). Emergency medical preparedness and response in disasters: The need for interorganizational coordination. *Public Administration Review, 45,* 77–84.

Tierney, K.J. (1989). Improving theory and research on hazard mitigation: Political economy and organizational perspectives. *International Journal of Mass Emergencies and Disasters, 7,* 367–396.

Tierney, K.J. (1993). *Project summary: Disaster analysis: Delivery of emergency medical services in disasters.* Newark, DE: University of Delaware, Disaster Research Center.

Tierney, K.J. (1994). Research overview: Emergency response. In P. Vaziri (Compiler), *Proceedings of the NEHRP conference and workshop on the Northridge earthquake of January 17, 1994—Volume IV: Social science and emergency management* (pp. IV-9–IV-15). Richmond, CA: California Universities for Research in Earthquake Engineering.

Tierney, K. (1997). Business impacts of the Northridge earthquake. *Journal of Contingencies and Crisis Management, 5,* 87–97.

Tierney, K.J. (1999). Toward a critical sociology of risk. *Sociological Forum, 14*, 215–242.

Tierney, K.J. (2000). Controversy and consensus in disaster mental health research. *Prehospital and Disaster Medicine, 15*, 181–187.

Tierney, K.J. (2002a). *Lessons learned from research on group and organizational responses to disasters.* Paper presented at Countering Terrorism: Lessons Learned from Natural and Technological Disasters. National Academy of Sciences.

Tierney, K.J. (2002b). The field turns fifty: Social change and the practice of disaster fieldwork. In R. A. Stallings, (Ed.), *Methods of disaster research* (pp. 349–374). Philadelphia: Xlibris.

Tierney, K.J. (2003). Disaster beliefs and institutional interests: Recycling disaster myths in the aftermath of 9–11. In L. Clarke (Ed.), *Terrorism and disaster: New threats, new ideas: Research in social problems and public policy* (pp. 33–51). New York, Elsevier .

Tierney, K.J. (2005a). *Recent developments in the US homeland security policies and their implications for the management of extreme events.* 1st International conference on urban disaster reduction, Kobe.

Tierney, K.J. (2005b). The 9/11 Commission and disaster management: Little depth, less context, not much guidance. *Contemporary Sociology, 34*, 115–121.

Tierney, K.J., & Dahlhamer, J.M. (1997). Earthquake vulnerability and emergency preparedness among businesses. In M. Shinozuka, A. Rose, & R. T. Eguchi (Eds.), *Engineering and socioeconomic impacts of earthquakes: An analysis of electricity lifeline disruptions in the New Madrid area* (pp. 53–73). Buffalo, NY: State University of New York at Buffalo, Multidisciplinary Center for Earthquake Engineering Research.

Tierney, K.J., Lindell, M.K., & Perry, R.W. (2001). *Facing the unexpected: Disaster preparedness and response in the United States.* Washington, DC: Joseph Henry Press.

Tierney, K.J., Nigg, J.M., & Dahlhamer, J.M. (1996). The impact of the 1993 Midwest floods: Business vulnerability and disruption in Des Moines. In R.T. Sylves & W.L. Waugh, Jr. (Eds.), *Disaster management in the U.S. and Canada: The politics, policymaking, administration and analysis of emergency management.* (pp. 214–233). Springfield, IL: Charles C Thomas.

Tierney, K.J. & Webb, G.R. (Forthcoming). Business vulnerability to earthquakes and other disasters. In E. Rovai & C.M. Rodrigue (Eds.), *Earthquakes.* New York: Routledge.

Timmerman, P. (1981). *Vulnerability, resilience and the collapse of society.* Toronto: Institute of Environmental Studies.

Tinker, I. (Ed.) (1990). *Persistent inequalities: Women and world development.* Oxford: Oxford University Press.

Titan Systems Corporation (2002). *Arlington County after action report on the response to the September 11 terrorist attack on the Pentagon.* Retrieved 10 October 2005, http://www.co.arlington.va.us/departments/Fire/edu/about/docs/after_report.pdf.

Tobin, G.A., & Montz, B.E. (1997). *Natural hazards: Explanation and integration.* New York: Guilford Press.

Topping, K. (1991). *Key laws, codes and authorities affecting recovery and reconstruction.* Los Angeles: Consultant Report No. 1.

Toulmin, L.M., Bivans, C.J., & Steel, D.L. (1989). The impact of intergovernmental distance on disaster communications. *International Journal of Mass Emergencies and Disasters, 7*, 116–132.

Townsend, A., & Moss, M. (2005). Telecommunications infrastructure in disasters: Preparing cities for crisis communication. Retrieved October 10, 2005; http://hurricane. wagner.nyu.edu/pcikup/report1.pdf.

Trainor, J., & Aguirre, B. (2005). *The origins and organizational features of the Federal Urban Search and Rescue system.* Forthcoming.

Traube, E.G. (1996). The "popular" in American culture. *Annual Review of Anthropology, 25*, 127–151.

Trichopoulos, D., Katsouyanni, K., Zavilsanos, X., Tzonou, A., & Dalla-Vorgia, P. (1981). Psychological stress and fatal heart attack: The Athens 1981 natural experiment. *Lancet, 1*, 441–444.

Trout, D., Nimgade, A., Mueller, C., Hall, R., & Earnest, G.S. (2002). Health effects and occupational exposures among office workers near the World Trade Center disaster site. *Journal of Occupational and Environmental Medicine, 44*, 601–605.

Tsuchiya, Y., & Shuto, N. (1995). *Tsunami: Progress in prediction, disaster prevention and warning.* Norwell, MA: Kluwer Academic.

Tung X.B., & Siva, R.S. (2001). Design considerations for a virtual information center for humanitarian assistance/disaster relief using workflow modeling. *Decision Support Systems Archive, 31*(2), 165–179.

Turkel, G. (2002). Sudden solidarity and the rush to normalization: Toward an alternative approach. *Sociological Focus, 35*, 73–79.

Turker, M., & San, B.T. (2003). SPOT HRV data analysis for detecting earthquake-induced changes in Izmit, Turkey. *International Journal of Remote Sensing, 24*(2), 2439.

Turner, B.A. (1978). *Man-made disasters.* London: Wykeham.

Turner, B.A. (1994). Flexibility and improvisation in emergency response. *Disaster Management, 6*, 84–89.

Turner, B.A., & Pidgeon, N. (1997). *Man-made disasters*. London: Wykeham.

Turner, J.H. (1986). *The structure of sociological theory* (4th ed.). Belmont, CA: Wadsworth.

Turner, R.H. (1964). Collective behavior. In R.E.L. Faris (Ed.), *Handbook of Sociology* (pp. 382–425). Chicago: Rand McNally.

Turner, R.H. (1980a). Strategy for developing an integrated role theory. *Humboldt Journal of Social Relations, 7*, 123–139.

Turner, R.H. (1980b). The mass media and preparations for natural disaster. *Disasters and the mass media* (pp. 281–292). Washington: The National Research Council.

Turner, R.H. (1989). Aspects of role improvisation. In G. A. Kreps (Ed.), *Social structure and disaster* (pp. 207–213). Newark, Toronto, and London: University of Delaware and Associated University Presses.

Turner, R., Nigg, J., & Paz, D. (1980). *Community response to earthquake threat in Southern California*. Los Angeles: University of California Los Angeles, Institute for Social Research.

Turner, R., Nigg, J., & Paz, D. (1986). *Waiting for disaster: Earthquake watch in California*. Berkeley, CA: University of California Press.

Twigg, J. (2004). Disaster risk reduction: mitigation and preparedness in development and emergency programming. *Good Practice Review, 9*. London: Overseas Development Institute.

Tyler, K.A., & Hoyt, D.R. (2000). The effects of an acute stressor on depressive symptoms among older adults: The moderating effects of social support and age. *Research on Aging, 22*, 143–164.

Tzannatos, E. (2003). A decision support system for the promotion of security in shipping: Disaster prevention and management. *An International Journal, 12*(3), 222–229.

Ullberg, S. (2004). *The Buenos Aires blackout: Argentine crisis management across the public–private divide*. Stockholm: Crismart.

United Church of Christ (1987). *Toxic wastes and race in the United States: A national report on the racial and socio-economic characteristic with hazardous waste sites*. New York: United Church of Christ Commission for Racial Justice.

United Nations (2005). *Know risk*. Leicester: Tudor Rose.

United Nations Development Programme/Department of Humanitarian Affairs, Disaster Management Training Programme (1994). *Disasters and development*.

United Nations Development Programme. (2004). Reducing disaster risk: A challenge for development. Retrieved October 10, 2005; http://www.undp.org/bcpr/cpr_all/9_natural_disaster/9.2_risk_reduction/1_reducing_disaster_risk_report.p

United Nations Environment Programme (2002). *Global environment outlook 3*(3). Human vulnerability to environmental change. Nairobi: UNEP/London: Earthscan.

United Nations Environment Programme (2005). Retrieved October 1, 2005; http://maps.grid.unep.ch.

United Nations Environment Programme /Division of Early Warning and Assessment/ EUROPE/GRID–Geneva 1998–2004 (2005). Retrieved October 1, 2005; http://maps.grid.unep.ch/.

United Nations International Strategy for Disaster Reduction (2002). *Living with risk: A global review of disaster reduction initiatives*. Geneva.

United Nations International Strategy for Disaster Reduction (2003). *Women, disaster reduction, and sustainable development*. Paper prepared for the World Meteorological Organization Bulletin.Geneva: Switzerland. Retrieved June 2003; http://www.unisdr.org/unisdr /eng/risk–reduction/gender/Women,%20disaster%20reduction %20and%20SD.pdf.

UN Millennium Development Goals. Retrieved October, 2005; http://www.un.org/millenniumgoals.

Uphoff, N. (1986). *Local institutional development: An analytical sourcebook with cases*. West Hartford, CT: Kumarian.

Ural, D.N. (2005). *Disaster management perspective of terrorist attacks in Istanbul on November 15 & 20, 2003*. Istanbul, Turkey: ITU Press.

Ursano, R.J., Fullerton, C.S., & Norwood, A.E. (1995). Psychiatric dimensions of disaster: Patient care, community consultation, and preventive medicine. *Harvard Review of Psychiatry, 3*, 196–209.

U.S. Army Corps of Engineers. (2005). http://www.mvn.usace.army.mil/pao/response/HURPROJ.asp?prj=lkponl (August 2005).

U.S. Department of Commerce. (2001a). *Black-owned businesses: 1997. Census brief. Survey of minority-owned business enterprises*. Washington, DC: U. S. Census Bureau.

U.S. Department of Commerce. (2001b). *1997 Economic Census: Survey of minority owned business enterprises*. Washington, DC: U.S. Census Bureau.

U.S. Department of Commerce. (2001c). *Statistics about business size (including small business) from the U.S. Census Bureau: Table 2a Employment size of employer firms*. Washington, DC: U.S. Census Bureau.

U.S. Department of Commerce. (2002). *Survey of Business owners: Preliminary estimates of ownership by gender, hispanic origin, and race*. Washington, DC: U.S. Census Bureau.

U.S. Department of Energy. (1998). The wingspread principles: A community vision for sustainability. Retrieved October 10, 2005; http://www.sustainable.doe.gov/wingspread2/wingprin.html.

U.S. Department of Homeland Security. (2005). *National preparedness guidance: Homeland security presidential directive 8*. National preparedness.

U.S. Department of Labor. (2005). *Bureau of Labor Statistics, Occupational Employment Statistics*. Retrieved August 10, 2005; http://bls.gov/oco/oco20051.htm.

U.S. Department of State. (2004). *Patterns of global terrorism—2003*. Washington, DC: U.S. Department of State, May.

U.S. Department of State. (2005). *Country reports on terrorism 2004*. Washington: U.S. Department of State, Office of the Coordinator for Counterterrorism, April.

U.S. Environmental Protection Agency. (2005). Retrieved October 1, 2005; http://www.epa.gov/ceppo/cameo/.

U.S. General Accounting Office. (2003). *September 11: Overview of federal disaster assistance to the New York City area*. Washington, DC: USGAO, GAO–04–72.

U.S. Geological Survey. (2001). *Community-based research team begins to examine vog's health effects*. Retrieved November 11, 2004; http://hvo.wr.usgs.gov/ volcanowatch/2001/01_12_20.html.

U.S. Geological Survey. (2005a). Retrieved October 1, 2005; http://earthquake.usgs.gov/hazmaps/ov/viewer.htm.

U.S. Geological Survey. (2005b). Retrieved October 1, 2005; http://waterdata.usgs.gov/nwis/rt.

U.S. Geological Survey. (2005c). Retrieved October 1, 2005; http://www.usgs.gov/themes/hazpics.html.

U.S. Geological Survey. (2005d). Retrieved October 1, 2005; http://geode.usgs.gov/.

U.S. Geological Survey. (2005e). Retrieved October 1, 2005; http://nmviewogc.cr.usgs.gov/.

U.S. Geological Survey. (2005f). Retrieved October 1, 2005; http://earthquake.usgs.gov/networks/global.html.

U.S. Strategic Bombing Survey. (1947). *Reports*. Washington, DC: Government Printing Office.

Ustinov, V. (2005). *Pravda o "Kurske": The truth about Kursk disaster*. Moscow: Olma Press.

Vale, L., & Campanella, T. (2004). *The resilient city: How modern cities recover from disasters*. New York: Oxford University Press.

Van Gennep, A. (2004). The Rites of Passage. London: Routledge.

Van Willigen, M. (2001). Do disasters affect individuals' psychological well-being? An over-time analysis of the effect of Hurricane Floyd on men and women in eastern North Carolina. *International Journal of Mass Emergencies and Disasters, 19*, 59–83.

Varley, A. (1994a). The exceptional and the everyday: Vulnerability analysis in the international decade for natural disaster reduction. In A. Varley, (Ed.), *Disasters, development and environment*. London: Wiley.

Varley, A. (1994b). *Disasters, development and environment*. London: Wiley.

Vaughan, D. (1996). *The challenger launch decision: Risky technology, culture, and deviance at NASA*. Chicago: The University of Chicago Press.

Vaughan, D. (1999). The dark side of organizations: Mistake, misconduct, and disaster. *Annual Review of Sociology, 25*, 271–305

Veness, A. (1993). Neither homed nor homeless: Contested definitions and the personal worlds of the poor. *Political Geography, 12*(4), 319–340.

Vigo, G., & Wenger, D.E. (1994). Emergent behavior in the immediate response to the 1985 Mexico City earthquake and the 1994 Northridge earthquake in Los Angeles. In P. Vaziri (Compiler), *Proceedings of the NEHRP conference and workshop on the Northridge earthquake of January 17, 1994—Volume IV: Social science and emergency management* (pp. IV-237–IV-244). Richmond, CA: California Universities for Research in Earthquake Engineering.

Villagran De Leon, J.C. (2005). WCDR in Kobe and the way forward, the unspoken challenges. *International Journal of Mass Emergencies and Disasters, 23*(1), 141–160.

Vlahov, D., Galea, S., Resnick, H., Ahern, J., Boscarino, J.A., Bucuvalas, et al. (2002). Increased use of cigarettes, alcohol, and marijuana among Manhattan, New York, residents after the September 11th terrorist attacks. *American Journal of Epidemiology, 155*, 988–996.

Vogt, B. (1990). *Evacuation of institutionalized and specialized populations, ORNL/SUB–7685/1 & T23*. Oak Ridge, TN: Oak Ridge National Laboratory.

Vogt, B. (1991). Issues in nursing home evacuations. *International Journal of Mass Emergencies and Disasters, 9*, 247–265.

Vogt, B., & Sorensen, J. (1999). *Description of survey data regarding the chemical repackaging plant accident West, Helena, Arkansas, ORNL/TM–13722*. Oak Ridge, TN: Oak Ridge National Laboratory.

Vogt, B., & Sorensen, J. (2002). *How clean is safe—improving the effectiveness of decontamination of structures and people following chemical and biological incidents–ORNL/TM–2002/178*. Oak Ridge, TN: Oak Ridge National Laboratory.

Von Kotze, A., & Holloway, A. (1996). *Reducing risk: Participatory learning activities for disaster mitigation in Southern Africa.* Oxford: Oxfam International Federation.

Vorobiev, Y., Akimov, V., & Sokolov, Y. (2003). *Katastroficheskiye navodneniya nachala XXI veka: Uroki I Vivodi. (Catastrophic floods in the beginning of the 21st century: lessons and conclusions.)* Moscow: Deks-Express.

Wachtendorf, T. (2000). When disasters defy borders: What we can learn from the Red River flood about transnational disasters. *The Australian Journal of Emergency Management, 15*(3), 36–41.

Wachtendorf, T. (2004). Improvising 9/11 organizational improvisation following the World Trade Center disaster. Doctoral dissertation. Newark, DE: University of Delaware, Department of Sociology and Criminal Justice.

Wachtendorf, T., Connell, R., Tierney, K.J., & Kompanik, K. (2002). *Disaster resistant communities initiative: Assessment of the pilot phase—year 3.* Final Report No. 39. Newark, DE: Disaster Research Center, University of Delaware.

Wachtendorf, T., & Kendra, J.M. (2005). A typology of organizational response to disasters. Presentation to the American Sociological Association, Philadelphia, August 14.

Wachtendorf, T., & Tierney, K.J. (2001). *Disaster resistant communities initiative: Local community representatives share their views.* In Year 3 Focus Group final report (75 pp.). Newark, DE: University of Delaware, Disaster Research Center.

Waddell, E. (1983). Coping with frosts, governments and disaster experts: Some reflections based on a New Guinea experience and a perusal of the relevant literature. In K. Hewitt (Ed.), *Interpretations of calamity* (pp. 33–43). Boston: Allen & Unwin.

Waddington, D.P. (1992). *Contemporary issues in public disorder: A comparative and historical approach.* London: Routledge.

Wade, R. (1990). *Governing the market.* Princeton, NJ: Princeton University Press.

Wade, R. (1996). Japan, The World Bank, and the art of paradigm maintenance: The East Asian miracle in political perspective. *New Left Review, 217*, 3–36.

Wagman, D. (2003). Get out of town. *Homeland Protection Professional.* Retrieved October 1, 2005; www.hppmag.com.

Wald, M. (2005). Experts assess deregulation as factor in '03 blackout. *The New York Times,* September 16, 2005, A5, 20.

Walker, P. (1990). Coping with famine in southern Ethiopia. *International Journal of Mass Emergencies and Disasters, 8*(2), 103–116.

Wallace, A.F.C. (1956a). *Human behavior in extreme situations.* Washington, DC: National Research Council, National Academy of Sciences.

Wallace, A.F.C. (1956b). *Tornado in Worcester: An exploratory study of individual and community behavior in an extreme situation.* Disaster Study Number 3. Washington, DC: Committee on Disaster Studies, National Academy of Sciences, National Research Council.

Wallace, M., & Webber, L. (2004). *The disaster recovery handbook: A step-by-step plan to ensure business continuity and protect vital operations, facilities, and assets.* NewYork: American Management Association.

Wallerstein, L. (1995). Letter from the President. *International Sociological Association Newsletter,* 2.

Walsh, E.J. (1981). Resource mobilization and citizen protest in communities around three mile island. *Social Problems, 29*, 1–21.

Walsh, E.J. (1984). Local community vs. national industry: The TMI and Santa Barbara protests compared. *International Journal of Mass Emergencies and Disasters, 2*, 147–163.

Walter, T. (1990). *Funerals and how to improve them.* London: Hodder & Stoughton.

Walters, L.M., Wilkins, L., & Walters T. (Eds.). (1989). *Bad tidings communications and catastrophe.* Hillsdale, NJ: Erlbaum.

Wang, D., Sava, J., Sample, G., & Jordan, M. (2005). The Pentagon and 9/11. *Critical Care Medicine, 33*(Suppl.), S42–S47.

Warheit, G. (1972). Organizational differences and similarities in disasters and civil disturbances. In *Proceedings of the Japan–United States Research Seminar: Organizational and community responses to disasters* (pp. 130–141). Newark, DE: Disaster Research Center.

Warn, G., Berman, J., Whittaker, A., & Bruneau, M. (2003). Investigation of a damaged high–rise building near ground zero. In J. Monday (Ed.), *Beyond September 11th: An account of post-disaster research.* Special Publication No. 39. Boulder, CO: Natural Hazards Research and Applications Information Center, University of Colorado.

Warren, R.L., Rose, S.M., & Bergunder, A.F. (1974). *The structure of urban reform: Community decision organizations in stability and change.* Lexington, MA: D.C. Heath.

Warriner, C.K. (1981). Levels in the study of social structure. In P.M. Blau & R.K. Merton (Eds.), *Continuities in structural inquiry.* (pp. 179–190). Beverly Hills, CA: SAGE.

Waterbury, J. (1979). *Hydopolitics of the Nile Valley.* Syracuse, NY: Syracuse University Press.

Waterstone, M. (1978). *Hazard mitigation behavior of flood plain residents.* Natural hazard working paper no. 35. Boulder, CO: Institute of Behavioral Science, University of Colorado.

Watts, M.J. (1983). On the poverty of theory: Natural hazards research in context. In K. Hewitt, (Ed.), *Interpretations of calamity from the perspective of human ecology.* London: Allen and Unwin.

Watts, M.J. (1991). Heart of darkness: Reflections on famine and starvation in Africa. In R. Downs, D. Kerner, & S. Reyna (Eds.), *Political economy of an African famine* (pp. 23–70). Philadelphia: Gordon and Breach.

Watts, M.J., & Bohle, H. G. (1993). The space of vulnerability: The causal structure of hunger and famine. *Progress in Human Geography, 17,* 43–67.

Waugh, W.L., Jr. (1982). International terrorism: How nations respond to terrorists. Salisbury, NC: Documentary Publications.

Waugh, W.L., Jr. (1984). *Emergency management and mass destruction terrorism: A policy framework.* Report for the Federal Emergency Management Agency. Emmitsburg, MD: NASPAA/FEMA Workshop for Public Administration Faculty.

Waugh, W.L., Jr. (1988). Current policy and implementation issues in disaster preparedness. In L. K. Comfort (Ed.), *Managing disaster: Strategies and policy perspectives* (pp.111–125). Durham, NC: Duke University Press.

Waugh, W.L., Jr. (1990). *Terrorism and emergency management.* New York: Marcel Dekker.

Waugh, W.L., Jr. (1995). Geographic information systems: The case of disaster management. *Social Science Computer Review, 13*(4), 422–431.

Waugh, W.L., Jr. (2000a). *Living with hazards, dealing with hazards: An introduction to emergency management.* Armonk, NY: M. E. Sharpe.

Waugh, W.L., Jr. (2000b). *Terrorism and emergency management: Instructor guide.* Emmitsburg, MD: Federal Emergency Management Agency, Emergency Management Institute.

Waugh, W.L., Jr. (2001). Managing terrorism as an environmental hazard. In A. Farazmand (Ed.), *Handbook of crisis and emergency management* (pp. 659–676). New York: Marcel Dekker.

Waugh, W.L., Jr. (2003a). The global challenge of the new terrorism. *Journal of Emergency Management, 1*(1), 27–38.

Waugh, W.L., Jr. (2003b). Terrorism, homeland security and the national emergency management network. *Public Organization Review, 3,* 373–385.

Waugh, W.L., Jr. (2004a). Building a seamless homeland security: The cultural interoperability problem. Paper presented at the National Conference of the American Society for Public Administration, March 28–30, 2004. Portland, OR.

Waugh, W.L., Jr. (2004b). Securing mass transit: A challenge for homeland security. *Review of Policy Studies, 21*(3), 307–316.

Waugh, W.L., Jr. (2004c). The all-hazards approach must be continued. *Journal of Emergency Management, 2*(1), 11–12.

Waugh, W.L., Jr. (2005). Terrorism and the all-hazards model. *Journal of Emergency Management, 4*(2), 8, 10.

Waugh, W.L., & Hy, R. (Eds.). (1999). *Handbook of emergency management.* New York: Greenwood Press.

Waugh, W.L., Jr., & Sylves, R.T. (1996). The intergovernmental relations of emergency management. In R.T. Sylves & W.L. Waugh, Jr. (Eds.), *Disaster management in the U.S. and Canada* (2nd ed., pp. 46–68). Springfield, IL: Charles C Thomas.

Waugh, W.L., Jr., & Sylves, R.T. (2002). Organizing the war on terrorism. *Public Administration Review,* Special Issue (September): 145–153.

Waugh, W.L., & Tierney, K. (Forthcoming). *Emergency management: Principles and practice for local government* (2nd ed.). Washington, DC: International City Management Association.

Waxman, J. (1973). Local broadcast gatekeeping during natural disaster. *Journalism Quarterly, 50,* 751–758.

Weather Channel. (2005). Retrieved August 29, 2005; http://www.weather.com /aboutus/marketing/press/internet.

Webb, G.R. (1998). *Role enactment in disaster: Reconciling structuralist and interactionist conceptions of role.* Doctoral dissertation, University of Delaware. Ann Arbor, MI: UMI Dissertation Services.

Webb, G.R. (2002). Sociology, disasters and terrorism: Understanding threat of the new millennium. *Sociological Focus, 35*(1), 87–95.

Webb, G.R. (2004). Role improvising during crisis situations. *International Journal of Emergency Management, 2,* 47–61.

Weber, E.U., & Hsee, C.K. (1998). Cross-cultural differences in risk perception but cross–cultural similarities in attitudes towards risk. *Management Science, 44,* 1205–1217.

Weber, F.H., Jr., (October 1 & 4, 1987). Whittier narrow earthquakes—Los Angeles country. *California Geology, 40,* 275–281.

Webb, G.R., & Quarantelli, E.L. (Forthcoming). *The popular culture of disaster.* Philadelphia: Xlibris.

Webb, G.R., Tierney, K.J., & Dahlhamer, J.M. (2000). Businesses and disasters: Empirical patterns and unanswered questions. *Natural Hazards Review, 1*, 83–90.

Webb, G.R., Tierney, K.J., & Dahlhamer, J.M. (2002). Predicting long-term business recovery from disaster: A comparison of the Loma Prieta Earthquake and Hurricane Andrew. *Environmental Hazards, 4*, 45–58.

Webb, G.R., Wachtendorf, T., & Eyre, A. (2000). Bringing culture back in: Exploring the cultural dimensions of disaster. *International Journal of Mass Emergencies and Disasters, 18*, 5–19.

Weber, M. (1947). *The theory of social and economic organization*. New York: Macmillan.

Weber, M. (1949). *The methodology of the social sciences*. New York: Free Press.

Weber, M. (1958). *The Protestant ethic and the spirit of capitalism*. New York: Charles Scribner's Sons.

Wedel, K.R., & Baker, D.R. (1998). After the Oklahoma City bombing: A case study of the resource coordination committee. *International Journal of Mass Emergencies and Disasters, 16*, 333–362.

Weichselgartner, J. (2001). Disaster mitigation: The concept of vulnerability revisited. *Disaster Prevention and Management, 10*(2), 85–94.

Weick, K. (1981). Evolutionary theory as a backdrop for administrative practice. In H. D. Stein (Ed.), *Organization and the human services: Cross disciplinary reflections* (pp. 107–141). Philadelphia: Temple University Press.

Weick, K.E. (1993). The collapse of sensemaking in organizations: The Mann Gulch Disaster. *Administrative Science Quarterly, 38*, 628–652.

Weick, K.E. (1995). *Sensemaking in organizations*. Thousand Oaks, CA: SAGE.

Weick, K.E. (1998). Improvisation as a mindset for organizational analysis. *Organization Science, 9*, 543–555.

Weick, K.E., & Sutcliffe, K.M. (2002). *Managing the unexpected: Assuring high performance in an age of complexity*. San Francisco: Jossey-Bass.

Weick, K., Sutcliffe, K., & Obstfeld, D. (2005). Organizing and the process of sensemaking. *Organization Science, 16*(4), 409–421.

Weidner, N. (2004). *Neighborhood emergency networks in Corvallis, Oregon and Uzhhorod, Ukraine*. Paper prepared for the Gender Equality and Disaster Risk Reduction Workshop. Honolulu, Hawaii. Retrieved August 11, 2004; http://www.ssri.hawaii.edu/research/GDWwebsite/pages/proceeding.html.

Weinberg, A. (1985). Science and its limits: The regulator's dilemma. *Issues in Science and Technology, 2*, 59–72.

Weisbrot, M.D., Baker, D., Kraev, E., & Chen, J. (2001). *The scorecard on globalization 1980–2000*. London: Center for Economic Policy Research.

Weiss, J. (2002). *Industrialisation and globalization*. London: Routledge.

Weller, C. (2001). Financial crisis after financial liberalization: Exceptional circumstances or structural weakness? *Journal of Development Studies, 1*, 98–127.

Weller, J.M., & Quarantelli, E.L. (1973). Neglected characteristics of collective behavior. *American Journal of Sociology, 75*, 665–685.

Wenger, D.E. (1972). *DRC Studies of community functioning*. Proceedings of the Japan–United States disaster research seminar: Organizational and community responses to disasters. Columbus, OH: Disaster Research Center, Ohio State University.

Wenger, D.E. (1978). Community response to disaster: Functional and structural alternations. In E.L. Quarantelli (Ed.), *Disasters: Theory and research* (pp. 18–47). London: SAGE.

Wenger, D.E. (1985). *Mass media and disasters*. Preliminary Paper No. 98. Newark, DE: Disaster Research Center.

Wenger, D.E. (1987). Collective behavior and disaster research. In R. R. Dynes, B. De Marche, & C. Pelanda (Eds.), *Sociology of disasters: Contributions of sociology to disaster research* (pp. 213–239). Milano, Italy: Franco Angelo.

Wenger, D.E. (1990). *Volunteer and organizational search and rescue activities following the Loma Prieta Earthquake: An integrated emergency and sociological analysis*. College Station, TX: Texas A&M University, Hazard Reduction and Recovery Center.

Wenger, D.E., Dykes, J.D., Sebok, T.D., & Neff, J.L. (1975). It's a matter of myths: An empirical examination of individual insight into disaster response. *Mass Emergencies, 1*, 33–46.

Wenger, D.E., Dyke, J.D., Sebok, T.D., & Neff, J.L. (1980). It's a matter of myths: An empirical examination of individual insight into disaster response. In M. D. Pugh (Ed.), *Collective behavior: A source book* (pp. 65–78). New York: West.

Wenger, D.E., & Friedman, B. (1986). Local and national media coverage of disaster: A content analysis of the print media's treatment of disaster myths. *International Journal of Mass Emergencies and Disasters, 4*, 27–50.

Wenger, D.E., & James, T. (1990). *Convergence of volunteers in a consensus crisis: The case of the 1985 Mexico City earthquake*. HRRC Publication 13P. College Station, TX: Hazard Reduction and Recovery Center, Texas A&M University.

Wenger, D.E., James, T.F., & Faupel, C.E. (1980). *Disaster beliefs and emergency planning*. Newark, DE: Disaster Research Center.

Wenger, D.E., James, T.F., & Faupel, C.E. (1985). *Disaster beliefs and emergency planning*. New York: Irvington.

Wenger, D.E., & Quarantelli, E. L. (1989). *Local mass media operations, problems and products in disasters* (62 pp.). Report Series No. 19. Newark, DE: Disaster Research Center.

Wenger, D.E., Quarantelli, E.L., & Dynes, R.R. (1987). *Disaster analysis: Emergency management offices and arrangements*. Final Report on Phase I. Newark, DE: Disaster Research Center, University of Delaware.

Wenger, D.E., Quarantelli, E.L., & Dynes, R.R. (1989). Disaster analysis: Police and fire departments. Final Project Report. Newark, DE: University of Delaware, Disaster Research Center.

Wenger, D.E., & Weller, J.M. (1973). *Disaster subcultures: The cultural residues of community disasters*. Newark, DE: Disaster Research Center, University of Delaware.

West, C., & Lenze, D. (1994). Modeling the regional impact of natural disaster and recovery. *International Regional Science Review, 17*, 121–150.

West, P. (2004). *Conspicuous compassion: Why sometimes it really is cruel to be kind*. Trowbridge: Institute for the Study of Civil Society, Civitas.

Wettenhall, R.L. (1975). *Bushfire disaster: An Australian community in crisis*. Sydney: Angus & Robertson.

White, G.F. (1945). *Human adjustment to floods: A geographical approach to the flood problems in the United States*. Research Paper No. 29. Chicago: Department of Geography, The University of Chicago.

White, G.F. (1973). Natural hazards research. In R. J. Chorley (Ed.), *Directions in geography* (pp. 193–216). London: Methuen.

White, G.F. (Ed.). (1974). *Natural hazards: Local, national global*. Oxford: Oxford University Press.

White, G.F., & Haas, J. (1975). *Assessment of research on natural hazards*. Cambridge, MA: MIT Press.

Whitehead, J.C., Edwards, B., Van Willigan, M., Maiolo, J.R., Wilson, K., & Smith, K.T. (2000). Heading for higher ground: Factors affecting real and hypothetical hurricane evacuation behavior. *Environmental Hazards, 2*, 133–142.

White House. (2003). *The national strategy for the physical protection of critical infrastructure and key assets*. Washington, DC: Executive Office of the President.

Wicker, T. (1966). The assassination. In R. Adler (Ed.), *The working press*. New York: G. P. Putman and Sons.

Wiest, R.E. (1998). A comparative perspective on household, gender, and kinship in relation to disaster. In E. Enarson & B.H. Morrow (Eds.), *The gendered terrain of disaster: Through women's eyes* (pp. 63–80). Westport, CT: Praeger.

Wiest, R.E., Mocellin, J.S.P., & Motsisi, D.T. (1994). *The needs of women in disasters and emergencies*. Report prepared for the United Nations Development Programme and the Office of the United Nations Disaster Relief coordinator. Winnipeg, Manitoba (June 20, 1994); http://online.northumbria.ac.uk/geography_research/gdn/resources/women-in-disaster-emergency.pdf.

Wijkman, A., & Timberlake, L. (1988). *Natural disasters: Acts of God or acts of man?* Philadelphia: New Society Publishers.

Wildavsky, A. (1979). *Speaking the truth to power: The art and craft of policy analysis*. Boston: Little Brown.

Wildavsky, A.B. (1988). *Searching for safety*. Berkeley, CA: University of California Press.

Wilkins, L. (1986). Media coverage of the Bhopal disaster: A cultural myth in the making. *International Journal of Mass Emergencies and Disasters, 4*, 7–33.

Wilkinson, K., & Ross, P. (1970) *Citizens response to warnings of Hurricane Camille*. Report No. 35. Starkville, MS: Mississippi State University, Social Science Research Center.

Wilkinson, P. (2005). Welcome to Nowhere: Pop. 1,062. *Rolling Stone, 987* (November 17, 2005):58–64.

Wilkinson, S. (2005). *Mission findings in Thailand, Indian Ocean Tsunami preliminary field mission report*. Presented to the Institution of Structural Engineers. Retrieved July 15, 2005; http://www.istructe.org.uk/eefit/index.asp?bhcp=1.

Williams, H.B. (1954). Fewer disasters, better studied. *Journal of Social Issues, 10*, 11.

Williams, H.B. (1964). Human factors in the warning and response systems. In G. Grosser et al. (Eds.), *The threat of impending disaster* (pp. 79–104). Cambridge, MA: MIT Press.

Williams, H.B. (1989). A class act: Anthropology and the race to nation across ethnic terrain. *Annual Review of Anthropology, 18*, 401–444.

Williams, J. (1994). Responding to women in emergencies and disasters: The role of community services development. *Australian Journal of Emergency Management, 8*(4), 32–36.

Williams, R.M. (1970) *American society: A sociological interpretation*. New York: Alfred A. Knopf.

Williams, R.M. (1983). *Keywords*. London: Fontana.

Williamson, J. (Ed.). (1990). *Latin American adjustment: How much has happened?* Washington, DC: Institute for International Economics.

Wilson, J. (1999). Professionalization and gender in local emergency management. *International Journal of Mass Emergencies and Disasters, 17*(1), 111–122.

Wilson, J. (2005). Ethnic minorities to form majority by 2050. *The Guardian*. Retrieved August 13, 2005; http://guardian.co.uk/usastory/0,12271,154825,00/html.

Wilson, J., & Oyola-Yemaiel, A. (1998). *Emergent coordinative groups and women's response roles in the Central Florida tornado disaster, February 23, 1998*. Quick Response Report No. 110. Boulder, CO: Natural Hazards Research and Applications Information Center, University of Colorado at Boulder.

Wilson, J., & Oyola-Yemaiel, A. (2000). The historical origins of emergency management professionalization in the United States. *The Journal of the American Society of Professional Emergency Planners, 7*, 125–153.

Wilson, J., Phillips, B.D., & Neal, D.M. (1998). Domestic violence after disaster. In E. Enarson & B.H. Morrow (Eds.), *The gendered terrain of disaster: Through women's eyes* (pp. 115–122). Westport, CT: Praeger.

Wilson, R. (1991). *Rebuilding after the Loma Prieta Earthquake in Santa Cruz*. Washington, DC: International City Management Association.

Winant, H. (2001). *The world is a ghetto: Race and democracy since World War II*. New York: Basic Books.

Windham, G., Posey, E., Ross, P., & Spencer, B. (1977). *Reaction to storm threat during Hurricane Eloise*. Report No. 35. Starkville, MS: Mississippi State University, Social Science Research Center.

Windrem, R. (2001). They are trying to kill us. *Columbia Journalism Review, November/December*, 18–19.

Winslow, Frances E. (1999). The first responder's perspective. In S.D. Drell, A.D. Sofaer, & G.D. Wilson (Eds.), *The new terror: Facing the threat of biological and chemical weapons* (pp. 375–389). Stanford, CA: Hoover Press.

Wisner, B. (1998). Marginality and vulnerability: Why the homeless of Tokyo don't 'count' in disaster preparations, *Applied Geography, 18*, 25–53.

Wisner, B. (1999). There are worse things than earthquakes: Hazard vulnerability and mitigation capacity in Greater Los Angeles. In J.K. Mitchell (Ed.), *Crucibles of hazard: Mega-cities and disasters in transition* (pp. 375–427). Tokyo: United Nations University Press.

Wisner, B. (2004). The societal implications of a comet/asteroid impact on earth: A perspective from international development studies. Unpublished paper.

Wisner, B. (2005). Circus of hope. *International Journal of Mass Emergencies and Disasters, 23*(1), 141–160.

Wisner, B. (n.d.) *Disaster risk reduction in megacities: Making the most of human and social capital*. London: Hazard Research Centre, University College London & London School of Economics.

Wisner, B., Blaikie, P., Cannon, T., & Davis, I. (2004). *At risk: Natural hazards, people's vulnerability, and disaster* (2nd ed.). London: Routledge.

Wisner, B., & Walker, P. (2005). The world conference on disaster viewed through the lens of political ecology: A dozen big questions for Kobe and beyond. *Capitalism, Nature, Socialism, 16*(2), 89–95.

Withey, S.B. (1962). Reaction to uncertain threat. In G. Baker, & D. Chapman (Eds.), *Man and society in disaster* (pp. 93–123). New York: Basic Books.

Witt, J.L. (2004). Testimony before the Subcommittee on National Security, Emerging Threats and International Relations and the Subcommittee on Energy Policy, Natural Resources and Regulatory Affairs, March 24, 2004.

Witzig, W.F., & Shillenn, J.K. (1987). *Evaluation of protective action risks*. Washington, DC: Office of Nuclear Regulatory Research, U.S. Nuclear Regulatory Commission.

Wolensky, R.P. (1977). Comment: How do community officials respond to major catastrophes? *Disasters, 1*(4), 272–274.

Wolensky, R.P., & Miller, E.J. (1981). The everyday versus the disaster role of local officials—citizen and official definitions. *Urban Affairs Quarterly, 16*, 483–504.

Wolensky, R.P., & Wolensky, K.C. (1990). Local government's problem with disaster management: A literature review and structural analysis. *Policy Studies Review, 9*, 703–725.

Wolshon, B., Hamilton, E.U., Levitan, M., & Wilmot, C. (2005) Review of policies and practices for hurricane evacuation II: Traffic operations, management, and control. *Natural Hazards Review, 6*, 143–161.

Wood, N.J., & Good, J.W. (2004). Vulnerability of port and harbor communities to earthquake and tsunami hazards: The use of GIS in community hazard planning. *Coastal Management, 32*, 243–269.

Woodman, R.W., Sawyer, J.E., & Griffin, R.W. (1993). Toward a theory of organizational creativity. *The Academy of Management Review, 18*(2), 293–321.

Woolcock, M., & Narayan, D. (2000). Social capital: Implications for development theory, research, and policy. *The World Bank Research Observer, 15*(2), 225–249.

Worden, W. (1982). Grief counseling and grief therapy. *A handbook for the mental health practitioner*. New York: Springer.

World Bank (2001). *Globalization, growth and poverty*. Washington, DC: World Bank.

World Bank (2004). Enhancing poverty alleviation through disaster reduction. Manila: World Bank.

World Bank (2005). *Natural disaster hotspots: A global risk analysis.* Washington, DC: Hazard Management Unit.

World Commission on Environment and Development. (1987). *Our common future.* New York: Oxford University Press.

Wraith, R. (1997). Women in emergency management: Where are they? *Australian Journal of Emergency Management, 12,* 9–11.

Wright, J.D., & Rossi, P.H. (Eds.). (1981). *Social science and natural hazards.* Cambridge, MA: Abt Books.

Wright, J.D., Rossi, P.H., Wright, S.R., & Weber-Burdin, E. (1979). *After the clean-up: Long-range effects of natural disasters.* Beverly Hills, CA: SAGE.

Writers, S. (2005). *FEMA: A legacy of waste.* South Florida Sun–Sentinal Miami. Retrieved December 5, 2005;-http://www.sun-sentinel.com/news/local/southflorida/sfl-femareport,0,7651043.storygallery?coll=sfla–home–headlines.

Wu, J.Y., & Lindell, M.K. (2004). Housing reconstruction after two major earthquakes: The 1994 Northridge Earthquake in the United States and the 1999 Chi-Chi Earthquake in Taiwan. *Disasters, 28,* 63–81.

Wyllie, L.A., & Lew, H.S. (1989). Performance of engineered structures. *Earthquake Spectra* (Special Supplement), 70–92.

Yamin, F., & Huq, S. (Eds.). (2005). Vulnerability, adaptation & climate disasters. *IDS Bulletins, 36*(4).

Yardley, J. (2005). After its epidemic arrival, SARS vanishes. Retrieved May 5, 2005; http://www.nytimes.com.

Yates, C. (2000). They're floody heroes. *The Sun,* October, p. 6.

Yates, M. (2005). A statistical portrait of the working class. *Monthly Review, 56*(11), 12–31.

Yelvington, K. (1997). Coping in a temporary way: The tent cities. In W. Peacock, B. Morrow, & H. Gladwin (Eds.), *Hurricane Andrew: Ethnicity, gender, and the sociology of disaster* (pp. 92–115). New York: Routledge.

Yerolympos, A. (2002). Urban space as "field" aspects of late Ottoman town planning after fire. In G. Massard-Guilbaud, H. Platt, & D. Schott (Eds.), *Cities and catastrophes: Coping with emergency in European history* (pp. 223–236). Frankfurt: Peter Lang.

Yin, R., & Moore, G.B. (1985). *Utilization of research: Lessons from the natural hazards field.* Washington, DC: Cosmos Corporation.

Yonder, A., Akcar, S., & Gopalan, P. (2005). *Women's participation in disaster relief and recovery.* Seeds Series Report. New York: The Population Council.

Zerger, A., & Smith, D.I. (2003). Impediments to using GIS for real-time disaster decision support. *Computers, Environment and Urban Systems, 27*(2), 123–141.

Zetterberg, H. (1965). *On theory and verification in sociology.* Totowa, NJ: Bedminister Press.

Zimmerman, E. (1983). *Political violence, crises and revolutions: Theories and research.* Cambridge: Schenkman.

Zlatanova, S., Van Oosterom, P., & Verbree, E. (2004). 3D technology for improving disaster management: Geo-DBMS and positioning. In *Proceedings of the XXth ISPRS Congress* (p. 6). Istanbul: Turkey.

Zmud, J. (2005). *Technical documentation for survey administration: Questionnaires, interviews, and focus groups (draft).* Federal building and fire safety investigations into the world trade center disaster. NIST NCSTAR 1–7B, Draft. Gaithersburg, MD: National Innstitute of Standards and Technology.

Index

CPSIA information can be obtained at www.ICGtesting.com
Printed in the USA
LVOW091746091012

302147LV00001B/3/A